Systems Medicine and Network-Based Pharmacology

Systems Medicine and Network-Based Pharmacology

Editor: Lida Murdock

AMERICAN
MEDICAL PUBLISHERS
www.americanmedicalpublishers.com

AMERICAN
MEDICAL PUBLISHERS
www.americanmedicalpublishers.com

Cataloging-in-Publication Data

Systems medicine and network-based pharmacology / edited by Lida Murdock.
p. cm.
Includes bibliographical references and index.
ISBN 979-8-88740-484-4
1. Developmental pharmacology. 2. Pharmacology--Data processing. 3. System analysis.
4. Medical informatics. 5. Systems biology. 6. Medicine--Data processing. I. Murdock, Lida.
RM301.35 .S97 2023
615.7--dc23

American Medical Publishers,
41 Flatbush Avenue,
1st Floor, New York,
NY 11217, USA

ISBN 979-8-88740-484-4 (Hardback)

Contents

Preface

I am honored to present to you this unique book which encompasses the most up-to-date data in the field. I was extremely pleased to get this opportunity of editing the work of experts from across the globe. I have also written papers in this field and researched the various aspects revolving around the progress of the discipline. I have tried to unify my knowledge along with that of stalwarts from every corner of the world, to produce a text which not only benefits the readers but also facilitates the growth of the field.

Systems medicine refers to the study of the human body by incorporating environmental, physiological and biochemical interactions. It evaluates disease by the integration of large volumes of patient datasets, while offering the scope for personalizing healthcare strategies by developing a novel classification of disease. The redefinition of disease is done on the basis of mechanisms in place of analyzing the symptoms, which provide therapeutic targets, involving network pharmacology and drug repurposing. Network pharmacology is an interdisciplinary science based on pharmacology, network biology, systems biology, bioinformatics, computational science, and other related scientific disciplines. The usage of network-based insight allows network pharmacology to systematically reflect and uncover the biological foundation of complex diseases and medication. It uses a systems approach to generate significant insights for drug development and has the capability to serve as a foundation for developing drugs for complicated diseases. This book discusses the fundamentals as well as modern approaches of systems medicine and network-based pharmacology. Those in search of information to further their knowledge will be greatly assisted by it.

Finally, I would like to thank all the contributing authors for their valuable time and contributions. This book would not have been possible without their efforts. I would also like to thank my friends and family for their constant support.

Editor

1

Krukovine Suppresses KRAS-Mutated Lung Cancer Cell Growth and Proliferation by Inhibiting the RAF-ERK Pathway and Inactivating AKT Pathway

Huanling Lai[1,2], Yuwei Wang[1,2], Fugang Duan[1,2], Ying Li[1,2], Zebo Jiang[1,2], Lianxiang Luo[1,2], Liang Liu[1,2], Elaine L. H. Leung[1,2]* and Xiaojun Yao[1,2]**

[1] State Key Laboratory of Quality Research in Chinese Medicines, Macau University of Science and Technology, Taipa, Macau, [2] Macau Institute for Applied Research in Medicine and Health, Macau University of Science and Technology, Taipa, Macau

***Correspondence:**
Liang Liu
lliu@must.edu.mo
Elaine L. H. Leung
lhleung@must.edu.mo
Xiaojun Yao
xjyao@must.edu.mo

Oncogenic activation of the KRAS gene via point mutations occurs in 20–30% of patients with non-small cell lung cancer (NSCLC). The RAS-RAF-ERK and RAS-PI3K-AKT pathways are the major hyper-activated downstream pathways in RAS mutation, which promotes the unlimited lifecycle of cancer cells and their metastasis in humans. However, the success of targeted therapy is restricted by many factors. Herein, we show a new pharmacological KRAS signaling inhibitor krukovine, which is a small molecular bisbenzylisoquinoline alkaloid, isolated from the bark of *Abuta grandifolia* (Mart.) Sandw. (Menispermaceae). This alkaloid targets the KRAS downstream signaling pathways in different NSCLC cell lines, such as H460 and A549, which are established by KRAS mutations. In the present study, we initially investigated the anti-cancer activities of krukovine in KRAS-mutated NSCLC cell lines, as well as KRAS wild type cancer cell line and normal lung cell. Results indicated that krukovine can inhibit the growth and dose-dependently inhibit the colony formation capacity and wound healing ability of H460 and A549. This cytotoxic effect is associated with the induction of cell apoptosis and G1 arrest in those cell lines. Krukovine treatment also suppressed the C-RAF, ERK, AKT, PI3K, p70s6k, and mTOR phosphorylation in H460 and A549. This finding suggests that krukovine represses the growth and proliferation of KRAS-mutated cells by inactivating AKT signaling pathway and downregulating the RAF-ERK signaling pathway. This study provides detailed insights into the novel cytotoxic mechanism of an anti-cancer compound from an herbal plant and promotes the anti-cancer potential of krukovine in NSCLC with KRAS mutation.

Keywords: krukovine, KRAS, non-small cell lung cancer, natural products, inhibitor, RAF, ERK, AKT

INTRODUCTION

Lung cancer has long been a highly common cancer and the leading cause of cancer-related mortality globally, and its incidence is still increasing (Cancer Genome Atlas Research Network, 2012, 2014). About 85% of lung cancer cases are non-small cell lung cancer (NSCLC), and almost 30% of this proportion were diagnosed at an advanced stage (Abacioglu et al., 2005).

In most patients with NSCLC, proto-oncogenes, such as KRAS (Kirsten rat sarcoma viral oncogene homolog), and the AKT (also named PKB, protein kinase B) and ERK (extracellular signal-regulated kinase) signaling pathways are constitutionally activated. Aberrant activation of these signaling pathways in cells leads to uncontrolled cell proliferation, apoptotic resistance, and other oncogenic cascades in many cancer types (Brognard and Dennis, 2002; Papadimitrakopoulou and Adjei, 2006; Dutta et al., 2014; Yip, 2015). Therefore, increasing research efforts have targeted these oncogenic signaling pathways to develop novel agents or therapeutics that will effectively treat NSCLC (Harada et al., 2014; Stinchcombe and Johnson, 2014).

Actually, effective inhibitors specific for many key constituents of the RAS-PI3K (phosphatidylinositol 3-kinase)-AKT and RAS-RAF-MEK-ERK pathways have been developed. Many of these inhibitors have been used or evaluated in clinical trials. A study involving 3,620 patients with NSCLC reported that KRAS is a prominent prognostic marker for the survival of patients with lung adenocarcinoma but ineffective for patients with lung small cell carcinoma (Brose et al., 2002). Patients with KRAS mutation show reduced progression-free survival, and the mutation has been adopted for biomarker analyses in NSCLC (De Grève et al., 2012; Yasuda et al., 2012). However, the development of RAS inhibitors, such as farnesyltransferase inhibitors, has been unsuccessful to date (Mazières et al., 2013). Although several AKT inhibitors have been developed and subjected to clinical trials for NSCLC treatment, their adverse side effects, such as severe hyperglycemia and other potential metabolic abnormalities, hinder their applications (Heavey et al., 2014; Yip, 2015). Side effects also limit the clinical use of the ERK inhibitor (Gioeli et al., 2011). In this regard, novel targeted drug therapy that can suppress these oncogenic pathways has attracted much research interest.

Given their low toxicity and high effectiveness, natural products have been studied and used worldwide recently as potential anti-cancer agents. Our current study identified krukovine, a novel anti-NSCLC compound from natural products. Krukovine is a small molecular bisbenzylisoquinoline alkaloid derived from *Abuta grandifolia* (Mart.) Sandw. (Menispermaceae). Menispermaceae is a well-known family of flowering plants serving as folk herbal medicine for various diseases, including gastrointestinal diseases, such as diarrhea, genitourinary tract diseases, and respiratory tract diseases (e.g., asthma) (Corrêa, 1984). Several compounds, such as bisbenzylisoquinolinic, morphinic, aporphinic, and oxoaporphinic alkaloids, have been isolated from the roots and leaves of this species (Thomas et al., 1997; de Lira et al., 2002; De Sales et al., 2015). Krukovine was first isolated from the bark of *A. grandifolia* (Mart.) Sandw. and showed potent anti-plasmodial activity decades ago (Steele et al., 1999). In the present study, krukovine exhibited a cytotoxic effect and inhibited the growth and proliferation of two KRAS-mutated lung cancer cell lines. Krukovine also inhibited the proliferation of these cancer cells by inducing G1 arrest and apoptosis. Krukovine downregulates the activity of phospho-C-RAF, phospho-AKT, phospho- p70s6k, phospho-mTOR, and phospho-ERK and modulates the PI3K-AKT-mTOR and RAF-ERK signaling pathways. Krukovine may be an alternative candidate for the development of combined targeted therapy against the abnormal expression of RAS oncogenic downstream signaling pathways in NSCLC.

RESULTS

Krukovine Shows a Cytotoxic Effect Toward KRAS-Mutated Cells

To evaluate the potential anti-cancer effect of krukovine (**Figure 1A** shows the chemical structure), we subjected the KRAS-mutated cell lines H460 and A549 to cytotoxicity tests. These cell lines were treated with krukovine at 0, 5, 10, and 20 μM for 48 or 72 h. Results showed that krukovine inhibited the growth of H460 and A549 in a time-dependent manner, while have less cytotoxicity effect on non-KRAS mutation lung cancer cell line H1299 and normal lung cell CCD19-Lu (**Figure 1B**). IC_{50} values revealed the potent cytotoxicity of krukovine to KRAS-mutated cancer cells, as summarized in **Table 1**. The IC_{50} values were much lower in the H460 and A549 cell lines treated with krukovine for 72 h (9.80 ± 0.13 and 8.40 ± 0.37 μM, respectively) than in those treated for 48 h (19.89 ± 0.19 and 13.69 ± 0.15 μM, respectively).

Krukovine Inhibits Cell Colony Formation and Wound Healing Ability in H460 and A549 Cells

Long-term colony formation assays of H460 and A549 cells verified the growth inhibiting effect of krukovine. Krukovine significantly inhibited the colony formation capacities (**Figure 2**) and wound healing ability (**Figure 3**) of the H460 and A549 cells in a dose-dependent manner.

Krukovine Significantly Induces Apoptosis in H460 and A549 Cells

To explore the anti-cancer properties of krukovine, we measured the level of cell apoptosis by flow cytometry using Annexin V-FITC/propidium iodide (PI) staining. The results are shown in **Figure 4**. Krukovine caused limited apoptosis in H460 and A549 cells in low dosage. With increased treatment dosage, the cells experienced extensive apoptosis. Krukovine inhibits caspase-3 expression while increases cleaved PARP (poly ADP ribose polymerase) expression level. This result indicated that cell apoptosis induction also contributes to the krukovine-mediated inhibition of H460 and A549 cell proliferation.

Krukovine Induces Cell Cycle Arrest at the G1 Phase in H460 and A549 Cells

To explain the decreased cell viability, we treated H460 and A549 cells with krukovine, and their cell cycles were detected by flow cytometry through PI staining. **Figure 5** show that krukovine induced a moderate accumulation in the G1 phases and a reduction in the sub-G1 phase.

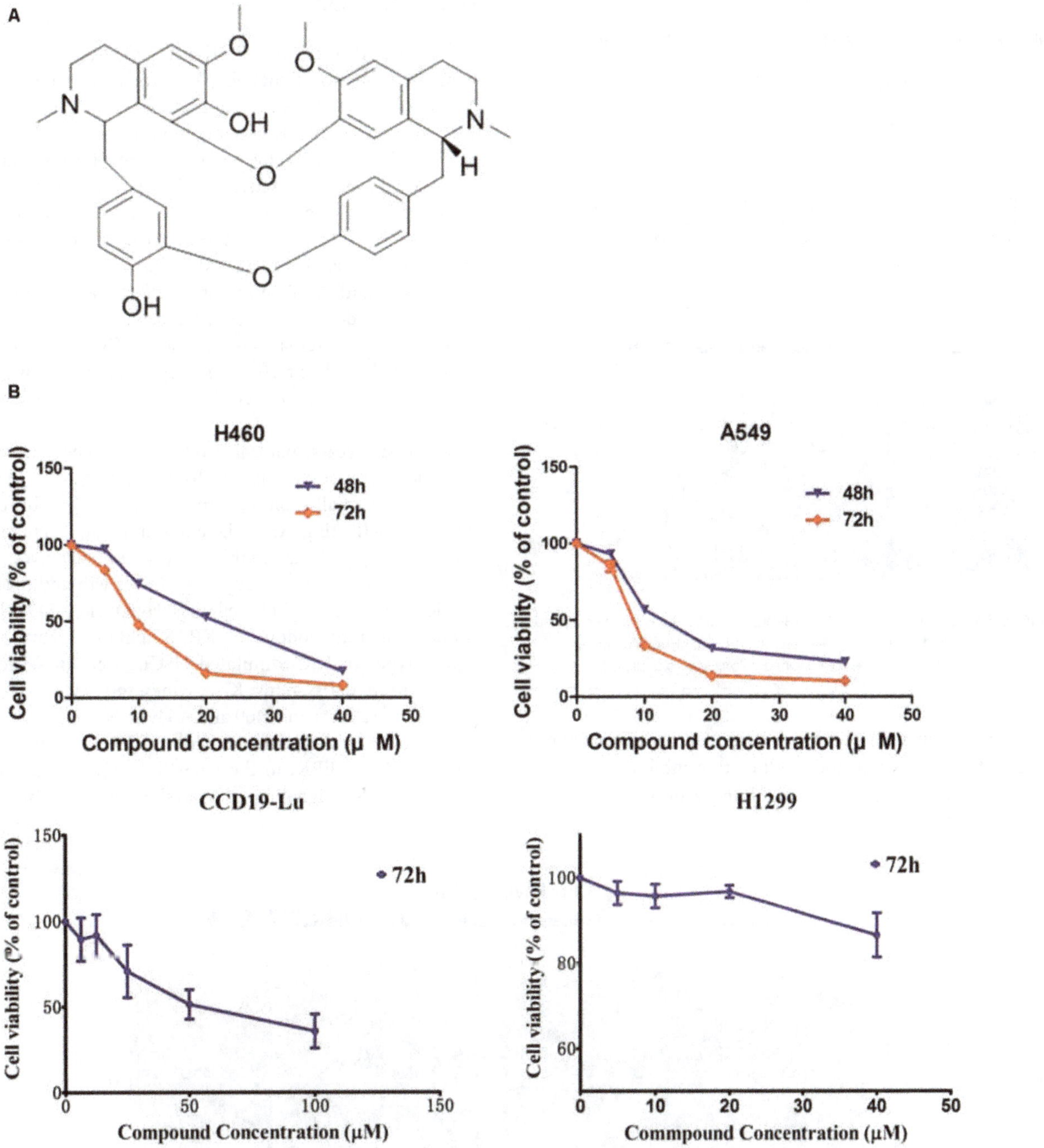

FIGURE 1 | (A) The structure of krukovine. **(B)** Cytotoxic effect of krukovine. Cancer cell lines A549 and H460 were treated with varying concentrations of krukovine and detected by MTT assay after 48 or 72 h. Cancer cell lines H1299 and normal cell CCD19-Lu were treated with varying concentrations of krukovine and detected by MTT assay after 72 h.

Krukovine Inhibits the RAF-ERK Pathway and Inactivates AKT

We next evaluated the effect of krukovine on mediating the PI3K-AKT and RAF-MEK-ERK signaling pathways. These two pathways can be activated by KRAS (Turke et al., 2012; Tomasini et al., 2016). The expression levels of phospho-C-RAF, phospho-AKT (Ser473), phospho-ERK (Thr202/Thy204), phospho-PI3K, phospho-p70s6k, phospho-mTOR, total-C-RAF, total-ERK, total-p70s6k, total-mTOR, total-PI3K, and total-AKT were determined by Western blot. Results indicated that krukovine decreased the levels of phospho-C-RAF, phospho-AKT, phospho-p70s6k, phospho-mTOR, phospho-PI3K, and phospho-ERK but did not significantly affect the levels of total-C-RAF, total-ERK, total-p70s6k, total-mTOR, total-PI3K, and

TABLE 1 | IC_{50} of KRAS-mutated cell lines after treatment with krukovine.

Cell line	IC_{50} (μM)		KRAS mutation states
	48 h	72 h	
H460	19.89 ± 0.19	9.80 ± 0.13	Q61H
A549	13.69 ± 0.15	8.40 ± 0.37	G12S
H1299	–	>40	WT
CCD19-Lu	–	56.34 ± 6.56	WT

IC_{50} is presented as mean ± SEM. CCD19-Lu is normal cell.

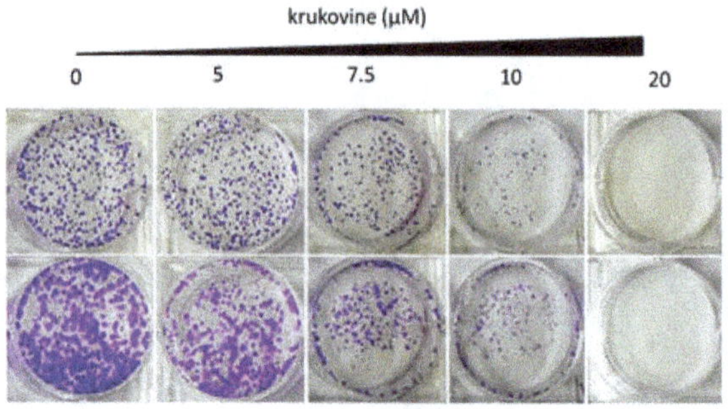

FIGURE 2 | Colony formation of KRAS-mutated cells treated with krukovine (0, 5, 7.5, 10, and 20 μM) and monitored for 14 days. Representative photomicrographs of crystal violet-stained colonies were depicted.

total-AKT (**Figure 6**). These data suggests that krukovine exerts its growth-suppressing and proliferation-inhibiting effects by regulating KRAS downstream signaling pathways.

DISCUSSION

The RAS-RAF-ERK and PI3K-AKT-mTOR pathways are two main downstream signaling pathways involved in the KRAS genes (Gioeli et al., 2011; Tomasini et al., 2016; Matikas et al., 2017). About 20–30% KRAS mutation (Prior et al., 2012; Stephen et al., 2014), 50–70% overexpression of phosphorylated AKT (Yip, 2015), and 70% activated ERK expression (Heavey et al., 2014) were found in patients with NSCLC. The relatively limited subset of NSCLC carrying these genetic mutations should be effectively treated by mediated target therapy, such as using RAF, ERK, and AKT inhibitors. Unfortunately, most patients with NSCLC do not harbor these genomic events, and the 5-year survival rate remains unsatisfactory (Nussinov et al., 2018). Moreover, the side effects of the target inhibitors have hindered their clinical use (Gioeli et al., 2011; Heavey et al., 2014; Yip, 2015).

For many years, natural products have been considered as potential resources for novel drug discovery. We identified a new class of small-molecule from herbs that exhibit effects on directly inactivating AKT signaling and downregulating RAF-ERK signaling pathway. In this study, we initially investigated the potential of krukovine to suppress the growth and proliferation of KRAS-mutated NSCLC cell lines. H460 and A549 cells, which contain different codons of KRAS mutation, have served as typical types of KRAS-mutated NSCLC cell lines widely used as *in vitro* model systems. Krukovine exerts cytotoxic and anti-proliferative effects on H460 and A549 cells.

We also found that the activities of pivotal proteins, such as AKT, RAF, and ERK, in the RAS-PI3K-AKT-mTOR and RAS-RAF-MEK-ERK signaling pathways are inhibited by krukovine

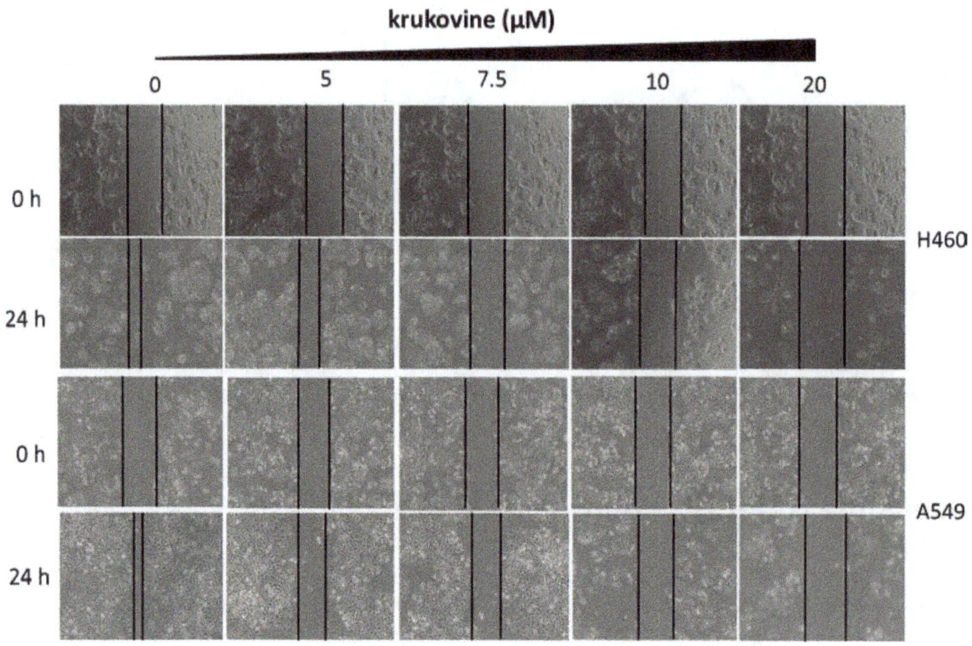

FIGURE 3 | Scratch wound healing assay of KRAS-mutated cells treated with krukovine (0, 5, 7.5, 10, and 20 μM) and monitored for 24 h.

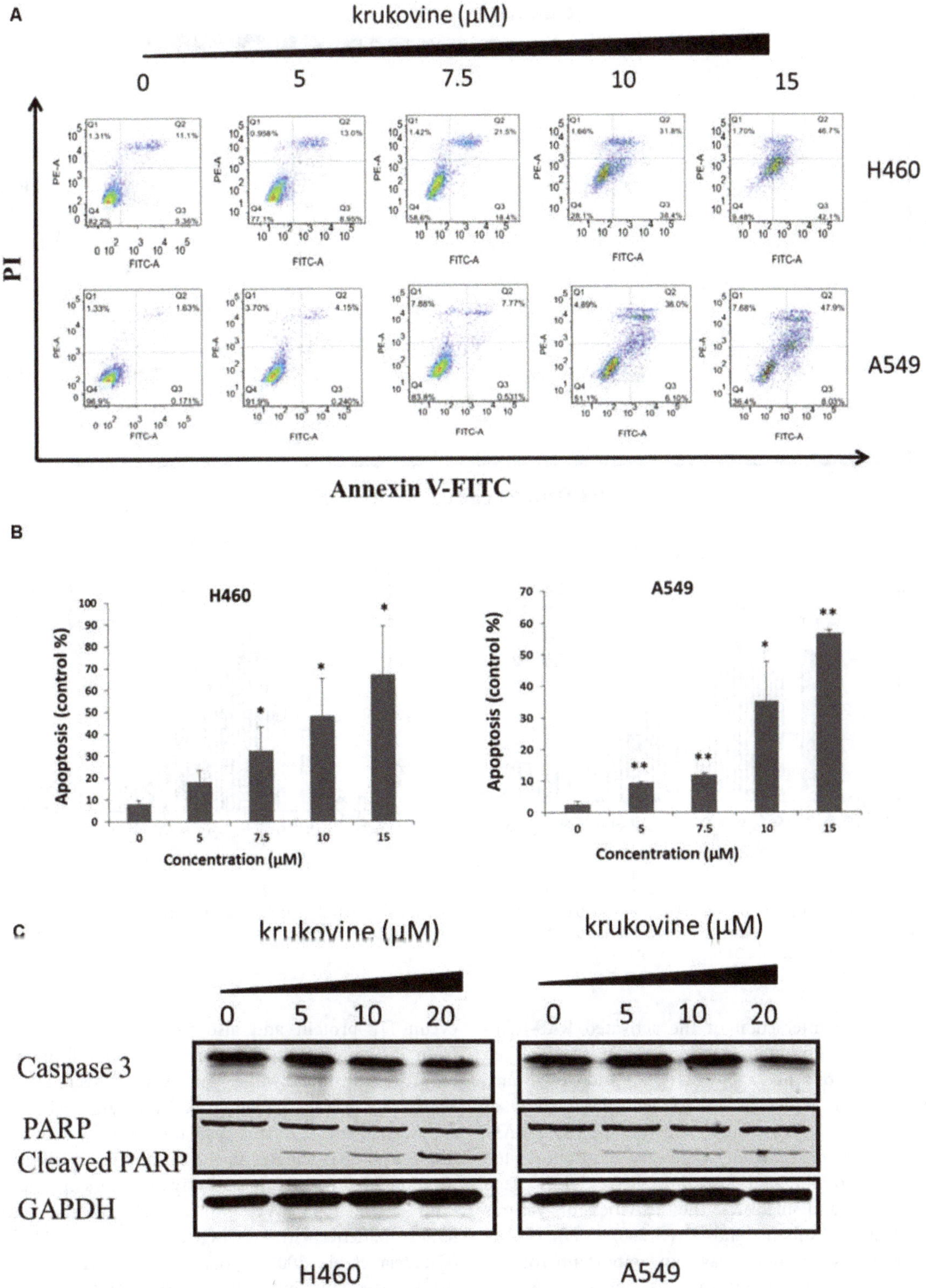

FIGURE 4 | Krukovine-induced cell apoptosis in H460 and A549 cells. Two cells were treated with krukovine at different concentrations (0, 5, 7.5, 10, and 15 μM) for 48 h. **(A)** Cell apoptosis was measured by flow cytometry using Annexin V-FITC/PI staining. **(B)** Statistical analysis of the cell apoptosis rate at 48 h. All data are presented as mean ± SEM ($n = 3$, *$p < 0.05$, **$p < 0.01$). **(C)** Krukovine inhibits caspase-3 expression while increases PARP expression level.

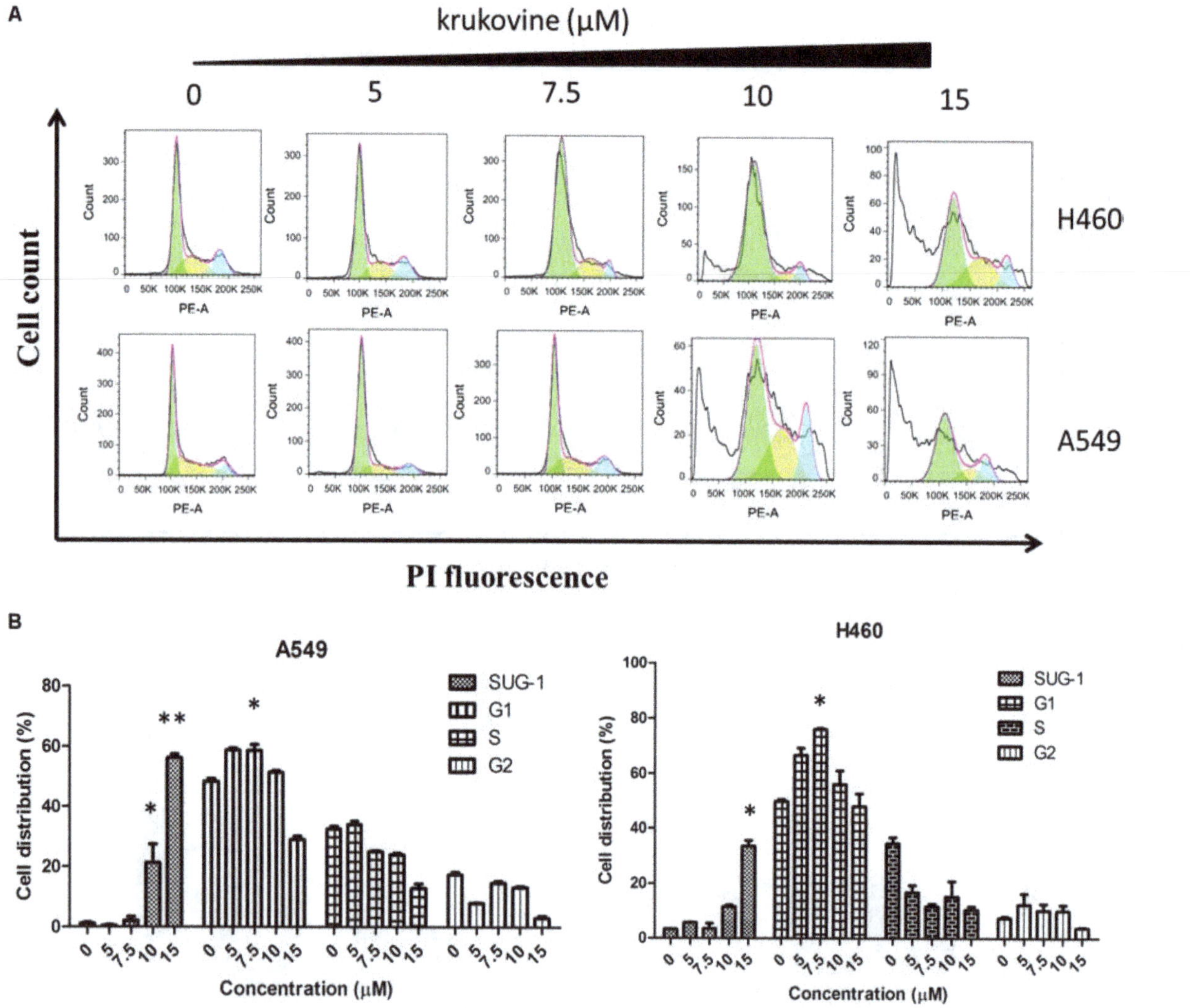

FIGURE 5 | Krukovine-induced cell cycle arrest in H460 and A549 cells. Three cells were treated with krukovine at different concentrations (0, 5, 7.5, 10, and 15 μM) for 48 h. **(A)** Cells were stained with PI, and cell cycle arrest was detected by flow cytometry. **(B)** Statistical analysis of the cell apoptosis rate at 48 h. All data are presented as mean ± SEM ($n = 3$, *$p < 0.05$, **$p < 0.01$).

in NSCLC cells. The interaction of the activated RAS-RAF-MEK-ERK pathway with multiple effectors can regulate cell growth, cell differentiation, and apoptosis (Cully and Downward, 2008; Montagut and Settleman, 2009). Phosphorylation of the ERK protein is a key component of the RAS-RAF-MEK-ERK downstream signaling pathway. Phosphorylated ERK translocates to the nucleus and then causes gene expression changes and mediates the activities of various transcription factors (Roberts and Der, 2007). The PI3K-AKT-mTOR signaling pathway plays an important role in cell growth, cell proliferation, angiogenesis, and cell survival; these processes determine treatment resistance against systemic chemotherapy and radiation (Pal et al., 2008). AKT is a crucial factor in this pathway. Phosphorylation of AKT downregulates various downstream substrates, such as Bad, and can result in malignant transformation (Chang et al., 2003). During cancer cell proliferation, AKT phosphorylation can accumulate the cyclin D1 protein and also prevent the release of calcium from the mitochondria and hence avert cell apoptosis (Diehl et al., 1998). Meanwhile, inactivating AKT can inhibit the PI3K-AKT-mTOR signaling pathway and achieve a tumor-suppressive effect. In this case, the feedback activation of AKT importantly participates in the unsatisfactory clinical results of several RAS downstream pathway inhibitors in cancer treatment (Sun et al., 2005; Wei et al., 2015). In the clinics, up to 45% of patients with NSCLC show increased AKT expression (Okudela et al., 2007; Spoerke et al., 2012). In our present study, krukovine induced G1 arrest and apoptosis in H460 and A549 cells; such effects can lead to cell growth inhibition. This action can be associated with the inhibitory effect of krukovine by AKT phosphorylation and RAF-ERK pathway downregulation, which can lead to cancer cell death (Cully and Downward, 2008; Pal et al., 2008; Montagut and Settleman, 2009).

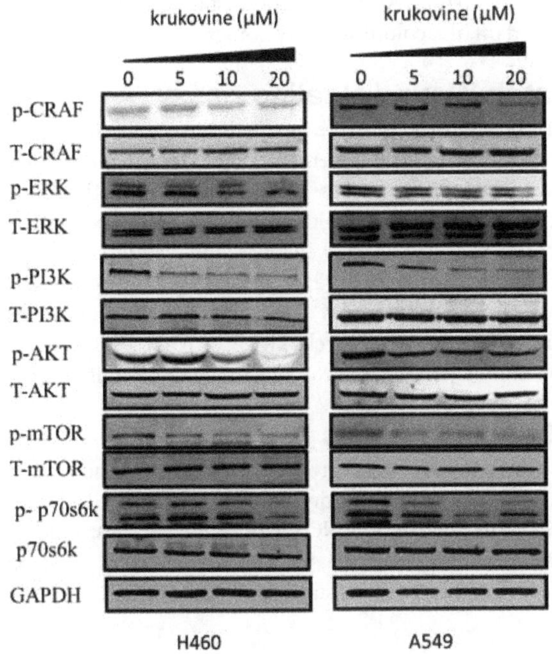

FIGURE 6 | Krukovine inhibits the KRAS signaling pathway. The effect of krukovine treatment mediates the inhibition of signaling in two KRAS-mutated lung cancer cell lines. Untreated cells were used as control. A representative of at least three independent experiments for each cell line is shown.

The RAF-ERK and PI3K-AKT pathways are the two major hyper-activated downstream pathways in RAS mutation; these pathways promote the uncontrolled growth of abnormal cells and their metastasis in humans. These signaling pathways have been identified as promising targets in cancer therapy in recent years (Asati et al., 2016). However, the success of targeted therapy can be limited by the developed resistance of cancer cells through the mutation of target kinases, redundancy in signaling, feedback activation of pathway components, and compensatory activation of parallel circuits (Shamma et al., 1967). Use multi-targeting synthetic signaling pathway inhibitor to treat NSCLC has been proposed by some studies (Logue and Morrison, 2012; Cheng et al., 2014). In this light, targeting two or more constituents of the same pathway or two different pathways simultaneously, for example, AKT and ERK, has been suggested to improve the success of NSCLC-targeted therapy (Meng et al., 2010; Heavey et al., 2014).

In our study, we identified krukovine as a novel KRAS signaling inhibitor and evaluated its anti-cancer activity in NSCLC cell lines. Krukovine effectively inhibited KRAS downstream signaling and induced G1 arrest and apoptosis to exert a cytotoxic effect on KRAS-mutated lung cancer cells lines.

MATERIALS AND METHODS

Reagents and Antibodies

Krukovine was purchased from Top Science (Shanghai, China) and dissolved in dimethyl sulfoxide (DMSO). The Annexin V/PI staining kit was produced by BD Biosciences (San Jose, United States). The antibodies for Western blot are as follows. Primary antibodies against phospho-C-RAF, total-C-RAF, phospho-ERK(Thr202-Thy204), total-ERK, phospho-AKT(Ser473), phospho-PI3K, total-PI3K, phospho-p70s6k, total-p70s6k, phospho-mTOR, total-mTOR, caspase-3, PARP, and GAPDH were produced by CST (Cell Signaling Technology, United States). The primary antibody against AKT was produced by Santa Cruz Biotechnology (Santa Cruz, United States). Fluorescein-conjugated goat anti-rabbit and -mouse secondary antibodies were produced by Odyssey (Belfast, United States).

Cell Lines and Cell Culture

The KRAS mutant NSCLC cell lines used in this study (H460 and A549) were purchased from the ATCC (American Type Culture Collection, United States). All cells were cultured in RPMI-1640 medium containing 10% fetal bovine serum with 100 μg/mL streptomycin and 100 U/mL penicillin. Cells were cultured in an incubator with 5% CO_2 at 37°C.

Cell Growth Inhibition Assay

The standard MTT (3-(4,5-dimethylthiazol-2-yl)-2,5-diphenyltetrazolium bromide) assay was carried out to evaluate the cell growth inhibition effect of krukovine. In brief, H460, A549, H1299, and CCD19-Lu cells were each planted at 4×10^3 cells or 3×10^3 cells per well in a 96-well plate and cultured for 12 h to allow cell adhesion. Different concentrations (0, 5, 10, and 20 μM) of krukovine were applied as treatment for another 48 or 72 h. DMSO treatment served as a vehicle control. Every dosage was repeated three times, and at least three independent experiments were performed. At the end of the treatment, MTT solution (5 mg/mL) was added to each well (10 μL per well), and each plate was placed back to the incubator. After further culture for 4 h, the supernatant was carefully removed, and 100 μL of DMSO, as resolved solution, was added to each well while lightly shaking for 10 min to dissolve the MTT crystals. The absorbance was measured by a Tecan microplate reader at 570 nm and used as a reference at 650 nm. The percentages obtained from the absorbance of the treated cells divided by the absorbance of untreated cells were presented as the cell viabilities. The IC_{50} of krukovine was calculated by the GraphPad Prism 5.0 software.

Cell Apoptosis and Cell Cycle Analysis

H460 and A549 cells were each planted on a six-well plate with a density of 1×10^5 cells per well overnight. The cells were cultured for over 12 h to allow cell adhesion and then exposed to various concentrations of krukovine for 48 h. At the end of treatment, cells were harvested using trypsin, washed with PBS, and then collected after centrifugation. For cell apoptosis analysis, cells were treated with 5 μL of PI (1 mg/mL) and 5 μL of Annexin V fluorescein dye and stained for 15 min; this step must be performed away from light and at room temperature. The cells were then resuspended in 300–500 μL of Annexin binding buffer and filtered before analysis by a BD FACSAriaIII flow cytometer (BD Biosciences). The percentage of apoptotic cells was quantitatively determined. For cell cycle assay, the cells were fixed with 70% (v/v) ethanol for at least 30 min at 4°C. Thereafter, the cells were washed with PBS before treatment with 5 μL of PI (1 mg/mL). The percentages of cells at different cell cycle phases (sub-G, S, G1, and G2) were quantitatively measured by the same equipment in the corresponding process.

Western Blot

Total-cell protein lysates and Western blot materials were prepared as follows. Then, 48 h after drug treatment, the cells were rinsed with lysed ice-cold PBS and lysed in RIPA buffer (150 mmol/L NaCl, 50 mmol/L Tris–HCl, pH 8.0, 1% deoxycholate, 0.1% SDS, and 1% Triton X-100) containing protease and phosphatase inhibitors (Roche, United Kingdom) for at least 30 min and then centrifuged at 14,000 × *g* for 10 min at 4°C. The concentration of total protein for each sample was measured by DCTM protein assay kit (Bio-Rad). Then, equal amounts of total protein of each sample were resuspended in loading buffer and denatured for 5 min in 100°C. The total protein (30 μg) of each sample was separated by 10% SDS-PAGE and then transferred to PVDF membranes (Millipore, United States). The protein membranes were blocked by 5% non-fat milk in 1× TBST for 1 h at room temperature. The samples were incubated with different primary antibodies [phospho-C-RAF, phospho-AKT (Ser473), phospho-ERK (Thr202/Thy204), total-C-RAF, total-ERK, total-AKT, total-p70s6k, phospho-p70s6k, total-mTOR, phospho-mTOR, phospho-PI3K, total-PI3K, caspase-3, PARP, and GAPDH] at 4°C overnight. The above-mentioned primary antibodies were diluted in 1:1,000. Protein membranes were subsequently incubated with secondary fluorescent antibodies for 2 h and then washed in 1× TBST three times for 5 min each time. All secondary antibodies (anti-rabbit or anti-mouse) were diluted in 1:10,000. All membranes were analyzed by an LI-COR Odyssey scanner (Belfast, United States).

Colony Formation Assay

H460 and A549 cells were planted into six-well plates (500 cells/well), respectively. After attachment overnight, the cells were treated with various concentrations (0, 5, 7.5, 10, and 20 μM) of krukovine, and the medium was changed every 3 days. When colony formation was visible, the medium was discharged. The colonies were washed with ice-cold PBS gently, fixed in 4% paraformaldehyde (PFA) for 15 min, and then stained with 0.5% crystal violet (20% methanol, 0.5% crystal violet, and 1% PFA in ddH_2O) for 30 min. After the extra crystal violet was washed away and dried off, the colonies were photographed and analyzed.

Scratch Wound Healing Assay

H460 and A549 cells were planted into six-well plates (500 cells/well), respectively. After attachment overnight, they should reach ∼70% confluence as a monolayer, then, the confluent monolayer was scratched with a 200 μL sterile pipette tip. After scratching, gently wash the well twice with medium to remove the detached cells. The cells were treated with various concentrations (0, 5, 7.5, 10, and 20 μM) of krukovine. After growing for additional 24 h, wash the cells twice with 1× PBS, take photos for the monolayer on a microscope in the same configurations.

Statistical Analysis

Statistical analysis was carried out by GraphPad Prism 5.0 software. The results were presented as (mean ± SEM) of three individual experiments. ANOVA or Student's *t*-test followed by Bonferroni's test was used to compare all pairs of columns. *p*-Values <0.05 were set as statistically significant.

AUTHOR CONTRIBUTIONS

LLi, EL, and XY conceived the study, participated in the design and coordination of the whole study, and helped in critically revising the draft for important intellectual content. HL carried out the cell culture studies, molecular biology experiments, data collection, statistical analysis, and manuscript drafting. YW participated in the data collection and performed the statistical analysis. ZJ and FD participated in the molecular biology experiments. YL and LLu helped in critically revising the draft for important intellectual content. All authors have checked and approved the final manuscript and agreed to be accountable for all aspects of the work by ensuring that questions related to the accuracy or integrity of any part of the work are appropriately investigated and resolved.

FUNDING

This work was supported by Macao Science and Technology Development Fund (Project Nos. 046/2016/A2, 086/2015/A3, 005/2014/AMJ, and FDCT-16-010-SKL).

REFERENCES

Abacioglu, U., Yumuk, P. F., Caglar, H., Sengoz, M., and Turhal, N. S. (2005). Concurrent chemoradiotherapy with low dose weekly gemcitabine in stage III nonsmallcell lung cancer. *BMC Cancer* 5:71. doi: 10.1186/1471-2407-5-71

Asati, V., Mahapatra, D. K., and Bharti, S. K. (2016). PI3K/Akt/mTOR and Ras/Raf/MEK/ERK signaling pathways inhibitors as anticancer agents: structural and pharmacological perspectives. *Eur. J. Med. Chem.* 109, 314–341. doi: 10.1016/j.ejmech.2016.01.012

Brognard, J., and Dennis, P. A. (2002). Variable apoptotic response of NSCLC cells to inhibition of the MEK/ERK pathway by small molecules or dominant negative mutants. *Cell Death Differ.* 9, 893–904. doi: 10.1038/sj.cdd.4401054

Brose, M. S., Volpe, P., Feldman, M., Kumar, M., Rishi, I., Gerrero, R., et al. (2002). BRAF and RAS mutations in human lung cancer and melanoma. *Cancer Res.* 62, 6997–7000.

Cancer Genome Atlas Research Network. (2012). Comprehensive genomic characterization of squamous cell lung cancers. *Nature* 489, 519–525. doi: 10.1038/nature11404

Cancer Genome Atlas Research Network. (2014). Comprehensive molecular profiling of lung adenocarcinoma. *Nature* 511, 543–550. doi: 10.1038/nature13385

Chang, F., Lee, J. T., and Navolanic, P. M. (2003). Involvement of PI3K/Akt pathway in cell cycleprogression, apoptosis, and neoplastic transformation: a target for cancer chemotherapy. *Leukemia* 17, 590–603. doi: 10.1038/sj.leu.2402824

Cheng, H., Shcherba, M., Pendurti, G., Liang, Y., Piperdi, B., and Perez-Soler, R. (2014). Targeting the PI3K/AKT/mTOR pathway: potential for lung cancer treatment. *Lung Cancer Manag.* 3, 67–75. doi: 10.2217/lmt.13.72

Corrêa, M. P. (1984). *Dicionário de PlantasÚteis do Brasil e das ExóticasCultivadas.* Rio de Janeiro: InstitutoBrasileiro de DefesaFlorestal.

Cully, M., and Downward, J. (2008). SnapShot: ras signaling. *Cell* 133, 1292–1292. doi: 10.1016/j.cell.2008.06.020

De Grève, J., Teugels, E., Geers, C., Decoster, L., Galdermans, D., De Mey, J., et al. (2012). Clinical activity of afatinib (BIBW 2992) in patients with lung adenocarcinoma with mutations in the kinase domain of HER2/neu. *Lung Cancer* 76, 123–127. doi: 10.1016/j.lungcan.2012.01.008

de Lira, G. A., de Andrade, L. M., Florêncio, K. C., da Silva, M. S., Barbosa-Filho, J. M., and Leitão da-Cunha, E. V. (2002). Roraimine: a bisbenzylisoquinoline alkaloid from Cissampelos sympodialis roots. *Fitoterapia* 73, 356–358. doi: 10.1016/S0367-326X(02)00089-8

De Sales, I. R. P., Machado, F. D. F., Marinho, A. F., Lúcio, A. S. S. C., Filho, J. M. B., and Batista, L. M. (2015). Cissampelos sympodialis Eichl. *(Menispermaceae)*, a medicinal plant, presents antimotility and antidiarrheal activity in vivo. *BMC Complement. Altern. Med.* 15:253. doi: 10.1186/s12906-015-0578-7

Diehl, J. A., Cheng, M., Roussel, M. F., and Sherr, C. J. (1998). Glycogen synthase kinase-3β regulatescyclin D1 proteolysis and subcellular localization. *Genes Dev.* 15, 3499–3511. doi: 10.1101/gad.12.22.3499

Dutta, P., Sabri, N., Li, J., and Li, W. X. (2014). Role of STAT3 in lung cancer. *JAKSTAT.* 3:e999503. doi: 10.1080/21623996.2014.999503

Gioeli, D., Wunderlich, W., Sebolt-Leopold, J., Bekiranov, S., Wulfkuhle, J. D., Petricoin, E. F. III, et al. (2011). Compensatory pathways induced by MEK inhibition are effective drug targets for combination therapy against castration-resistant prostate cancer. *Mol. Cancer Ther.* 10, 1581–1590. doi: 10.1158/1535-7163.MCT-10-1033

Harada, D., Takigawa, N., and Kiura, K. (2014). The role of STAT3 in non-small cell lungcancer. *Cancers* 6, 708–722. doi: 10.3390/cancers6020708

Heavey, S., O'Byrne, K. J., and Gately, K. (2014). Strategies for co-targeting the PI3K/AKT/mTOR pathway in NSCLC. *Cancer Treat. Rev.* 40, 445–456. doi: 10.1016/j.ctrv.2013.08.006

Logue, J. S., and Morrison, D. K. (2012). Complexity in the signaling network: insights from the use of targeted inhibitors in cancer therapy. *Genes Dev.* 26, 641–650. doi: 10.1101/gad.186965.112

Matikas, A., Mistriotis, D., Georgoulias, V., and Kotsakis, A. (2017). Targeting KRAS mutated non-small cell lung cancer: a history of failures and a future of hope for a diverse entity. *Crit. Rev. Oncol. Hematol.* 110, 1–12. doi: 10.1016/j.critrevonc.2016.12.005

Mazières, J., Peters, S., Lepage, B., Cortot, A. B., Barlesi, F., Beau-Faller, M., et al. (2013). Lung cancer that harbors an HER2 mutation: epidemiologic characteristics and therapeutic perspectives. *J. Clin. Oncol.* 31, 1997–2003. doi: 10.1200/JCO.2012.45.6095

Meng, J., Dai, B., Fang, B., Bekele, B. N., Bornmann, W. G., Sun, D., et al. (2010). Combination treatment with MEK and AKT inhibitors is more effective than each drug alone in human non-small cell lung cancer in vitro and in vivo. *PLoS One* 5:e14124. doi: 10.1371/journal.pone.0014124

Montagut, C., and Settleman, J. (2009). Targeting the RAF-MEK-ERK pathway in cancer therapy. *Cancer Lett.* 283, 125–134. doi: 10.1016/j.canlet.2009.01.022

Nussinov, R., Tsai, C.-J., and Jang, H. (2018). Oncogenic ras isoforms signaling specificity at the membrane. *Cancer Res.* 78, 593–602. doi: 10.1158/0008-5472.CAN-17-2727

Okudela, K., Suzuki, M., Kageyama, S., Bunai, T., Nagura, K., Igarashi, H., et al. (2007). PIK3CA mutation and amplification in human lung cancer. *Pathol. Int.* 57, 664–671. doi: 10.1111/j.1440-1827.2007.02155.x

Pal, S. K., Figlin, R. A., and Reckamp, K. L. (2008). The role of targeting mammalian target of rapamycin in lung cancer. *Clin. Lung Cancer* 9, 340–345. doi: 10.3816/CLC.2008.n.049

Papadimitrakopoulou, V., and Adjei, A. A. (2006). The Akt/mTOR and mitogen-activated protein kinase pathways in lung cancer therapy. *J. Thorac. Oncol.* 1, 749–751.

Prior, I. A., Lewis, P. D., and Mattos, C. (2012). A comprehensive survey of Ras mutations in cancer. *Cancer Res.* 72, 2457–2467. doi: 10.1158/0008-5472.CAN-11-2612

Roberts, P. J., and Der, C. J. (2007). Targeting the Raf-MEK-ERK mitogen-activated protein kinasecascade for the treatment of cancer. *Oncogene* 26, 3291–3310. doi: 10.1038/sj.onc.1210422

Shamma, M., Shine, R. J., and Dudock, B. S. (1967). Thalictrum alkaloids-IV. *Tetrahedron* 23, 2887–2892. doi: 10.1016/S0040-4020(01)83344-5

Spoerke, J. M., O'Brien, C., Huw, L., Koeppen, H., Fridlyand, J., Brachmann, R. K., et al. (2012). Phosphoinositide 3-kinase (PI3K) pathway alterations are associated with histologic subtypes and are predictive of sensitivity to PI3K inhibitors in lung cancer preclinical models. *Clin. Cancer Res.* 18, 6771–6783. doi: 10.1158/1078-0432.CCR-12-2347

Steele, J. C., Simmonds, M. S., Veitch, N. C., and Warhurst, D. C. (1999). Evaluation of the anti-plasmodial activity of bisbenzylisoquinoline alkaloids from Abutagrandifolia. *Planta Med.* 65, 413–416. doi: 10.1055/s-1999-14017

Stephen, A. G., Esposito, D., Bagni, R. K., and McCormick, F. (2014). Dragging ras back in the ring. *Cancer Cell* 25, 272–281. doi: 10.1016/j.ccr.2014.02.017

Stinchcombe, T. E., and Johnson, G. L. (2014). MEK inhibition in non-small cell lungcancer. *Lung Cancer* 86, 121–125. doi: 10.1016/j.lungcan.2014.09.005

Sun, S. Y., Rosenberg, L. M., Wang, X., Zhou, Z., Yue, P., Fu, H., et al. (2005). Activation of Akt and eIF4E survival pathways by rapamycin-mediated mammalian target of rapamycin inhibition. *Cancer Res.* 65, 7052–7058. doi: 10.1158/0008-5472.CAN-05-0917

Tomasini, P., Walia, P., Labbe, C., Jao, K., and Leighl, N. B. (2016). Targeting the KRAS pathway in non-small cell lung cancer. *Oncologist* 21, 1450–1460. doi: 10.1634/theoncologist.2015-0084

Turke, A. B., Song, Y., Costa, C., Cook, R., Arteaga, C. L., Asara, J. M., et al. (2012). MEK inhibition leads to PI3K/AKT activation by relieving a negative feedback on ERBB receptors. *Cancer Res.* 72, 3228–3237. doi: 10.1158/0008-5472.CAN-11-3747

Thomas, G., Burns, F., Pyne, S., and Pyne, N. J. (1997). Characterization of an extract from the leaves of *Cissampelos sympodialis* Eichl. on the spontaneous tone of isolated trachea. *Phytother. Res.* 11, 496–499. doi: 10.1002/(SICI)1099-1573(199711)11:7<496::AID-PTR137>3.0.CO;2-7

Wei, F., Zhang, Y., Geng, L., Zhang, P., Wang, G., and Liu, Y. (2015). mTOR inhibition induces EGFR feedback activation in association with its resistance to human pancreatic cancer. *Int. J. Mol. Sci.* 16, 3267–3282. doi: 10.3390/ijms16023267

Yasuda, H., Sng, N. J., Yeo, W. L., Figueiredo-Pontes, L. L., Kobayashi, S., and Costa, D. (2012). Sensitivity of EGFR exon 20 insertion mutations to EGFR inhibitors is determined by their location within the tyrosine kinase domain of EGFR. *Cancer Res.* 72, 23. doi: 10.1158/1538-7445.AM2012-23

Yip, P. Y. (2015). Phosphatidylinositol 3-kinase-AKT-mammalian target of rapamycin (PI3K-Akt-mTOR) signaling pathway in non-small cell lung cancer. *Transl. Lung Cancer Res.* 4, 165–176. doi: 10.3978/j.issn.2218-6751.2015.01.04

2

Integrated Metabolomics and Network Pharmacology Revealed Hong-Hua-Xiao-Yao Tablet's Effect of Mediating Hormone Synthesis in the Treatment of Mammary Gland Hyperplasia

Ziqing Gao[1], Rui Mi[2], Zhaoxi Cheng[2], Xiaofeng Li[3], Huawu Zeng[2], Gaosong Wu[1], Jing Zhao[1], Weidong Zhang[1,2]* and Ji Ye[2]**

[1]Institute of Interdisciplinary Integrative Medicine Research, Shanghai University of Traditional Chinese Medicine, Shanghai, China, [2]School of Pharmacy, Second Military Medical University, Shanghai, China, [3]School of Pharmacy, Fudan University, Shanghai, China

***Correspondence:**
Jing Zhao
Zhaojanne@gmail.com
Weidong Zhang
wdzhangy@hotmail.com
Ji Ye
catheline620@163.com

Hong-Hua-Xiao-Yao Tablet (HHXYT) is a traditional Chinese medicine (TCM) formula that has been approved for the treatment of mammary gland hyperplasia (MGH), but its mechanism of action is unclear. In this study, a strategy that integrated metabolomics and network pharmacology was applied to systemically reveal the mechanism of HHXYT in the treatment of MGH. Our pharmacodynamic study indicated that the proliferation of mammary gland was inhibited in rats, and serum-level disorder of estradiol and progesterone was reversed after HHXYT treatment. 54 compounds absorbed in rat plasma were identified after administration of HHXYT. The serum metabolome revealed 58 endogenous differential metabolites, of which 31% were steroid lipids metabolites, with steroid hormone biosynthesis being the most significant metabolic module. 7 targets, 6 herbs, and 17 ingredients were found to play key roles in HHXYT's treatment of MGH. 3 of the 7 key targets (CYP11A1, HSD3B2, and CYP17A1) were directly involved in androgen synthesis, while 2 targets (AR and ESR1) were receptors for the direct action of androgens and estrogens. Molecular docking was utilized to confirm the bindings between the 5 targets and their corresponding compounds. In an *in vitro* test, HHXYT (50 μg/ml) and its ingredient formononetin (3.2, 6.3, and 12.5 μM) were found to significantly reduce the increase of testosterone level induced by dexamethasone (10 μM) in thecal cells. In summary, this study illustrated that the mechanism of HHXYT's treatment of MGH was to regulate hormone disorder. HHXYT could reduce estrogen-stimulated hyperplasia by inhibiting the production of its precursor androgen.

Keywords: Hong-Hua-Xiao-Yao tablet, mammary gland hyperplasia, traditional medicine, metabolomics, network pharmacology, pharmacological effects

1 INTRODUCTION

The most common breast disease, mammary gland hyperplasia (MGH), is a proliferative lesion of mammary tissue accompanying by the lumps and pain symptoms of the breast. It has overtly interfered with the patient's daily life (You et al., 2017; Li et al., 2018). In the past few years, it has been increasingly reported that the incidence of breast cancer in MGH patients is remarkably higher than that in average person (Hartmann et al., 2005), since the pathogenesis of MGH is similar to that of breast cancer, both of which are closely related to endocrine and hormone level disorders (Coussens and Pollard, 2011; Arendt and Kuperwasser, 2015). Hormone drugs are currently applied to the therapy of MGH to regulate internal hormone levels. However, due to its obvious side effects, such as gastrointestinal and cardiovascular problems, the safety and effectiveness of this approach are not optimistic (Wibowo et al., 2016).

As a traditional Chinese medicine (TCM) formula on MGH treatment in the clinic for years, Hong-Hua-Xiao-Yao Tablet (HHXYT) was composed of nine herbal medicines, including *Carthamus tinctorius* L. (Honghua), *Angelica sinensis* (Oliv.) Diels (Danggui), *Paeonia lactiflora* Pall. (Baishao), *Gleditsia sinensis* Lam. (Zaojiaoci), *Atractylodes macrocephala* Koidz. (Baizhu), *Wolfiporia cocos* (F.A. Wolf) Ryvarden & Gilb (Fuling), *Mentha canadensis* L. (Bohe), *Bupleurum marginatum* Wall. ex DC. (Zhuye Chaihu), and *Glycyrrhiza uralensis* Fisch. ex DC. (Gancao). Chemical profiling of HHXYT has been previously elucidated by high-performance liquid chromatography combined with mass spectrometry technique, and 55 constituents were characterized. Moreover, in our earlier study, 14 components that were identified as potential HHXYT quality markers were quantified using high-performance liquid chromatography-tandem triple quadrupole mass spectrometry (HPLC-QQQ-MS) technique (Mi et al., 2020). In clinical trials, HHXYT was found to be effective in the treatment of perimenopausal syndrome, ovarian syndrome, menstrual disorders, as well as mammary gland hyperplasia (Wang, 2012; Pei et al., 2016; Chen et al., 2020). However, the mechanism of its therapy was still unelucidated.

Metabolomics could integrally focus on alterations of endogenous metabolites to monitor and analyze metabolic disturbances for elucidating therapeutic mechanisms (Nicholson and Wilson, 2003). Moreover, compared with other omics techniques, it is more in line with the change of disease phenotype (Newgard, 2017). Network pharmacology performs network analysis of complex biological systems by constructing network models (Hopkins, 2007; Li and Zhang, 2013). The combined analysis of metabolomics and network pharmacology can characterize the overall changes of biological systems, which is in accordance with the holistic therapeutic concept of TCM. This strategy has been increasingly applied in the study of TCM pharmacology and has contributed to elucidating the mechanism of multi-pathway and multi-target of TCM (Xu et al., 2018; Wu, Zhang and Li, 2019; Zhao et al., 2019).

In this study, the integrated metabolomics and network pharmacology strategy were used to reveal the mechanism of HHXYT in the treatment of MGH on a systemic level. Rat model of MGH was established and the metabolomics approach based on the HPLC-QTOF-MS/MS analysis was operated to search for serum endogenous differential metabolites. The ingredients and putative targets of HHXYT were then analyzed using the network pharmacology method. Next, an integrated analysis of differential metabolites and targets identified HHXYT's key targets and substances against MGH. Ultimately, the cell-based assay on the synthesis of sex hormones was performed to validate HHXYT's effects *in vitro* (**Figure 1**).

2 MATERIALS AND METHODS

2.1 Chemicals and Reagents

Reagents of the LC-MS purity grade were acquired from Fisher Scientific (Fair Lawn, NJ, United Staes), including formic acid (purity >98%), acetonitrile, and methanol. Estradiol benzoate and progesterone injection were purchased from Zhejiang Xianju Pharmaceutical Co., Ltd. (Taizhou, China). ELISA kits of estradiol (E_2), testosterone (T), and progesterone (P) were obtained from Boster Biological Technology Co., Ltd. (Shanghai, China). McCoy's 5A medium was provided by Gibco® (Grand Island, NY, United States). Follicle-stimulating hormone (FSH) and luteinizing hormone (LH) were acquired from Shanghai Linc-Bio Science Co. Ltd. (Shanghai, China). Dexamethasone (DEX) and formononetin (FT) were supplied by Chengdu Must Biotechnology Co., Ltd. (Chengdu, China). The purity of FT was above 98%. Cell Counting Kit-8 (CCK-8) was purchased from Shanghai Beyotime Biotechnology Co., Ltd. (Shanghai, China). HHXYT (batch number: 190106), the same batch named as "PZ-5" in our previous study (Mi et al., 2020), was supplied by Puzheng Pharmaceutical Co., Ltd. (Jiangxi, China). The contents of fourteen quality marker compounds of HHXYT were quantified by HPLC-QQQ-MS (**Table 1**). The chromatograms and chemical structure were shown in **Supplementary Figure S1**.

2.2 Animal Experiment and Sample Preparation

All sexually mature and non-pregnant female Sprague-Dawley rats were obtained from Shanghai Xipuer-Bikai Experimental Animal Co. Ltd., Shanghai, China (License No.: SCXK-Shanghai-2018-0006). They were bred in a stabilized environment for 1 week with room temperature 25 ± 2°C, relative humidity 55 ± 5%, 12 h each of light and dark, and free access to drinking water and feed. All procedures were approved by the Animal Care and Use Committee of Second Military Medical University and abided by the Guide for the Care and Use of Laboratory Animals.

2.2.1 Prototypes of HHXYT and Related Metabolites in Plasma

The animal experiment used to study the chemicals absorbed in rat plasma was previously described (Mi et al., 2020). Briefly, the HHXYT sample was suspended in 0.5% carboxymethylcellulose

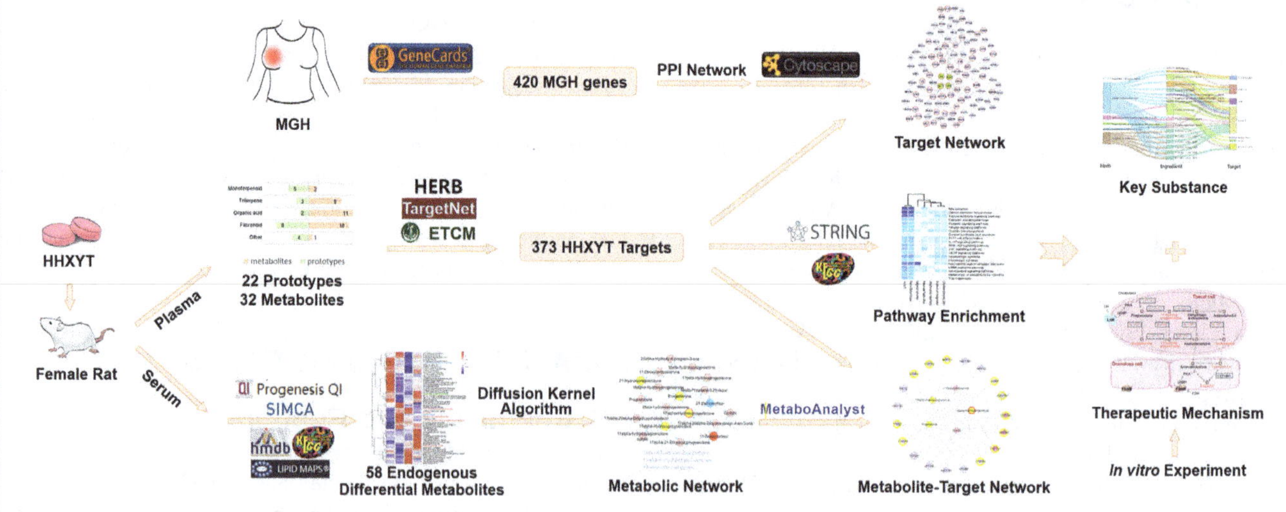

FIGURE 1 | Integrated workflow for exploring the potential mechanisms of HHXYT against MGH.

TABLE 1 | The contents of fourteen quality marker components of HHXYT (batch number: 190106, mg/g, Mean ± SD, *n* = 3).

Number	Analytes	Structure class	Contents
1	Protocatechuic acid	Organic acid	0.296 ± 0.015
2	Paeoniflorin	Monoterpenoid	8.360 ± 0.589
3	Liquiritin	Flavonoid	0.693 ± 0.037
4	Senkyunolide I	Other	0.110 ± 0.007
5	Isoliquiritin	Flavonoid	0.301 ± 0.020
6	Liquiritigenin	Flavonoid	0.143 ± 0.004
7	Isoliquiritigenin	Flavonoid	0.085 ± 0.005
8	Formononetin	Flavonoid	0.028 ± 0.005
9	Glycyrrhizic acid	Triterpene	9.840 ± 0.312
10	Glycyrrhetinic acid 3-*O*-glucuronide	Triterpene	0.037 ± 0.008
11	Licoricone	Flavonoid	0.009 ± 0.001
12	Z-ligustilide	Other	5.013 ± 0.303
13	Licoisoflavone B	Flavonoid	0.022 ± 0.002
14	Glycyrrhetinic acid	Triterpene	0.015 ± 0.002

sodium (CMC-Na) and administered orally to twenty-five female rats at five time-set points of 0.5, 1, 2, 4, and 6 h, at a dose of 8.82 g/kg (the optimal dose among 4 different doses in the amount and intensity of target compounds, Supplementary Figure S2), respectively ($n = 5$). Five other rats received oral administration of an equivalent volume of 0.5% CMC-Na. The blood samples were gathered from the hepatic portal vein, and all the samples were centrifuged at 3,500 rpm for 10 min at 4°C. A four-fold volume of methanol was used to extract the supernatants by the protein precipitation approach. After centrifuging at 13,000 rpm for 10 min at 4°C, the supernatants were blow-dried and reconstituted with 100 μL of 75% methanol for further analysis.

2.2.2 Pharmacodynamics and Metabolomics Study

Twenty-four female Rats were haphazardly and equally divided into four groups: sham operation group (Sham), the mammary gland hyperplasia model group (MGH), low dose group of HHXYT (HHXYT-L), and high dose group of HHXYT (HHXYT-H). The MGH model was achieved by injecting intramuscularly with estradiol benzoate (0.5 mg/kg/d) for 25 days and then with progesterone (5 mg/kg/d) for 5 days (Wang et al., 2011). Meanwhile, the Sham group was injected with saline injection (0.5 mg/kg/d). After modeling, the HHXYT-L group and HHXYT-H group were administrated HHXYT orally with suspending in 0.5% CMC-Na aqueous solution, at a dosage of 0.5 g/kg/d (clinical equivalent dose) and 4.5 g/kg/d for 3 weeks, respectively. The Sham group and MGH group were given oral administration of 0.5% CMC-Na.

Rats were injected intraperitoneally with 10% chloral hydrate for anesthesia after 3 weeks of administration, and the diameter of the second pair of nipples was measured. The blood samples were obtained from the abdominal aorta, centrifuged at 3,500 rpm at 4°C for 15 min. The serum was separated from the upper layer and stored at −80°C. The left mammary gland of the second pair of breasts was collected and fixed in tissue fixative for 24 h, then sectioned in paraffin and stained with Hematoxylin-Eosin (HE) for optical microscopy. The contents of estradiol (E_2) and progesterone (P) in serum were determined by ELISA kits.

300 μL of methanol was put in 100 μL of serum, which was eddied for 1 min to ensure complete mingling before centrifugation at 14,000 rpm for 15 min at 4°C. The supernatant was aspirated and stored overnight at −80°C, followed by centrifugation under the same conditions for 15 min to remove proteins once again. The final supernatant was pipetted into the inner tube of vials and allowed to stand for LC-MC analysis. The quality control samples (QC) were prepared by pooling 20 μL of 6 random samples (containing all groups) from all samples.

2.3 Instrument Parameters

2.3.1 UPLC-QTOF-MS/MS for Identifying Prototypes of HHXYT and Related Metabolites in Plasma

The compounds absorbed in rat plasma were detected using a Waters Acquity UPLC I-class system (Waters Corp., Milford, MA, United States) and Q-tof Synapt G2-Si mass spectrometry system (Waters, Manchester, United Kingdom). A Waters Acquity UPLC BEH reverse-phase C18 analytical column (1.7 μm, 3.0 × 100 mm, Waters) was used to separate the compounds. The column temperature was set at 35°C and the injection volume was 5 μL. The mobile phase was made up of 0.1% formic acid in water (*v/v*) (A) and acetonitrile (B). At a flow rate of 0.4 ml/min, the elution gradient was processed in 37 min. The base peak chromatograms of both positive and negative ion modes were acquired under multiple detection modes of MS^E and Fast DDA. The parameters were set following the previous report (Mi et al., 2020).

2.3.2 HPLC-QTOF-MS/MS for Metabolomics Analysis

LC system was considered to apply with a Shimadzu HPLC system (Nexera XR LC-20AD, Japan) and use an ACQUITY UPLC® HSS T3 (2.1 × 100 mm, 1.8 μm, Waters, Milford, MA, United States) as the chromatographic column. Mass spectrometric detection was carried out on a SCIEX Triple TOF 5600⁺, using the electrospray ion (ESI) source and information-dependent acquisition (IDA) mode. The column temperature was set at 40°C and the injection volume was 2 μL. The mobile phase was made up of mass spectrometric grade 0.1% formic acid in water (*v/v*) (A) and acetonitrile (B). The calibration deliver system (CDS) was applied to calibrate the mass spectrometric acquisitions automatically. Additional parameter settings are provided in the Supplementary Materials.

2.4 Data Processing for Metabolomics Results

The raw data files were imported into the Progenesis QI 2.0 software (Waters, Milford, MA, United States) for data preprocessing, including alignment, peak picking, and compound identification. StatTarget was utilized to remove system errors as well as signal drift (Luan et al., 2018). The data was then imported into SICMA 14.1 (Umetric, Umeå, Sweden) for multivariable statistical analysis. Variates with *p*-values < 0.05, fold change (FC) ≥1.2 or FC ≤ 0.8, and VIP >1 (variable importance in the projection), were considered as endogenous differential metabolites, and further identified with online databases of HMDB (Wishart et al., 2018), LIPID MAPS (Liebisch et al., 2020) and KEGG (Kanehisa et al., 2017).

2.5 Identification and Analysis of Metabolic Modules

We applied the diffusion kernel algorithm to detect metabolites that locate at the proximity of the endogenous differential metabolites in the genome-scale metabolic network of rats (Luan et al., 2018). The diffusion parameter was set as 0.1. All endogenous differential metabolites of the MGH, HHXYT-L, and HHXYT-H groups were input as seed nodes to perform the diffusion kernel algorithm. The nodes with high diffusion scores were taken as compounds close to the endogenous differential metabolites in the genome-scale metabolic network. Then, the metabolic network affected by mammary glands hyperplasia and HHXYT treatment was constructed by extracting these nodes and links between them from the background network.

2.6 Putative Targets for HHXYT's Plasma Absorbed Compounds

For prototypes and their metabolites in the plasma of rats after intragastric administration of HHXYT, we collected or predicted their putative targets from 3 databases and web servers: ETCM (Encyclopaedia of Traditional Chinese Medicine) (Xu et al., 2019), HERB (High-throughput Experiment- and Reference-guided dataBase of traditional Chinese medicine) (Fang et al., 2021), and TargetNet (Yao et al., 2016). Target information in HERB was collected by manual reference mining and from multiple TCM databases, including SymMap (Wu, Zhang, Yang et al., 2019), TCMID (Xue et al., 2013), TCMSP (Ru et al., 2014), and TCM-ID (Chen et al., 2006). The threshold of confidence score was set as 0.9 to filter the compound-protein interactions predicted by TargetNet.

2.7 Collection of MGH Associated Genes and Functional Enrichment Analysis

Disease genes of MGH were collected from the GeneCards database (Stelzer et al., 2016). Inputting the keyword "mammary gland hyperplasia" generated 4,251 results with relevance scores in the area [0.53, 248.35]. We set the threshold of relevance score as 20 to filter the results and obtained 420 top-ranked genes with high relevance to MGH, taking about 10% of the results. These 420 genes were considered as MGH associated genes for further analysis.

We used the STRING platform to conduct functional enrichment analysis for gene groups under study (Szklarczyk et al., 2019).

2.8 Network Construction, Analysis, and Visualization

The genomic scale protein-protein interaction (PPI) network of human beings was downloaded from the HINT (High-quality INTeractomes) database (Das and Yu, 2012), whose PPI data was integrated from 8 databases (BioGRID, MINT, iRefWeb, DIP, IntAct, HPRD, MIPS, and the PDB) and filtered both systematically and manually to keep high-confidence and -quality interactions. It was used as a background network for the construction of HHXYT's target network. We used Cytoscape version 3.6.0 to construct, analysis and visualize networks (Shannon et al., 2003). The Cytohubba app of Cytoscape was applied to compute topological measures of nodes (Chin et al., 2014).

Metabolite-gene network was constructed by the Network Analysis module of MetaboAnalyst platform version 5.0 (Chong et al., 2019).

2.9 Molecular Docking

The SDF file for a ligand's structure was downloaded from the PubChem database (Kim et al., 2021). The PDB file for a protein receptor's crystal structure was obtained from RCSB Protein Data Bank (PDB) database (Burley et al., 2021). For proteins without known crystal structures, the predicted crystal structures were downloaded from AlphaFold Protein Structure Database (Jumper et al., 2021). The preprocessing and preparing of ligands and receptors were conducted by AutoDock Tools (Tanchuk et al., 2016) following the tutorial and manual (http://vina.scripps.edu/manual.html). Each ligand was docked with corresponding receptors by AutoDock Vina (Trott and Olson, 2010), and a compound-target pair with the docking score of less than −5 kcal/mol was considered as a binding pair. PLIP platform was used to analyze the binding sites of the binding compound-target pair (Adasme et al., 2021). PyMol was applied for visualizing the results of AutoDock Vina and PLIP (Alexander et al., 2011).

2.10 Cell-Based Assay Evaluation of HHXYT *In Vitro*

Thecal cells were extracted and purified from the ovaries of female rats at 3–4 weeks old (Li and Hearn, 2000). 5×10^3 thecal cells per well were seeded into 96-well plates and set as the control group and experimental groups. The control group was McCoy's 5A medium containing thecal cell. The experimental groups were based on the control group supplemented with different concentrations of luteinizing hormone (LH), follicle-stimulating hormone (FSH), HHXYT, and its ingredient formononetin (FT). After 36 h of adherent culture at 37°C and 5% CO_2, these drugs were supplemented according to different groups and cultured for another 24 h. Then 10 μL of CCK-8 reagent was added to each well in the dark, and the absorbance was measured at a wavelength of 450 nm 2 h later to calculate the cell survival rate (Chen et al., 2021).

4×10^4 Cells were added to each well of 48-well plates containing McCoy's 5A medium, which consisted of 10% FBS and 1% penicillin-streptomycin. After culturing at 37°C and 5% CO_2 for 36 h, different concentrations of LH, dexamethasone (DEX), HHXYT, and FT were added into different groups of wells and cultured for another 24 h (Ong et al., 2019). ELISA kits were used to detect the levels of estradiol (E_2) or testosterone (T) in cell media.

3 RESULTS

3.1 Pharmacodynamic Results of HHXYT on MGH Model

To evaluate the therapeutic effect of HHXYT on MGH, we detected variations of nipple diameter and serum sex hormone level. After establishing the MGH model, the nipple diameter grew significantly ($p < 0.01$, MGH vs. Sham) from 0.858 ± 0.068 mm to 1.230 ± 0.086 mm, compared to the Sham group. Different doses of HHXYT, on the other hand, could significantly ($p < 0.01$, HHXYT vs. MGH) reduce nipple enlargement (**Figure 2A**). Meanwhile, in the MGH group, the estradiol level in serum increased prominently ($p < 0.01$, MGH vs. Sham) while the progesterone level decreased notably ($p < 0.01$, MGH vs. Sham). After treatment with different doses of HHXYT, the serum level of estradiol and progesterone was reversed, respectively (**Figures 2B,C**).

According to Hematoxylin-Eosin (HE) staining, mammary tissue in the Sham group had no aberrant proliferation, a tiny number of the acinus, nearly no dilatation, and no secretion of mammary ducts and lumens (**Figure 2D**). The mammary tissue in the MGH group showed distinct proliferation; the volume of mammary lobules was increased; the number of glandular bubbles was also increased and became close to fusion; the acinus and lumens were revealed dilatation and excessive secretions (**Figure 2E**). However, after HHXYT treatment, mammary gland hyperplasia was prominently alleviated due to a considerable reduction in the account of the volume of mammary lobules, the number of glandular vesicles, and the secretion of lumens (**Figure 2F**).

3.2 Characterization of Prototypes and Metabolites in HHXYT, and Functional Enrichment Analysis of Putative Targets

It is widely accepted that prototypes and their metabolites in blood after oral TCM intake have a therapeutic effect (Ye et al., 2019). In order to determine the active components of HHXYT, we comprehensively analyzed the prototypes and their metabolites of HHXYT in rat plasma. A total of 54 components were identified, comprising 22 prototypes (**Figures 3A,B; Supplementary Table S1**) and 32 metabolites (**Supplementary Table S2**). After HHXYT treatment, three prototype components, named desbenzoylpaeoniflorin, 1-*O*-*β*-D–glucopyranosylpaeonisuffrone, and bohenoside A, as well as 32 metabolites, were identified in rat plasma for the first time. These 32 metabolites include 2 monoterpenoids, 8 triterpenes, 11 organic acids, 10 flavonoids, and 1 other metabolite (**Figure 3C; Supplementary Table S4-S7**).

Based on 54 active ingredients identified in the rat plasma, we predicted their potential target through network pharmacology (hydroxysafflower yellow A was also added to the analysis because it was reported to be an active ingredient of *Carthami Flos* (Honghua) (Li et al., 2021)). Using 3 databases and web servers (ETCM, HERB, and TargetNet), 373 distinct protein targets were predicted as HHXYT's putative targets regulated by the 55 active ingredients (**Supplementary Table S3**).

The STRING platform was utilized to analyze the 373 targets for functional enrichment. Setting FDR<10^{-4} as the threshold, we identified 93 statistically enriched KEGG pathways. The top enriched pathways were presented in **Table 2**, and these pathways were mainly involved in the biological processes of the endocrine, immune, and nervous system.

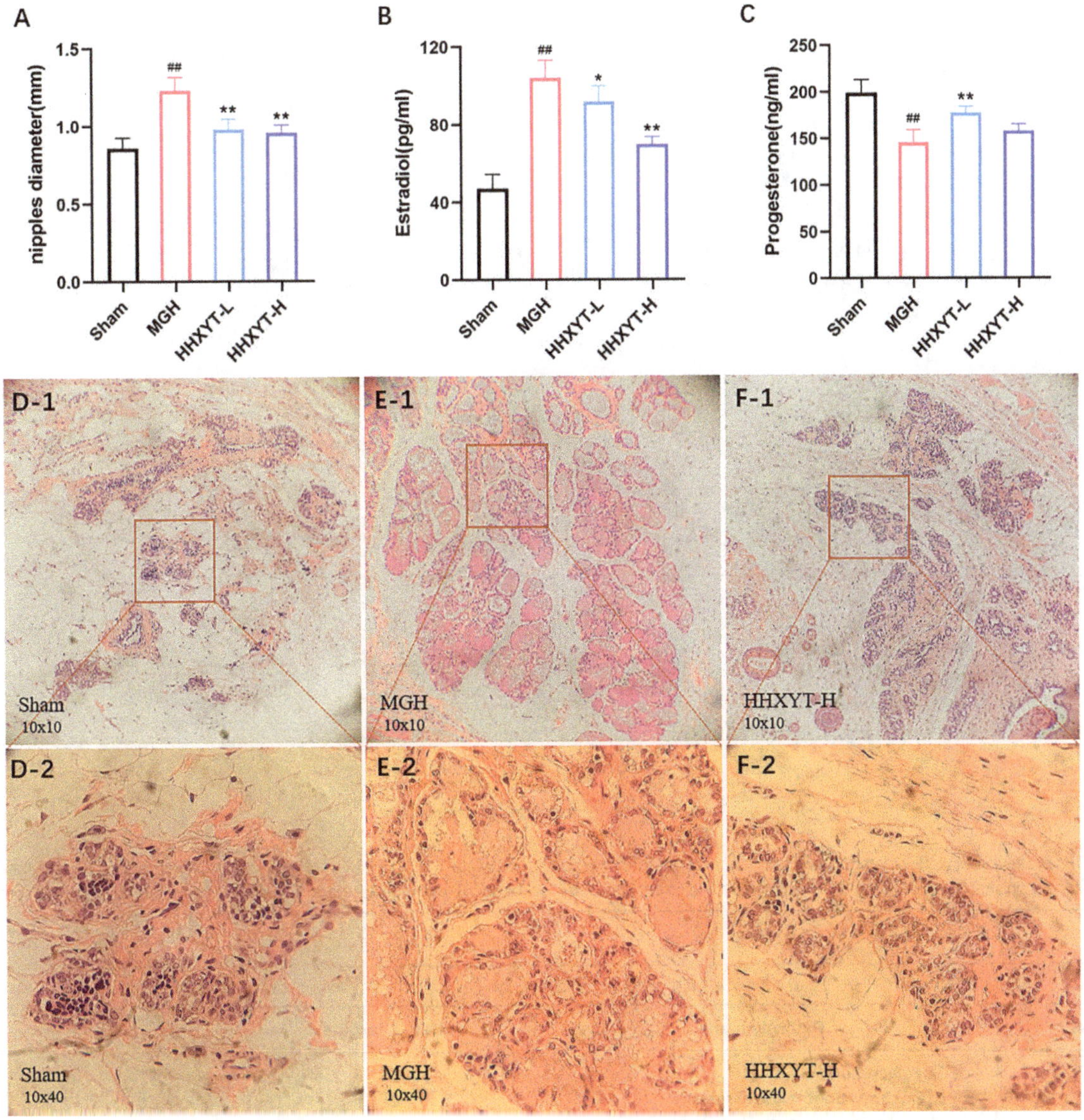

FIGURE 2 | The effect of HHXYT on pharmacodynamic results of the MGH model. **(A)** The diameter of nipples. The serum levels of sex hormone estradiol **(B)** and progesterone **(C)**. $n = 6$ per group, ##$p < 0.01$, compared to Sham; *$p < 0.05$, **$p < 0.01$, compared to MGH. HE staining results for mammary gland sections in Sham **(D)**, MGH **(E)**, HHXYT-H **(F)** group (10 × 10: D-1, E-1, and F-1; 10 × 40: D-2, E-2, and F-2).

Then, based on the KEGG pathways in **Table 2**, we performed enrichment analysis for targets of HHXYT's herbs and prototypes. When conducting enrichment analysis, we combined targets of metabolites derived from its prototype with targets of the prototype. The threshold for statistical significance was set as FDR<10^{-4}. As shown in **Figure 4**, targets of 6 herbs and 9 prototypes from HHXYT were enriched in at least 3 of the 20 KEGG pathways in **Table 2**, respectively. These results suggested that the 6 herbs and 9 prototypes could play key roles in HHXYT's treatment of MGH.

3.3 HHXYT Alters the Serum Metabolome

On the basis of research on prototypes and their metabolites of HHXYT, the metabolomics analysis was used to further identify the serum endogenous differential metabolites of rats intervened by HHXYT. The PLS-DA model was applied to characterize the metabolic disturbances. As shown in **Figures 5A,B**, the serum samples of Sham, MGH, HHXYT-L, and HHXYT-H groups were distinctly separated in both positive and negative modes. Based on the criteria of *p*-values < 0.05, FC ≥ 1.2 or FC ≤ 0.8, and VIP >1, 58 endogenous differential metabolites in serum were screened and identified, including 29 metabolites in the Sham/MGH group, 19 metabolites in the MGH/HHXYT-L group, and 18 metabolites in the MGH/HHXYT-H group (**Figure 5C**). There were 5 same endogenous differential metabolites between HHXYT-H and MGH (**Figure 5D**, red compound names), as well as 2 overlaps between HHXYT-L and MGH (blue compound names). Furthermore, the regulatory trends of

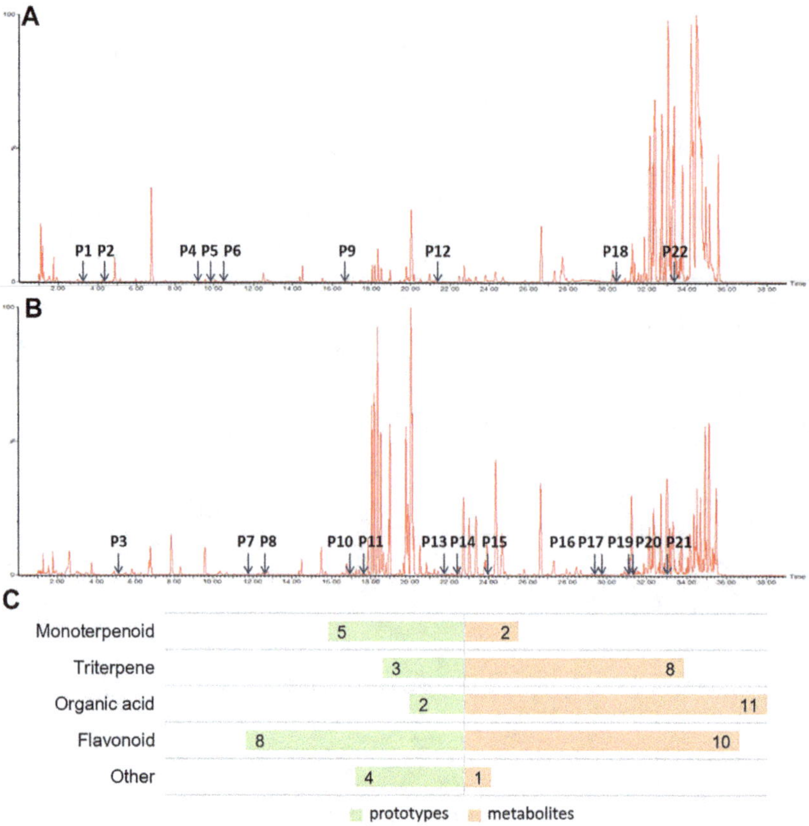

FIGURE 3 | The prototypes and their metabolites in the plasma of rats after intragastric administration of HHXYT. Total ion chromatograms of rat plasma samples after intragastric administration of HHXYT and the distribution of 22 prototypes, positive mode **(A)** and negative mode **(B)**. **(C)** Categories of prototypes and metabolites.

TABLE 2 | Enriched KEGG pathways of HHXYT's targets. The pathways with bold type are associated with metabolic modules affected by HHXYT.

Pathway class	Pathway name	HHXYT targets	Total genes	FDR
Endocrine	**Bile secretion**	30	71	1.08E-25
	Steroid hormone biosynthesis	28	58	1.85E-25
	Thyroid hormone signaling pathway	29	115	2.59E-20
	Estrogen signaling pathway	24	133	2.01E-14
	Prolactin signaling pathway	19	69	2.42E-14
	Relaxin signaling pathway	22	130	6.79E-13
	Ovarian steroidogenesis	15	49	3.65E-12
	Cortisol synthesis and secretion	8	63	8.24E-05
Immune	Th17 cell differentiation	21	102	1.09E-13
	IL-17 signaling pathway	20	92	1.74E-13
	PI3K-Akt signaling pathway	37	348	3.66E-15
	TNF signaling pathway	23	108	4.18E-15
	VEGF signaling pathway	16	59	3.10E-12
Nervous system	Serotonergic synapse	24	112	1.06E-15
	Cholinergic synapse	20	111	2.97E-12
	Neuroactive ligand-receptor interaction	36	272	2.74E-17
	cAMP signaling pathway	30	195	4.60E-16
	Sphingolipid signaling pathway	23	116	1.39E-14
Other	Metabolism of xenobiotics by cytochrome P450	18	70	2.81E-13
	Thermogenesis	30	228	1.37E-14

HHXYT-H on the 5 same differential metabolites were all opposite to that of MGH. Meanwhile, only one differential metabolite had been oppositely regulated between HHXYT-L and MGH groups. These results indicated that the HHXYT-H group had more pronounced alterations in metabolites endogenous on treating MGH. The majority of these endogenous differential metabolites

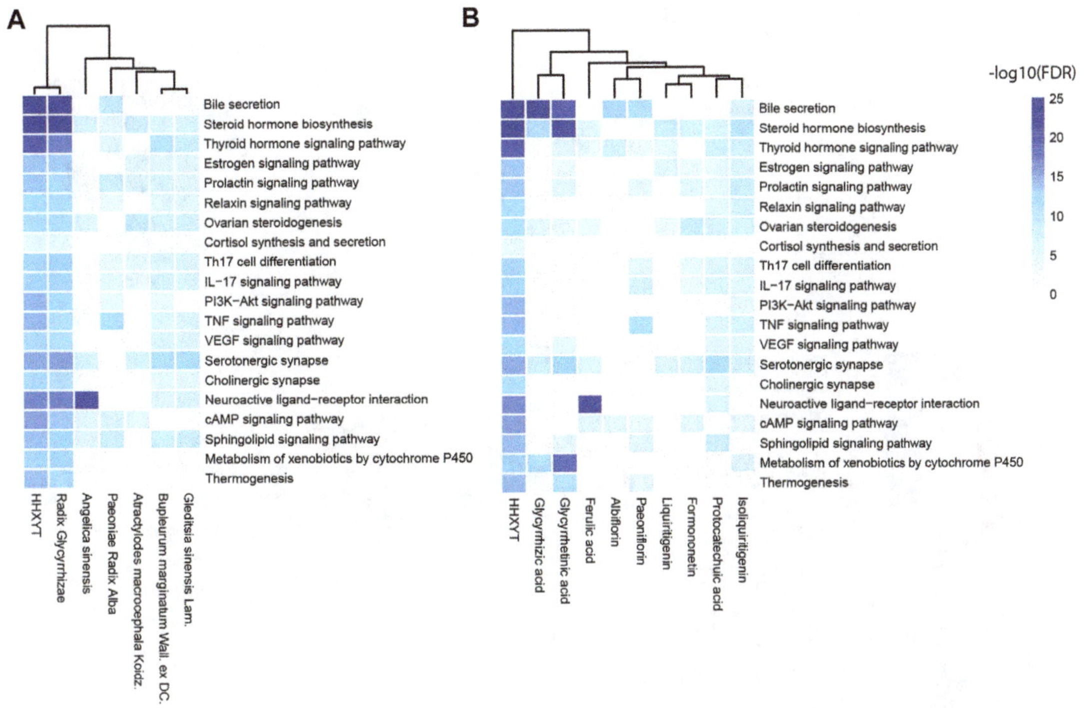

FIGURE 4 | KEGG pathway enrichment analysis for the targets of herbs and prototypes of HHXYT. Targets of 6 herbs **(A)** and 9 prototypes **(B)** from HHXYT were enriched in at least 3 of the top 20 KEGG pathways regulated by HHXYT, respectively.

are lipid metabolites, accounting for 68%, including 31% steroids lipid (12% bile acids, 8% pregnane steroids, 7% hydroxysteroids, etc.), 8% fatty acids, 7% fatty acid esters, 8% prenol lipids, 8% glycerophospholipids and so on (**Figure 5E**). The above results suggested that HHXYT could prominently regulate lipid metabolism, especially hormone disorder in rats with hyperplasia of mammary glands.

3.4 Metabolic Modules Affected by the Treatment of HHXYT

To reveal the underlying significance of metabolites variation *in vivo,* we proceeded with metabolic module establishment and pathway analysis of endogenous differential metabolites. Inputting all the endogenous differential metabolites as seed nodes, we ran the diffusion kernel algorithm to score all nodes in the genome-scale metabolic network of rats. The metabolic network influenced by MGH and HHXYT therapy was then constructed by extracting the nodes with diffusion scores at least 0.05 and the links between them (**Figure 6**). This network consists of 19 isolated modules, in which only the first three large modules include endogenous differential metabolites affected by both MGH and HHXYT treatment, suggesting that they could be key metabolic modules by which HHXYT exerts its therapeutic effect on MGH.

We searched the KEGG database (Kanehisa et al., 2017) to annotate the first 3 modules in **Figure 6**. It was found that metabolites in the first module were mainly involved in pathways of steroid hormone biosynthesis, cortisol synthesis and secretion, and ovarian steroidogenesis; the compounds in the second module participated in primary bile acid biosynthesis and bile secretion; the third module was associated with glycerophospholipid metabolism and biosynthesis of unsaturated fatty acids. Notably, all the 3 pathways associated with the first metabolic module and 1 pathway of the second metabolic module, were also found in the pathways listed in **Table 2**, which were enriched by 373 HHXYT's predicted targets. It demonstrated that the pathways involved by HHXYT's putative targets discovered by network pharmacology were consistent with the analyzed regulation of metabolic disturbances in rat serum by metabolomics.

3.5 Network Pharmacological Analysis for HHXYT's Putative Targets and Metabolic Modules

The first step was to conduct a network analysis of HHXYT's potential targets. We calculated the intersections of HHXYT's 373 target genes with the 420 diseases genes for MGH (**Supplementary Table S4; Figure 7A**). It could be seen that one-fourth of HHXYT's targets were disease genes. Then we constructed the protein-protein interaction (PPI) network between the targets based on the human genomic-scale PPI network from the HINT database. As shown in **Figure 7B,** 114 of the 373 targets interacted with each other to form HHXYT's target network, with 53 of them being disease genes associated with MGH.

The centrality measures for nodes in the target network were computed using the Cytohubba App of the Cytoscape software. The centrality of nodes was then ranked applying 3 global parameters based on shortest paths (Closeness, EcCentricity, and Radiality). As shown in **Figure 7C,** the 4 nodes with the

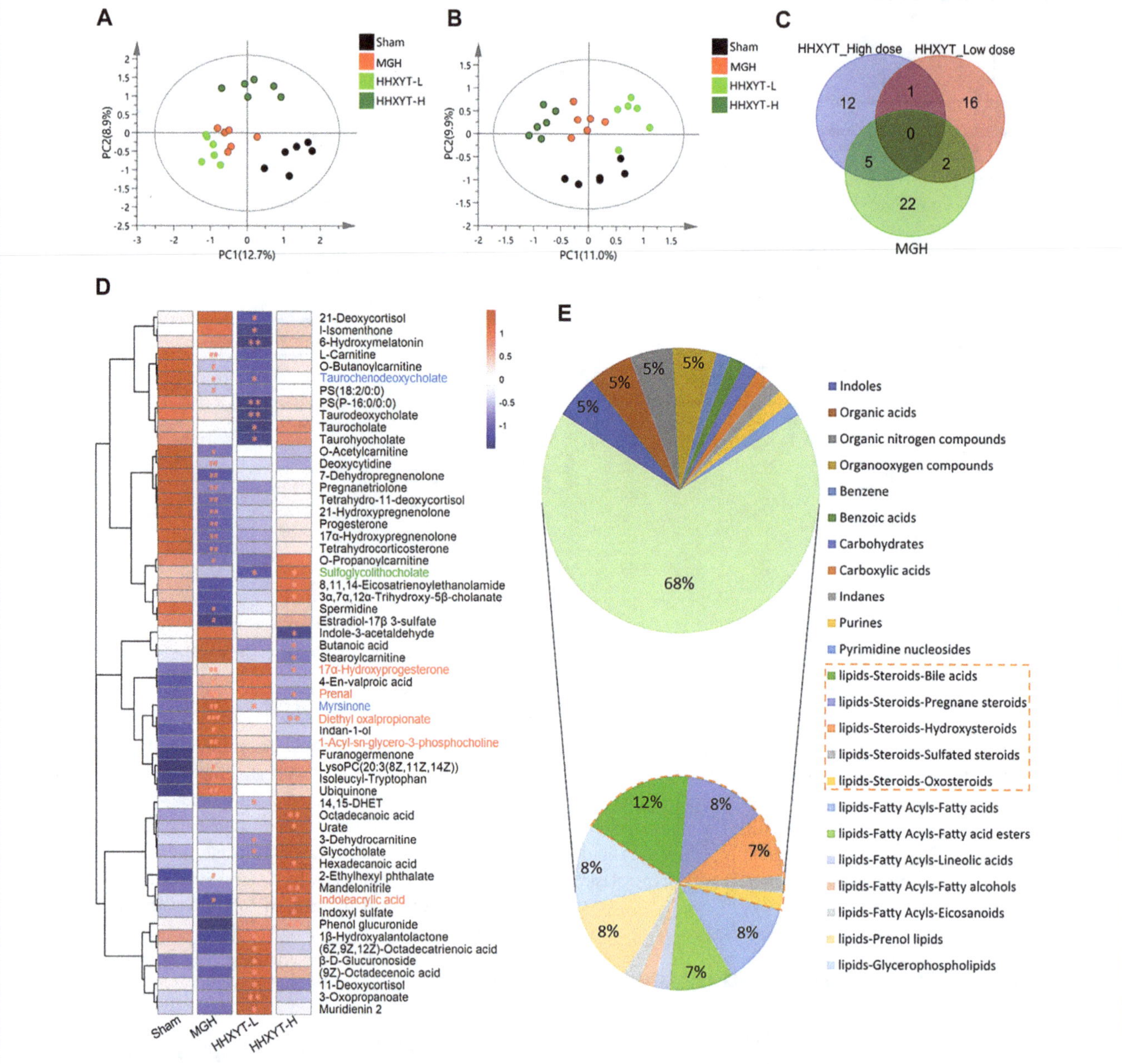

FIGURE 5 | Endogenous differential metabolites were identified from the metabolomics experiment. PLS-DA score plots of Sham, MGH HHXYT-L, and HHXYT-H, in positive mode **(A)** and negative mode **(B)**. **(C)** The intersection of endogenous differential metabolites in the 3 groups. **(D)** Heatmap of 58 endogenous differential metabolites. $n = 6$, #$p < 0.05$, ##$p < 0.01$, compared to Sham; *$p < 0.05$, **$p < 0.01$, compared to MGH. The red compound name means the common differential metabolites between HHXYT-H and MGH; Blue: the common differential metabolites of HHXYT-L/MGH; Green: the common differential metabolites of HHXYT-H/HHXYT-L. **(E)** Categories of endogenous differential metabolites. 31% of steroids were marked with the orange border.

highest global centrality were AR, ESR1, AKT1, and JUN, suggesting that they were central nodes whose impacts were easy to reach out into the whole target network.

The Network Analysis module of the MetaboAnalyst platform version 5.0 was then utilized to construct metabolite-gene networks corresponding to the metabolic modules affected by HHXYT. We input the endogenous differential metabolites in the first and second modules of **Figure 6**, together with HHXYT's targets enriched in the corresponding pathways of the modules, respectively. Then we got the metabolite-gene interaction modules for the first and second metabolite module affected by HHXYT (**Figures 7D,E**). As shown in **Figure 7D**, the first module included 3 hub genes, i.e., CYP11A1, HSD3B2, and CYP17A1, which linked to all the metabolites in the network, implying that they performed a key role in HHXYT's treatment to MGH.

The key targets of HHXYT for treating MGH were then obtained by combining the 4 central genes of the target network and the 3 hub

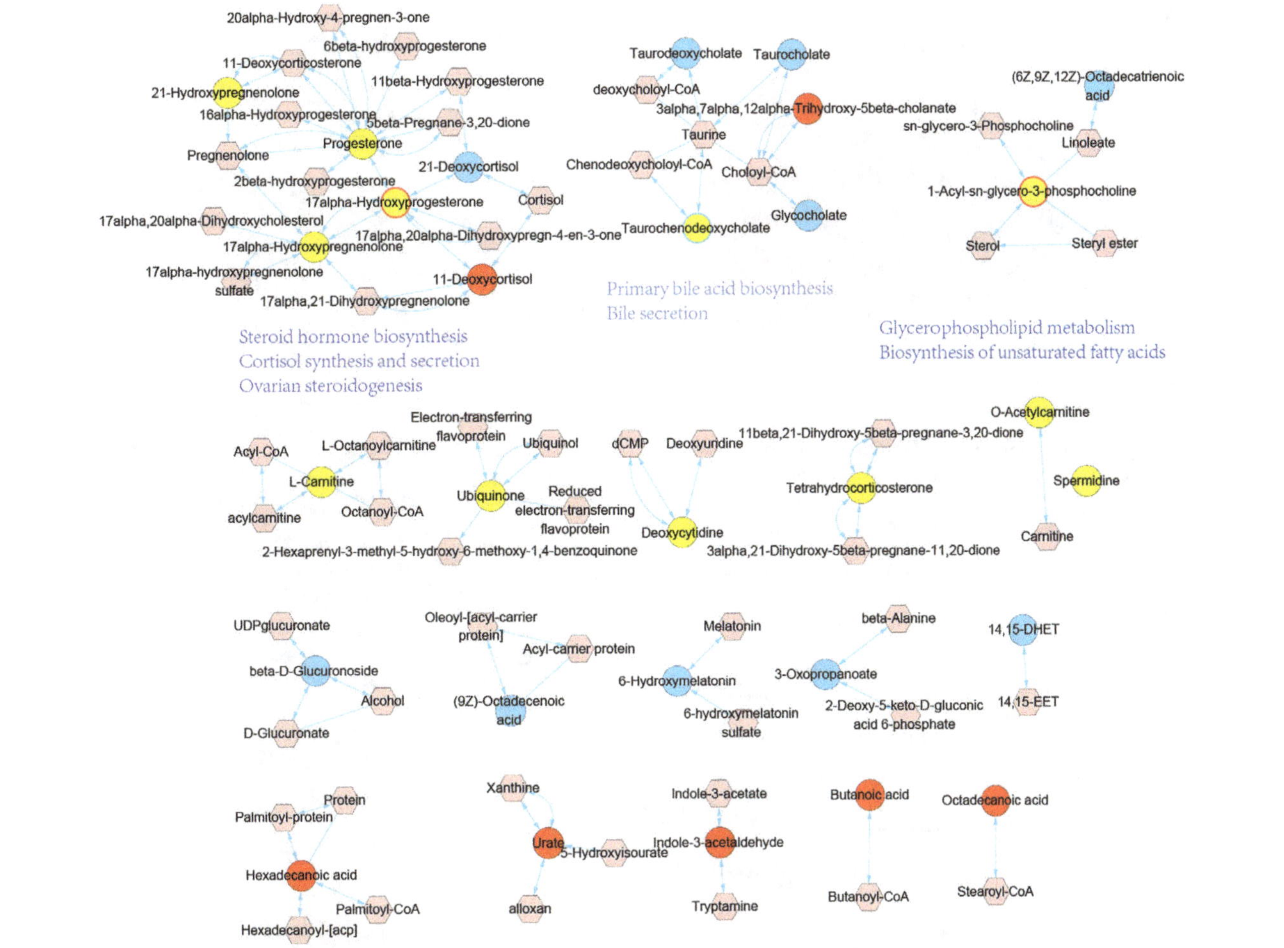

FIGURE 6 | Metabolic modules affected by HHXYT treatment and their functions. Circle nodes are endogenous differential metabolites identified in metabolomics, and hexagonal nodes are metabolites close to the endogenous differential metabolites in the genomic metabolic network which were identified by the diffusion kernel algorithm. Yellow circles are endogenous differential metabolites in MGH, while circles with blue and red colors or borders were in HHXYT-L and HHXYT-H, respectively.

genes in the first metabolite-gene module. We integrated the 7 key targets with the key herbs, prototypes (**Figure 4**), and their metabolites on HHXYT's treatment to MGH, to construct the herb-ingredient-target network as shown in **Figure 8A**. There were 7 targets, 6 herbs, and 17 ingredients in this network. 8 of 17 ingredients were HHXYT's prototypes absorbed in plasma, and 9 were metabolites derived from them. These herbs, ingredients, and targets constitute key substances for HHXYT to exert therapeutic effects on MGH.

At last, to verify the binding between 5 of HHXYT's key targets and corresponding prototypes, we utilized AutoDock Vina software to conduct molecular docking. The crystal structures of 4 targets, i.e., AR (PDB ID:2q7i), CYP11A1 (PDB ID:3n9y), CYP17A1 (PDB ID:6ciz), ESR1 (PDB ID: 2qgw), which have higher resolution, were downloaded from RCSB Protein Data Bank. The predicted structure of HSD3B2 (ID: AF-P26439-F1) was downloaded from AlphaFold Protein Structure Database. The SDF files for chemical structures of the compounds (ferulic acid, formononetin, glycyrrhetinic acid, glycyrrhizic acid, isoliquiritigenin, liquiritigenin, and protocatechuic acid) were downloaded from the PubChem database. The docking scores between 14 pairs of compound-target are less than −5 kcal/mol (**Table 3**), suggesting that the corresponding compounds and targets have a higher binding affinity. Binding poses and binding sites for 5 pairs of compound-target interactions were shown in **Figures 8B–F**.

3.6 Effects of HHXYT and its Ingredient on the Testosterone Synthesis in Thecal Cells

Firstly, the cell-based assay was performed to demonstrate that the extracted and purified cells *in vitro* were thecal cells. After LH (50 ng/ml) was added, the cell proliferation rate (maximum ratio 147%) and testosterone (T) level (from 1965.15 ± 96.65 to 2,329.43 ± 87.93 pg/ml) both increased prominently (**Figures 9A,B**). However, after the addition of FSH, no significant changes in cell quantity were observed, and estradiol (E_2) was not detected. It indicated that the purified cells were primarily thecal cells, with no obvious interference from granulosa cells, which were also presented in follicles of the ovary. The cell survival rate results of HHXYT and its ingredient formononetin (FT, **Figure 9C**) were shown in **Supplementary Figure S9**.

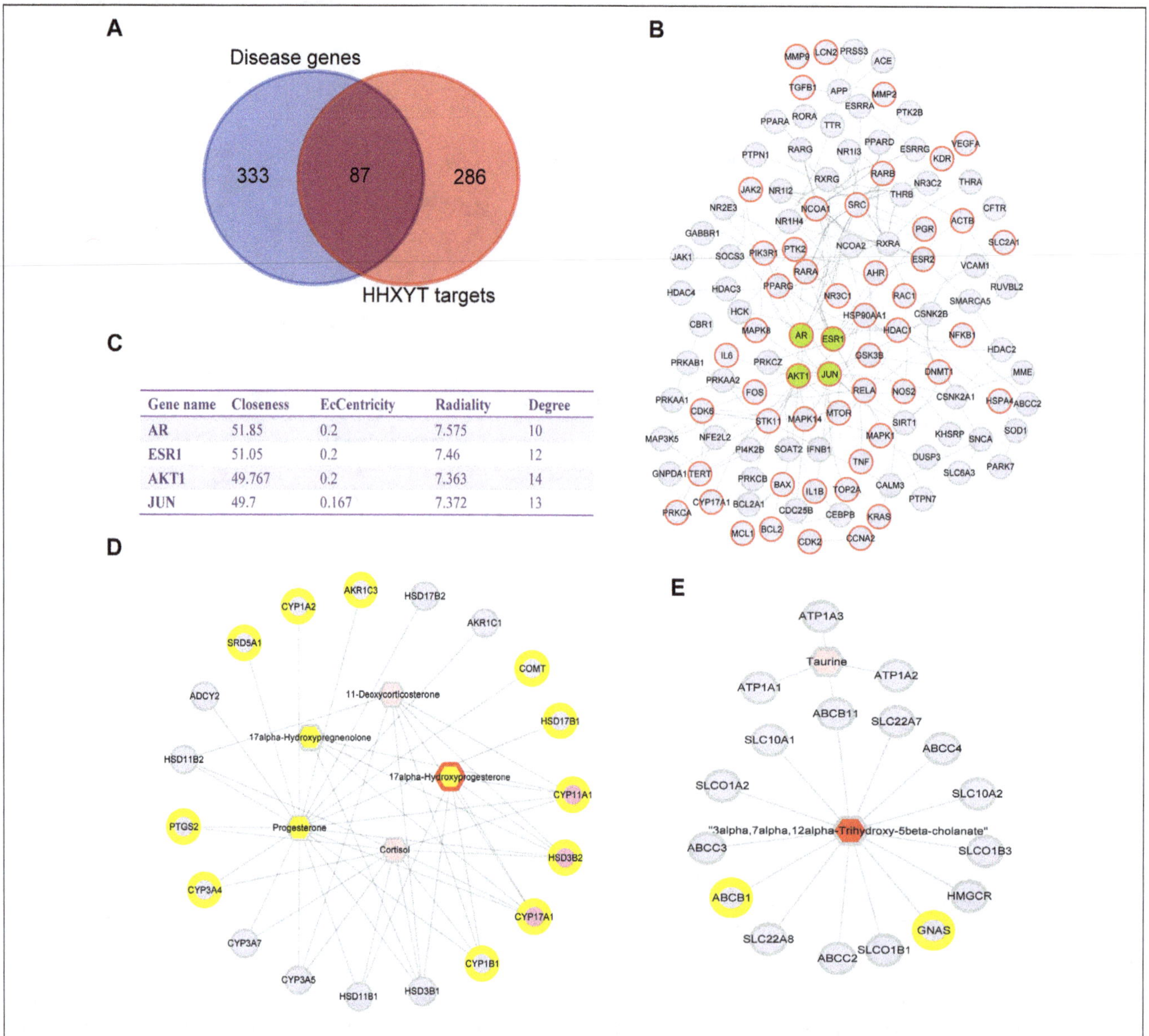

Gene name	Closeness	EcCentricity	Radiality	Degree
AR	51.85	0.2	7.575	10
ESR1	51.05	0.2	7.46	12
AKT1	49.767	0.2	7.363	14
JUN	49.7	0.167	7.372	13

FIGURE 7 | Network pharmacological analysis for HHXYT's putative targets and integrated analysis of metabolic modules. **(A)** The intersection between HHXYT's putative targets and MGH disease genes from GeneCards. **(B)** HHXYT's putative target network, where the nodes with red borders are MGH disease genes and the green nodes are central nodes with the highest global centrality. **(C)** Global (Closeness, EcCentricity, Radiality) and local centrality measures (Degree) of the four central nodes in the target network. Metabolite-gene networks for the first **(D)** and second metabolic module **(E)** affected by HHXYT, respectively. Hexagons were endogenous differential metabolites identified from the metabolomics analysis and circles were HHXYT's target and genes. Yellow represented in MGH disease conditions, while red represented in HHXYT-H. Pink circles were the hub genes of the network.

To evaluate the effect of HHXYT and its ingredient formononetin (FT) on the production of testosterone in thecal cells, thecal cells were stimulated with different concentrations of dexamethasone (DEX) and then treated with different concentrations of HHXYT and FT. The results showed that testosterone levels were markedly elevated at the DEX concentration of 10, 20, 25 μM (**Figure 9D**). Whereas, HHXYT (50 μg/ml) and FT (3.2, 6.3, and 12.5 μM) could distinctly inhibit the increase of testosterone level caused by DEX (10 μM) in thecal cells, suggesting that HHXYT and FT have an inhibitory effect on testosterone production in thecal cells.

4 DISCUSSION

MGH is the most prevalent breast disease and the incidence of breast cancer in MGH patients is remarkably higher than that in the average person (Basree et al., 2019). However, in the current clinical treatment of MGH, hormone therapy such as tamoxifen is not suitable for long-term use with apparent ill effects and complications (Wibowo et al., 2016); operative treatment is unacceptable for patients because of its complexity. Fortunately, HHXYT has been applied in the treatment of

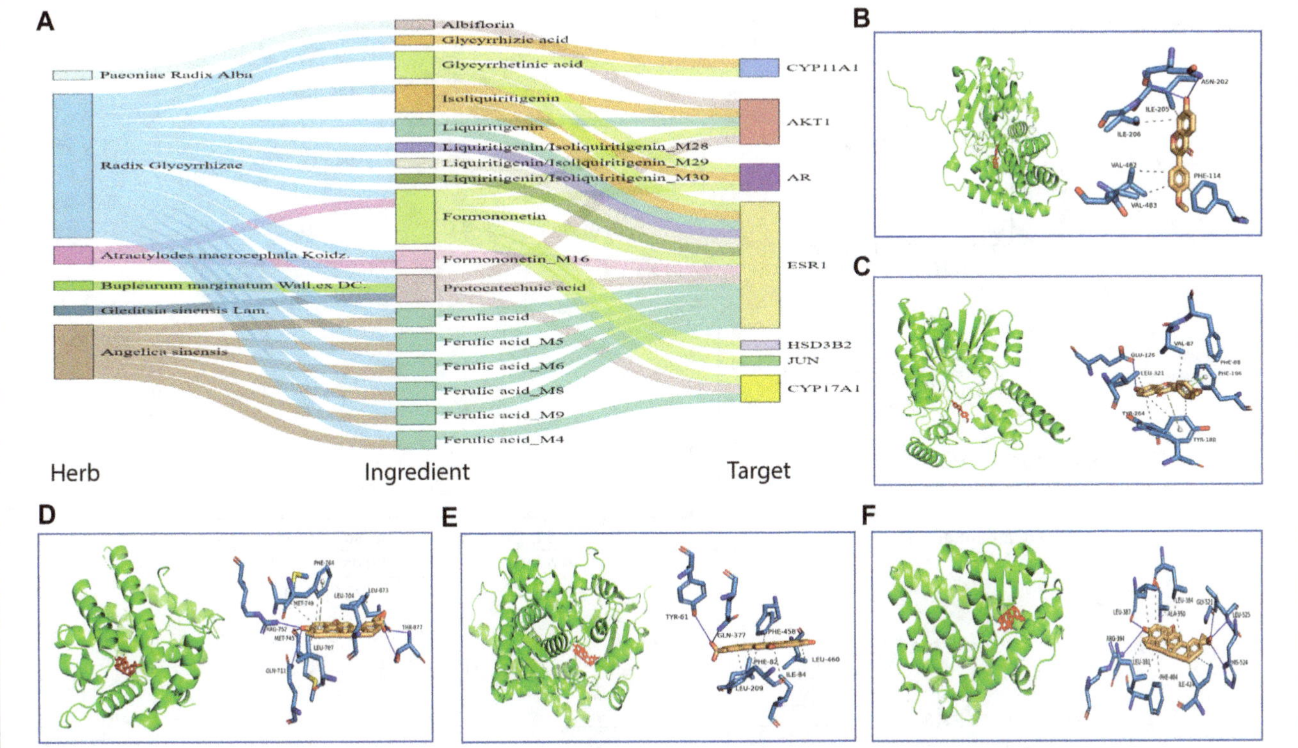

FIGURE 8 | The key substances for HHXYT to exert therapeutic effects on MGH. **(A)** Herb-ingredient-target relationships for key targets, herbs, and ingredients of HHXYT. The integrated name of prototypes and their metabolite ID means that the metabolite is derived from the corresponding prototypes. **(B–F)** Molecular docking of HHXYT's five key targets with corresponding compounds. The binding poses and binding sites of formononetin complexed with CYP17A1 **(B)** and HSD3B2 **(C)**; The binding poses and binding sites of glycyrrhetinic acid complexed with AR **(D)**, CYP11A1 **(E)**, and ER **(F)**.

TABLE 3 | The docking scores between HHXYT's key targets and compounds (kcal/mol).

Target	Target structure ID	Compound	Binding score
AR	2q7i	Formononetin	−9.3
		Glycyrrhetinic acid	−17.4
		Isoliquiritigenin	−8.2
CYP11A1	3n9y	Glycyrrhetinic acid	−15.7
		Glycyrrhizic acid	−14.7
CYP17A1	6ciz	Formononetin	−8.6
		Protocatechuic acid	−5.8
ESR1	2qgw	Ferulic acid	−6.2
		Formononetin	−9.3
		Glycyrrhetinic acid	−16.6
		Isoliquiritigenin	−8.1
		Liquiritigenin	−9.5
		Protocatechuic acid	−6.1
HSD3B2	AF-P26439-F1-model_v1	Formononetin	−9.4

MGH for years and its efficacy has been validated clinically (Meng et al., 2014; Pei et al., 2016).

In this study, the integrated metabolomics and network pharmacology strategy were applied to systemically reveal the mechanism of HHXYT in the treatment of MGH. Firstly, the rat model of MGH was established to reconfirm the therapeutic effect of HHXYT. HHXYT effectively inhibited the abnormal proliferation of mammary lobules, glandular bubbles, and lumens in mammary glands, according to HE staining of mammary tissue. Meanwhile, the abnormal levels of estradiol (E_2) and progesterone (P) in serum were reversed after treatment with HHXYT. In fact, the mammary gland is closely regulated by sex hormones (Li et al., 2017). Furthermore, it has been reported that the disturbance of sex hormones, particularly estrogen and progesterone, is the primary cause and defining feature of MGH: estrogen stimulation can accelerate breast proliferation, whereas progesterone can facilitate the growth and maturation of breast acinous cells and resist the proliferation impact of estrogen (Kleinberg et al., 2011; Chang et al., 2014). In other words, high levels of E_2 or a lack of P cause estrogen to stimulate breast epithelium for an extended period without the protection of progesterone, resulting in significant mammary tissue hyperplasia (Liu et al., 2020). As a result, the above results confirmed that HHXYT could inhibit the symptoms of MGH visibly.

To figure out active compounds which exert therapeutic effects in HHXYT, we studied the plasma of rats after oral administration of HHXYT and identified 22 prototypes and their 32 metabolites. Following that, these compounds were used for HHXYT's putative target prediction and functional enrichment analysis by network pharmacology. 373 putative targets, 93 pathways, 6 key herbs, and 9 key prototypes of HHXYT were sought out and the most relevant of these

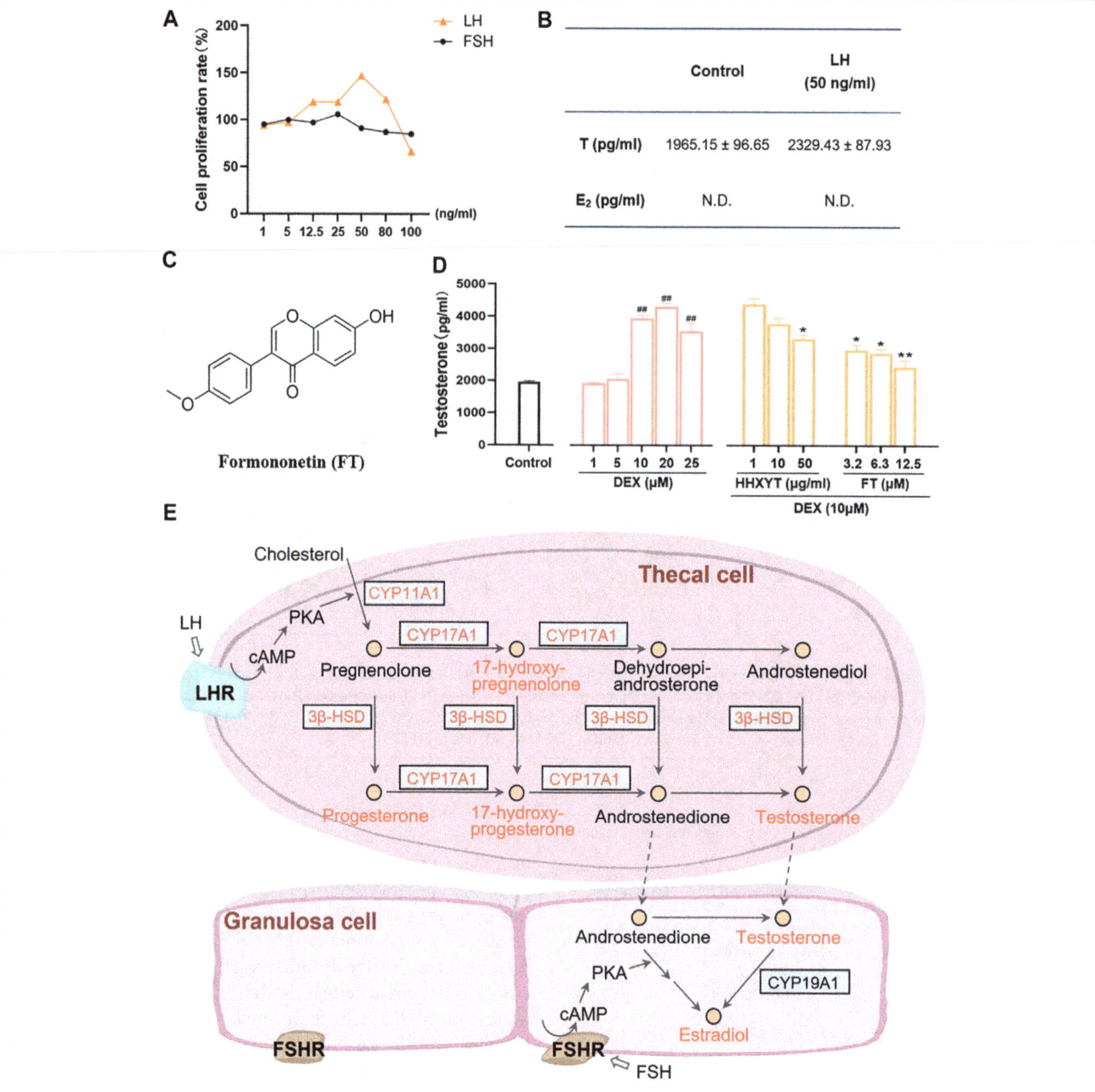

FIGURE 9 | Cell-based assay to evaluate the HHXYT's effects on testosterone synthesis in thecal cells. **(A)** The proliferation effect of luteinizing hormone (LH) and follicle-stimulating hormone (FSH) on thecal cells. **(B)** Effects of LH on the production of testosterone (T) and estradiol (E_2) in thecal cells. **(C)** The chemical structures of formononetin (FT). **(D)** Effects of dexamethasone (DEX), HHXYT, and FT on the production of testosterone by thecal cell. $n = 4$, ##$p < 0.01$, to the Control group; *$p < 0.05$, **$p < 0.01$, compared to the DEX (10 μM) group. **(E)** Pathways for the synthesis of testosterone and estradiol by thecal cells and granulosa cells in follicles. The compounds and targets involved in this study were marked by orange-red colors.

pathways was biological processes of the endocrine, especially the synthesis of hormones (**Table 2**). To further explore the therapeutic mechanism of HHXYT, the analysis of serum metabolomics was performed to intuitively characterize changes in endogenous metabolites. 58 endogenous different metabolites were identified, of which 31% were steroid lipids. In addition, the most significant metabolic modules were primarily involved in steroid hormone biosynthesis, cortisol synthesis and secretion, and ovarian steroidogenesis pathways. The compounds in the second module participated in primary bile acid biosynthesis and bile secretion. Notably, all these 4 pathways were also found to be enriched by HHXYT's putative targets. It demonstrated that metabolomic confirmed the regulation of metabolic disturbances similar to network pharmacology's prediction results, both of which were related to hormones and bile acid biosynthesis.

Actually, bile acid was closely related to the synthesis, absorption, and metabolism of cholesterol, which was the precursor of all hormone synthesis (Capponi, 2002). As shown in **Figure 9E**, in the pathway of sex hormone synthesis, cholesterol was applied as a raw material to synthesize androgens, and estrogens and androgens were precursors for the production of estrogen (Williams et al., 2001). The superiority of network pharmacology is that biological networks can be constructed to assist in elucidating drug treatment mechanisms from a holistic perspective (Zhao et al., 2019; Zhao et al., 2021). Ultimately, the herb-ingredient-target network was established as the substance basis for HHXYT to exert therapeutic effects on mammary gland hyperplasia. Among the 7 key targets of HHXYT, CYP11A1, HSD3B2, and CYP17A1 were directly involved in androgen synthesis and played vital roles, meanwhile, AR and ESR1 were receptors for the direct action of androgens and estrogens, respectively. In detail, estrogen was principally generated by the synergistic effects of thecal and granulosa cells of the ovary in females. Cholesterol was converted to pregnenolone in thecal cells by CYP11A1, which was turned into androgen under the catalysis of HSD3B2 and CYP17A1, especially CYP17A1. Then androgen was generated to estrogen in granulosa cells by CYP19A1 (Imamichi et al., 2017; Burris-Hiday and Scott, 2021). According to the above results, the synthesis of sex hormones, especially androgens, was significantly regulated by HHXYT.

Therefore, it was speculated that HHXYT may reduce the level of estrogen *in vivo* by inhibiting androgen synthesis, consequently protecting the mammary gland from excessive proliferation stimulated by estrogen. There were thecal cells and granulosa cells in the follicles of the ovary. Thecal cells possessed the luteinizing hormone (LH) receptor and synthesized testosterone (T), while granulosa cells owned follicle-stimulating hormone (FSH) receptors and produced E_2. In addition, thecal cells would promote cell proliferation and testosterone production after being stimulated by LH (Li and Hearn, 2000). To evaluate the HHXYT's effects on the synthesis of testosterone, we extracted thecal cells from the ovaries and experimented *in vitro*. Since dexamethasone (DEX) would promote the synthesis of T in thecal cells (Ong et al., 2019), DEX was added as the model group to observe the effects of HHXYT on testosterone synthesis. The results displayed that HHXYT (50 μg/ml) could distinctly inhibit the increase of T level caused by DEX (10 μM) in thecal cells. Meanwhile, formononetin (3.2, 6.3, and 12.5 μM), a prototype of HHXYT, also exhibited the inhibiting effect on testosterone levels rising. It demonstrated that they have an inhibitory effect on testosterone production in thecal cells. In summary, these findings contribute to elucidating the treatment mechanism of HHXYT on MGH and provide data and theoretical support for the in-depth study of its mechanism.

5 CONCLUSION

In this study, through integrating metabolomics and network pharmacology analysis, our results revealed the key substances for HHXYT to exert therapeutic effects on MGH, which included 7 targets, 6 herbs, and 17 ingredients. This study illustrated that HHXYT could regulate the hormone disorder prominently and the results suggested that HHXYT might reduce estrogen-stimulated mammary gland hyperplasia by inhibiting the production of its precursor androgen. The data and theoretical support were provided for the in-depth study of HHXYT's mechanism. In addition, this study provides new ideas for the research of the mechanism of the multi-component TCM formula.

AUTHOR CONTRIBUTIONS

WZ, JZ and ZG designed the study. ZG and RM performed the experiments. ZG, ZC and JZ analyzed the data. HZ and XL directed the design of animal and *in vitro* experiments. ZG and JZ wrote the manuscript. GW, JZ, JY, and WZ revised the manuscript. All the authors approved its final version and agreed to be accountable for all aspects of the work.

FUNDING

The work was supported by the National Key Research and Development Program of China (No. 2017YFC1700200), Professor of Chang Jiang Scholars Program, National Natural Science Foundation of China (Nos. 81520108030, 81572378, and 81973706), Shanghai Engineering Research Center for the Preparation of Bioactive Natural Products (No. 16DZ2280200), the Scientific Foundation of Shanghai China (No. 13401900103 and 13401900101).

SUPPLEMENTARY MATERIAL

Supplementary Table S1 | Original compounds identified in the rat plasma after the treatment of HHXYT.

Supplementary Table S2 | Metabolites identified in the rat plasma after the treatment of HHXYT.

Supplementary Table S3 | Putative targets of HHXYT's active ingredients.

Supplementary Table S4 | Diseases genes for mammary gland hyperplasia collected from GeneCards.

REFERENCES

Adasme, M. F., Linnemann, K. L., Bolz, S. N., Kaiser, F., Salentin, S., Haupt, V. J., et al. (2021). PLIP 2021: Expanding the Scope of the Protein-Ligand Interaction Profiler to DNA and RNA. *Nucleic Acids Res.* 49, W530–W534. doi:10.1093/nar/gkab294

Alexander, N., Woetzel, N., and Meiler, J. (2011). "bcl: Cluster: A Method for Clustering Biological Molecules Coupled with Visualization in the Pymol Molecular Graphics System," in IEEE Int. Conf. Comput. Adv. Bio Med. Sci. 2011, Orlando, FL, USA, 3-5 Feb. 2011, 13–18. doi:10.1109/iccabs.2011.5729867

Arendt, L. M., and Kuperwasser, C. (2015). Form and Function: How Estrogen and Progesterone Regulate the Mammary Epithelial Hierarchy. *J. Mammary Gland Biol. Neoplasia* 20, 9–25. doi:10.1007/s10911-015-9337-0

Basree, M. M., Shinde, N., Koivisto, C., Cuitino, M., Kladney, R., Zhang, J., et al. (2019). Abrupt Involution Induces Inflammation, Estrogenic Signaling, and Hyperplasia Linking Lack of Breastfeeding with Increased Risk of Breast Cancer. *Breast Cancer Res.* 21, 80. doi:10.1186/s13058-019-1163-7

Burley, S. K., Bhikadiya, C., Bi, C., Bittrich, S., Chen, L., Crichlow, G. V., et al. (2021). RCSB Protein Data Bank: Powerful New Tools for Exploring 3D Structures of Biological Macromolecules for Basic and Applied Research and Education in Fundamental Biology, Biomedicine, Biotechnology, Bioengineering and Energy Sciences. *Nucleic Acids Res.* 49, D437–D451. doi:10.1093/nar/gkaa1038

Burris-Hiday, S. D., and Scott, E. E. (2021). Steroidogenic Cytochrome P450 17A1 Structure and Function. *Mol. Cel Endocrinol* 528, 111261. doi:10.1016/j.mce.2021.111261

Capponi, A. M. (2002). Regulation of Cholesterol Supply for Mineralocorticoid Biosynthesis. *Trends Endocrinol. Metab.* 13, 118–121. doi:10.1016/s1043-2760(01)00538-0

Chang, X. J., Zhou, J., Zhang, S., Chen, J., Chen, C. M., Wang, Z. Z., et al. (2014). Effects of Guizhi Fuling Capsule on Sex Hormone Levels and Breast Issue Morphology of Mammary Gland Hyperplasia Model Rats. *Chin. J. Chin. Mater. Med.* 39, 4139–4142. doi:10.4268/cjcmm20142111

Chen, X., Zhou, H., Liu, Y. B., Wang, J. F., Li, H., Ung, C. Y., et al. (2006). Database of Traditional Chinese Medicine and its Application to Studies of Mechanism and to Prescription Validation. *Br. J. Pharmacol.* 149, 1092–1103. doi:10.1038/sj.bjp.0706945

Chen, Y., Yang, X., Qi, M., Yu, H., Du, Q., and Zhao, H. (2020). Observation on the Effect of Honghua Xiaoyao Tablets Assisted Western Medicine in the Treatment of Mastitis Guided by Real-Time Monitoring of Color Doppler Ultrasound. *Mod. J. Integr. Tradit. West Med.* 29, 2227–2229+2233. doi:10.3969/j.issn.1008-8849.2020.20.01

Chen, Z. M., Hu, J., Xu, Y. M., He, W., Meng, L., Huang, T., et al. (2021). Cryptotanshinone Inhibits Cytotoxin-Associated Gene A-Associated Development of Gastric Cancer and Mucosal Erosions. *World J. Gastrointest. Oncol.* 13, 693–705. doi:10.4251/wjgo.v13.i7.693

Chin, C. H., Chen, S. H., Wu, H. H., Ho, C. W., Ko, M. T., and Lin, C. Y. (2014). cytoHubba: Identifying Hub Objects and Sub-networks from Complex Interactome. *BMC Syst. Biol.* 8 (Suppl. 4), S11. doi:10.1186/1752-0509-8-s4-s11

Chong, J., Wishart, D. S., and Xia, J. (2019). Using MetaboAnalyst 4.0 for Comprehensive and Integrative Metabolomics Data Analysis. *Curr. Protoc. Bioinformatics* 68, e86. doi:10.1002/cpbi.86

Coussens, L. M., and Pollard, J. W. (2011). Leukocytes in Mammary Development and Cancer. *Cold Spring Harb Perspect. Biol.* 3, a003285. doi:10.1101/cshperspect.a003285

Das, J., and Yu, H. (2012). HINT: High-Quality Protein Interactomes and Their Applications in Understanding Human Disease. *BMC Syst. Biol.* 6, 92. doi:10.1186/1752-0509-6-92

Fang, S., Dong, L., Liu, L., Guo, J., Zhao, L., Zhang, J., et al. (2021). HERB: a High-Throughput experiment- and Reference-Guided Database of Traditional Chinese Medicine. *Nucleic Acids Res.* 49, D1197–D1206. doi:10.1093/nar/gkaa1063

Hartmann, L. C., Sellers, T. A., Frost, M. H., Lingle, W. L., Degnim, A. C., Ghosh, K., et al. (2005). Benign Breast Disease and the Risk of Breast Cancer. *N. Engl. J. Med.* 353, 229–237. doi:10.1056/NEJMoa044383

Hopkins, A. L. (2007). Network Pharmacology. *Nat. Biotechnol.* 25, 1110–1111. doi:10.1038/nbt1007-1110

Imamichi, Y., Sekiguchi, T., Kitano, T., Kajitani, T., Okada, R., Inaoka, Y., et al. (2017). Diethylstilbestrol Administration Inhibits Theca Cell Androgen and Granulosa Cell Estrogen Production in Immature Rat Ovary. *Sci. Rep.* 7, 8374. doi:10.1038/s41598-017-08780-7

Jumper, J., Evans, R., Pritzel, A., Green, T., Figurnov, M., Ronneberger, O., et al. (2021). Highly Accurate Protein Structure Prediction with AlphaFold. *Nature* 596, 583–589. doi:10.1038/s41586-021-03819-2

Kanehisa, M., Furumichi, M., Tanabe, M., Sato, Y., and Morishima, K. (2017). KEGG: New Perspectives on Genomes, Pathways, Diseases and Drugs. *Nucleic Acids Res.* 45, D353–D361. doi:10.1093/nar/gkw1092

Kim, S., Chen, J., Cheng, T., Gindulyte, A., He, J., He, S., et al. (2021). PubChem in 2021: New Data Content and Improved Web Interfaces. *Nucleic Acids Res.* 49, D1388–D1395. doi:10.1093/nar/gkaa971

Kleinberg, D. L., Ameri, P., and Singh, B. (2011). Pasireotide, an IGF-I Action Inhibitor, Prevents Growth Hormone and Estradiol-Induced Mammary Hyperplasia. *Pituitary* 14, 44–52. doi:10.1007/s11102-010-0257-0

Li, S., and Zhang, B. (2013). Traditional Chinese Medicine Network Pharmacology: Theory, Methodology and Application. *Chin. J. Nat. Med.* 11, 110–120. doi:10.1016/s1875-5364(13)60037-0

Li, S. K., and Hearn, M. T. (2000). Isolation of Thecal Cells: an Assessment of Purity and Steroidogenic Potential. *J. Biochem. Biophys. Methods* 45, 169–181. doi:10.1016/s0165-022x(00)00107-x

Li, T., Zhang, W., Hu, E., Sun, Z., Li, P., Yu, Z., et al. (2021). Integrated Metabolomics and Network Pharmacology to Reveal the Mechanisms of Hydroxysafflor Yellow A against Acute Traumatic Brain Injury. *Comput. Struct. Biotechnol. J.* 19, 1002–1013. doi:10.1016/j.csbj.2021.01.033

Li, H. T., Liu, H. H., Yang, Y. X., Wang, T., Zhou, X. L., Yu, Y., et al. (2018). Therapeutic Effects of a Traditional Chinese Medicine Formula Plus Tamoxifen vs. Tamoxifen for the Treatment of Mammary Gland Hyperplasia: A Meta-Analysis of Randomized Trials. *Front. Pharmacol.* 9, 45. doi:10.3389/fphar.2018.00045

Li, X., Xin, P., Wang, C., Wang, Z., Wang, Q., and Kuang, H. (2017). Mechanisms of Traditional Chinese Medicine in the Treatment of Mammary Gland Hyperplasia. *Am. J. Chin. Med.* 45, 443–458. doi:10.1142/s0192415x17500276

Liebisch, G., Fahy, E., Aoki, J., Dennis, E. A., Durand, T., Ejsing, C. S., et al. (2020). Update on LIPID MAPS Classification, Nomenclature, and Shorthand Notation for MS-derived Lipid Structures. *J. Lipid Res.* 61, 1539–1555. doi:10.1194/jlr.S120001025

Liu, J., Zhang, J. F., Gong, G. H., Zhang, B., and Wei, C. X. (2020). Therapeutic Effect of Mongolian Medicine RuXian-I on Hyperplasia of Mammary Gland Induced by Estrogen/Progesterone through CRYAB-Promoted Apoptosis. *Evid. Based Complement. Alternat Med.* 2020, 5707106. doi:10.1155/2020/5707106

Luan, H., Ji, F., Chen, Y., and Cai, Z. (2018). statTarget: A Streamlined Tool for Signal Drift Correction and Interpretations of Quantitative Mass Spectrometry-Based Omics Data. *Anal. Chim. Acta* 1036, 66–72. doi:10.1016/j.aca.2018.08.002

Meng, Q., Liu, S., and Wu, X. (2014). Clinical Observation on 215 Cases of Mammary Gland Hyperplasia Treated with Honghua Xiaoyao Tablets. *Hebei J. TCM* 36, 1536–1537.

Mi, R., Li, X., Zhang, Z., Cheng, T., Tian, S., Xu, X., et al. (2020). Chemical Profiling of Honghua Xiaoyao Tablet and Simultaneous Determination of its Quality Markers by Liquid Chromatography-Tandem Mass Spectrometry Combined with Chemometrics Methods. *J. Sep. Sci.* 43, 4263–4280. doi:10.1002/jssc.202000689

Newgard, C. B. (2017). Metabolomics and Metabolic Diseases: Where Do We Stand?. *Cell Metab* 25, 43–56. doi:10.1016/j.cmet.2016.09.018

Nicholson, J. K., and Wilson, I. D. (2003). Opinion: Understanding 'global' Systems Biology: Metabonomics and the Continuum of Metabolism. *Nat. Rev. Drug Discov.* 2, 668–676. doi:10.1038/nrd1157

Ong, M., Cheng, J., Jin, X., Lao, W., Johnson, M., Tan, Y., et al. (2019). Paeoniflorin Extract Reverses Dexamethasone-Induced Testosterone Over-secretion through Downregulation of Cytochrome P450 17A1 Expression in Primary Murine Theca Cells. *J. Ethnopharmacol* 229, 97–103. doi:10.1016/j.jep.2018.09.006

Pei, S., Zhang, Q., and Yang, J. (2016). Clinical Observation of Honghua Xiaoyao Tables in the Treatment of Delayed Menstrual Cycle of Liver-Depression and Qi-Blood Stagnation. *China Pharm.* 27, 245–247. doi:10.6039/j.issn.1001-0408.2016.02.3210.1353/jod.2016.0057

Ru, J., Li, P., Wang, J., Zhou, W., Li, B., Huang, C., et al. (2014). TCMSP: a Database of Systems Pharmacology for Drug Discovery from Herbal Medicines. *J. Cheminform* 6, 13. doi:10.1186/1758-2946-6-13

Shannon, P., Markiel, A., Ozier, O., Baliga, N. S., Wang, J. T., Ramage, D., et al. (2003). Cytoscape: a Software Environment for Integrated Models of Biomolecular Interaction Networks. *Genome Res.* 13, 2498–2504. doi:10.1101/gr.1239303

Stelzer, G., Rosen, N., Plaschkes, I., Zimmerman, S., Twik, M., Fishilevich, S., et al. (2016). The GeneCards Suite: From Gene Data Mining to Disease Genome Sequence Analyses. *Curr. Protoc. Bioinformatics* 54, 1.30.1–1.30.33. doi:10.1002/cpbi.5

Szklarczyk, D., Gable, A. L., Lyon, D., Junge, A., Wyder, S., Huerta-Cepas, J., et al. (2019). STRING V11: Protein-Protein Association Networks with Increased Coverage, Supporting Functional Discovery in Genome-wide Experimental Datasets. *Nucleic Acids Res.* 47, D607–D613. doi:10.1093/nar/gky1131

Tanchuk, V. Y., Tanin, V. O., Vovk, A. I., and Poda, G. (2016). A New, Improved Hybrid Scoring Function for Molecular Docking and Scoring Based on AutoDock and AutoDock Vina. *Chem. Biol. Drug Des.* 87, 618–625. doi:10.1111/cbdd.12697

Trott, O., and Olson, A. J. (2010). AutoDock Vina: Improving the Speed and Accuracy of Docking with a New Scoring Function, Efficient Optimization, and Multithreading. *J. Comput. Chem.* 31, 455–461. doi:10.1002/jcc.21334

Wang, J. (2012). 35 Cases of Perimenopausal Syndrome Treated with Honghua Xiaoyao Tablets. *Chin. J. Exp. Tradit Med. Form* 18, 312–313. doi:10.13422/j.cnki.syfjx.2012.18.01510.1007/s11655-012-1064-4

Wang, L., Zhao, D., Di, L., Cheng, D., Zhou, X., Yang, X., et al. (2011). The Anti-hyperplasia of Mammary Gland Effect of Thladiantha Dubia Root Ethanol Extract in Rats Reduced by Estrogen and Progestogen. *J. Ethnopharmacol* 134, 136–140. doi:10.1016/j.jep.2010.11.071

Wibowo, E., Pollock, P. A., Hollis, N., and Wassersug, R. J. (2016). Tamoxifen in Men: a Review of Adverse Events. *Andrology* 4, 776–788. doi:10.1111/andr.12197

Williams, K., Mckinnell, C., Saunders, P. T., Walker, M., Fisher, J. S., Turner, K. J., et al. (2001). Neonatal Exposure to Potent and Environmental Oestrogens and Abnormalities of the Male Reproductive System in the Rat: Evidence for Importance of the Androgen-Oestrogen Balance and Assessment of the Relevance to Man. *Hum. Reprod. Update* 7, 236–247. doi:10.1093/humupd/7.3.236

Wishart, D. S., Feunang, Y. D., Marcu, A., Guo, A. C., Liang, K., Vázquez-Fresno, R., et al. (2018). HMDB 4.0: the Human Metabolome Database for 2018. *Nucleic Acids Res.* 46, D608–D617. doi:10.1093/nar/gkx1089

Wu, G., Zhang, W., and Li, H. (2019). Application of Metabolomics for Unveiling the Therapeutic Role of Traditional Chinese Medicine in Metabolic Diseases. *J. Ethnopharmacol* 242, 112057. doi:10.1016/j.jep.2019.112057

Wu, Y., Zhang, F., Yang, K., Fang, S., Bu, D., Li, H., et al. (2019). SymMap: an Integrative Database of Traditional Chinese Medicine Enhanced by Symptom Mapping. *Nucleic Acids Res.* 47, D1110–D1117. doi:10.1093/nar/gky1021

Xu, H. Y., Zhang, Y. Q., Liu, Z. M., Chen, T., Lv, C. Y., Tang, S. H., et al. (2019). ETCM: an Encyclopaedia of Traditional Chinese Medicine. *Nucleic Acids Res.* 47, D976–D982. doi:10.1093/nar/gky987

Xu, W., Zhang, Y., Yu, Y., Li, B., Liu, J., Wang, P., et al. (2018). Dose-dependent Target Diversion of Danhong Injection on the Glu-GLT-1/Gly-GlyRα Dynamic Balance Module of Cerebral Ischemia. *Pharmacol. Res.* 135, 80–88. doi:10.1016/j.phrs.2018.07.020

Xue, R., Fang, Z., Zhang, M., Yi, Z., Wen, C., and Shi, T. (2013). TCMID: Traditional Chinese Medicine Integrative Database for Herb Molecular Mechanism Analysis. *Nucleic Acids Res.* 41, D1089–D1095. doi:10.1093/nar/gks1100

Yao, Z. J., Dong, J., Che, Y. J., Zhu, M. F., Wen, M., Wang, N. N., et al. (2016). TargetNet: a Web Service for Predicting Potential Drug-Target Interaction Profiling via Multi-Target SAR Models. *J. Comput. Aided Mol. Des.* 30, 413–424. doi:10.1007/s10822-016-9915-2

Ye, J., Li, R., Zeng, H., Liu, R., and Zhang, W. (2019). Discovery and Research Advances in Quality Markers of Chinese Material Medica Based on Holistic Characteristics. *Chin. Tradit Herbal Drugs* 50, 4529–4537. doi:10.7501/j.issn.0253-2670.2019.19.002

You, Z., Sun, J., Xie, F., Chen, Z., Zhang, S., Chen, H., et al. (2017). Modulatory Effect of Fermented Papaya Extracts on Mammary Gland Hyperplasia Induced by Estrogen and Progestin in Female Rats. *Oxid. Med. Cell. Longev.* 2017, 8235069. doi:10.1155/2017/8235069

Zhao, J., Lv, C., Wu, Q., Zeng, H., Guo, X., Yang, J., et al. (2019). Computational Systems Pharmacology Reveals an Antiplatelet and Neuroprotective Mechanism of Deng-Zhan-Xi-Xin Injection in the Treatment of Ischemic Stroke. *Pharmacol. Res.* 147, 104365. doi:10.1016/j.phrs.2019.104365

Zhao, J., Tian, S., Lu, D., Yang, J., Zeng, H., Zhang, F., et al. (2021). Systems Pharmacological Study Illustrates the Immune Regulation, Anti-infection, Anti-inflammation, and Multi-Organ protection Mechanism of Qing-Fei-Pai-Du Decoction in the Treatment of COVID-19. *Phytomedicine* 85, 153315. doi:10.1016/j.phymed.2020.153315

3

The Anti-Inflammatory Effect of a Combination of Five Compounds from Five Chinese Herbal Medicines Used in the Treatment of COPD

Jiansheng Li[1,2,3]**, *Peng Zhao*[1,2,4], *Yange Tian*[1,2,4], *Kangchen Li*[1,2], *Lanxi Zhang*[1,2], *Qingzhou Guan*[1,2,4], *Xiaofeng Mei*[1,2] *and Yanqin Qin*[1,2,4]

[1]*Henan Key Laboratory of Chinese Medicine for Respiratory Disease, Henan University of Chinese Medicine, Zhengzhou, China,* [2]*Collaborative Innovation Center for Chinese Medicine and Respiratory Diseases Co-constructed by Henan Province and Education Ministry of P.R. China, Zhengzhou, China,* [3]*Department of Respiratory Diseases, The First Affiliated Hospital of Henan University of Chinese Medicine, Zhengzhou, China,* [4]*Academy of Chinese Medical Sciences, Henan University of Chinese Medicine, Zhengzhou, China*

***Correspondence:**
Jiansheng Li
li_js8@163.com

Effective compound combination (ECC; i.e, 20-S-ginsenoside Rh1, astragaloside, icariin, nobiletin, and paeonol), derived from Chinese herbal medicine, significantly ameliorates chronic obstructive pulmonary disease (COPD) in rats; however, the underlying mechanisms of ECC remain largely unclear. In this study, network pharmacology analysis integrated with experimental validation was used to explore the therapeutic mechanisms of ECC against COPD. ECC targets and COPD genes and targets were identified from multiple databases, and then used for an analysis of protein–protein interaction (PPI) networks, Kyoto Encyclopedia of Genes and Genomes (KEGG) pathways, and biological functioning. BisoGenet was used to comprehensively analyze the hub-network. We validated the therapeutic effect and mechanisms of ECC both *in vivo* and *in vitro*. We identified 45 ECC targets, which were mainly related to inflammatory processes, such as the NOD-like and NF-kappa B signaling pathways, hematopoietic cell lineage, Th17 cell differentiation, cellular response to lipopolysaccharide, and interleukin-8 secretion. In addition, 1180 COPD genes and 70 COPD targets were identified as being involved in the biological functions associated with COPD development, such as cytokine–cytokine receptor interaction, the TNF signaling pathway, the mitogen-activated protein kinase (MAPK) signaling pathway, regulation of lymphocyte proliferation, and positive regulation of leukocyte migration. Integrative analysis of COPD genes and targets and ECC target networks revealed that 54 genes were mainly involved in the inflammatory process, such as IL-17 signaling, NF-kappa B signaling, innate immune response–activating signal transduction, and macrophage cell differentiation. Six targets (AR, ESR1, HNRNPA1, PAPR1, TP53, and VCAM1) contained in the hub-network and their four related compounds were obtained and recognized as the key molecules associated with the effects of ECC. Molecular docking validation demonstrated that four compounds could bind to six targets that interact with COPD genes. Finally, *in vivo* and *in vitro* experiments verified that ECC treatment ameliorated the symptoms of COPD in rats by improving their lung function, reducing pathological changes, and suppressing oxidative responses and pro-inflammatory cytokine secretion, while inhibiting inflammation in LPS-induced macrophages, which may be associated with NF-kappa B and MAPK signaling regulation. This study demonstrates the therapeutic mechanisms and effects of ECC on COPD *via* regulation of the underlying inflammatory process.

Keywords: effective compound combination, chronic obstructive pulmonary disease, network pharmacology, inflammatory process, macrophage

INTRODUCTION

Chronic obstructive pulmonary disease (COPD) is a major respiratory disorder that is characterized by persistent airflow limitation and an abnormal inflammation response to noxious particles such as cigarette smoke (Wang et al., 2018). COPD is a leading cause of mortality, causing a significant economic and social burden in many countries worldwide (Zhou et al., 2019). However, to date, no drugs have been developed to specifically treat this disorder (Global Initiative for Choric Obstructive Lung Disease, 2020). The traditional Chinese medicine (TCM) has been shown to have a beneficial effect in the treatment of COPD patients. The Bufei Yishen formula (BYF; patent: ZL.201110117578.1) is a representative formula for the treatment of COPD patients with lung kidney qi deficiency syndrome, which is characterized by labored breathing, shortness of breath, fatigue, dizziness and tinnitus, frequent urination and nocturia, and weakness of the waist and knees (Li et al., 2012; Li et al., 2015). Our previous clinical study showed that COPD patients treated using BYF fared better, including a reduced frequency and duration of acute exacerbation COPD and an improved rate of decline in FVE1, than those treated with conventional Western medicine, while simultaneously demonstrating improved modified Medical Research Council dyspnea scale scores, six-minute walk distance (6MWD), and exercise tolerance (Li et al., 2021). In a previous study, the critical compounds derived from BYF were combined into a new effective compound combination (ECC) consisting of 20-S-ginsenoside Rh1, astragaloside IV, icariin, nobiletin, and paeonol (at a proportion of 25:5:100:4:6.25), which had a potential bioactive equivalence to BYF (Li et al., 2020). 20-S-Ginsenoside Rh1 and astragaloside IV have been reported to show anti-inflammatory, antioxidant, and immunomodulatory effects, and are widely used to treat inflammatory diseases (Ren et al., 2013; Chen et al., 2016; Tam et al., 2018). In addition, icariin, nobiletin, and paeonol have a wide range of pharmacological effects, such as anti-inflammatory, antitumor, immunomodulatory, and anti-lung injury effects (Liu et al., 2017; Li et al., 2018; Sun et al., 2018; Sun et al., 2020). However, the action mode and the underlying mechanisms of ECC for the treatment of COPD remain unclear, and it is difficult to gain a greater insight into these mechanisms while using traditional experimental approaches.

Network pharmacology was first constructed to identify systematic targets and explore the synergistic mechanism of multiple compounds. More recently, network pharmacology, which integrates target prediction, statistical analysis, network-based algorithms, and bioinformatics analysis with pharmacological validation, has been used to uncover the details of system interrelationships within "drug–target–pathway" diseases. Furthermore, we have previously applied system pharmacology to successfully predict the active compounds from BYF and their associated targets; their functions are mainly related to the activation of inflammatory and immune responses, and matrix metalloproteinases (Li et al., 2016). Nonetheless, the mechanisms of the five BFY effective compounds for treating COPD have not yet been demonstrated. Thus, we applied a network pharmacological analysis, based on both clinical and experimental data, to explore the potential mechanism of ECC for the treatment of COPD.

In this work, we systematically explored the underlying mechanisms of ECC for the treatment of COPD using integrative network pharmacology strategies (**Figure 1**). In brief, we identified the putative targets of ECC from ingenuity pathway analysis (IPA), a list of COPD-related genes and targets from well-established databases. The network and pathway analyses were then employed to illustrate the molecular function, immune processes, and signaling regulation of ECC for the treatment of COPD. We further identified the important targets and pathways for ECC treatment, and used molecule docking to validate compound–target bindings. Consequently, we validated the therapeutic effect of ECC for the treatment of COPD in rats. *In vitro* experiments were also performed to validate the molecular mechanisms of the pharmacological action of ECC.

MATERIALS AND METHODS

ECC–Target Prediction

ECC consists of 20-S-Ginsenoside Rh1 (PubChem CID: 12855920), astragaloside IV (PubChem CID: 13943297), icariin (PubChem CID: 5318997), nobiletin (PubChem CID: 72344), and paeonol (PubChem CID: 11092). The putative targets of these five compounds were identified using the following steps. First, we collected the putative targets of the compounds from the QIAGEN IPA, which was performed by the Beijing Computing Center. We then verified the reliability of the interactions of the compound–putative targets in the literature (**Supplementary Table S1**).

COPD-Related Genes and Putative Targets

To identify COPD related genes, we initially used the keyword "chronic obstructive pulmonary disease" to search in three

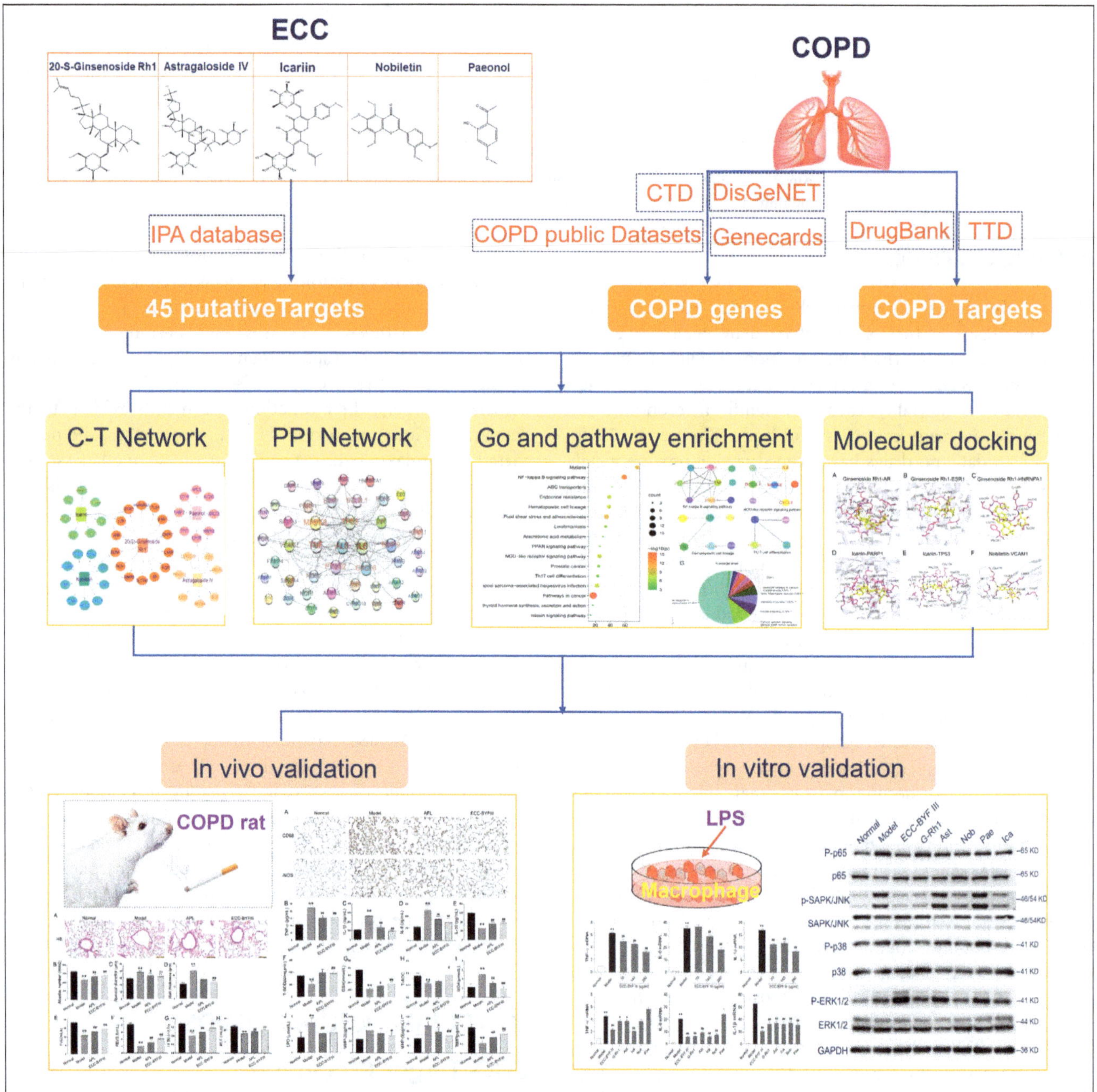

FIGURE 1 | Integrative network pharmacology strategies to investigate the mechanism of ECC for the treatment of COPD.

databases: the Comparative Toxicogenomics Database (CTD; http://ctdbase.org/), the MalaCards (https://www.malacards.org/), and DisGeNET (http://www.disgenet.org/). We also identified COPD genes based on public data: a total of 137 human COPD samples and 119 normal lung tissue samples from the GSE38974, GSE57148, and GSE8581 datasets were obtained from the GEO database, as shown in **Table 1**. For the data assessed *via* sequence-based platforms, gene symbols were converted to Entrez gene IDs using the Biological Database Network (bioDBnet). Furthermore, differential gene expression analysis was performed using the significance analysis of microarrays algorithm (Tusher et al., 2001) and the Wilcoxon rank-sum test for array- and sequence-based data, respectively. A total of 422 genes, including 80 upregulated and 342 downregulated genes, were considered to be COPD-related genes and included in the subsequent analysis. The potential genes were screened according to their scores in the respective databases; when repeated at least three times in the four databases, they were considered COPD-related genes. COPD-associated targets were identified from the Therapeutic Target Database (http://db.

TABLE 1 | Human COPD data used in this study.

	Platform	Normal	COPD
GSE38974	Agilent GPL4133	9	23
GSE8581	Affymetrix GPL570	19	16
GSE57148[a]	Illumina GPL11154	91	98

[a]*These samples were measured by the RNA-seq platform.*

idrblab.net/ttd/) and DrugBank (https://go.drugbank.com/) (**Supplementary Table S2**).

Functional enrichment analysis

The Metascape analysis resource (https://metascape.org) was used for the KEGG signaling pathway enrichment analysis. Molecular function, immune system, and biological processes were analyzed using ClueGo and Cluepedia in Cytoscape 3.7.2.

Network construction and analysis

The ECC compounds and targets were used to construct the ECC–target network using Cytoscape 3.7.2. Protein–protein interaction (PPI) data were obtained from STRING 11.0 (https://www.string-db.org/) and applied for the construction of the PPI network.

BisoGenet, a Cytoscape plugin, was used to search for the molecular interactions of ECC targets, COPD genes, or COPD targets from "SysBiomics," thus constructing three networks within Cytoscape, respectively (Martin et al., 2010). Consequently, the networks of ECC targets, COPD genes, or COPD targets that had been constructed in BisoGenet were merged, and a subnetwork was extracted according to node topological features, including degree, betweenness centrality, and closeness centrality (≥ 2 x median values).

Molecular Docking

We downloaded the 3D structures (SDF file) of the compounds from the PubChem website (https://pubchem.ncbi.nlm.nih.gov/), whereas the protein crystal structures were extracted from the Protein Data Bank (http://www.rcsb.org/pdb). PyMol 2.3.4 was used to remove the waters, hydrogens, ions, and original ligands from the proteins. Finally, the proteins and ligands were saved using the AutoDock Tools, and each compound was docked into the target proteins.

Chemicals and Animals

Klebsiella pneumoniae (strain ID: 46,114) was obtained from the National Center for Medical Culture Collection (Beijing, China). Tobacco was purchased from the Henan Tobacco Industry (Hongqi Canal® Filter tip cigarette; tobacco type, tar: 10 mg; nicotine content: 1.0 mg; carbon monoxide: 12 mg; Zhengzhou, China). Aminophylline (APL) was purchased from Shandong Xinhua Pharmaceutical (Shandong, China). Rat IL-6, IL-10, MMP-2, MMP-9, and the TIMP-1 ELISA kits were obtained from Boster Biological Engineering (Wuhan, China). Total superoxide dismutase (T-SOD), malondialdehyde (MDA), glutathione (GSH), total antioxidant capacity (T-AOC), and lipid peroxidation (LPO) were obtained from Elabscience Biotechnology (Guangdong, China). Antibodies for mouse p65, p-p65, JUN N-terminal kinase (JNK), p-JNK, p38, and p-p38 were obtained from Proteintech (Wuhan, China). Qiazol lysis reagent was obtained from Qiagen (Valencia, CA, United States). HiScriptIIQ RT SuperMix for qPCR and SYBR Green Master Mix were obtained from Vazyme Biotech (Nanjing, China). Fifty Sprague–Dawley rats (25 males and 25 females; 200 ± 20 g) were purchased from Jinan Pengyue Experimental Animal (Jinan, China).

ECC Compounds and Ratios

ECC was composed of 20-S-ginsenoside Rh1 (Cas, 63,223-86-9), astragaloside (Cas, 84,687-43-4), icariin (Cas, 489-32-7), nobiletin (Cas, 478-01-3), and paeonol (Cas, 552-41-0) (**Table 2**). These compounds were purchased from Chengdu Must Bio-Technology (Chengdu, China). A purity of greater than 99% was determined using high-performance liquid chromatography, which was provided by Chengdu Must Bio-Technology. The ratio of these compounds in ECC was as follows: 25 20-S-ginsenoside Rh1: 5 astragaloside: 100 icariin: 4 nobiletin: 6.25 paeonol.

Animal Experiments

The COPD rat model was developed as previously described (Li et al., 2012). The cigarette smoke exposure system primarily consisted of a closed chamber with a cigarette smoke producer. The rats were exposed to smoke in this smoke exposure system from 1 to 12 weeks and were repeatedly intranasally inoculated with *K. pneumonia* from 1 to 8 weeks.

Rats with COPD were randomly split into three groups: model group, ECC group, and APL group, which were orally administered normal saline, ECC (5.5 mg/ kg/ d), and APL (54 mg/ kg/ d) from 13 weeks of age, respectively. The normal rats were also orally treated with saline. At week 20, rats were anesthetized and sacrificed to collect lung tissue, blood, and bronchoalveolar lavage fluid (BALF). All animal experiments were approved by the Experimental Animal Care and Ethics Committee of the First Affiliated Hospital, Henan University of Chinese Medicine.

Pulmonary Function, Histopathology, Cytokine, MMP, and Oxidative Factor Analysis

Peak expiratory flow (PEF), forced expiratory volume (FEV), and forced vital capacity (FVC) were detected using computer-controlled unrestrained pulmonary function testing plethysmography (Buxco Inc., Wilmington, NC, United States). The left lower lobe was fixed in formalin, and then embedded in paraffin. Paraffin sections were stained with Mayer's hematoxylin and 1% eosin (H&E staining) or CD68, iNOS.

Lung tissue levels of TNF-α, IL-1β in BALF, IL-6, IL-10, MMP-9, and MMP-12 were determined using ELISA kits, according to the manufacturer instructions. MDA, LPO, T-SOD, GSH, and T-AOC were also assessed using ELISA kits, according to the manufacturer instructions.

TABLE 2 | Plant source of five chemical compounds.

No.	Chemical compounds	CAS	Herbal drug	Latin scientific name	Plant part(s)
1	20-S-Ginsenoside Rh1	63223-86-9	Ginseng Radix et Rhizoma	*Panax ginseng* C.A. Mey	Radix et Rhizoma
2	Astragaloside IV	84687-43-4	Astragali Radix	*Astragalus tibetanus* Bunge	Radix
3	Icariin	489-32-7	Epimedii Folium	*Epimedium acuminatum* Franch	Folium
4	Nobiletin	Cas, 478-01-3	Citri Reticulatae Pericarpium	*Citrus sinensis* (L.) Osbeck	Pericarpium
5	Paeonol	552-41-0	Paeoniae Rubra Radix	*Paeonia anomala* L	Radix

TABLE 3 | Primers used in the cellular experiments.

Gene	Primer 5'→3'
TNF-α	Forward-CAGGCGGTGCCTATGTCTC Reverse-CGATCACCCCGAAGTTCAGTAG
IL-6	Forward-CTGCAAGAGACTTCCATCCAG Reverse-AGTGGTATAGACAGGTCTGTTGG
IL-1β	Forward-GAAATGCCACCTTTTGACAGTG Reverse-TGGATGCTCTCATCAGGACAG
GAPDH	Forward-AGGTCGGTGTGAACGGATTTG Reverse-GGGGTCGTTGATGGCAACA

Cell Culture and Treatment

A mouse macrophage MH-S cell line was purchased from Shanghai Zishi Bio-Technology (Shanghai, China). MH-S cells were cultured in RPMI 1640 medium (Solarbio Life Science), which contained 10% fetal bovine serum (FBS), 100 U/ mL penicillin, and 100 µg/ ml streptomycin in a humidified 95% air/5% CO_2 incubator at 37°C.

MH-S cells were seeded into six-well plates and cultured overnight. Cells were treated with different concentrations of ECC or its compounds for 3 h, and then exposed to LPS (100 ng/ ml) for 6 or 12 h. The concentrations of the compounds were as follows: 20-S-ginsenoside Rh1 (G-Rh1, 50 µg/ ml, 78.26 µM), astragaloside IV (Ast, 10 µg/ ml, 12.74 µM), icariin (Ica, 200 µg/ ml, 295.55 µM), nobiletin (Nob, 8 µg/ ml, 19.88 µM), and paeonol (Pae, 12.5 µg/ ml, 75.22 µM).

Real-Time Polymerase Chain Reaction Assay

Cells were lysed with Qiazol lysing buffer, and total RNA was extracted according to the manufacturer instructions. RNA was reverse-transcribed into cDNA, and then used for Q-PCR with HiScriptIIQ RT SuperMix and SYBR Green Master Mix (Vazyme; Nanjing, China). The primer sequences of the target gene are shown in **Table 3**. Last, gene expression was calculated using the $2^{\Delta\Delta}$Ct method.

Western Blot Assay

After treatment with ECC and its compounds, macrophages were lysed with RIPA buffer in ice. Protein samples with equal concentrations were separated using 10% SDS-PAGE gel and electro-transferred to PVDF membranes. Membranes with proteins were blocked with 5% nonfat milk, and then incubated with primary and secondary antibodies. Detection was performed using the Bio-Rad Imaging System.

Statistical Analysis

All values are expressed as means ± standard errors of the means. Statistical differences were assessed using a one-way analysis of variance, followed by a *post hoc* Tukey's test. P values < 0.05 were considered statistically significant. All statistical analyses were performed using SPSS 22.0 (IBM Corporation, Armonk, NY, United States).

RESULTS

Functional Analysis of ECC Targets

The five compounds contained in ECC may exert a synergistic effect through multiple targets (**Figure 2A**). Thus, an accurate evaluation of the ECC targets was necessary. Based on the IPA database, we identified 45 targets for ECC, and then constructed the respective compound–target network (**Figure 2B**). The number of potential targets connected by 20-S-ginsenoside Rh1, astragaloside IV, icariin, nobiletin, and paeonol was 14, 9, 10, 11, and 9, respectively. As seen in **Figure 2C**, 42 of these 45 targets interacted with each other to construct a PPI network, in which inflammatory mediators and their regulators (e.g., TNF, IL-6, CXXL8, PTGS2, VCAM1, ICAM1, NOS2, and MAPK8) were contained.

The KEGG pathway enrichment analysis identified the signaling pathways associated with the 45 targets. As shown in **Figure 2D**, the top 20 KEGG pathways were markedly enriched with 45 targets, which were mainly involved in cancer, inflammatory, and immune system processes. Consequently, the regulation of immune and inflammation responses, including the NOD-like and NF-kappa B signaling pathways, hematopoietic cell lineage, Th17 cell differentiation, and PPAR signaling pathway, may be the major mechanism of ECC (**Figure 2E**). In addition, the molecular function and immune system process analysis demonstrated that the targets could regulate multiple biological functions, including oxidoreductase activity, cellular responses to lipopolysaccharide, interleukin-8 secretion, acute inflammatory responses, and leukocyte adhesion to vascular endothelial cells; these can effectively regulate inflammatory processes (**Figures 2F,G**).

Functional Analysis of COPD-Associated Genes and Therapeutic Targets

COPD pathogenesis is associated with innate and adaptive immune responses as a result of the inhalation of toxic particles and gases (Barnes, 2016); however, details regarding

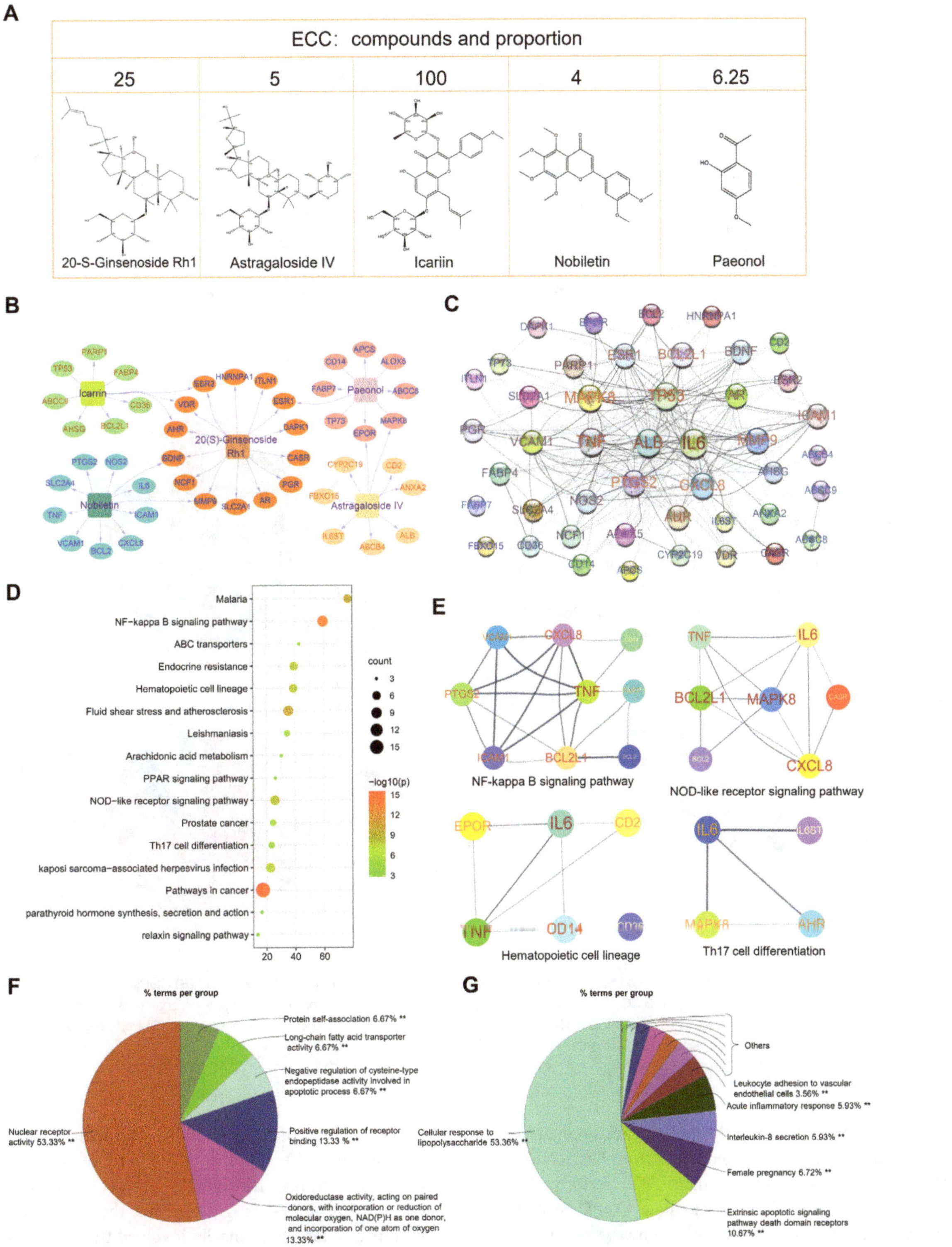

FIGURE 2 | Bioinformatics analysis of ECC targets. **(A)** Compound–target network of ECC constructed using Cytoscape. **(B)** Protein–protein network of ECC targets constructed using STRING. The size of the label is proportional to its strength. **(C)** The top 20 enriched KEGG pathways of ECC targets constructed using Metascape. **(D, E)** Protein–protein interactions of the proteins contained in the top pathways. **(F)** Molecular function analysis and **(G)** biological process analysis for 45 targets constructed using ClueGo in Cytoscape.

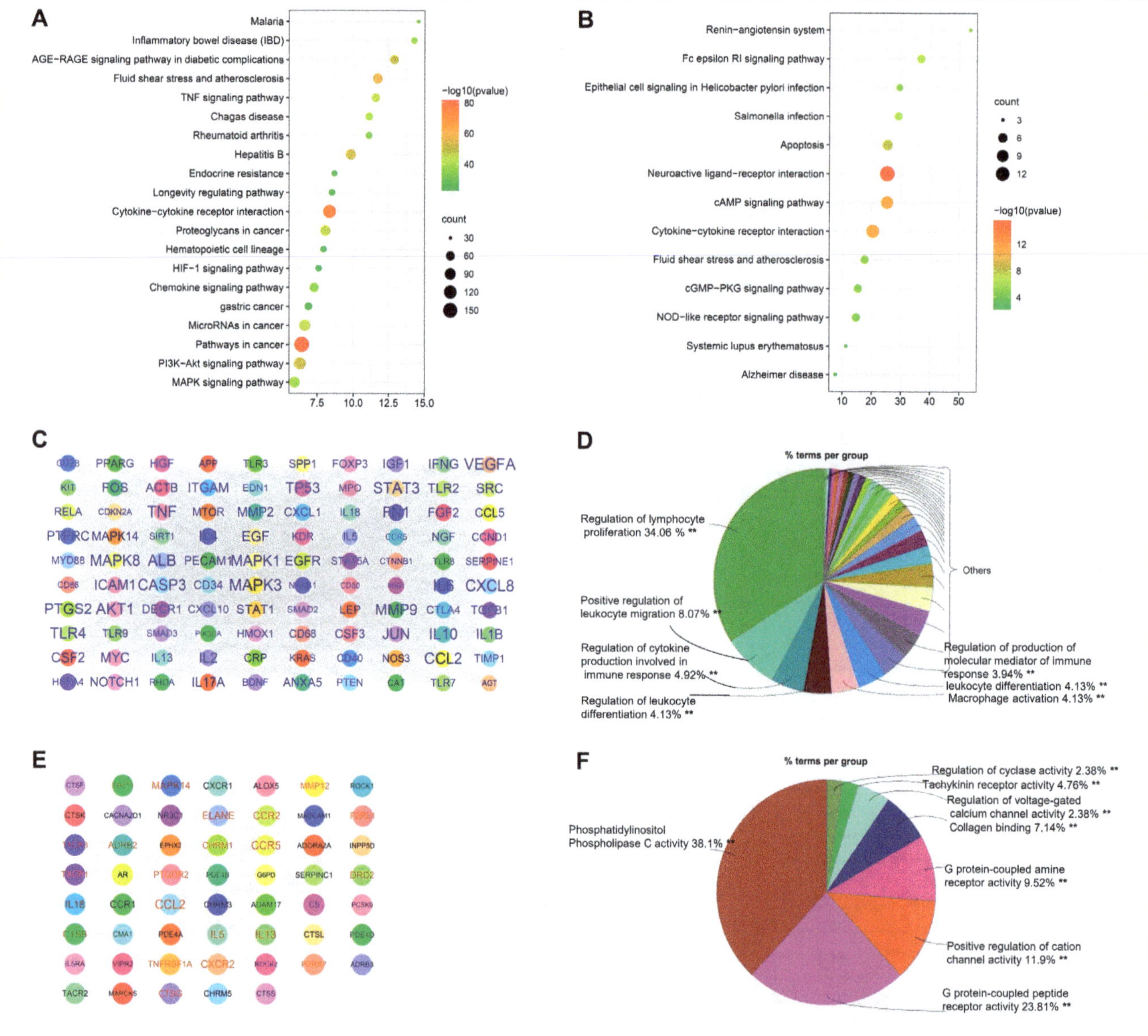

FIGURE 3 | Bioinformatics analysis of COPD genes and targets. **(A)** Top 20 enriched KEGG pathways of COPD genes and **(B)** COPD targets, constructed using Metascape. **(C)** Protein–protein network of top 100 COPD genes constructed by Cytoscape. The size of the label is proportional to its strength. **(D)** Immune system process analysis of the top 100 COPD genes using ClueGo in Cytoscape. The size of the label is proportional to its strength. **(E)** Protein–protein network of COPD targets. **(F)** Immune system process analysis of COPD targets.

the mechanisms that dictate COPD pathogenesis remain unclear. We identified 1180 COPD-related genes from DisGeNET, CTD, GeneCard, and COPD public data. We performed KEGG pathway enrichment analysis using these COPD-related genes and noted that the top 20 KEGG pathways were markedly enriched with COPD genes, which could be categorized as related to inflammation regulation (cytokine–cytokine receptor interaction, TNF signaling pathway, chemokine signaling pathway, hematopoietic cell lineage, HIF-1 signaling pathway, mitogen-activated protein kinase (MAPK) signaling pathway, and PI3K-Akt signaling pathway), cancer, and infections, among other roles (**Figure 3A**).

To analyze the main COPD therapeutic targets and their mechanisms, 70 therapeutic targets of COPD drugs were collected from therapeutic target databases. Pathway enrichment analysis suggested that the major functions of the therapeutic targets primarily involved the regulation of immune responses, such as cytokine–cytokine receptor interaction, the Fc epsilon RI signaling pathway, the NOD-like receptor signaling pathway, apoptosis, the cAMP signaling pathway, and the cGMP-PKG signaling pathway, but also included infections and other functions (**Figure 3B**).

As shown in **Figure 3C**, 100 hub genes (e.g., MAPK3, MAPK14, PTGS2, ICAM1, CXCL8, JUN, and IL17A) were

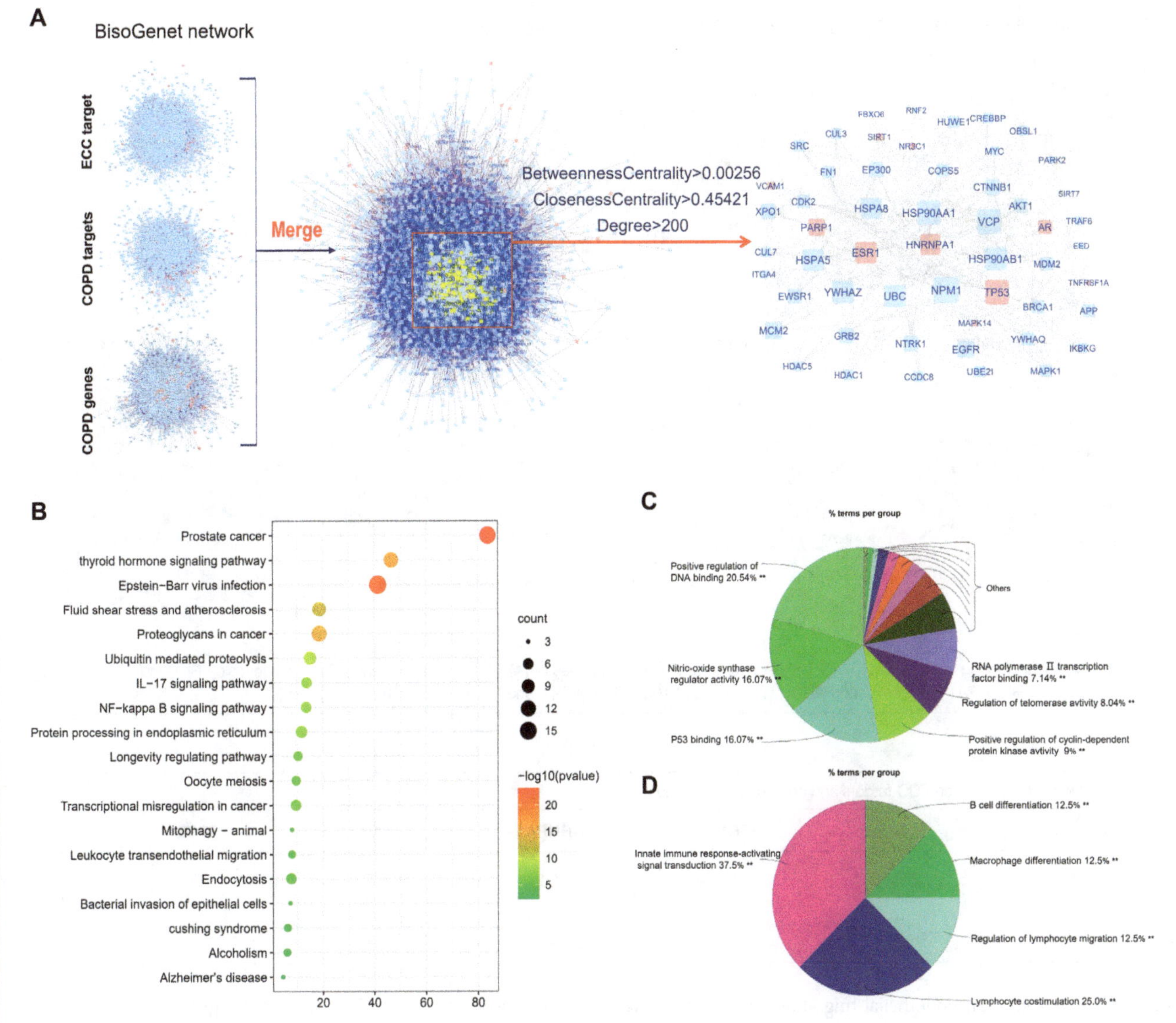

FIGURE 4 | Integrative analysis of ECC targets, and COPD genes and targets. **(A)** Hub-network extracted from the merged network of ECC targets, COPD genes, and targets. **(B)** Top 20 enriched KEGG pathways of genes contained in the hub-network constructed using Metascape. **(C)** Molecular function and **(D)** immune system process analysis for the genes contained in the hub-network.

extracted from a PPI network of 1180 COPD genes based on their degree value, and then their immune system processes were analyzed. As shown in **Figure 3D**, results indicated that the hub genes of COPD-related genes were mainly involved in the regulation of lymphocyte proliferation, positive regulation of leukocyte migration, and macrophage activation, among other roles. Similarly, COPD targets were used to construct PPI networks for an analysis of their immune system processes. The collected data suggested that the hub genes, including CCL2, IL13, MAPK14, and ALOX5, were mainly associated with phosphatidylinositol phospholipase C activity, G protein-coupled peptide receptor activity, and the positive regulation of cation channel activity, which are regulated by COPD drugs (**Figures 3E,F**).

Intersection Analysis Among ECC Targets, COPD Targets, and Genes

Similar to the above analysis, the ECC targets, COPD targets, and COPD genes were mainly associated with inflammatory responses, immune responses, and cancer, respectively; however, this analysis did not reveal the mechanisms of ECC with respect to the treatment of COPD. Consequently, we performed an intersection analysis among the ECC targets, COPD targets, and COPD genes; the obtained hub-network comprised 54 proteins that contained six ECC and three COPD–drug targets, respectively (**Figure 4A**). These 54 proteins were then analyzed to obtain a pathway from the KEGG database. As shown in **Figure 4B**, the top 20 KEGG signaling pathways were mainly involved in cancer, viral infections, and inflammatory processes, such as IL-17 and NF-kappa

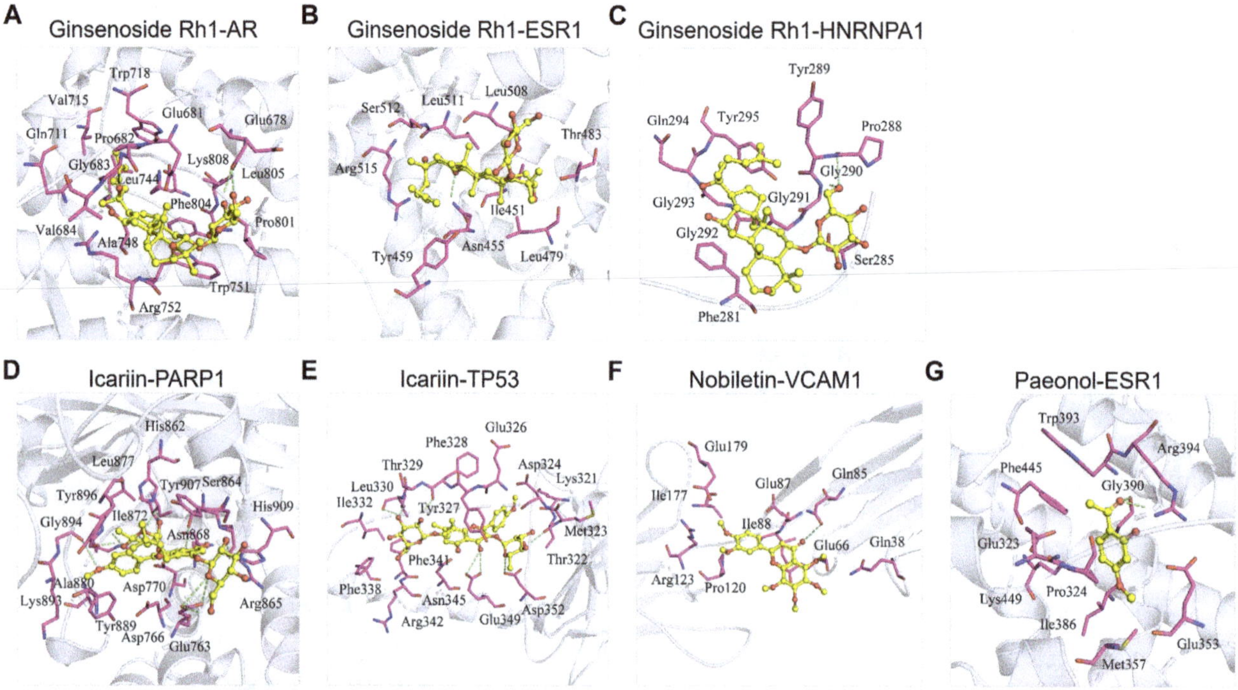

FIGURE 5 | Molecular docking of ECC compounds with their targets. The binding poses of **(A)** ginsenoside Rh1 and AR, **(B)** ginsenoside Rh1 and ESR1, **(C)** ginsenoside Rh1 and HNRNPA1, **(D)** icariin and PARP1, **(E)** icariin and TP53, **(F)** nobiletin and VCAM1, and **(G)** paeonol and ESR1.

TABLE 4 | Docking scores between ECC targets and compounds (kcal/mol).

Target compound	AR	ESR1	HNRNPA1	PAPR1	TP53	VCAM1
20(S)-GinsenosideRh1	−8.6	−6.3	−6.4	–	–	–
Icariin	–	–	–	−10	−7.6	–
Nobiletin	–	–	–	–	–	−6
Paeonol	–	−5.5	–	–	–	–

B signaling, leukocyte transendothelial migration, and the bacterial invasion of epithelial cells. To obtain a more comprehensive view of the therapeutic mechanisms of ECC, the 54 proteins were analyzed with respect to their molecular functions and immune system processes. Our findings revealed that the molecular functions of these proteins mainly involved the positive regulation of DNA binding and cyclin-dependent protein kinase activity, nitric-oxide synthase regulator activity, and p53 binding (**Figure 4C**). In addition, the immune system processes of these proteins were mainly associated with innate immune response–activating signal transduction, lymphocyte co-stimulation, regulation of lymphocyte migration, and macrophage and B-cell differentiation (**Figure 4D**). Therefore, our data suggest that ECC may have a critical impact as a treatment for COPD *via* intervention with the underlying inflammatory processes.

Validation of ECC Targets by Molecular Docking

Among the 45 targets of the ECC compounds, six targets were included in the BisoGenet networks of the COPD genes and the COPD-drug's targets. As a result, a subsequent molecular docking analysis was performed to verify whether the ECC compounds bind to these targets.

We collected the crystal structures of these six targets [i.e., AR (PDBID: 5V8Q), ESR1 (PDBID: 4XI3), HNRNPA1 (PDBID: 7BX7), PAPR1 (PDBID: 7KK2), TP53 (PDBID: 3Q05), and VCAM1 (PDBID: 1VSC)] from the Protein Data Bank, and obtained the chemical structures of these compounds from PubChem. The molecular docking score represented the affinity between the target protein and compounds. As shown in **Figure 5**; **Table 4**, the docking scores for the seven protein–ligand pairs were lower than −5 kcal/ mol, indicating that four compounds could bind to six targets. As shown in **Figure 5A**, the binding pattern between receptor protein AR and 20(S)-ginsenosideRh1 ligand, where the amino acid residues Glu678, Gly683, and Trp751 form hydrogen bonds with the ligand, and the amino acid residues Val715, Gln711, Pro682, Leu744, Val684, Ala748, Arg752, Trp751, Phe804, Pro801, and Leu805 form hydrophobic interactions with the ligand.

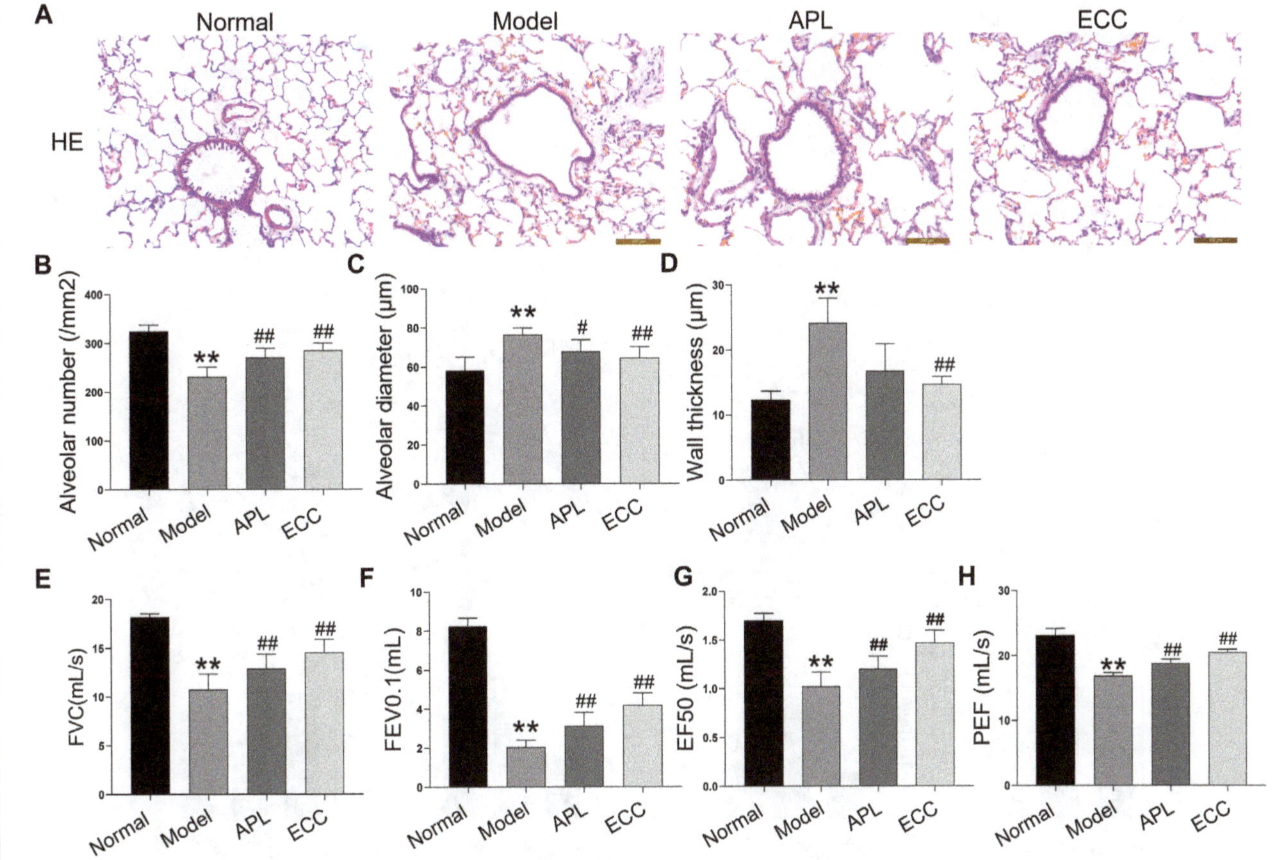

FIGURE 6 | Effects of ECC on pathological changes and lung functioning in rats with COPD. COPD rats were treated with ECC (5.5 mg/ kg) and aminophylline (APL; 54 mg/ kg) for 8 weeks (weeks 12–20). **(A)** H&E staining (magnification, × 100), **(B)** alveolar number, **(C)** alveolar diameter, **(D)** wall thickness, **(E)** FVC, **(F)** FEV at 0.1 s, **(G)** peak expiratory flow, and expiratory flow at 50% tidal volume (EF50); and **(H)** PEF were assessed at week 20. All data are presented as the mean ± SEM ($n = 6$ for each group) *vs.* normal, $^{**}p < 0.01$; *vs.* model, $^{\#}p < 0.05$, $^{\#\#}p < 0.01$.

As shown in **Figure 5B**, the amino acid residue Asn455 forms hydrogen bond with the 20(S)-ginsenosideRh1 ligand, and the amino acid residues Trp459, Arg515, Ser512, Leu511, Leu508, Thr483, Ile451, and Leu479 form hydrophobic interactions with the ligand. As shown in **Figure 5C**, the amino acid residues Gly290 and Pro288 form hydrogen bonds interactions with the ligand, and the amino acid residues Trp289, Gly291, Tyr295, Gln294, Gly293, Gly292, Phe281, and Ser285 form hydrophobic interactions with the ligand. As shown in **Figure 5D**, the amino acid residues Ser864, Asn868, His862, Arg878, Glu763, Ala880, Gly894, and His909 form hydrogen bonds with the ligand, and the amino acid residues Lys893, Trp896, Ile872, Leu877, His862, Tyr907, Ser864, Arg865, Asp770, Asp766, and Tyr889 form hydrophobic interactions with the ligand. As shown in **Figure 5E**, the amino acid residues Thr322, Asp352, Glu349, Phe328, and Leu330 form hydrogen bonds with the ligand, and the amino acid residues Ile332, Thr329, Tyr327, Glu326, Asp324, Lys321, Met323, Asn345, Phe341, and Phe338 form hydrophobic interactions with the ligand. As shown in **Figure 5F**, the amino acid residues Gln85 form hydrogen bonds with the ligand, and the amino acid residues Glu179, Ile177, Arg123, Pro120, Ile88, Glu87, Glu66, and Gln38 form hydrophobic interactions with the ligand. As shown in 5G, the amino acid residues Gly390 and Arg394 form hydrogen bonds with ligand small molecules, and the amino acid residues Trp393, Phe445, Glu323, Lys449, Pro324, Ile386, Met357, and Glu353 form hydrophobic interactions with the ligand. Thus, the ECC compounds may target these six proteins to regulate the activation of COPD genes and targets.

ECC Alleviates the Severity of COPD in Rats

To verify the therapeutic effect of ECC on COPD, we established a COPD rat model based on the simultaneous exposure of cigarette smoke and *Klebsiella pneumonia*. The rats with COPD were treated with ECC and APL on a daily basis for eight consecutive weeks, as opposed to the positive control. As shown in **Figures 6A–D**, hematoxylin and eosin (H&E) staining analysis of lung tissues demonstrated that ECC can increase the alveolar number while decreasing the alveolar diameter and wall thickness. There was a decrease in

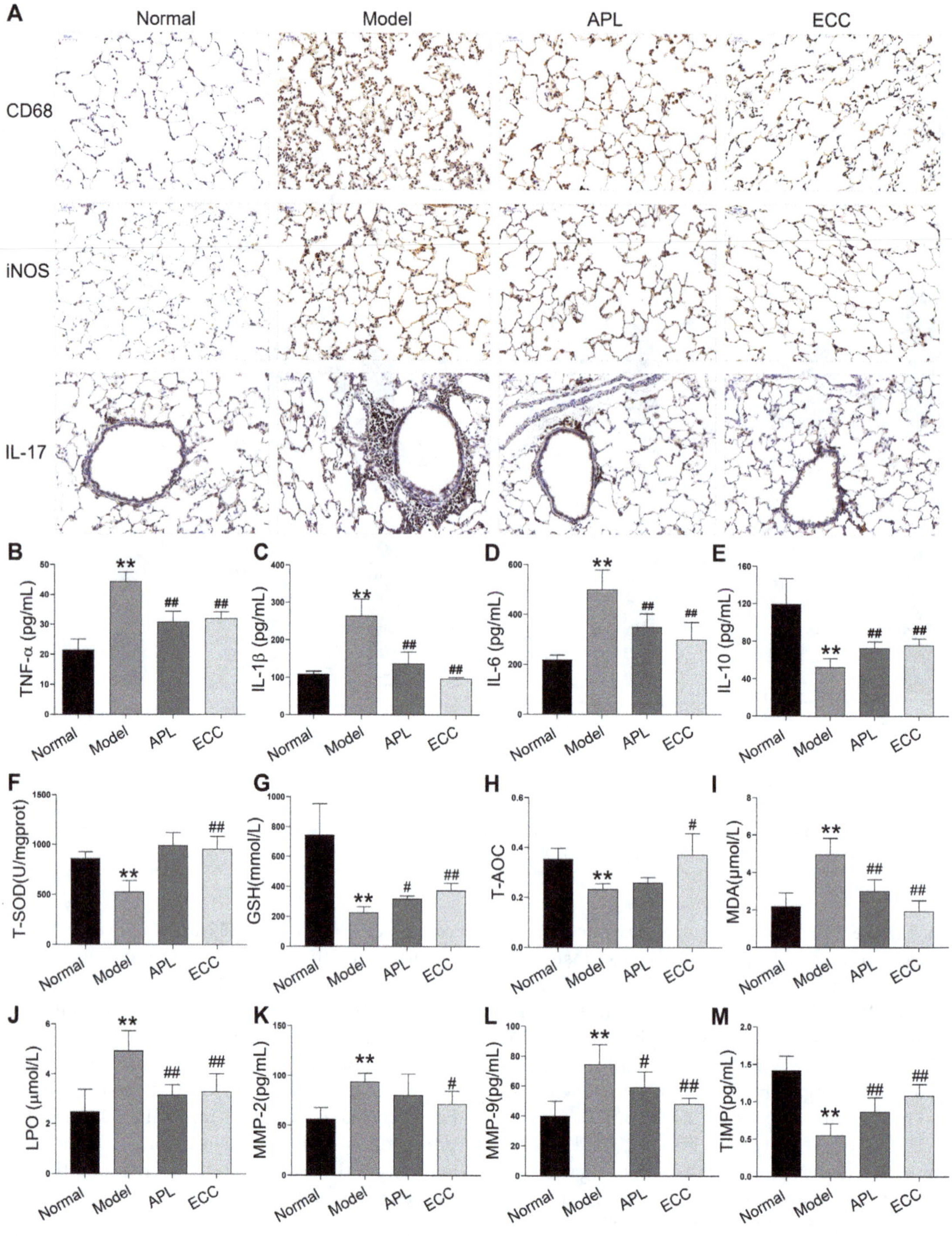

FIGURE 7 | Effect of ECC on inflammation, oxidative stress, and proteinase/anti-proteinase in rats with COPD. Rats with COPD were treated with ECC (5.5 mg/ kg) and aminophylline (APL; 54 mg/ kg) for 8 weeks (weeks 12–20). **(A)** Macrophage marker, CD68, and iNOS were tested in lung tissue *via* immunohistochemistry. Levels of **(B)** TNF-α, **(C)** IL-1β, **(D)** IL6, and **(E)** IL-10 cytokines were detected using ELISA. Serum levels of **(F)** T-SOD, **(G)** GSH, **(H)** T-AOC, **(I)** MDA, and **(J)** LPO were detected using kits. In lung tissue, **(K)** MMP-2, **(L)** MMP-9, and **(M)** TIMP-1 were detected using ELISA. All data are presented as the mean ± SEM ($n = 6$ for each group) *vs*. normal, $^{**}p < 0.01$, *vs*. model, $^{\#}p < 0.05$, $^{\#\#}p < 0.01$.

the pulmonary functioning of COPD rats, indicating a distinct airflow limitation. In contrast, ECC and APL treatment resulted in an increase in FVC, FEV0.1, EF50, and PEF (**Figures 6E–H**). Thus, our data suggest that daily treatment with ECC can attenuate the progression and severity of COPD.

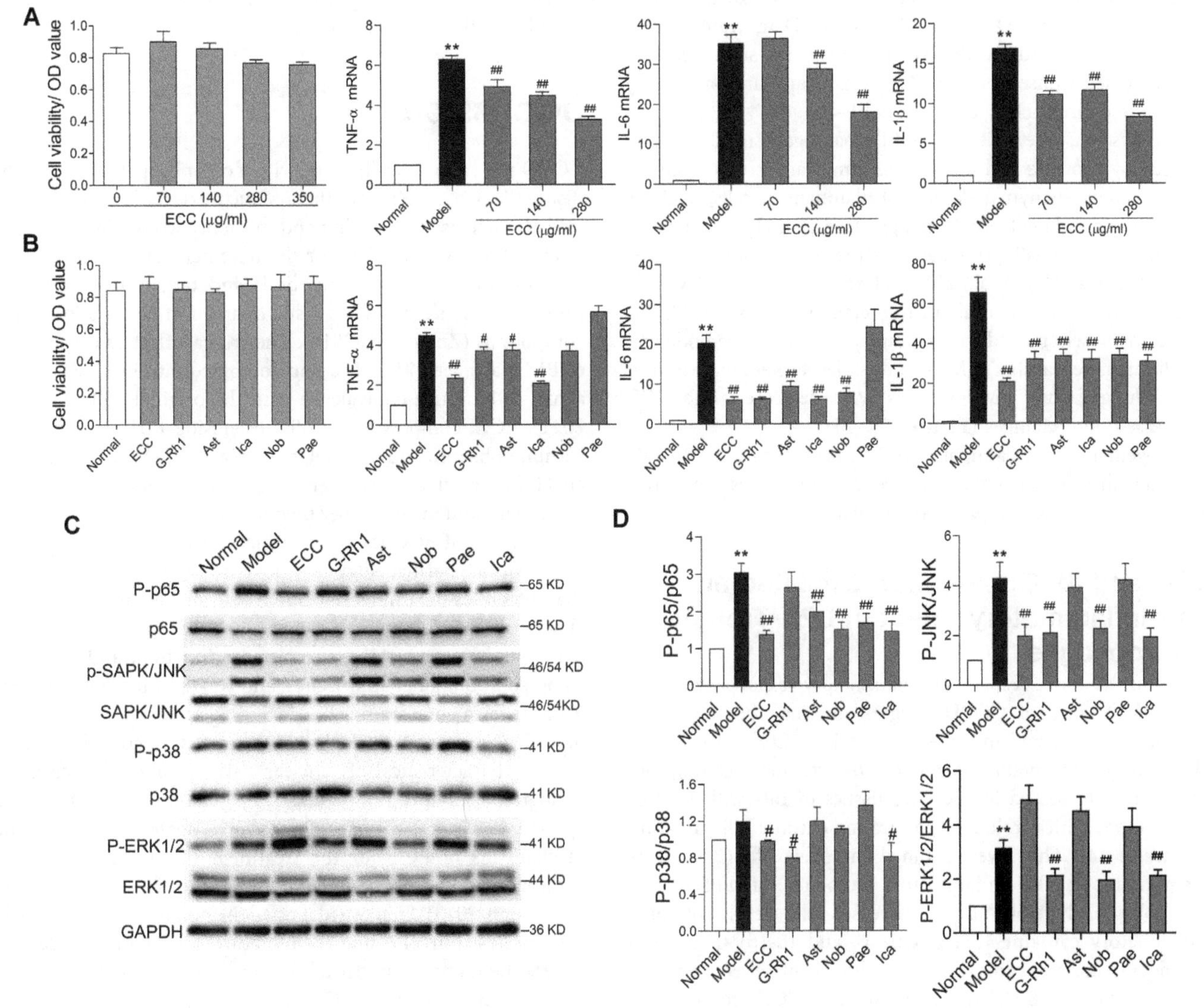

FIGURE 8 | ECC suppressed cytokine levels and activation of NF-κB and MAPK signaling. Macrophages were treated with LPS (100 ng/ ml) and/or ECC (70, 140, and 280 μg/ ml), 20-S-ginsenoside Rh1 (G-Rh1, 78.26 μM), astragaloside IV (Ast, 12.74 μM), icariin (Ica, 295.55 μM), nobiletin (Nob, 19.88 μM), and paeonol (Pae, 75.22 μM) for 6 h. **(A)** Effect of ECC on cell viability and mRNA levels of TNF-α, IL-6, and IL-β. **(B)** Effect of ECC and compounds on cell viability and cytokine mRNA. **(C)** Detection of p-p65, p65, p-p38 (T180/Y182), p38, p-SAPK/JNK, SAPK/JNK, p-ERK1/2 (T202/185), and ERK1/2 *via* Western blotting. Data are presented as the mean ± SEM, $n = 3$. *vs*. normal $^{**}p < 0.01$, *vs*. model $^{\#\#}p < 0.01$, $^{\#}p < 0.05$. **(D)** Quantification of p-p65/p65, p-p38/p38, p-JNK/JNK, p-ERK1/2/ERK1/2.

ECC Inhibits the Inflammatory Response, Oxidative Stress, and Protease Imbalance *In Vivo*

COPD is associated with systemic inflammation, which predominantly affects the airways and lung parenchyma (Hogg, 2009). Inflammation increases further in acute exacerbations of COPD, which represent a sudden worsening in airway functioning and respiratory symptoms (Bafadhel et al., 2011). Based on the above analysis, the ECC targets and COPD genes were mainly associated with inflammatory processes. Thus, we examined the inhibitory effect of ECC on inflammatory responses in rats with COPD. In the lung tissue of these rats, the macrophage number and pro-inflammatory cytokines, including IL-17, TNF-α, IL-1β, and IL-6, were all increased, whereas IL-10 was decreased. Therefore, ECC may reduce the inflammatory changes induced in rats with COPD (**Figures 7A–E**).

Noxious particles expose airways and lung parenchyma to reactive oxygen species, resulting in oxidative stress, which in turn causes injury and subsequent inflammation (Wiegman et al., 2020). Oxidative stress is a critical predisposing factor in COPD pathogenesis. Several markers of oxidative stress, such as MDA and LPO, have consistently been shown to be higher in COPD patients, whereas many antioxidant markers are lower (Singh et al., 2017). Thus, we assessed the levels of antioxidant markers, including T-SOD, GSH, and T-AOC, and oxidative stress markers, including MDA and LPO. In COPD rats, antioxidant marker levels were decreased, whereas oxidative stress markers were increased. Consequently, ECC treatment appears to markedly inhibit these serum changes (**Figures 7F–J**).

Emphysema, the critical COPD pathogenesis, is mainly induced by protease and antiprotease imbalances that result in pulmonary parenchymal damage. Inflammatory cells, such as macrophages and neutrophils, can produce a variety of proteases, such as matrix metalloproteinases (MMPs), neutrophil elastase, and cathepsins (Haq et al., 2011). Here, we tested the levels of MMP-2, -9, and tissue inhibitor of metalloproteinase (TIMP) 1, which are closely related to lung injury and airway remodeling. Our findings reveal that MMP-2 and -9 levels were increased in COPD lung tissue, TIMP-1 levels were decreased, and ECC suppressed both changes (**Figures 7K–M**).

Altogether, daily treatment with ECC may alleviate COPD *via* reducing the subsequent inflammatory responses, oxidative stress, and protease–antiprotease imbalance.

ECC and Its Compounds Exhibited an Anti-Inflammatory Effect in LPS-Treated Macrophages

Based on the above results, an inflammatory response, which is the critical cause of COPD progression, may be the major therapeutic mechanism involved with ECC treatment. Macrophages, the main contributors of cytokine secretion, are significantly increased in the lung tissues of rats with COPD, which play a critical role in orchestrating chronic inflammation (Barnes, 2014). Thus, we examined the effect of ECC and its compounds on the inflammatory response of LPS-treated macrophages. Notably, ECC decreased the levels of pro-inflammatory cytokines (TNF-α, IL-6, and IL-1β) in a dose-dependent manner and had no significant effect on cell viability (**Figure 8A**). In addition, the ECC compounds, including 20-S-ginsenoside Rh1, astragaloside IV, icariin, and nobiletin, downregulated the expression of TNF-α, IL-6, and IL-1β, and had no effect on cell viability; however, paeonol markedly decreased the levels of IL-1β only (**Figure 8B**).

According to the network pharmacology results, inflammatory processes, such as IL-17 and NF-kappa B signaling, were associated with the therapeutic mechanism of ECC. Furthermore, the IL-17 signaling pathway is mainly activated by the NF-kB and MAPK pathways, which include p38, extracellular signal–regulated kinase (ERK), and JNK (Le Rouzic et al., 2017). Thus, we assessed whether ECC and its compounds could regulate the activation of the NF-kB and MAPK pathways. As shown in **Figures 8C,D**, our results indicate that ECC decreased the levels of p-p65, p-JNK, and p-p38, but had no effect on p-ERK1/2. Five compounds were found to induce different effects on this signaling. For instance, 20-S-ginsenoside Rh1 significantly decreased the levels of p-JNK, p-p38, and p-ERK1/2, whereas astragaloside IV and paeonol only decreased p-p65 levels, and nobiletin and icariin suppressed the levels of p-p65, p-JNK, and p-ERK1/2; however, icariin also had an effect on p-p38 levels. These results suggest that ECC can inhibit inflammatory responses *via* suppression of the NF-kappa B and MAPK signaling pathways.

DISCUSSION

COPD is a serious health issue with a complex pathogenesis; the distinct lack of an effective therapeutic treatment for this disease leads to increased morbidity and mortality worldwide (Maigeng et al., 2019). BYF, a TCM for the treatment of COPD patients, contains thousands of compounds and targets from different proteins, and its efficacy is a result of an effective combination of compounds (Zhao et al., 2018). The critical effective compounds of BYF have been identified and combined into ECC, which has achieved bioactive equivalence with the original BYF (Li et al., 2021). ECC, composed of 20-S-ginsenoside Rh1, astragaloside, icariin, nobiletin, and paeonol, may treat COPD *via* a synergistic effect. In the current study, we integrated network pharmacology and *in vivo* and *in vitro* experiments to investigate the therapeutic mechanisms of ECC for the treatment of COPD.

Network pharmacology is a novel multidisciplinary method that integrates the immense volume of available information and allows for new discoveries. It usually predicts potential active compounds, protein targets, molecular function, and pathways using computational approaches, and validates these predictions using experimental approaches, including omics technologies and biological and pharmacological experiments. In consideration of ECC's characteristics of unclear targets, and the complex biological activities and holistic regulation of COPD, we applied network pharmacology to investigate the therapeutic mechanisms of ECC for the treatment of COPD using both computational and experimental approaches (Li et al., 2014; Li and Zhang, 2013). First, we identified the putative targets for ECC compounds from IPA and the literature. 20-S-Ginsenoside Rh1 targets the highest number of proteins; thus, it may be the main active compound in ECC. In addition, PPI and pathway enrichment analysis suggested that the inflammatory response may be the critical biological process regulated by ECC compounds. For instance, the compounds' hub targets, including IL6, TNF, MAPK8, PTGS2, CXCL8, and TP53, are closely related to inflammation. The top pathways, such as the NF-kappa B signaling pathway, Th17 cell differentiation, hematopoietic cell lineage, and the NOD-like receptor signaling pathway, were important in signaling for the regulation of the inflammatory response. Furthermore, the top immune system processes, including cellular responses to lipopolysaccharide, the extrinsic apoptotic signaling pathway *via* death domain receptors, interleukin-8 secretion, acute inflammatory response, and leukocyte adhesion to vascular endothelial cells, were the typical inflammatory processes. These results suggest that ECC targets multiple proteins, which collectively participate in the regulation of the inflammatory process.

Inflammation is a major biological process in the development of COPD (Barnes, 2016); however, it is unclear whether inflammatory response regulation is the underlying therapeutic mechanism of ECC in the treatment of COPD. Thus, we first collected 1180 COPD genes and 69 therapeutic targets from public databases, which were then used to analyze the molecular functions and pathways, thus uncovering the molecular mechanisms of COPD. The top pathways of the COPD genes and targets, such as the TNF signaling pathway, cytokine–cytokine receptor, MAPK signaling, the Fc epsilon RI signaling pathway, and epithelial cell signaling in helicobacter pylori infection, were mainly related to immune regulation. For instance, elevated levels of TNFα, and phosphorylation levels of p38 MAPK and ERK1/2, have been observed in COPD patients, and the inhibitors of p38 MAPK and TNFα have been shown to exhibit inhibitory effects on the inflammatory responses of COPD (Lemire et al., 2012; Zhang et al., 2019). Thus, the molecular mechanisms of inflammation may be critical in the subsequent pathogenesis of COPD.

ECC targets, COPD genes, and COPD targets were comprehensively analyzed with BisoGenet, from which the hub-network was extracted. Functional enrichment analysis showed that the genes contained in the hub-network were mainly associated with the IL-17 and NF-kappa B signaling pathways, nitric-oxide synthase regulator activity, innate immune response–activating signal transduction, and macrophage differentiation, which are closely related to the inflammatory response. IL-17 can activate the inflammatory transcription factor NF-κB and the MAPK pathways (i.e., p38, ERK, and JNK), which regulate the expression of pro-inflammatory cytokines in COPD (AudreeshbanerjeeKoziol-White and Jr, 2012; Schuliga, 2015; Le Rouzic et al., 2017). According to the network pharmacology analysis, PARP1, TP53, ESR1, HNRNPA1, VCAM1, and AR, which are contained in the hub PPI network of ECC targets, COPD genes, and targets, were considered important targets of ECC; in addition, molecular docking demonstrated that the compounds could bind to these targets, which are involved in the inflammatory response. Thus, our findings suggest that the inflammatory process is the critical therapeutic mechanism for both ECC and COPD progression.

We thus validated the anti-COPD and anti-inflammatory effect of ECC both *in vivo* and *in vitro*. Our results highlight that ECC treatment can ameliorate the symptoms of COPD in rats by improving lung function, reducing pathological changes, and suppressing the respective oxidative response and pro-inflammatory cytokine secretion. The IL-17 and NF-kappa B signaling pathways were the main inflammatory pathways related to both the ECC targets and COPD genes. In addition, the IL-17 signaling pathway was found to activate the inflammatory transcription factors to increase inflammatory genes, mainly through the regulation of NF-κB and MAPK (i.e., p38, ERK, and JNK; Li et al., 2019). Thus, we validated the anti-inflammatory and regulatory effects of ECC *via* NF-kappa B and MAPK signaling pathway effects in LPS-induced macrophages. Our results demonstrate that ECC can inhibit the inflammatory response by decreasing the expression of pro-inflammatory cytokines and suppressing the activation of MAPK (p38 and JNK) and NF-kappa B signaling. However, ECC can also increase the levels of p-ERK1/2 in LPS-induced macrophages. Overall, in this experiment, ECC treatment led to an alleviation of COPD, although an increase of p-ERK1/2 was found in LPS-induced macrophages. Additionally, 20-S-ginsenoside Rh1 (78.26 μM), astragaloside IV (12.74 μM), icariin (295.55 μM), nobiletin (19.88 μM), and paeonol (75.22 μM) exerted different effects on the inflammatory response in macrophages. More specifically, low concentrations of 20-S-ginsenoside Rh1, astragaloside IV, and nobiletin had the same anti-inflammatory effects as icariin. Thus, we speculate that as part of ECC, 20-S-ginsenoside Rh1 and astragaloside IV may play an important role in inhibiting inflammation. We previously evaluated the effect of ECC at three different doses on COPD rats, and found that ECC at middle dose could exert the best efficacy and presented with bioactive equivalence to the original BYF. Here, we only treated COPD rat with ECC at single dose, which showed significant beneficial effects on COPD rats. However, evaluation of therapeutic effect and underlying mechanisms of ECC at different doses is helpful to optimize the safe and effective use of the drug. Thus, the anti-COPD effect of ECC at different doses will be examined in the next work. Altogether, ECC appears to ameliorate the effects of COPD through suppression of the inflammatory response *via* MAPK and NF-kappa B signaling regulation.

CONCLUSION

This work revealed the therapeutic mechanisms of ECC for the treatment of COPD using an integrative analysis of network pharmacology and *in vivo* and *in vitro* experiments. ECC appears to exhibit protective effects against COPD through the regulation of inflammatory responses *via* MAPK and NF-kappa B signaling.

AUTHOR CONTRIBUTIONS

JL designed the outline of the study. PZ and YT conceived the study and drafted the manuscript. KL, LZ, QG, XM, and YQ performed experiments and data analysis. All authors contributed toward data analysis, drafting and critically revising the paper, gave final approval of the version to be published, and agree to be accountable for all aspects of the work.

FUNDING

The research was supported by the National Natural Science Foundation of China (Grant Number: 81973822, 81603473).

REFERENCES

Bafadhel, M., Mckenna, S., Terry, S., Mistry, V., Reid, C., Haldar, P., et al. (2011). Acute Exacerbations of Chronic Obstructive Pulmonary Disease: Identification of Biologic Clusters and Their Biomarkers. *Am. J. Respir. Crit. Care Med.* 184 (6), 662–671. doi:10.1164/rccm.201104-0597OC

BanerjeeKoziol-White, A., Koziol-White, C., and Panettieri, R. (2012). p38 MAPK Inhibitors, IKK2 Inhibitors, and TNFα Inhibitors in COPD. *Curr. Opin. Pharmacol.* 12, 287–292. doi:10.1016/j.coph.2012.01.016

Barnes, P. J. (2014). Cellular and Molecular Mechanisms of Chronic Obstructive Pulmonary Disease. *Clin. Chest Med.* 35 (1), 71–86. doi:10.1016/j.ccm.2013.10.004

Barnes, P. J. (2016). Inflammatory Mechanisms in Patients with Chronic Obstructive Pulmonary Disease. *J. Allergy Clin. Immunol.* 138 (1), 16–27. doi:10.1016/j.jaci.2016.05.011

Chen, T., Wang, R., Jiang, W., Wang, H., Xu, A., Lu, G., et al. (2016). Protective Effect of Astragaloside IV Against Paraquat-Induced Lung Injury in Mice by Suppressing Rho Signaling. *Inflammation* 39 (1), 483–492. doi:10.1007/s10753-015-0272-4

Global Initiative for Chronic Obstructive Lung Disease (2020). Global Strategy for the Diagnosis, Management, and Prevention of Chronic Obstructive Pulmonary Disease. Available at: http://www.goldcopd.org. 2020.

Haq, I., Lowrey, G. E., Kalsheker, N., and Johnson, S. R. (2011). Matrix Metalloproteinase-12 (MMP-12) SNP Affects MMP Activity, Lung Macrophage Infiltration and Protects against Emphysema in COPD. *Thorax* 66 (11), 970–976. doi:10.1136/thx.2011.159087

Hogg, J. C., and Timens, W. (2009). The Pathology of Chronic Obstructive Pulmonary Disease. *Annu. Rev. Pathol. Mech. Dis.* 4:435-59. doi:10.1146/annurev.pathol.4.110807.092145

Le Rouzic, O., Pichavant, M., Frealle, E., Guillon, A., Si-Tahar, M., and Gosset, P. (2017). Th17 Cytokines: Novel Potential Therapeutic Targets for COPD Pathogenesis and Exacerbations. *Eur. Respir. J.* 50 (4), 1602434. doi:10.1183/13993003.02434-2016

Lemire, B. B., Debigaré, R., Dubé, A., Thériault, M. E., Côté, C. H., and Maltais, F. (2012). MAPK Signaling in the Quadriceps of Patients with Chronic Obstructive Pulmonary Disease. *J. Appl. Physiol. (1985)* 113 (1), 159–166. doi:10.1152/japplphysiol.01518.2011

Li, J., Xie, Y., Zhao, P., Qin, Y., Oliver, B. G., Tian, Y., et al. (2021). A Chinese Herbal Formula Ameliorates COPD by Inhibiting the Inflammatory Response via Downregulation of P65, JNK, and P38. *Phytomedicine* 83, 153475. doi:10.1016/j.phymed.2021.153475

Li, J., Zhao, P., Li, Y., Tian, Y., and Wang, Y. (2015). Systems Pharmacology-Based Dissection of Mechanisms of Chinese Medicinal Formula Bufei Yishen as an Effective Treatment for Chronic Obstructive Pulmonary Disease. *Sci. Rep.* 5, 15290. doi:10.1038/srep15290

Li, J., Zhao, P., Yang, L., Li, Y., Tian, Y., and Li, S. (2016). System Biology Analysis of Long-Term Effect and Mechanism of Bufei Yishen on COPD Revealed by System Pharmacology and 3-omics Profiling. *Sci. Rep.* 6 (1), 25492. doi:10.1038/srep25492

Li, J. S., Liu, X. F., Dong, H. R., Zheng, W. C., Feng, S. X., Tian, Y. G., et al. (2020). Effective-constituent Compatibility-Based Analysis of Bufei Yishen Formula, a Traditional Herbal Compound as an Effective Treatment for Chronic Obstructive Pulmonary Disease. *J. Integr. Med.* 18 (4), 351–362. doi:10.1016/j.joim.2020.04.004

Li, S., Fan, T. P., Jia, W., Lu, A., and Zhang, W. (2014). Network Pharmacology in Traditional Chinese Medicine. *Evid. Based Complement. Alternat Med.* 2014, 138460–138462. doi:10.1155/2014/138460

Li, S. Y., Li, J. S., Wang, M. H., Xie, Y., Yu, X. Q., Sun, Z. K., et al. (2012). Effects of Comprehensive Therapy Based on Traditional Chinese Medicine Patterns in Stable Chronic Obstructive Pulmonary Disease: a four-center, Open-Label, Randomized, Controlled Study. *BMC Complement. Altern. Med.* 12, 197. doi:10.1186/1472-6882-12-197

Li, W., Zhao, R., Wang, X., Liu, F., Zhao, J., Yao, Q., et al. (2018). Nobiletin-Ameliorated Lipopolysaccharide-Induced Inflammation in Acute Lung Injury by Suppression of NF-Kb Pathway *In Vivo* and Vitro. *Inflammation* 41, 996–1007. doi:10.1007/s10753-018-0753-3

Li, X., Bechara, R., Zhao, J., Mcgeachy, M. J., and Gaffen, S. L. (2019). IL-17 Receptor-Based Signaling and Implications for Disease. *Nat. Immunol.* 20 (12), 1594–1602. doi:10.1038/s41590-019-0514-y

Li, Y., Li, S. Y., Li, J. S., Deng, L., Tian, Y. G., Jiang, S. L., et al. (2012). A Rat Model for Stable Chronic Obstructive Pulmonary Disease Induced by Cigarette Smoke Inhalation and Repetitive Bacterial Infection. *Biol. Pharm. Bull.* 35 (10), 1752–1760. doi:10.1248/bpb.b12-00407

Liu, M. H., Lin, A. H., Ko, H. K., Perng, D. W., Lee, T. S., and Kou, Y. R. (2017). Prevention of Bleomycin-Induced Pulmonary Inflammation and Fibrosis in Mice by Paeonol. *Front. Physiol.* 8, 193. doi:10.3389/fphys.2017.00193

Maigeng, Z., Haidong, W., Xinying, Z., Yin, P., and Jun, Z. (2019). Mortality, Morbidity, and Risk Factors in China and its Provinces, 1990-2017: a Systematic Analysis for the Global Burden of Disease Study 2017. *Lancet* 394 (10204), 1145–1158. doi:10.1016/S0140-6736(19)30427-1

Martin, A., Ochagavia, M. E., Rabasa, L. C., Miranda, J., Fernandez-De-Cossio, J., and Bringas, R. (2010). BisoGenet: a New Tool for Gene Network Building, Visualization and Analysis. *BMC Bioinformatics* 11 (1), 91. doi:10.1186/1471-2105-11-91

Ren, S., Zhang, H., Mu, Y., Sun, M., and Liu, P. (2013). Pharmacological Effects of Astragaloside IV: a Literature Review. *J. Tradit. Chin. Med.* 33 (3), 413–416. doi:10.1016/S0254-6272(13)60189-2

Schuliga, M. (2015). NF-kappaB Signaling in Chronic Inflammatory Airway Disease. *Biomolecules* 5 (3), 1266–1283. doi:10.3390/biom5031266

Singh, S., Verma, S. K., Kumar, S., Ahmad, M. K., Nischal, A., Singh, S. K., et al. (2017). Evaluation of Oxidative Stress and Antioxidant Status in Chronic Obstructive Pulmonary Disease. *Scand. J. Immunol.* 85 (2), 130–137. doi:10.1111/sji.12498

Sun, X., Cheng, H., Liu, B., Du, Y., Dong, J., and Huang, J. (2020). Icariin Reduces LPS-Induced Acute Lung Injury in Mice Undergoing Bilateral Adrenalectomy by Regulating GRα. *Eur. J. Pharmacol.* 876, 173032. doi:10.1016/j.ejphar.2020.173032

Sun, X., Deng, X., Cai, W., Li, W., Shen, Z., Jiang, T., et al. (2018). Icariin Inhibits LPS-Induced Cell Inflammatory Response by Promoting GRα Nuclear Translocation and Upregulating GRα Expression. *Life Sci.* 195, 33–43. doi:10.1016/j.lfs.2018.01.006

Tam, D., Truong, D., Nguyen, T., Quynh, L., Tran, L., Nguyen, H., et al. (2018). Ginsenoside Rh1: A Systematic Review of its Pharmacological Properties. *Planta Med.* 84 (03), 139–152. doi:10.1055/s-0043-124087

Tusher, V. G., Tibshirani, R., and Chu, G. (2001). Significance Analysis of Microarrays Applied to the Ionizing Radiation Response. *Proc. Natl. Acad. Sci. USA* 9 (98), 5116–5121. doi:10.1073/pnas.091062498

Wang, C., Xu, J., Yang, L., Xu, Y., Zhang, X., Bai, C., et al. (2018). Prevalence and Risk Factors of Chronic Obstructive Pulmonary Disease in China (The China Pulmonary Health [CPH] Study): a National Cross-Sectional Study. *The Lancet* 391 (10131), 1706–1717. doi:10.1016/S0140-6736(18)30841-9

Wiegman, C. H., Li, F., Ryffel, B., Togbe, D., and Chung, K. F. (2020). Oxidative Stress in Ozone-Induced Chronic Lung Inflammation and Emphysema: A Facet of Chronic Obstructive Pulmonary Disease. *Front. Immunol.* 11. doi:10.3389/fimmu.2020.01957

Zhang, J. L., Yang, C. Q., and Deng, F. (2019). MicroRNA-378 Inhibits the Development of Smoking-Induced COPD by Targeting TNF-Alpha. *Eur. Rev. Med. Pharmacol. Sci.* 23 (20), 9009–9016. doi:10.26355/eurrev_201910_19302

Zhao, P., Li, J., Tian, Y., Mao, J., and Liu, X. (2018). Restoring Th17/Treg Balance via Modulation of STAT3 and STAT5 Activation Contributes to the Amelioration of Chronic Obstructive Pulmonary Disease by Bufei Yishen Formula. *J. Ethnopharmacol.* 2018 (217), 152–162. doi:10.1016/j.jep.2018.02.023

Zhou, M., Haidong, fnm., Wang, X., Zeng, X., Peng, Y., and Zhu, J. (2019). The Global burden of Falls: Global, Regional and National Estimates of Morbidity and Mortality from the Global Burden of Disease Study 2017. *Lancet* 2019 (394), 1145–1158. doi:10.1136/injuryprev-2019-043286

4

Diosgenin from Dioscorea Nipponica Rhizoma Against Graves' Disease—On Network Pharmacology and Experimental Evaluation

Jingxin Xin[1,2,3,4], *Wencong Cheng*[1,3,4], *Yongbing Yu*[1,2,3,4], *Juan Chen*[1,3,4], *Xinhuan Zhang*[2*] *and Shanshan Shao*[1,3,4*]

[1]*Department of Endocrinology, Shandong Provincial Hospital Affiliated to Shandong First Medical University, Jinan, China,* [2]*Department of Endocrinology, The Second Affiliated Hispital of Shandong First Medical University, Taian, China,* [3]*Shandong Clinical Research Center of Diabetes and Metabolic Diseases, Jinan, China,* [4]*Shandong Key Laboratory of Endocrinology and Lipid Metabolism, Jinan, China*

***Correspondence:**
Shanshan Shao
shaoshanshan11@126.com
Xinhuan Zhang
kathy0418@163.com

Dioscorea nipponica rhizoma (DNR) is commonly used for the cure of hyperthyroidism resulting from Graves' disease (GD) or thyroid nodules. However, its therapeutic mechanism remains unclear. This study aimed to utilize network pharmacology integrated molecular docking and experimental verification to reveal the potential pharmacological mechanism of DNR against GD. First, the active componds of DNR were collected from the HERB database and a literature search was conducted. Then, according to multisource database, the predicted genes of DNR and GD were collected to generate networks. The analysis of protein–protein interaction and GO enrichment and KEGG pathway were employed to discover main mechanisms associated with therapeutic targets. Moreover, molecular docking simulation was applied in order to verify the interactions between the drug and target. Finally, our experiments validated the ameliorated effects of diosgenin, the main component of DNR, in terms of phosphorylation deactivation in IGF-1R, which in turn inhibited the phosphorylation and activation of PI3K-AKT and Rap1-MEK signaling pathways, promoting cell apoptosis and GD remission. Our present study provided a foundation for further investigation of the in-depth mechanisms of diosgenin in GD and will provide new scientific evidence for clinical application.

Keywords: dioscorea nipponica rhizoma, diosgenin, graves' disease, network pharmacology, IGF-1R, apoptosis, traditional chinese medicine

1 INTRODUCTION

Graves' disease (GD) is an organ-specific autoimmune disease featured by hyperthyroidism, diffuse goiter and thyroid-associated ophthalmopathy (Bahn et al., 2011). Hyperthyroidism of GD is due to the liganding of thyrotropin receptor (TSHR) on thyroid cells by stimulatory autoantibodies, which act as a TSHR agonist and induce excessive secretion of thyroid hormones, causing the thyroid to escape the control of the pituitary gland (Ross et al., 2016). GD is the most common cause of hyperthyroidism in iodine-sufficient regions, with 20–30 GD patients per 100,000 people per year (Kahaly et al., 2018). Female patients are reported to be more likely to develop GD, with a population prevalence of 1–1.5% (Nyström et al., 2013). The primary role of currently used drugs for GD is to inhibit thyroid hormones synthesis by interfering with thyroid peroxidase expression rather than promoting apoptosis or inhibiting excessive proliferation of thyrocytes (Cooper, 2005). Therefore, these antithyroid drugs cannot effectively alleviate goiter, resulting in a heavy financial burden and mental stress on GD patients with large goiters. Proapoptotic and antiproliferative approaches might be potential therapies for the treatment of GD goiter.

According to traditional Chinese medicine (TCM) theory, Dioscorea nipponica rhizoma (DNR), the rhizome of Dioscorea nipponica Makino (DNM), is rich in a variety of steroidal saponins. DNR exhibits various pharmacological activities, such as anti-inflammatory (Yao et al., 2012), analgesic (Vasanthi et al., 2010), antitumor (X. Li et al., 2017) hypoglycemic (Tang et al., 2015), and hypolipidemic (Vasanthi et al., 2012) activities. In the treatment of thyroid disease, DNR is used for thyroid tumors and hyperthyroidism. Wang et al. used the DNM to treat established GD rat model and concluded that DNM could inhibit the process of iodine capture and improve the morphological structure disorder of thyroid in GD (Q. H. Wang and Chen, 2007). However, it was reported that diosgenin produced from the metabolism of intestinal flora is the major bioactive compound and plays a vital role after the oral administration of dioscin (Ou-Yang et al., 2018). Its main component, diosgenin (Yan et al., 2013; Yi et al., 2014), has also been reported to inhibit proliferation and cell progress (Bian et al., 2011), promote apoptosis (Mu et al., 2012) of thyrocytes, and relieve goiter (Cai et al., 2014). Nevertheless, its pharmacodynamic mechanism remains unclear.

With the widely application of bioinformatics, network pharmacology has emerged as effective tool toward TCM research (Hao and Xiao, 2014). Based on omics data analysis, high-performance virtual computing and network database retrieval, network pharmacology could not only build the priority of disease-associated genes, but also predict the target information and pharmacological effects of TCM compounds systematically (Hopkins, 2008; S.; Li and Zhang, 2013; T. T.; Luo et al., 2020). It is believed to a new original discipline of cost-effective drug development in the era of artificial intelligence and Big Data (S. Li, 2021). In the current results, we adopted a network pharmacology approach coupled with molecular docking to screen the putative targets and signaling pathways of DNR against GD and then conducted experimental verification on a rat model of GD goiter to further illustrate the pharmacological mechanism of DNR against GD.

2 MATERIALS AND METHODS

2.1 Database-Based Network Pharmacology Analysis

2.1.1 Screening of the Active Chemical Constituents of DNR

To collect the pharmacologically active ingredients of DNR, the term "DNR and DN" was searched first in the HERB database (http://herb.ac.cn/) (Fang et al., 2021). The database links 12,933 targets and 28,212 diseases with 7,263 Chinese herbal medicines and 49,258 Chinese medicine ingredients, providing six pairing relationships between them. The ingredients of DNR searched from HERB are mainly from the TCMSP, SymMap, TCMID, and TCM-ID databases. Then, the BATMAN database (http://bionet.ncpsd.org/batman-tcm) (Z. Liu et al., 2016), domestic as well as foreign literature (Guo et al., 2016; Lin et al., 2007) supplemented the search. According to the absorption, distribution, metabolism, excretion, and toxicity characteristics of ADME (Daina et al., 2017) (http://www.swissadme.ch/), the Lipinski rules (Omran and Rauch, 2014) were used to screen the active ingredients of DNR. It has four rules: MW $\leq$ 500; nON$\leq$10; nOHNH$\leq$5; MLogP$\leq$4.15. A compound that met at least two conditions was determined to be an orally active drug. If the compound in the database does not meet the Lipinski rules, it can also be included if there is a compound in relevant reports clearly described as the active ingredient of DNR (https://pubchem.ncbi.nlm.nih.gov/).

2.2 Prediction and Screening of the Related Targets of DNR

To prepare for predicting the target of the active ingredient, the 2D structural formulas of the active ingredients were downloaded from PubChem database (Kim et al., 2021). Using the method of matching reversed pharmacophores from the Pharm Mapper database (http://www.lilab-ecust.cn/pharmmapper/) (X. Wang et al., 2016; X. Wang et al., 2017), we can predict the targets of each compound. The advantage of this method is that it uses active small molecules as probes to explore qualified putative targets and then predicts the biological activity of the compound. Then, we screened the human target genes of each component according to the score value. The Swiss Target Prediction database (http://www.swisstargetprediction.ch/) (Daina et al., 2019) is another way to predict the target. This method is based on the similarity of ligand 2D and 3D structures. The credibility of the composites was generally poor using this approach. Therefore, we added target genes with a credibility of one to the corresponding compound. After screening, we standardized the protein target information using the UniProt protein database (https://www.uniprot.org/) (UniProt, 2019).

2.3 Screening the Related Targets for GD

Using "Graves' disease" as the key word, we obtained a large number of targets from the Gene Cards (Stelzer et al., 2016) (https://www.genecards.org), DisGeNET (Pinero et al., 2020) (http://www.disgenet.org/home/), CTD (Davis et al., 2021) (ctdbase.org), and GAD (Becker et al., 2004) (https://geneticassociationdb.nih.gov/) databases. Then, the therapeutic target of clinical first-line western medicine of GD was identified through the OMIM (Boyadjiev and Jabs, 2000) (http://www.omim.org), TTD (Y. Wang et al., 2020) (http://db.idrblab.net/ttd/), and DRUGBANK (Wishart et al., 2008) (https://www.drugbank.ca) (https://www.drugbank.ca) databases. In database analysis, the criteria for screening targets have little difference in databases. Briefly, they are generally judged by score value. If the target has a high score value, it indicates that the target is highly correlated to the disease. To be specific, the targets from the CTD and Gene Card databases were selected by median screening of the score value. The targets from the DisGeNET database were selected according to score values greater than the average value. In the OMIM database, the gene targets were selected with * in front of the number. After merging the targets obtained from the seven disease databases and deleting the duplicate GD target, the screened targets of disease were collected.

2.4 The Mapping Relation of Overlapping Targets of DNR in GD

To clarify the interaction between the predicted targets of DNR and the targets of GD, a Venn diagram was drawn with the Venn diagram website (http://www.bioinformatics.com.cn/plot_basic_proportional_2_or_3_venn_diagram_028) (W. Luo and Brouwer, 2013) to identify the intersection of the two targets. Then, the intersection target was submitted to the STRING database (https://string-db.org/) (Szklarczyk et al., 2017). To generate the protein interaction network, the organism type was set to "Homo Sapiens", the minimum interaction threshold was set to "highest confidence" (>0.4), and the other settings were the default settings. Topological property analysis was carried out to identify important targets of diosgenin in GD.

2.5 GO and KEGG Analyses

To further elucidate the potential pharmacological mechanism of DNR against GD, we put common targets on DAVID 6.8 (https://david.ncifcrf.gov/) (Huang da et al., 2009) to perform GO biological process (BP), molecular function (MF), cell component (CC) and KEGG pathway analysis (Shi et al., 2017) The items with correction $p \le 0.01$, the top ten pathways with the most enriched targets were selected to visualize the data by bioinformatics (W. Luo and Brouwer, 2013) (http://www.bioinformatics.com.cn/). The information enrichments genes were analyzed using R-Studio.

2.6 Network Construction Analyses

To understand the interaction relationship of each target more intuitively, the targets were imported into the String database (https://string-db.org/cgi/input.pl) to construct a PPI network. Then, the PPI network was imported into Cytoscape 3.7.2 to perform network analysis. The following networks were constructed: 1) DNR component target network; 2) The target network of GD; 3) PPI network of DNR's compound-GD targets; and 4) compound-core target-pathway network. The nodes in each network represent interacting molecules. An edge refers to the line connecting two nodes, which represents the interaction between nodes. Usually, three indicators are used to evaluate the topological properties of each node. The first is "Degree", which means the number of directly connected nodes of one node in a network, and its level is proportional to the betweenness centrality of this node. This means that the more pathways that depend on this node, the more important this node is. The second is "betweenness centrality", which means the proportion of nodes that as a shortest route in a network. The more times a node acts as an "intermediary", the greater its degree of intermediary centrality. The third is "closeness centrality", which means the average length of the shortest path between each two nodes. In other words, for a node, the shorter distance it is to other nodes, the higher its degree of closeness centrality. In short, if these three parameters have higher score values, the node is more important in this network.

2.7 Target-Compound Molecular Docking

The IGF-1R protein crystal structures were obtained from the RCSB Protein Data Bank (http://www.rcsb.org/pdb/) (Goodsell et al., 2020) and saved in pdb format. Diosgenin structures were downloaded through PubChem converted to. pdb format files via Open Babel (O'Boyle et al., 2011). Auto Dock Tools 1.5.6 software (Cosconati et al., 2010) was used to remove water molecules, to add nonpolar hydrogen bonds, to calibrate the Gasteiger charge and to save them as pdbqt format files. Diosgenin was performed with energy minimization, assigned the ligand atom type, calculated the charge, and saved in pdbqt format. Then, Auto Dock Tools 1.5.6 software was used to calculate the docking score to evaluate the matching degree and docking activity between a target and its ligand. A docking score < -4.25 can be considered as having binding activity; a score < -5.0 can be considered as having better binding activity; and a score < -7 can be considered as representing a strong docking activity between the ligand and the target. The binding model was visualized using PyMol2.3.0 software (Seeliger and de Groot, 2010).

2.8 Experimental Validation

2.8.1 Animals and Treatments

Forty-eight male Sprague–Dawley (SD) rats (170–190 g, 6 weeks old) were purchased from Vital River Laboratory Animal Technology Co., Ltd (Beijing, China). After making adaption of 1 week, all rats were randomly distributed into four groups (n = 12 per group): Norm (normal control group), (methimazole group), MMI + L-Dio (methimazole plus diosgenin 20 mg kg^{-1} d^{-1} treatment group), and MMI + H-Dio (methimazole plus diosgenin 80 mg kg^{-1} d^{-1} treatment group). Briefly, 0.04% MMI was added to the drinking water for the three groups. One week later, rats were treated with 20 mg kg^{-1} d^{-1} or 80 mg kg^{-1} d^{-1} diosgenin by intraperitoneal injection. Correspondingly, the Norm and MMI groups were injected with the same amount of solvent (4% Tween-80) for 3 weeks (Han et al., 2009). All animals were anesthetized, and the thyroid glands were collected and fixed in 4% paraformaldehyde for hematoxylin-eosin (H&E) and immunohistochemistry staining. All animal operations were performed according to the animal guidelines and were approved by the Animal Ethics Committee of Shandong Provincial Hospital.

2.9 H&E Staining

The rats thyroid tissues were fixed in 4% paraformaldehyde and enclosed in paraffin. 4 μM slides were stained with hematoxylin and eosin (Shao et al., 2014). The histological changes were observed by upright microscopy (Axio Imager A2; Zeiss, Germany).

2.10 Immunohistochemical Analysis

Immunohistochemical staining was carried out for p-IGF-1R (AF3125; Affinity, China). Sections were incubated with the p-IGF-1R primary antibody at 4°C overnight, followed by incubation with HRP-conjugated secondary antibody. Finally, immunohistochemical reactions were visualized using DAB (Cai et al., 2014).

2.11 TUNEL Staining

A TUNEL apoptosis detection kit (KGA7071; KeyGEN, China) was used to discover cell nuclear DNA breakage during the late stage of apoptosis (He et al., 2019; Ma et al., 2020). Tissue sections were deparaffinized according to conventional methods. The sections were emulsified with proteinase K. After that, the paraffin sections were sequentially incubated in the dark with TdT buffer solution at 37°C for 1 h, streptavidin-fluorescein labeling solution was added for 30 min, and the sections were covered with DAPI containing an anti-fluorescence quenching mounting plate for 10 min. Finally, the apoptosis reaction of thyroid tissues were uncovered by a microimaging system (Axio Imager Z2, Zeiss, Germany).

2.12 Cells Culture and Processing

Nthy-ori 3-1 cells (obtain from ATCC, Manassas, VA, United States) were cultured with RPMI (HyClone, United States) supplemented with 10% FBS (Gibco, United States) and 1% penicillin/streptomycin at 37°C and 5% CO2. When the thyrocytes were 70–80% confluent, they were starved in serum-free medium for 2 h and then preincubated with or without 100 ng/ml IGF-1 (cat. no. I1271, Sigma, United States; purity 95%) for 24 h. Then, cells were added with 10 μM diosgenin (cat. no. D1634, Sigma, United States; purity 93%) for another 24 h.

2.13 CCK-8 Assay

The cytotoxicity of IGF-1 and diosgenin was determined by CCK-8 assay. Briefly, *Nthy-ori 3-1* cells were seeded onto 96-well plates and cultured until they adhered completely. Then, the thyrocytes were induced by IGF-1, diosgenin or IGF-1 plus diosgenin at different concentrations for 24 or 48 h. Finally, 10 μl of CCK-8 solution was added and incubated at 37°C for 1 h. The absorbance at 450 nm was determined.

2.14 Western Blot Analysis

Nthy-ori 3-1 cells were lysed in RIPA buffer containing protease and phosphatase inhibitors (Bimake, Houston, United States). The BCA protein quantitative analysis was used to determine the protein concentration. Proteins were resolved on 10% SDS–PAGE, and transferred to 0.22 μm PVDF membranes (Millipore, United States). Subsequently, the membranes were blocked with 5% skim milk for 1 h and were then probed with the

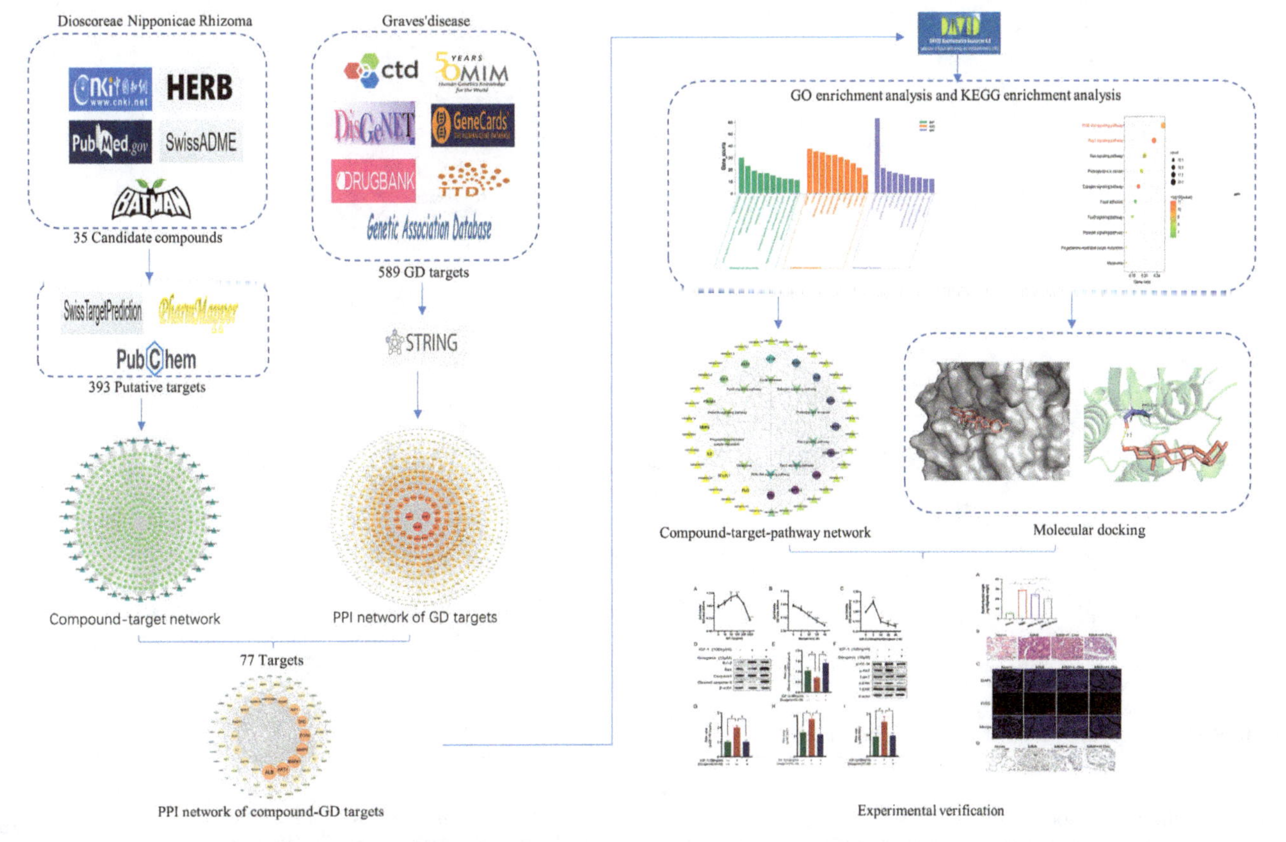

FIGURE 1 | Workflow for investigating the mechanism of DNR in GD treatment.

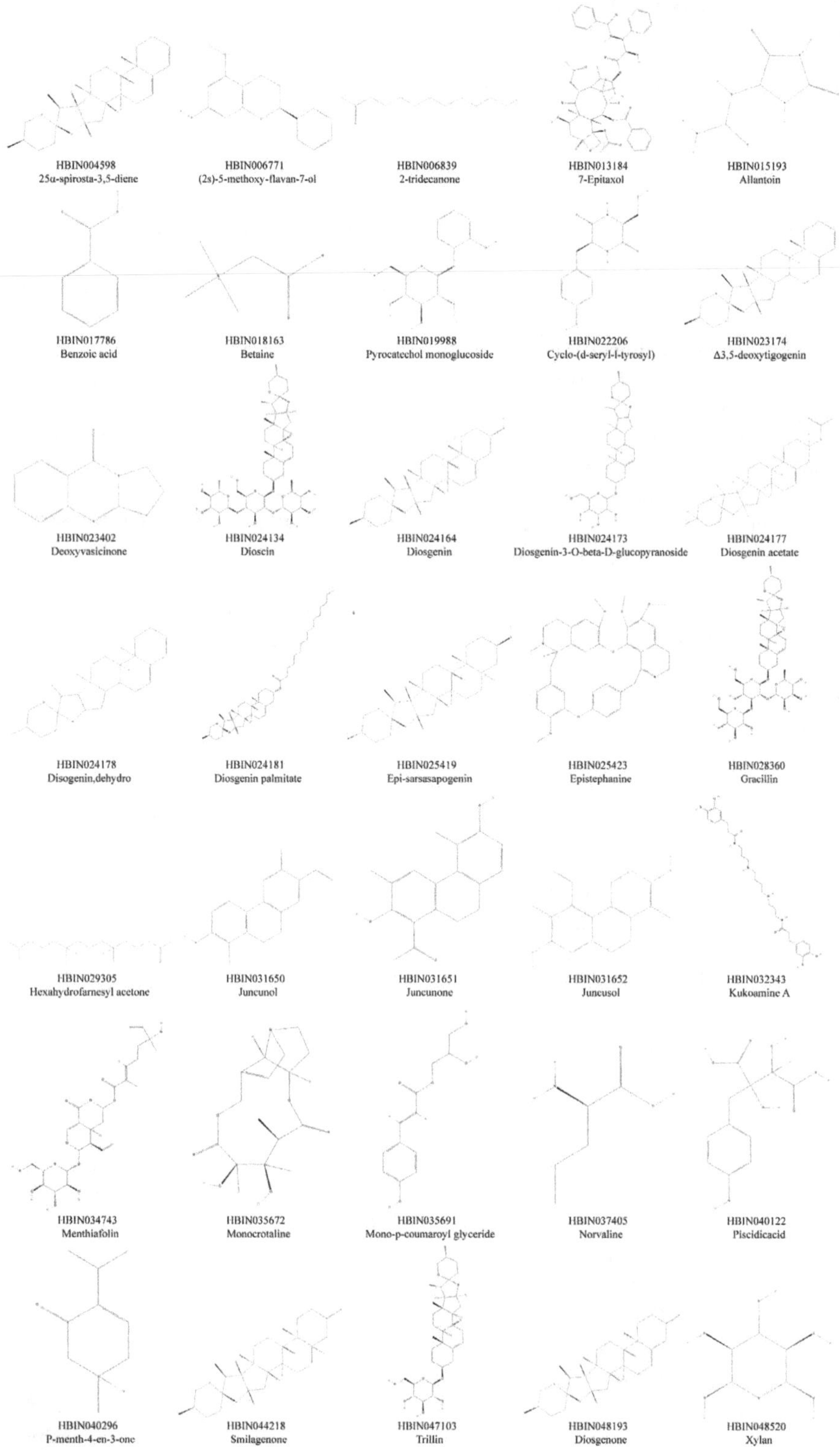

FIGURE 2 | The chemical structure of active componds in DNR.

following primary antibodies: p-IGF-1R (1:1,000; cat. no.3024; CST), P-IGF-1R (1:1,000; cat. no. AF3125; Affinity), p-ERK (1: 1,000; cat. no. ab201015; Abcam), ERK (1:1,000; cat. no. ab184699; Abcam), p-AKT (1:1,000; cat. no. 66444-1-Ig; Proteintech), AKT (1:1,000; cat. no. 10176-2-AP; Proteintech), CASPASE3 (1:1,000; cat. no. 19677-1-AP; Proteintech), BCL2 (1:

1,000; cat. no. 26593-1-AP; Proteintech), BAX (1:1,000; cat. no. 50599-2-AP; Proteintech), GAPDH (1:1,000; cat. no. 60004-1-Ig; Proteintech), and ß-actin (1:1,000; cat. no.66009-1-Ig; Proteintech). The membranes were gently incubated overnight at 4°C followed by incubation with HRP-conjugated secondary antibodies at room temperature for 1 h. The Alpha Q detection system was used for visualization.

2.15 Statistical Analysis

GraphPad Prism 8.0 software was used for Statistical analysis. Data are expressed as mean ± standard deviation (x ± s). For statistical analysis, means were compared using one-way ANOVA for multiple comparisons. A two-tailed $p < 0.05$ indicates that the difference is statistically significant.

3 RESULT

3.1 Compounds and Targets of DNR

A workflow of our study was summarized in **Figure 1**. We obtained 30 active compounds in DNR based on HERB database. Another five active compounds were incorporated into study after literature searching, including benzoic acid, pyrocatechol monoglucoside, cyclo-(d-seryl-l-tyrosyl), gracillin, and diosgenone. Ultimately, the structure of thirty-five active compounds of DNR were obtained and are presented in **Figure 2**, and their chemical information are showed in **Table 1**. We mainly counted the predicted targets of each component based on PharmMapper and obtained 394 potential targets of DNR. To further illustrate the correlationship between the 35 compounds and their predicted targets, we conducted a compound-target network (**Figure 3A**). A network topology analysis revealed that saponins account for approximately 40% of DNR, and the other ingredients are sterols, allantoin, resins, polysaccharides, starches, amino acids, flavonoids, and a small amount of 25α-Spirosta-3,5-diene. The composition is essentially the same as that reported in the literature (L. J. Zhang et al., 2012). Top six compounds were identified using the average degree (99.6) as threshold value: diosgenin (degree = 238), dioscin (degree = 198), mono-p-coumaroyl glyceride (degree = 102), hexahydrofarnesyl acetone (degree = 101), 7-epitaxol (degree = 101), and menthiafolin (degree = 100) (**Supplementary Table S1**). The targets enriched by diosgenin and dioscin were presented in significantly higher levels than other components, and the last four

TABLE 1 | Chemical information for the active compounds of DNR.

Number	HBIN ID	Compond	Composition	PubChem CID	MW	nON	nOHNH	MLogP
1	HBIN004598	25α-spirosta-3,5-diene	$C_{27}H_{40}O_2$	337494	396.61	2	0	5.71
2	HBIN006771	(2s)-5-methoxy-flavan-7-ol	$C_{16}H_{16}O_3$	14885875	256.3	3	1	2.45
3	HBIN006839	2-tridecanone	$C_{13}H_{26}O$	11622	198.34	1	0	3.54
4	HBIN013184	7-Epitaxol	$C_{47}H_{51}NO_{14}$	184492	853.91	14	4	1.7
5	HBIN015193	Allantoin	$C_4H_6N_4O_3$	204	158.12	3	4	−1.85
6	HBIN017786	Benzoic acid	$C_7H_6O_2$	243	122.12	2	1	1.6
7	HBIN018163	Betaine	$C_5H_{11}NO_2$	247	117.15	2	0	−3.67
8	HBIN019988	Pyrocatechol monoglucoside	$C_{12}H_{16}O_7$	9900144	272.25	7	5	−1.49
9	HBIN022206	Cyclo-(d-seryl-l-tyrosyl)	$C_{12}H_{14}N_2O_4$	3082196	250.25	4	4	−0.73
10	HBIN023174	Δ3,5-deoxytigogenin	$C_{27}H_{40}O_2$	131751534	396.61	2	0	5.71
11	HBIN023402	Deoxyvasicinone	$C_{11}H_{10}N_2O$	68261	186.21	2	0	2.04
12	HBIN024134	Dioscin	$C_{45}H_{72}O_{16}$	119245	869.04	16	0	2.01
13	HBIN024164	Diosgenin	$C_{27}H_{42}O_3$	99474	414.62	3	1	4.94
14	HBIN024173	Diosgenin-3-O-beta-D-glucopyranoside	$C_{33}H_{52}O_8$	129716073	576.76	8	4	2.41
15	HBIN024177	Diosgenin acetate	$C_{29}H_{44}O_4$	225768	456.66	4	0	5.18
16	HBIN024178	Disogenin,dehydro	$C_{27}H_{40}O_2$	587211	396.61	2	0	5.71
17	HBIN024181	Diosgenin palmitate	$C_{43}H_{72}O_4$	21159048	653. 02	4	0	7
18	HBIN025419	Epi-sarsasapogenin	$C_{27}H_{44}O_3$	12304430	416.64	3	1	5.08
19	HBIN025423	Epistephanine	$C_{37}H_{38}N_2O_6$	5317122	606.71	8	0	3.48
20	HBIN028360	Gracillin	$C_{45}H_{72}O_{17}$	159861	885.04	17	9	−1.46
21	HBIN029305	Hexahydrofarnesyl acetone	$C_{18}H_{36}O$	10408	268.48	1	0	4.79
22	HBIN031650	Juncunol	$C_{18}H_{18}O$	85926875	250.33	1	1	4.12
23	HBIN031651	Juncunone	$C_{18}H_{18}O_3$	327720	282.33	3	2	2.58
24	HBIN031652	Juncusol	$C_{18}H_{18}O_2$	72740	266.33	2	2	3.46
25	HBIN032343	Kukoamine A	$C_{28}H_{42}N_4O_6$	5318865	530.66	8	8	0.76
26	HBIN034743	Mentdiafolin	$C_{26}H_{36}O_{12}$	76960104	540.56	12	5	−0.44
27	HBIN035672	Monocrotaline	$C_{16}H_{23}NO_6$	9415	325.36	7	2	0.24
28	HBIN035691	Mono-p-coumaroyl glyceride	$C_{12}H_{14}O_5$	5319874	238.24	5	3	0.48
29	HBIN037405	Norvaline	$C_5H_{11}NO_2$	439575	117.15	3	2	−2.2
30	HBIN040122	Piscidicacid	$C_{11}H_{12}O_7$	120693	256.21	7	5	−0.6
31	HBIN040296	P-menth-4-en-3-one	$C_{10}H_{16}O$	107372	152.23	1	0	2.2
32	HBIN044218	Smilagenone	$C_{27}H_{42}O_3$	160498	414.62	3	0	4.94
33	HBIN047103	Trillin	$C_{33}H_{52}O_8$	11827970	576.76	8	4	2.41
34	HBIN048193	Diosgenone	$C_{27}H_{40}O_3$	10251134	412.6	3	0	4.83
35	HBIN048520	Xylan	$C_5H_{10}O_6$	50909243	166.13	6	5	−2.73

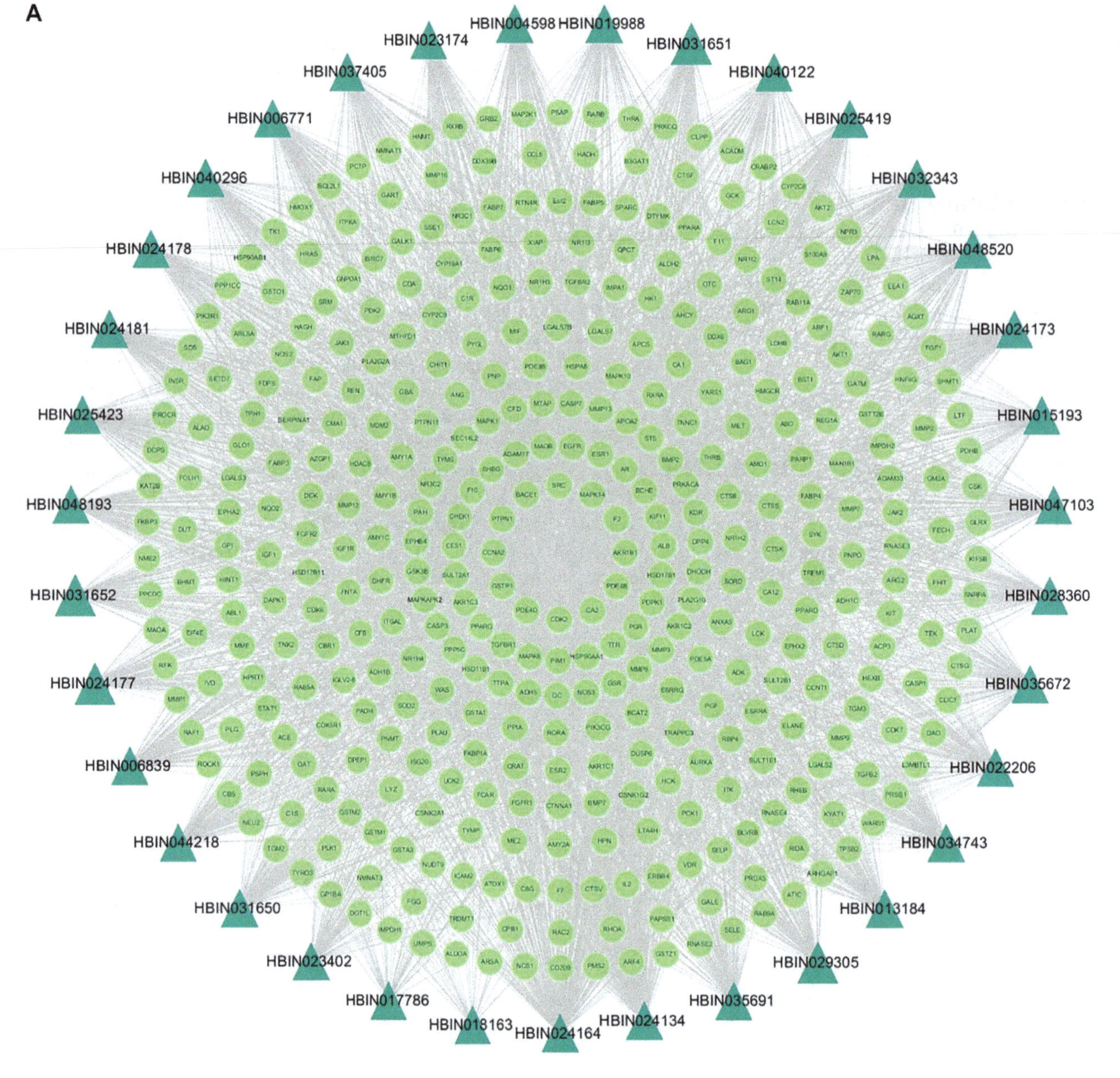

FIGURE 3 | Compound-target network and protein-protein Interaction (PPI) network of GD targets. **(A)** The compound-target network of DNR. Active compounds were represented by bottle green triangle nodes, and targets were represented by pale green circular nodes. **(B)** The PPI network of GD targets. The nodes size and color depth image are proportional to their degree values.

components are lipids and ketones, which are the basic components of DNR.

3.2 The Target Network of GD

In our study, 589 targets were taken as potential disease genes of GD (**Supplementary Table S2**) and their interaction relationship was shown in PPI network (**Figure 3B**). Eight targets were identified highly related to the pathological process of GD, including PIK3RI (degree = 105), STAT3 (degree = 105), MAPK1 (degree = 84), MAPK3 (degree = 73), NF-κB (degree = 67), SRC (degree = 67), IL6 (degree = 65), and AKT1 (degree = 65) (**Supplementary Table S3**). These eight targets played important roles in GD.

3.3 PPI Network of DNR's Compound-GD Targets

In order to discover overlapped targets, we mapped 393 predicted genes of DNR with 590 related genes of GD. 77 overlapped genes were taken as possible therapeutic targets against GD and

B

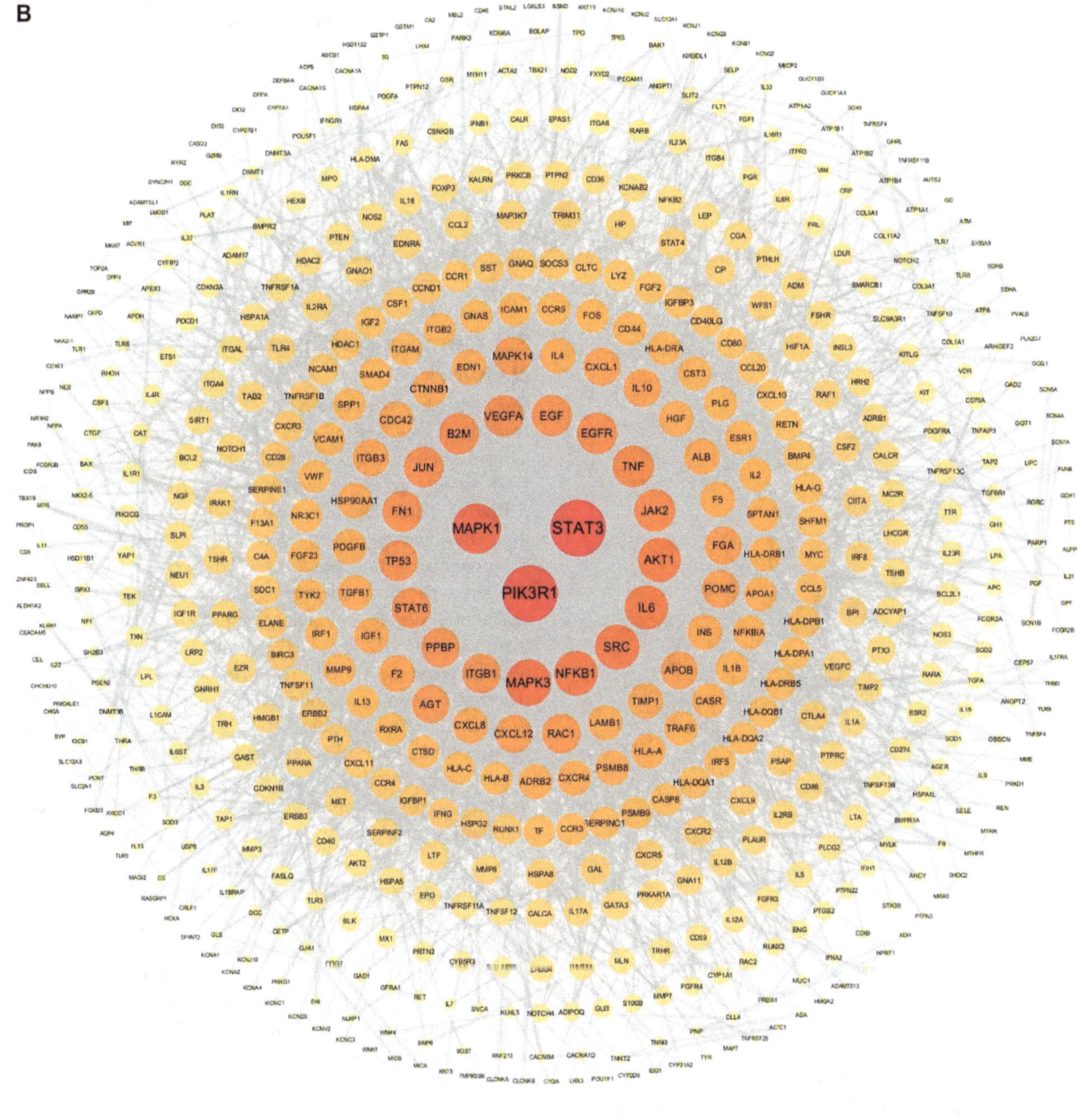

FIGURE 3 | Continued

expressed by a Venn diagram (**Figure 4A**). Based on PPI network topological analyzing, 77 targets were exhibited in descending order by their degree, as shown in **Supplementary Table S4**, and the average degree of 77 putative genes was 17.7. As shown in **Figure 4B**, the genes were exhibited in a concentric circle according to their degree, and the innercircle was comprised of 16 core targets: ALB (degree = 60), AKT1 (degree = 54), MAPK1 (degree = 50), MMP9 (degree = 47), EGFR (degree = 46), SRC (degree = 42), IGF-1 (degree = 40), ESR1 (degree = 36), MAPK14 (degree = 32), HSP90AA1 (degree = 32), NOS3 (degree = 31), PIK3R1 (degree = 28), IL2 (degree = 26), PLG (degree = 26), IGF-1R (degree = 24), and BCL2L1 (degree = 23). These targets are the hub targets of the network and the core targets of DNR to treat GD and will be used in subsequent molecular docking studies.

3.4 Enrichment Analyses of GO and KEGG

In order to further illustrate the potential pharmacological mechanism of DNR systematically, 77 common genes were enriched by DAVID. GO enrichment analysis screened out 84 biological processes (BP), 43 molecular functions (MF) and 36 cell components (CC) according to false discovery rate (FDR) <

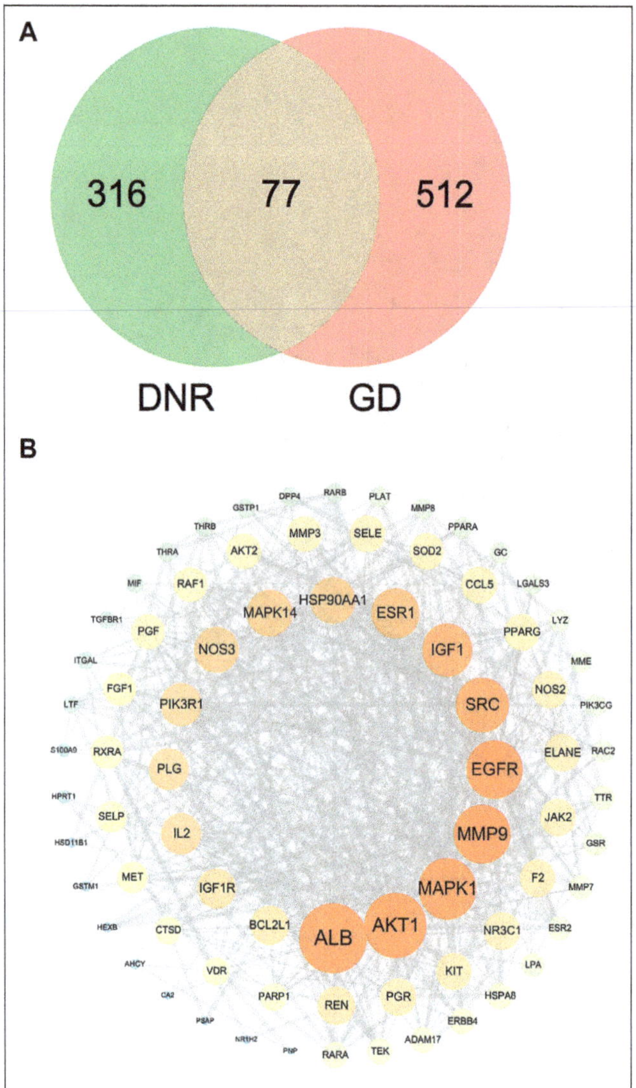

FIGURE 4 | Venn diagram and PPI network for overlapped targets. **(A)** Venn diagram of overlapping genes of DNR and GD. **(B)** PPI network of GD's active compounds and their related targets. The node size and color depth are proportional to their degree values.

0.05 and p value < 0.05. The top 10 GO items were selected based on counts of hit genes (**Figure 5A**). The interactions between the common targets of GD and DNR were mainly in the cytoplasm (GO:0005737) and nucleus (GO:0005634) and mainly through the interconnection between proteins (GO:0005515). For biological processes, the targets were mainly enriched in signal transduction (GO:0007165), apoptosis (GO:0043066), cell proliferation (GO:0008284), proteolysis (GO:0006508) and cell migration (GO:0030335). The top ten signal pathways are displayed in **Figure 5B** according to the number of targets enriched by KEGG and the p values. Two signaling pathways with the most enriched targets were obtained by analysis, namely, the PI3K signaling pathway (hsa04151) and the Rap1 signaling pathway (hsa04015) (**Table 2**). The results above illustrated the crucial mechanism of action underlying GD therapy.

TABLE 2 | Information for top 10 pathways.

Pathway ID	Pathway name	Count	*p* Value
hsa04151	PI3K-Akt signaling pathway	20	4.36E-10
hsa04015	Rap1 signaling pathway	18	1.04E-11
hsa04014	Ras signaling pathway	16	3.33E-09
hsa05205	Proteoglycans in cancer	15	6.06E-09
hsa04915	Estrogen signaling pathway	14	8.30E-12
hsa04510	Focal adhesion	13	6.29E-07
hsa04068	FoxO signaling pathway	12	6.05E-08
hsa05218	Melanoma	11	1.29E-09
hsa04917	Prolactin signaling pathway	11	1.29E-09
hsa04914	Progesterone-mediated oocyte maturation	11	9.88E-09

3.5 Compound-Core Target-Pathway Network

Through the connection of potential signaling pathways, compounds, as well as core targets, a compound-core target-pathway network was established. As exhibited in **Figure 6A**, DNR mainly acted through the PI3K-Akt and Rap1 signaling pathways. There were 23 components with degree values greater than the average (6.9). We selected the first four main components with degree ≥9: diosgenin (degree = 14), diosgenin palmitate (degree = 9), juncunol (degree = 9), and juncunone (degree = 9). Diosgenin is a crucial compond in the treatment of GD by DNR. Juncunol and juncunone are phenanthrene derivatives that play roles of clearing the heart, reducing fire, and promoting water and leaching. Subsequently, to observe the relationship between diosgenin and the first two pathways in more detail, we extracted a subnet to show the mapping path of diosgenin at key targets (**Figure 6B**). These results confirmed that there were six common targets of diosgenin, among which PI3K and Rap1 signaling pathways showing effects.

3.6 Molecular Docking Analysis

To test whether diosgenin acts on IGF-1R, we predicted that the core compound diosgenin and the hub target IGF-1R were molecularly docked. The greater the docking affinity, the better the binding ability of the compound to its target. In the molecular docking results, IGF-1R and diosgenin are connected to each other through hydrogen bonds, and they have high binding affinity (-8.66 kcal/mol) (**Figure 7**).

3.7 Diosgenin Induces Apoptosis in Nthy-ori 3-1 Cells by Inhibiting the Phosphorylation of IGF-1R *in vitro*

To verify the mechanism of diosgenin's treatment of GD, we first investigated the effective concentration of diosgenin. The CCK8 results showed that IGF-1 significantly promoted cell proliferation in the concentration range of 0–100 ng/ml but showed obvious toxicity to *Nthy-ori 3-1 cells* at a concentration greater than 100 ng/ml (**Figure 8A**); therefore, 100 ng/ml IGF-1 was used for follow-up experiments. Diosgenin significantly inhibited the viability of thyrocytes in a dose-dependent manner (**Figure 8B**). Moreover, at concentrations of 5–40 μM, diosgenin had an increasingly

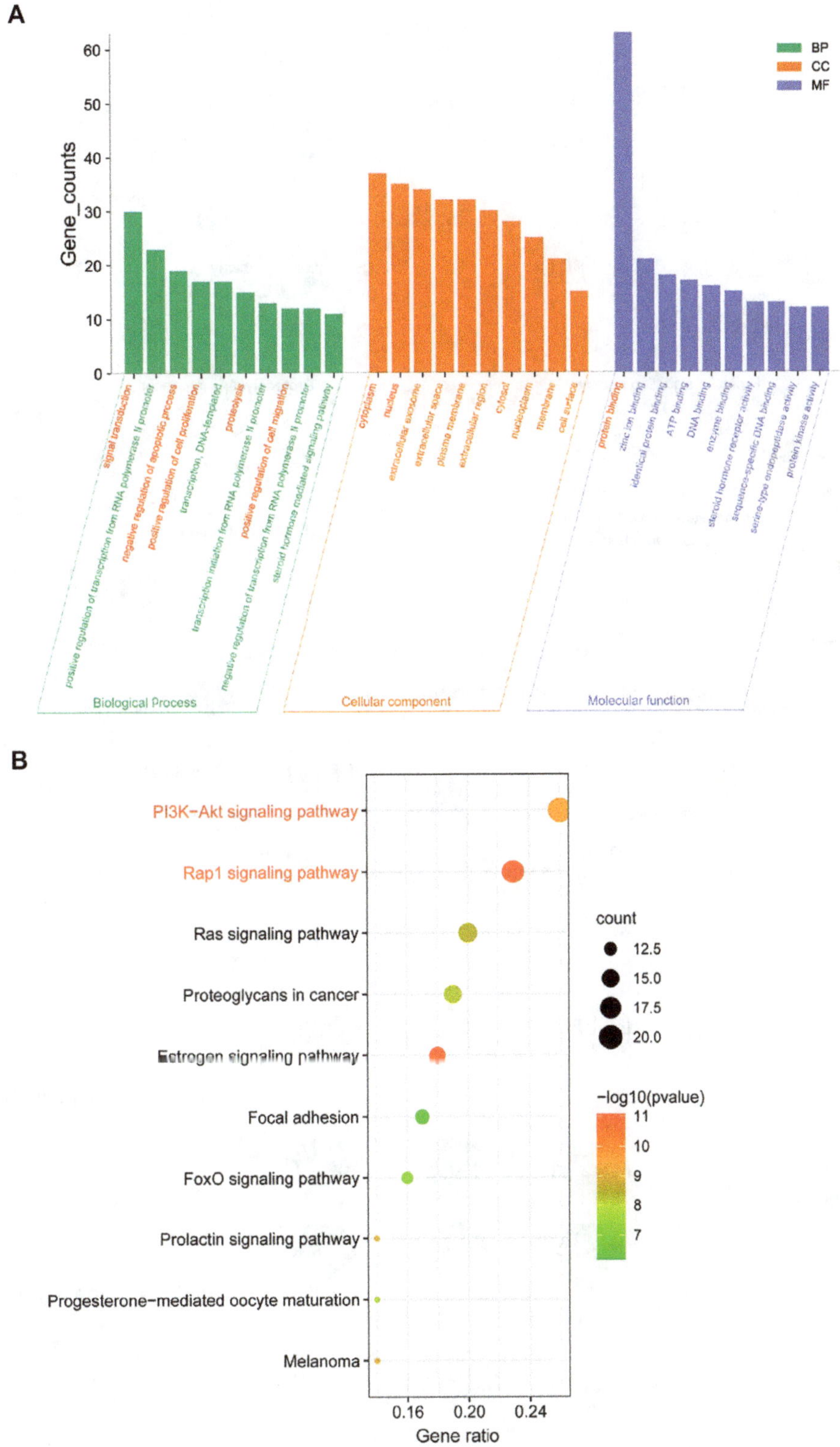

FIGURE 5 | Enrichment analysis for key targets. **(A)** The GO enrichment analysis of key targets. BP means biological processes, CC means cell component, MF means molecular function. **(B)** The KEGG pathway analysis of key targets. Nodes size and color depth are proportional to the gene ratio involved in the pathways.

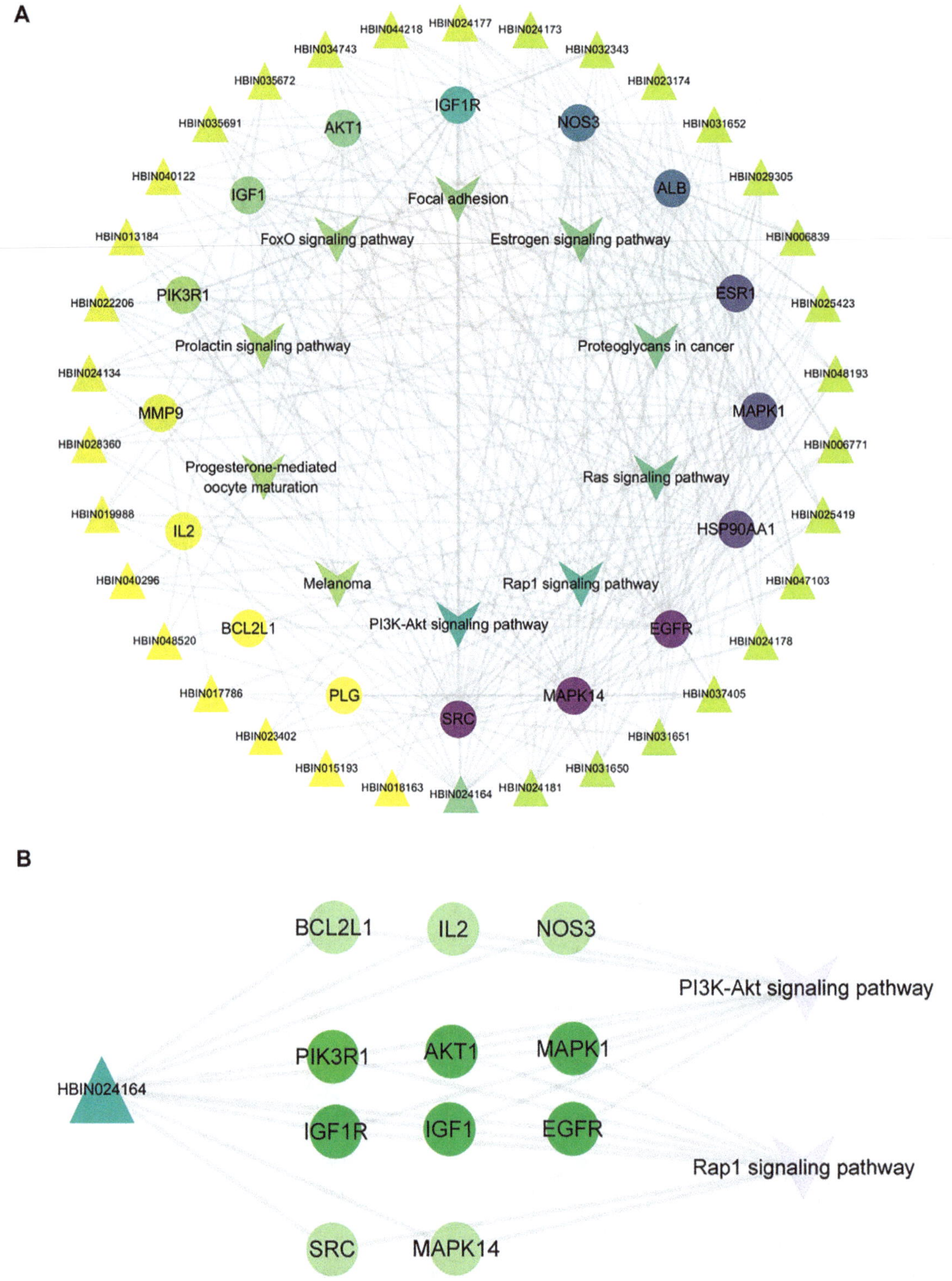

FIGURE 6 | Compound-target-pathway network of DNR against GD. **(A)** Compound-core-target-pathway network. Triangle nodes represent active compounds, whose colors are proportional to their degree. Circular nodes represent core targets. The nodes color are showed from purple to yellow in descending order of degree values. Inverted triangle nodes represent signaling pathways. **(B)** The targets of diosgenin enrichment in the PI3K and Rap1 signaling pathways. The dark green targets enriched by diosgenin and two pathways together.

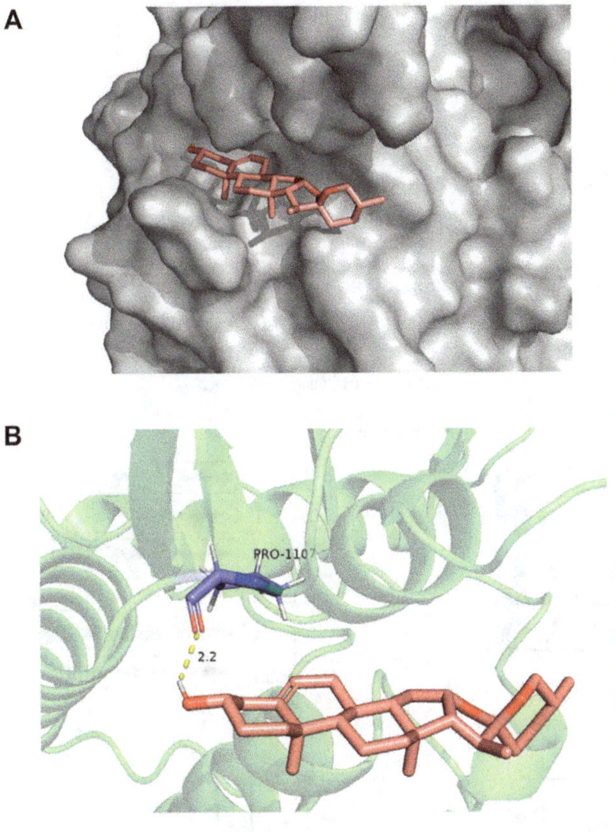

FIGURE 7 | The molecular docking of IGF-1R and diosgenin is shown. **(A)** The picture shows that the structure of diosgenin in 3D is located in the binding pocket of IGF-1R. The pink image on the right represents diosgenin. **(B)** The protein target that binds to diosgenin is in the shape of a blue rod, and the binding sites are connected by yellow hydrogen bonds. The length of the hydrogen bonds is indicated next to the bond.

stronger inhibitory effect on *Nthy-ori 3-1* cells pretreated with 100 ng/ml IGF-1. When we added 20 μM or even 40 μM diosgenin to IGF-1-induced cells, we found that *Nthy-ori 3-1* cell vability were obviously decreased. Thus, we chose 10 μM diosgenin as our treatment concentration in the ensuing experiments (**Figure 8C**). To verify whether diosgenin contributes to the apoptosis of *Nthy-ori 3-1* cells induced by IGF-1, we detected the protein levels of BCL2, BAX and caspase-3 by Western blot (**Figures 8D,E**). The thyrocytes were exposed to diosgenin (10 μM) with or without 100 ng/ml IGF-1 for 48 h. The levels of BCL2 were increased, and BAX and cleaved-caspase3 were decreased after pretreatment with IGF-1. These results indicated that IGF-1 inhibited the activation of apoptosis. In contrast, diosgenin successfully promoted apoptosis in IGF-1-induced cells. To verify whether diosgenin contributes to thyrocytes apoptosis through the inhibition of IGF-1R phosphorylation, we observed the activation of IGF-1R and its downstream pathways (**Figures 8F–I**). We found that IGF-1R phosphorylation was greatly increased in IGF-1-pretreated thyrocytes. After treated with diosgenin (10 μM), the phosphorylation level of IGF-1R decreased significantly, as did the two downstream pathways AKT and ERK. While the expression of the antiapoptotic protein BCL2 decreased, the proapoptotic protein BAX increased. Ultimately, caspase-3 was completely cleaved to its terminal fragments (17 kD). These results implied that diosgenin initiated apoptosis by inhibiting the phosphorylation of IGF-1R.

3.8 Diosgenin Could Suppress Thyrocyte Proliferation in MMI-Induced Rats

To confirm the inhibition of GD by diosgenin *in vivo*, we constructed a rat model of GD goiter. Based on previous research (Han et al., 2009; Cai et al., 2014) and following the best practice in pharmacological research (Heinrich et al., 2020), the safe, effective and non-toxic concentration of MMI and diosgenin were selected. The relative thyroid weight of the MMI group was significantly higher than that of the Norm group. Compared with the MMI group, diosgenin reduced the thyroid weight in the MMI + L-Dio and MMI + H-Dio groups by 17% ($p < 0.05$) and 30% ($p < 0.05$), respectively. Overall, as the dose of diosgenin increased, the relative weight of the thyroid gland gradually decreased compared with the MMI group (**Figure 9A**). H&E staining revealed that the monolayer of thyroid follicular epithelial cells in the Norm group was neatly arranged in a cubic shape, the structure of the follicles was clear, and the cytoplasm was abundant. However, in the MMI group, diffuse hyperplasia of thyroid follicular epithelial cells showed high columnar hyperplasia, and some showed papillary hyperplasia. The shape of the follicles was irregular, smaller, or even locked. The glia in the follicle cavity were significantly reduced, and absorption vacuoles of epithelial cells of different sizes were present around the follicle. Microscopy also revealed that the interstitial blood vessels were abundant and congested. These morphological abnormalities were relieved through diosgenin treatment. Surprisingly, most of the thyroid follicle morphology was restored in the MMI + H-Dio group (**Figure 9B**). To verify the effects of diosgenin on thyrocyte apoptosis, a TUNEL fluorescence staining assay was performed (**Figure 9C**). Much stronger green fluorescence was observed in the MMI + H-Dio groups, which revealed higher cell necrosis and apoptosis after treatment with high-dose diosgenin. To investigate the potential mechanism underlying the proapoptotic effects of diosgenin, immunohistochemical staining was used to examined the protein expression of IGF-1R in thyroid tissue. As shown in **Figure 9D**, the phosphorylation level of IGF-1R in the MMI group was upregulated obviously compared with that in the Norm group. However, this increase obviously reduced after diosgenin treatment.

DISCUSSION

Dioscin is a water-soluble steroidal saponin component extracted from DNR that can be hydrolyzed into diosgenin (Yan et al., 2013). Diosgenin could be considered as an important basic natural material for producing steroid hormone drugs, and it has a hormone-like effect, but the side effects are far lower than

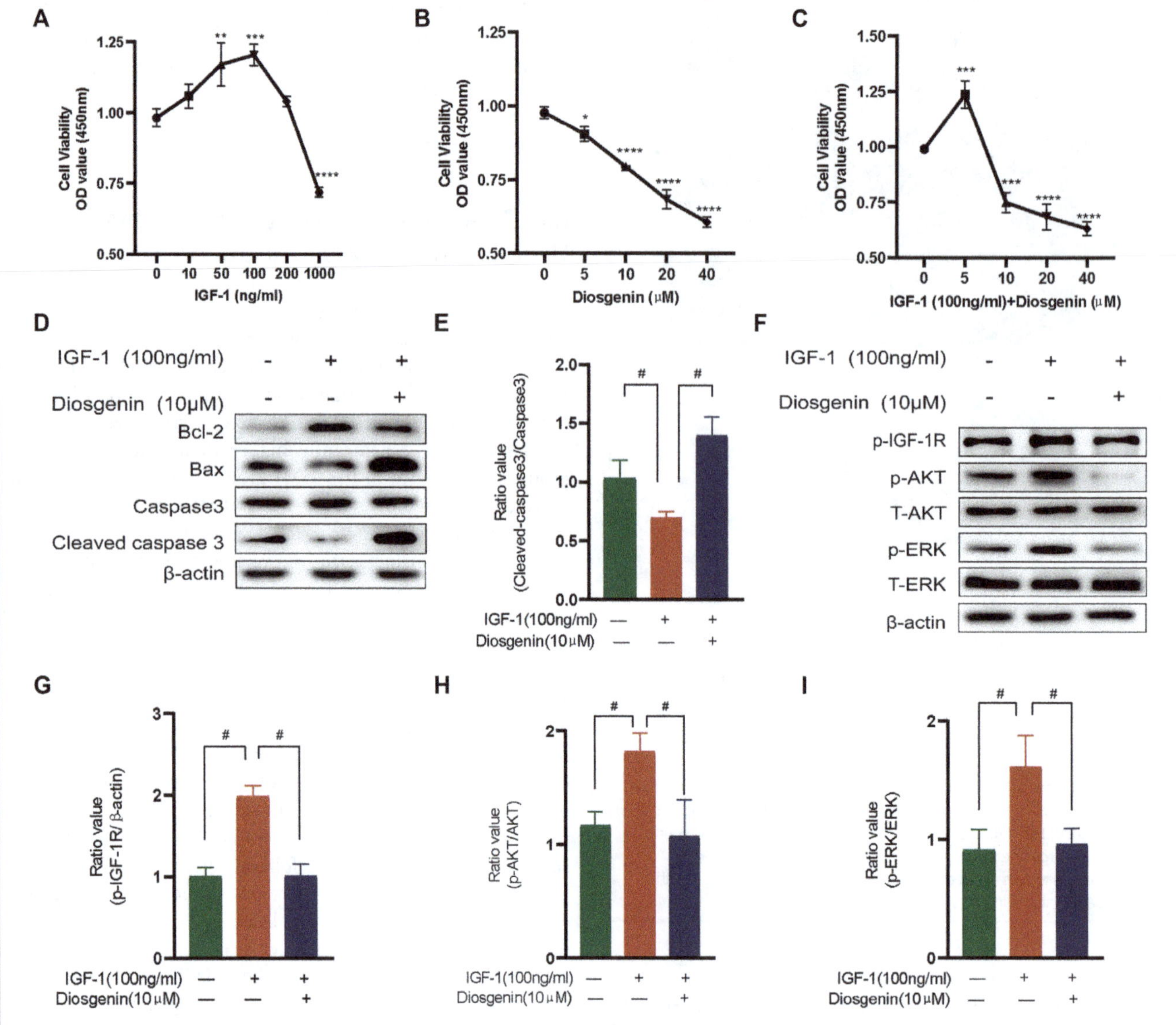

FIGURE 8 | Diosgenin induces apoptosis in *Nthy-ori 3-1* cells by inhibiting the phosphorylation of IGF-1R *in vitro* phosphorylation of IGF-1R *in vitro*. **(A)** Cell viability with IGF-1 (ng/ml) at increasing concentrations after culturing for 48 h. **(B)** Cell viability after 24 h of culture with diosgenin (μM) at different concentrations. **(C)** Cell viability with IGF1 (100 ng/ml) and diosgenin (μM) at different concentrations. **(D)** Apoptosis-related proteins were detected using WB as described above. *β*-actin was used as an internal reference. **(F)** Diosgenin devitalized the PI3K/AKT and Raf1/MEK signaling pathways by inhibiting p-IGF-1R. **(E, G–I)** Data are shown as the mean ± standard deviation of three independent experiments. $^{*}p < 0.05$, $^{**}p < 0.01$, $^{***}p < 0.001$ and $^{****}p < 0.0001$ compared with the 0 group. $\#p < 0.05$ compared with the IGF-1 group.

those of hormones (Parama et al., 2020). It could be absorbed quickly and its oral bioavailability reach up to 80.88% (Ru et al., 2014). In order to get diosgenin with better quality and purity from botanical sources, various techniques including elicitation, genetic transformations and bioconversions were employed (Nazir et al., 2021) (Chao et al., 2017; Qiao et al., 2018). The content of diosgenin in Medicinal Plants could be determinated accurately by enzyme-linked immunosorbent assay or a micellar electrokinetic capillary chromatographic (MECC) (J. Li et al., 2010; N. Wang et al., 2019), and the water contents in diosgenin could be assayed with high accuracy using the mathematical model of near-infrared spectroscopy technology (M. Zhang et al., 2019). For the past few years, the biological activities of diosgenin has drawn much attention by studied *in vivo* and *in vitro* (Leger et al., 2004; J.; Liagre et al., 2004; M. J.; Liu et al., 2005; Liagre et al., 2004; Srinivasan et al., 2009; Li et al., 2010; Ru et al., 2014; Chao et al., 2017; Qiao et al., 2018; Kessler et al., 2019; N.; Wang et al., 2019; M. Zhang et al., 2019; Mohamadi-Zarch et al., 2020). In previous studies, we found that diosgenin (Mu et al., 2012) promoted apoptosis of human primary thyroid cells under the action of IGF-1 through the caspase signaling pathway, but its specific mechanism is not clear. At the same time, it does not affect the serum TT4 level or the size of the thyroid gland in normal mice (Bian et al., 2011; Cai et al., 2014). Therefore, diosgenin may be a safe antithyroid drug to avoid hypothyroidism.

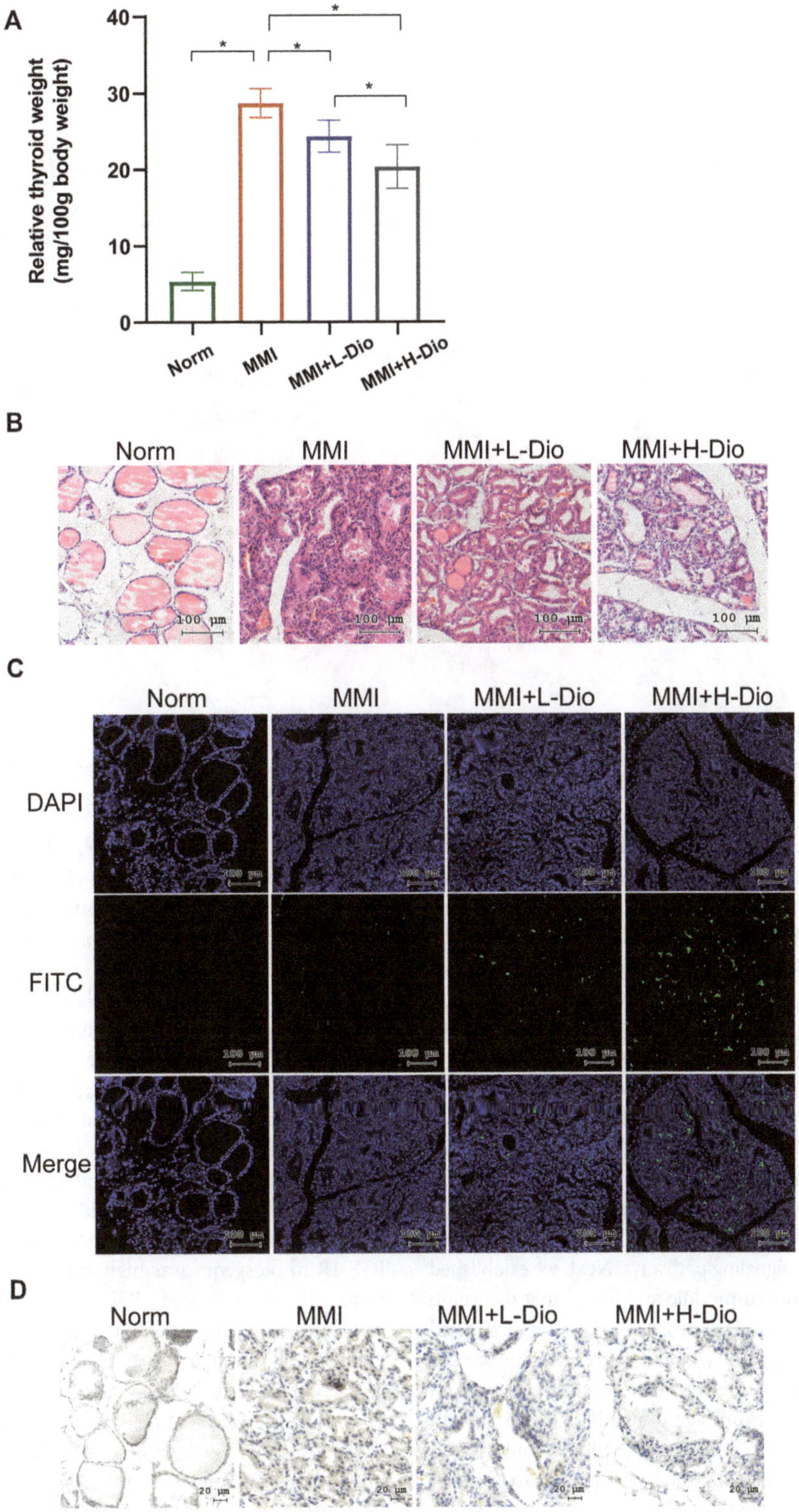

FIGURE 9 | Diosgenin could inhibit thyrocyte proliferation in MMI-induced rats. **(A)** The effects of diosgenin treatment on goiter. **(B)** After 3 weeks of diosgenin treatment, **(A–D)** refer to histological changes in thyroid glands stained with H&E (magnification, ×200). **(C)** The TUNEL kit allows apoptotic cells to emit green light through the FITC channel. The nucleus is stained by DAPI. **(D)** Immunohistochemical staining of p-IGF-1R in the thyroid after 3 weeks of diosgenin treatment.

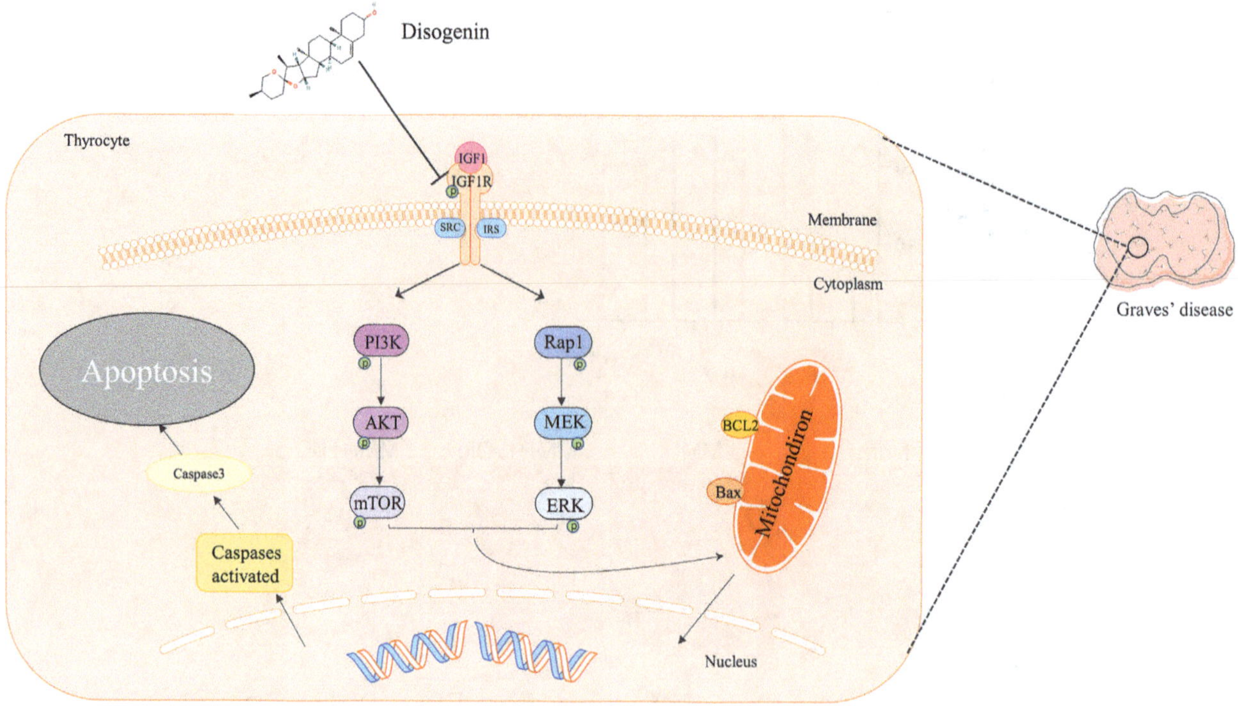

FIGURE 10 | Mechanism of diosgenin in the treatment of Graves' disease.

In this study, 589 targets of GD were collected from multiple databases, suggesting that the occurrence of GD may be caused by multiple targets. Through the HERB database and literature searches, 35 active components and 393 targets of DNR were screened, among which diosgenin was predicted as the most important compond. Then, the compond collected from GD and DNR were intersected to obtain 77 common targets, which can be speculated to be candidate therapeutic targets of DNR against GD. Based on topological property of PPI, 16 core targets for the treatment of GD by DNR were selected. Through GO and KEGG analyses of 77 common targets, it was found that the interaction between GD and DNR occurred mainly through the interconnection between proteins, and the main mechanisms were signal transduction, apoptosis and proliferation. KEGG analysis showed that DNR may play a role through the PI3K and Rap1 signaling pathways. Next, we established compond-core target-pathway co-module and found that diosgenin was enriches fourteen core targets in sixteen. Then, we extracted diosgenin, two key signaling pathways and corresponding targets from the PPI network, and we observed that most targets were in IGF-1, IGF-1R and its downstream pathways. IGF-1 is a growth factor that can promote cell proliferation, differentiation and angiogenesis. IGF-1R is a transmembrane tyrosine kinase protein with a tetramer structure composed of two subunits, *a* and *ß*. The combination of IGF-1 and IGF-1R can activate the PI3K/Akt and Raf1/MEK signaling pathways to suppress the apoptosis and promote the proliferation of tumor cells (Ryan and Goss, 2008; Weroha and Haluska, 2008; Bruchim et al., 2009). IGF-1 and IGF-1R also play important roles in the formation and development of GD (Minuto et al., 1989), thyroid carcinoma and thyroid nodules (Karagiannis et al., 2020; Y. J.; Liu et al., 2011; Y. J.; Liu et al., 2013). Transgenic mice overexpressing IGF-1 and IGF-1R could feedback the decrease of thyroid-stimulating hormone, suggesting that IGF-1 and IGF-1R could stimulate thyroid function to some extent (Clément et al., 2001). The expression of IGF-1R was significantly increased in thyroid cells and orbital fibroblasts in GD patients (Smith, 2003). Teprotumumab, a monoclonal antibody IGF-1 receptor antagonist, has achieved important curative effects in Graves' ophthalmopathy (Lanzolla et al., 2020). Therefore, IGF-1R plays vital part in the onset and development of GD (Tsui et al., 2008). This showed that drugs targeting the IGF-1 receptor can be very promising in the treatment of GD. Hence, we conducted validation experiments according to the standards of research in the field of pharmacology (Heinrich et al., 2018). The molecular docking showed that the binding activity of IGF-1R to diosgenin was high and that the structure was relatively stable. Then we used IGF-1 to induce excessive thyrocytes proliferation *in vitro* (Brandi et al., 1987; Bian et al., 2011; Mu et al., 2012; Yamanaka et al., 2012). Some predicted hub targets of diosgenin from network pharmacology were verified by Western blot. The results showed that diosgenin may inhibit the phosphorylation activation of IGF-1R compared with the IGF-1 group and then inhibit the PI3K and Raf1 pathways. This inhibition can lead to a decrease in the antiapoptotic protein BCL2 and an increase in the proapoptotic protein Bax, and finally activated caspase 3 to cleaved caspase 3, resulting in irreversible apoptosis. *In vivo*, we used MMI to compensate for thyroid enlargement in rats. The results showed that diosgenin reduced goiter in GD rats in a dose-dependent manner by promoting thyroid cell apoptosis. In addition, the phosphorylation of IGF-1R decreased with increasing thyroid cell apoptosis. This research confirmed that diosgenin could target and inhibit IGF-1R by molecular docking and *in vivo* and *in vitro* experiments. These results supported our prediction from network pharmacology. However, our study also had potential limitations. First, although network pharmacology could help us to realize the interactions between disease-specific molecules and drug-targeting proteins in the network target, it cannot tell whether the effect of the drug on the target is up-regulated or down-regulated (S. Li, 2021). Secondly, about the common targets of DNR and GD, we didn't analyze whether these targets have statistically significant. From another point of view, DNM has many componds related to saponins, it is also a good thought to explore their similarities and differences with network pharmacology. In the future, more extensive experiments are needed to reveal the above possibilities, such as proving the direct combined of diosgenin with IGF-1R. Based on the above results, we have drawn a simple diagram of the mechanism (**Figure 10**).

CONCLUSION

In conclusion, this work identified the mechanism of diosgenin on Graves' disease at the system level through network pharmacological analysis and biological verification. We confirmed that diosgenin can bind to IGF-1R and inhibit the activation of Akt and ERK pathways by inhibiting the phosphorylation of IGF-1R, resulting in increasing apoptosis of hyperproliferated thyroid cells in Graves' disease and alleviating goiter. Therefore, diosgenin plays an important role in the treatment of Graves' disease.

AUTHOR CONTRIBUTIONS

JX, XZ, and SS conceived and designed the study. JX collected the data, performed the data analysis, wrote the manuscript. JX, SS, and WC contributed to the data interpretation, YY and JC drafting and critical revision of the article and figures. All authors have read and approved the final manuscript.

FUNDING

This work was supported by the National Natural Science Foundation (82070818 and 81600604), the Natural Science Foundation of Shandong Province (ZR2017LH023), and Academic Promotion Program of Shandong First Medical University (Grant No. 2019QL017).

ACKNOWLEDGMENTS

The authors thank AJE company for providing language assistance and for proofreading the manuscript.

REFERENCES

Bahn, R. S., Burch, H. B., Cooper, D. S., Garber, J. R., Greenlee, M. C., Klein, I., et al. (2011). Hyperthyroidism and Other Causes of Thyrotoxicosis: Management Guidelines of the American Thyroid Association and American Association of Clinical Endocrinologists. *Endocr. Pract.* 17 (3), 456–520. doi:10.4158/ep.17.3.456

Becker, K. G., Barnes, K. C., Bright, T. J., and Wang, S. A. (2004). The Genetic Association Database. *Nat. Genet.* 36 (5), 431–432. doi:10.1038/ng0504-431

Bian, D., Li, Z., Ma, H., Mu, S., Ma, C., Cui, B., et al. (2011). Effects of Diosgenin on Cell Proliferation Induced by IGF-1 in Primary Human Thyrocytes. *Arch. Pharm. Res.* 34 (6), 997–1005. doi:10.1007/s12272-011-0617-y

Boyadjiev, S. A., and Jabs, E. W. (2000). Online Mendelian Inheritance in Man (OMIM) as a Knowledgebase for Human Developmental Disorders. *Clin. Genet.* 57 (4), 253–266. doi:10.1034/j.1399-0004.2000.570403.x

Brandi, M. L., Rotella, C. M., Mavilia, C., Franceschelli, F., Tanini, A., and Toccafondi, R. (1987). Insulin Stimulates Cell Growth of a New Strain of Differentiated Rat Thyroid Cells. *Mol. Cel Endocrinol* 54 (1), 91–103. doi:10.1016/0303-7207(87)90142-0

Bruchim, I., Attias, Z., and Werner, H. (2009). Targeting the IGF1 axis in Cancer Proliferation. *Expert Opin. Ther. Targets* 13 (10), 1179–1192. doi:10.1517/14728220903201702

Cai, H., Wang, Z., Zhang, H. Q., Wang, F. R., Yu, C. X., Zhang, F. X., et al. (2014). Diosgenin Relieves Goiter via the Inhibition of Thyrocyte Proliferation in a Mouse Model of Graves' Disease. *Acta Pharmacol. Sin* 35 (1), 65–73. doi:10.1038/aps.2013.133

Chao, Zhao., Yan, Cao., and Zhongqing, Ma. (2017). Optimization of Liquid Ammonia Pretreatment Conditions for Maximizing Sugar Release from Giant Reed (Arundo donax L.). *Biomass and Bioenergy* 98, 61–69. doi:10.1016/j.biombioe.2017.01.001

Clément, S., Refetoff, S., Robaye, B., Dumont, J. E., and Schurmans, S. (2001). Low TSH Requirement and Goiter in Transgenic Mice Overexpressing IGF-I and IGF-Ir Receptor in the Thyroid Gland. *Endocrinology* 142 (12), 5131–5139. doi:10.1210/endo.142.12.8534

Cooper, D. S. (2005). Antithyroid Drugs. *N. Engl. J. Med.* 352 (9), 905–917. doi:10.1056/NEJMra042972

Cosconati, S., Forli, S., Perryman, A. L., Harris, R., Goodsell, D. S., and Olson, A. J. (2010). Virtual Screening with AutoDock: Theory and Practice. *Expert Opin. Drug Discov.* 5 (6), 597–607. doi:10.1517/17460441.2010.484460

Daina, A., Michielin, O., and Zoete, V. (2017). SwissADME: a Free Web Tool to Evaluate Pharmacokinetics, Drug-Likeness and Medicinal Chemistry Friendliness of Small Molecules. *Sci. Rep.* 7, 42717. doi:10.1038/srep42717

Daina, A., Michielin, O., and Zoete, V. (2019). SwissTargetPrediction: Updated Data and New Features for Efficient Prediction of Protein Targets of Small Molecules. *Nucleic Acids Res.* 47 (W1), W357–W364. doi:10.1093/nar/gkz382

Davis, A. P., Grondin, C. J., Johnson, R. J., Sciaky, D., Wiegers, J., Wiegers, T. C., et al. (2021). Comparative Toxicogenomics Database (CTD): Update 2021. *Nucleic Acids Res.* 49 (D1), D1138–d1143. doi:10.1093/nar/gkaa891

Fang, S., Dong, L., Liu, L., Guo, J., Zhao, L., Zhang, J., et al. (2021). HERB: a High-Throughput experiment- and Reference-Guided Database of Traditional Chinese Medicine. *Nucleic Acids Res.* 49 (D1), D1197–d1206. doi:10.1093/nar/gkaa1063

Goodsell, D. S., Zardecki, C., Berman, H. M., and Burley, S. K. (2020). Insights from 20 years of the Molecule of the Month. *Biochem. Mol. Biol. Educ.* 48 (4), 350 355. doi:10.1002/bmb.21360

Guo, L., Zeng, S. L., Zhang, Y., Li, P., and Liu, E. H. (2016). Comparative Analysis of Steroidal Saponins in Four Dioscoreae Herbs by High Performance Liquid Chromatography Coupled with Mass Spectrometry. *J. Pharm. Biomed. Anal.* 117, 91–98. doi:10.1016/j.jpba.2015.08.038

Han, Y., Zhou, J., Yu, S. J., Cui, B., Zhang, H. Q., Gao, L., et al. (2009). Inhibitory Effect of Kangjia Pill on Thyrocyte Proliferation in Rat Goiter Model. *Chin. J. Integr. Med.* 15 (4), 284–288. doi:10.1007/s11655-009-0284-8

Hao, da. C., and Xiao, P. G. (2014). Network Pharmacology: a Rosetta Stone for Traditional Chinese Medicine. *Drug Dev. Res.* 75 (5), 299–312. doi:10.1002/ddr.21214

He, J., Xiao, H., Li, B., Peng, Y., Li, X., Wang, Y., et al. (2019). The Programmed Site-specific Delivery of the Angiostatin Sunitinib and Chemotherapeutic Paclitaxel for Highly Efficient Tumor Treatment. *J. Mater. Chem. B* 7 (32), 4953–4962. doi:10.1039/c9tb01159e

Heinrich, M., Appendino, G., Efferth, T., Fürst, R., Izzo, A. A., Kayser, O., et al. (2020). Best Practice in Research - Overcoming Common Challenges in Phytopharmacological Research. *J. Ethnopharmacol* 246, 112230. doi:10.1016/j.jep.2019.112230

Heinrich, M., Lardos, A., Leonti, M., Weckerle, C., Willcox, M., Applequist, W., et al. (2018). Best Practice in Research: Consensus Statement on Ethnopharmacological Field Studies - ConSEFS. *J. Ethnopharmacol* 211, 329–339. doi:10.1016/j.jep.2017.08.015

Hopkins, A. L. (2008). Network Pharmacology: the Next Paradigm in Drug Discovery. *Nat. Chem. Biol.* 4 (11), 682–690. doi:10.1038/nchembio.118

Huang, da. W., Sherman, B. T., and Lempicki, R. A. (2009). Systematic and Integrative Analysis of Large Gene Lists Using DAVID Bioinformatics Resources. *Nat. Protoc.* 4 (1), 44–57. doi:10.1038/nprot.2008.211

Kahaly, G. J., Bartalena, L., Hegedüs, L., Leenhardt, L., Poppe, K., and Pearce, S. H. (2018). 2018 European Thyroid Association Guideline for the Management of Graves' Hyperthyroidism. *Eur. Thyroid J.* 7 (4), 167–186. doi:10.1159/000490384

Karagiannis, A., Kassi, E., Chatzigeorgiou, A., and Koutsilieris, M. (2020). IGF Bioregulation System in Benign and Malignant Thyroid Nodular Disease: A Systematic Review. *In Vivo* 34 (6), 3069–3091. doi:10.21873/invivo.12141

Kessler, B. E., Mishall, K. M., Kellett, M. D., Clark, E. G., Pugazhenthi, U., Pozdeyev, N., et al. (2019). Resistance to Src Inhibition Alters the BRAF-Mutant Tumor Secretome to Promote an Invasive Phenotype and Therapeutic Escape through a FAK>p130Cas>c-Jun Signaling axis. *Oncogene* 38 (14), 2565–2579. doi:10.1038/s41388-018-0617-1

Kim, S., Chen, J., Cheng, T., Gindulyte, A., He, J., He, S., et al. (2021). PubChem in 2021: New Data Content and Improved Web Interfaces. *Nucleic Acids Res.* 49 (D1), D1388–D1395. doi:10.1093/nar/gkaa971

Lanzolla, G., Ricci, D., Nicolì, F., Sabini, E., Sframeli, A., Brancatella, A., et al. (2020). Putative Protective Role of Autoantibodies against the Insulin-like Growth Factor-1 Receptor in Graves' Disease: Results of a Pilot Study. *J. Endocrinol. Invest.* 43 (12), 1759–1768. doi:10.1007/s40618-020-01341-2

Léger, D. Y., Liagre, B., Cardot, P. J., Beneytout, J. L., and Battu, S. (2004). Diosgenin Dose-dependent Apoptosis and Differentiation Induction in Human Erythroleukemia Cell Line and Sedimentation Field-Flow Fractionation Monitoring. *Anal. Biochem.* 335 (2), 267–278. doi:10.1016/j.ab.2004.09.008

Li, J., Yang, D., Yu, K., He, J., and Zhang, Y. (2010). Determination of Diosgenin Content in Medicinal Plants with Enzyme-Linked Immunosorbent Assay. *Planta Med.* 76 (16), 1915–1920. doi:10.1055/s-0030-1250054

Li, S., and Zhang, B. (2013). Traditional Chinese Medicine Network Pharmacology: Theory, Methodology and Application. *Chin. J. Nat. Med.* 11 (2), 110–120. doi:10.1016/s1875-5364(13)60037-0

Li, S. (2021). Network Pharmacology Evaluation Method Guidance - Draft. *World J. Tradit Chin. Med.* 7 (1), 148–154. doi:10.4103/wjtcm.wjtcm_11_21

Li, X., Zhao, C., Jing, S., Sun, J., Li, X., Man, S., et al. (2017). Novel phenanthrene and isocoumarin from the rhizomes of Dioscorea nipponica Makino subsp. rosthornii (Prain et Burkill) C. T. Ting (Dioscoreaceae). *Bioorg. Med. Chem. Lett.* 27 (15), 3595–3601. doi:10.1016/j.bmcl.2017.03.095

Liagre, B., Vergne-Salle, P., Corbiere, C., Charissoux, J. L., and Beneytout, J. L. (2004). Diosgenin, a Plant Steroid, Induces Apoptosis in Human Rheumatoid Arthritis Synoviocytes with Cyclooxygenase-2 Overexpression. *Arthritis Res. Ther.* 6 (4), R373–R383. doi:10.1186/ar1199

Lin, S., Wang, D., Yang, D., Yao, J., Tong, Y., and Chen, J. (2007). Characterization of Steroidal Saponins in Crude Extract from Dioscorea Nipponica Makino by Liquid Chromatography Tandem Multi-Stage Mass Spectrometry. *Anal. Chim. Acta* 599 (1), 98–106. doi:10.1016/j.aca.2007.07.070

Liu, M. J., Wang, Z., Ju, Y., Wong, R. N., and Wu, Q. Y. (2005). Diosgenin Induces Cell Cycle Arrest and Apoptosis in Human Leukemia K562 Cells with the Disruption of Ca2+ Homeostasis. *Cancer Chemother. Pharmacol.* 55 (1), 79–90. doi:10.1007/s00280-004-0849-3

Liu, Y. J., Qiang, W., Liu, X. J., Xu, L., Guo, H., Wu, L. P., et al. (2011). Association of Insulin-like Growth Factor-1 with Thyroid Nodules. *Oncol. Lett.* 2 (6), 1297–1301. doi:10.3892/ol.2011.411

Liu, Y. J., Qiang, W., Shi, J., Lv, S. Q., Ji, M. J., and Shi, B. Y. (2013). Expression and Significance of IGF-1 and IGF-1R in Thyroid Nodules. *Endocrine* 44 (1), 158–164. doi:10.1007/s12020-012-9864-z

Liu, Z., Guo, F., Wang, Y., Li, C., Zhang, X., Li, H., et al. (2016). BATMAN-TCM: a Bioinformatics Analysis Tool for Molecular mechANism of Traditional Chinese Medicine. *Sci. Rep.* 6, 21146. doi:10.1038/srep21146

Luo, T. T., Lu, Y., Yan, S. K., Xiao, X., Rong, X. L., and Guo, J. (2020). Network Pharmacology in Research of Chinese Medicine Formula: Methodology, Application and Prospective. *Chin. J. Integr. Med.* 26 (1), 72–80. doi:10.1007/s11655-019-3064-0

Luo, W., and Brouwer, C. (2013). Pathview: an R/Bioconductor Package for Pathway-Based Data Integration and Visualization. *Bioinformatics* 29 (14), 1830–1831. doi:10.1093/bioinformatics/btt285

Ma, S., Song, W., Xu, Y., Si, X., Zhang, D., Lv, S., et al. (2020). Neutralizing Tumor-Promoting Inflammation with Polypeptide-Dexamethasone Conjugate for Microenvironment Modulation and Colorectal Cancer Therapy. *Biomaterials* 232, 119676. doi:10.1016/j.biomaterials.2019.119676

Minuto, F., Barreca, A., Del Monte, P., Cariola, G., Torre, G. C., and Giordano, G. (1989). Immunoreactive Insulin-like Growth Factor I (IGF-I) and IGF-I-Binding Protein Content in Human Thyroid Tissue. *J. Clin. Endocrinol. Metab.* 68 (3), 621–626. doi:10.1210/jcem-68-3-621

Mohamadi-Zarch, S. M., Baluchnejadmojarad, T., Nourabadi, D., Khanizadeh, A. M., and Roghani, M. (2020). Protective Effect of Diosgenin on LPS/D-Gal-induced Acute Liver Failure in C57BL/6 Mice. *Microb. Pathog.* 146, 104243. doi:10.1016/j.micpath.2020.104243

Mu, S., Tian, X., Ruan, Y., Liu, Y., Bian, D., Ma, C., et al. (2012). Diosgenin Induces Apoptosis in IGF-1-Stimulated Human Thyrocytes through Two Caspase-dependent Pathways. *Biochem. Biophys. Res. Commun.* 418 (2), 347–352. doi:10.1016/j.bbrc.2012.01.024

Nazir, R., Kumar, V., Gupta, S., Dwivedi, P., Pandey, D. K., and Dey, A. (2021). Biotechnological Strategies for the Sustainable Production of Diosgenin from Dioscorea Spp. *Appl. Microbiol. Biotechnol.* 105 (2), 569–585. doi:10.1007/s00253-020-11055-3

Nyström, H. F., Jansson, S., and Berg, G. (2013). Incidence Rate and Clinical Features of Hyperthyroidism in a Long-Term Iodine Sufficient Area of Sweden (Gothenburg) 2003-2005. *Clin. Endocrinol.* 78 (5), 768–776. doi:10.1111/cen.12060

O'Boyle, N. M., Banck, M., James, C. A., Morley, C., Vandermeersch, T., and Hutchison, G. R. (2011). Open Babel: An Open Chemical Toolbox. *J. Cheminform* 3, 33. doi:10.1186/1758-2946-3-33

Omran, Z., and Rauch, C. (2014). Acid-mediated Lipinski's Second Rule: Application to Drug Design and Targeting in Cancer. *Eur. Biophys. J.* 43 (4-5), 199–206. doi:10.1007/s00249-014-0953-1

Ou-Yang, S. H., Jiang, T., Zhu, L., and Yi, T. (2018). Dioscorea Nipponica Makino: a Systematic Review on its Ethnobotany, Phytochemical and Pharmacological Profiles. *Chem. Cent. J.* 12 (1), 57. doi:10.1186/s13065-018-0423-4

Parama, D., Boruah, M., Yachna, K., Rana, V., Banik, K., Harsha, C., et al. (2020). Diosgenin, a Steroidal Saponin, and its Analogs: Effective Therapies against Different Chronic Diseases. *Life Sci.* 260, 118182. doi:10.1016/j.lfs.2020.118182

Piñero, J., Ramírez-Anguita, J. M., Saüch-Pitarch, J., Ronzano, F., Centeno, E., Sanz, F., et al. (2020). The DisGeNET Knowledge Platform for Disease Genomics: 2019 Update. *Nucleic Acids Res.* 48 (D1), D845 D855. doi:10.1093/nar/gkz1021

Qiao, X., Zhao, C., and Qianjun, S. (2018). Structural Characterization of Corn Stover Lignin after Hydrogen Peroxide Presoaking Prior to Ammonia Fiber Expansion Pretreatment. *Energy and Fuels* 32 (5), 6022–6030. doi:10.1021/acs.energyfuels.8b00951

Ross, D. S., Burch, H. B., Cooper, D. S., Greenlee, M. C., Laurberg, P., Maia, A. L., et al. (2016). 2016 American Thyroid Association Guidelines for Diagnosis and Management of Hyperthyroidism and Other Causes of Thyrotoxicosis. *Thyroid* 26 (10), 1343–1421. doi:10.1089/thy.2016.0229

Ru, J., Li, P., Wang, J., Zhou, W., Li, B., Huang, C., et al. (2014). TCMSP: a Database of Systems Pharmacology for Drug Discovery from Herbal Medicines. *J. Cheminform* 6, 13. doi:10.1186/1758-2946-6-13

Ryan, P. D., and Goss, P. E. (2008). The Emerging Role of the Insulin-like Growth Factor Pathway as a Therapeutic Target in Cancer. *Oncologist* 13 (1), 16–24. doi:10.1634/theoncologist.2007-0199

Seeliger, D., and de Groot, B. L. (2010). Ligand Docking and Binding Site Analysis with PyMOL and Autodock/Vina. *J. Comput. Aided Mol. Des.* 24 (5), 417–422. doi:10.1007/s10822-010-9352-6

Shao, S. S., Zhao, Y. F., Song, Y. F., Xu, C., Yang, J. M., Xuan, S. M., et al. (2014). Dietary High-Fat Lard Intake Induces Thyroid Dysfunction and Abnormal Morphology in Rats. *Acta Pharmacol. Sin* 35 (11), 1411–1420. doi:10.1038/aps.2014.82

Shi, L., Yu, L., Zou, F., Hu, H., Liu, K., and Lin, Z. (2017). Gene Expression Profiling and Functional Analysis Reveals that P53 Pathway-Related Gene Expression Is Highly Activated in Cancer Cells Treated by Cold Atmospheric Plasma-Activated Medium. *PeerJ* 5, e3751. doi:10.7717/peerj.3751

Smith, T. J. (2003). The Putative Role of Fibroblasts in the Pathogenesis of Graves' Disease: Evidence for the Involvement of the Insulin-like Growth Factor-1 Receptor in Fibroblast Activation. *Autoimmunity* 36 (6-7), 409–415. doi:10.1080/08916930310001603000

Srinivasan, S., Koduru, S., Kumar, R., Venguswamy, G., Kyprianou, N., and Damodaran, C. (2009). Diosgenin Targets Akt-Mediated Prosurvival Signaling in Human Breast Cancer Cells. *Int. J. Cancer* 125 (4), 961–967. doi:10.1002/ijc.24419

Stelzer, G., Rosen, N., Plaschkes, I., Zimmerman, S., Twik, M., Fishilevich, S., et al. (2016). The GeneCards Suite: From Gene Data Mining to Disease Genome Sequence Analyses. *Curr. Protoc. Bioinformatics* 54, 1. doi:10.1002/cpbi.5

Szklarczyk, D., Morris, J. H., Cook, H., Kuhn, M., Wyder, S., Simonovic, M., et al. (2017). The STRING Database in 2017: Quality-Controlled Protein-Protein Association Networks, Made Broadly Accessible. *Nucleic Acids Res.* 45 (D1), D362–d368. doi:10.1093/nar/gkw937

Tang, Y. N., Pang, Y. X., He, X. C., Zhang, Y. Z., Zhang, J. Y., Zhao, Z. Z., et al. (2015). UPLC-QTOF-MS Identification of Metabolites in Rat Biosamples after Oral Administration of Dioscorea Saponins: a Comparative Study. *J. Ethnopharmacol* 165, 127–140. doi:10.1016/j.jep.2015.02.017

Tsui, S., Naik, V., Hoa, N., Hwang, C. J., Afifiyan, N. F., Sinha Hikim, A., et al. (2008). Evidence for an Association between Thyroid-Stimulating Hormone and Insulin-like Growth Factor 1 Receptors: a Tale of Two Antigens Implicated in Graves' Disease. *J. Immunol.* 181 (6), 4397–4405. doi:10.4049/jimmunol.181.6.4397

UniProt (2019). UniProt: a Worldwide Hub of Protein Knowledge. *Nucleic Acids Res.* 47 (D1), D506–d515. doi:10.1093/nar/gky1049

Vasanthi, H. R., Mukherjee, S., Ray, D., Pandian Jayachandran, K. S., Lekli, I., and Das, D. K. (2010). Protective Role of Air Potato (Dioscorea Bulbifera) of Yam Family in Myocardial Ischemic Reperfusion Injury. *Food Funct.* 1 (3), 278–283. doi:10.1039/c0fo00048e

Vasanthi, H. R., ShriShriMal, N., and Das, D. K. (2012). Retraction Notice: Phytochemicals from Plants to Combat Cardiovascular Disease. *Curr. Med. Chem.* 19 (14), 2242–2251. doi:10.2174/092986712800229078

Wang, N., He, F., Li, W., Fang, X., and Li, H. (2019). Purification of the Total Steroidal Saponins from Fenugreek Seeds (Trigonella Foenum- Graecum L.) Using Aqueous Two-phase System and Determination of Diosgenin Content Using Micellar Electrokinetic Chromatography Method. *Nat. Prod. Res.* 33 (3), 453–456. doi:10.1080/14786419.2018.1455047

Wang, Q. H., and Chen, R. (2007). *Effect of Dioscorea Nipponica Makine (DNM) on Thyroid Hormone of Rats with Graves Disease.*

Wang, X., Pan, C., Gong, J., Liu, X., and Li, H. (2016). Enhancing the Enrichment of Pharmacophore-Based Target Prediction for the Polypharmacological Profiles of Drugs. *J. Chem. Inf. Model.* 56 (6), 1175–1183. doi:10.1021/acs.jcim.5b00690

Wang, X., Shen, Y., Wang, S., Li, S., Zhang, W., Liu, X., et al. (2017). PharmMapper 2017 Update: a Web Server for Potential Drug Target Identification with a Comprehensive Target Pharmacophore Database. *Nucleic Acids Res.* 45 (W1), W356–W360. doi:10.1093/nar/gkx374

Wang, Y., Zhang, S., Li, F., Zhou, Y., Zhang, Y., Wang, Z., et al. (2020). Therapeutic Target Database 2020: Enriched Resource for Facilitating Research and Early Development of Targeted Therapeutics. *Nucleic Acids Res.* 48 (D1), D1031–D1041. doi:10.1093/nar/gkz981

Weroha, S. J., and Haluska, P. (2008). IGF-1 Receptor Inhibitors in Clinical Trials-Eearly Lessons. *J. Mammary Gland Biol. Neoplasia* 13 (4), 471–483. doi:10.1007/s10911-008-9104-6

Wishart, D. S., Knox, C., Guo, A. C., Cheng, D., Shrivastava, S., Tzur, D., et al. (2008). DrugBank: a Knowledgebase for Drugs, Drug Actions and Drug Targets. *Nucleic Acids Res.* 36, D901–D906. doi:10.1093/nar/gkm958

Yamanaka, D., Akama, T., Fukushima, T., Nedachi, T., Kawasaki, C., Chida, K., et al. (2012). Phosphatidylinositol 3-Kinase-Binding Protein, PI3KAP/XB130, Is Required for cAMP-Induced Amplification of IGF Mitogenic Activity in FRTL-5 Thyroid Cells. *Mol. Endocrinol.* 26 (6), 1043–1055. doi:10.1210/me.2011-1349

Yan, W., Ji, L., Hang, S., and Shun, Y. (2013). New Ionic Liquid-Based Preparative Method for Diosgenin from Rhizoma Dioscoreae Nipponicae. *Pharmacogn Mag.* 9 (35), 250–254. doi:10.4103/0973-1296.113282

Yao, L., Dong, W., Lu, F., and Liu, S. (2012). An Improved Acute Gouty Arthritis Rat Model and Therapeutic Effect of Rhizoma Dioscoreae Nipponicae on Acute Gouty Arthritis Based on the Protein-Chip Methods. *Am. J. Chin. Med.* 40 (1), 121–134. doi:10.1142/s0192415x12500103

Yi, T., Fan, L. L., Chen, H. L., Zhu, G. Y., Suen, H. M., Tang, Y. N., et al. (2014). Comparative Analysis of Diosgenin in Dioscorea Species and Related Medicinal Plants by UPLC-DAD-MS. *BMC Biochem.* 15, 19. doi:10.1186/1471-2091-15-19

Zhang, L. J., Yu, H. S., Kang, L. P., Feng, B., Quan, B., Song, X. B., et al. (2012). Two New Steroidal Saponins from the Biotransformation Product of the Rhizomes of Dioscorea Nipponica. *J. Asian Nat. Prod. Res.* 14 (7), 640–646. doi:10.1080/10286020.2012.682155

Zhang, M., Zhao, C., Zhao, C., Shao, Q., Yang, Z., Zhang, X., et al. (2019). Determination of Water Content in Corn stover Silage Using Near-Infrared Spectroscopy. *Int. J. Agric. Biol. Eng.* 12 (6), 143–148. doi:10.25165/j.ijabe.20191206.4914

5

A Combined Phytochemistry and Network Pharmacology Approach to Reveal the Potential Antitumor Effective Substances and Mechanism of *Phellinus igniarius*

Yu Dong[1,2†], Ping Qiu[2†], Rui Zhu[2], Lisha Zhao[1], Pinghu Zhang[3], Yiqi Wang[2], Changyu Li[2], Kequn Chai[1,2,4], Dan Shou[1] and Huajun Zhao[2*]*

[1] Department of Medicine, Zhejiang Academy of Traditional Chinese Medicine, Hangzhou, China, [2] College of Pharmaceutical Sciences, Zhejiang Chinese Medical University, Hangzhou, China, [3] Institute of Translational Medicine and Jiangsu Key Laboratory of Integrated Traditional Chinese and Western Medicine for Prevention and Treatment of Senile Diseases, Medical College, Yangzhou University, Yangzhou, China, [4] Zhejiang Key Laboratory of Tumor Diagnosis and Treatment with Integrated TCM and Western Medicine, Hangzhou, China

***Correspondence:**
Dan Shou
shoudanok@163.com
Huajun Zhao
zhj@zcmu.edu.cn

† These authors have contributed equally to this work

Phellinus igniarius (*P. igniarius*) is a medicinal fungus that is widely used in East Asia for the adjuvant treatment of cancer. To elucidate the antitumor effective substances and mechanism of *P. igniarius*, we designed an approach incorporating cytotoxicity screening, phytochemical analysis, network pharmacology construction, and cellular and molecular experiments. The dichloromethane extract of *P. igniarius* (DCMPI) was identified as the active portion in HT-29 cells. Nineteen constituents were identified, and 5 were quantified by UPLC-ESI-Q/TOF-MS. Eight ingredients were obtained in the network pharmacology study. In total, 473 putative targets associated with DCMPI and 350 putative targets related to colon cancer were derived from online databases and target prediction tools. Protein-protein interaction networks of drug and disease putative targets were constructed, and 84 candidate targets were identified based on topological features. Pathway enrichment analysis showed that the candidate targets were mostly related to reactive oxygen species (ROS) metabolic processes and intrinsic apoptotic pathways. Then, a cellular experiment was used to validate the drug-target mechanisms predicted by the system pharmacology analysis. Experimental results showed that DCMPI increased intracellular ROS levels and induced HT-29 cell apoptosis. Molecular biology experiments indicated that DCMPI not only increased Bax and Bad protein expression and promoted PARP and caspase-3/9 cleavage but also down-regulated Bcl-2 and Bcl-xl protein levels to induce apoptosis in HT-29 cells. In conclusion, our study provides knowledge on the chemical composition and antitumor mechanism of *P. igniarius*, which may be exploited as a promising therapeutic option for colon cancer.

Keywords: *Phellinus igniarius*, antitumor, phytochemistry, network pharmacology, effective substances, mitochondrial apoptosis pathway

INTRODUCTION

Cancer serves as a major public health problem worldwide and is expected to surpass heart disease as the leading cause of death in the next few years (Siegel et al., 2016). In the past decade, numerous significant advances in cancer research have revealed the genetics and pathologies of malignant tumors, which, in turn, facilitates the development of novel anticancer agents (Hare et al., 2017). Interestingly, multiple bioactive phytochemicals in consumed edible and medicinal fungi have recently attracted considerable attention as potential candidates for anticancer agents (Li et al., 2015).

Phellinus igniarius (*P. igniarius*), a well-known mushroom belonging to the genus *Phellinus* in the polyporaceae family, is a physiologically functional food and exemplary source of natural medicine that has been widely used in China, Japan, Korea, and other countries (Ma et al., 2016). *P. igniarius* possesses high anti-inflammatory, antioxidant and antitumor biological activities due to its accumulation of various secondary metabolites, including polysaccharides, flavonoids, polyphenols, steroids and organic acids (Dong et al., 2015; Shou et al., 2016). Notably, recent studies have creatively focused on the potential functions of *P. igniarius* extracts and their constituent compounds in the prevention and treatment of cancer (Zhou et al., 2014; Sangdee et al., 2017). A considerable amount of evidence indicates that *P. igniarius* extracts resulting from water, alcohol, ethyl acetate and other solvent extractions have a significant inhibitory effect on various tumor cells, such as S180, PC3, SK-HEP-1, and HT-29 cells (Yang et al., 2006; Song et al., 2008; Jeon et al., 2013). To date, no prior system reports on the chemical composition of *P. igniarius* contribute to its antitumor activity or functional mechanisms.

Network pharmacology is now popularly utilized to discover the basis of pharmacodynamic substances, explore their molecular mechanisms of action, and elucidate their scientific connotations (Kim et al., 2017). Especially, TCM network pharmacology focuses on the wholeness and systemicity of the interactions between components, targets and diseases of TCM (Cao et al., 2018; Huang et al., 2018), and is crucial to select the beneficial therapeutic targets of TCM, typical TCM syndromes and corresponding classic formulas (Zhang et al., 2017). At the same time, TCM network pharmacology substantially reduces the workload of follow-up experimental studies on TCM.

In the present study, we designed an approach incorporating cytotoxicity screening, phytochemical analysis, network pharmacology construction, and cellular and molecular biology validation to clarify the antitumor effective substance and mechanism of *P. igniarius*. Notably, this is the first integral study using multiple methods in combination to elucidate the antitumor efficacy substances and mechanism of this large medicinal fungus.

Abbreviations: BP, biological process; BPI, base peak intensity; CC, cellular component; DAPI, 4',6-diamidino-2-phenylindole; DEGs, differentially expressed genes; DMSO, dimethyl sulfoxide; ECL, enhanced chemiluminescence; GAD, genetic association database; GEO, gene expression omnibus database; GO, gene ontology; HMDB, Human Metablome Database; MF, molecular function; MMP, mitochondrial membrane potential; MTT, 3-[4,5-dimethylthiazol-2-yl]-2,5-diphenyltetrazolium bromide; OMIM, online mendelian inheritance in man; PARP, poly ADP-ribose polymerase; PBS, phosphate buffer saline; *P. igniarius*, *Phellinus igniarius*; *P. igniarius* DCM, dichloromethane extract of *Phellinus igniarius*; PPI, protein–protein interaction; ROS, reactive oxygen species; SDS-PAGE, sodium dodecyl sulfate polyacrylamide gel electrophoresis; SEA, similarity ensemble approach; TCM, traditional Chinese medicine; TCMSP, traditional Chinese medicine systems pharmacology; TTD, therapeutic target database; UPLC-ESI-Q/TOF-MS, ultra performance liquid chromatography-electrospray ionization- quadrupole/time-of-flight mass spectrometry.

MATERIALS AND METHODS

Chemicals and Materials

Phellinus igniarius sporocarps were purchased from Zhejiang Qingzheng Biotechnology Co. Ltd. (Hangzhou, China). Reference standards (purity > 98%) of protocatechuic aldehyde (671E-QHX2) and osmundacetone (RC5E-FH31) were purchased from the National Institute for the Control of Pharmaceutical and Biological Products (Beijing, China), and naringenin (170124), eriodictycol (170309) and sakuranetin (170124) were purchased from Beijing Century Aoke Biology Research Co., Ltd. (Beijing, China). HPLC grade methanol and acetonitrile were purchased from Merck (Darmstadt, Germany). Distilled water was purchased from Watson's Food & Beverage Co., Ltd. (Guangzhou, China). Leucine enkephalin and formic acid were purchased from Sigma-Aldrich (Darmstadt, Germany).

Human hepatoma carcinoma (HepG2, SMMC7721), human gastric carcinoma (BGC-823, SGC790, AGS), human colon carcinoma (HT-29) and human lung carcinoma (A549) cells were purchased from American Type Culture Collection (Rockefeller, MD, United States). DMEM and RPMI 1640 cell culture mediums were purchased from HyClone Corporation (Logan, UT, United States). Fetal bovine serum was purchased from Gibco Corporation (Grand Island, NE, United States). MTT was purchased from Sigma-Aldrich (Darmstadt, Germany). An AnnexinV-FITC/PI apoptosis detection kit was purchased from BD Biosciences (Franklin lakes, NJ, United States). A ROSs assay kit and JC-1 dye were purchased from Beyotime Biosciences (Nanjing, China). Antibodies against PARP (#9532), Caspase-3 (#9662), Caspase-8 (#6790), Caspase-9 (#9508), Bax (#5023), Bcl-2 (#2870), Bcl-xl (#2764), and β-actin (#4970) were purchased from Cell Signaling Technology (Boston, MA, United States). Antibody against Bad (ab32445) was purchased from Abcam (Cambridge, MA, United States). HRP-conjugated secondary antibody was purchased from Bio-Rad (Hercules, CA, United States).

P. igniarius Extract Preparation

The dried *P. igniarius* sporocarps were crushed into a powder (with an approximately 100 mesh screen) using a plant disintegrator. In total, 600 g of powder was weighed, immersed in 3 L of 95% (v/v) ethanol for 30 min, and extracted in an ultrasonic bath 3 times for 1 h each time. The extracted solution was merged and evaporated by a rotary evaporator, and distilled water was added to 1 L of the suspension (containing 20% ethanol). The suspension was then subjected to liquid-liquid extraction with petroleum ether, dichloromethane, ethyl acetate and *n*-butanol successively. Each extract fraction was merged, evaporated and then freeze-dried to obtain the petroleum ether extract (0.32 g), dichloromethane extract (0.51 g), ethyl acetate extract (2.23 g), and *n*-butanol extract (1.28 g).

Cell Culture

Human hepatoma carcinoma (HepG2) and human gastric carcinoma (BGC-823) cells were cultured in DMEM. Human gastric carcinoma (SGC790, AGS), human colon carcinoma (HT-29) and human lung carcinoma (A549) cells were maintained in RPMI 1640 medium. Human hepatoma carcinoma cells (SMMC7721) were cultured in DMEM/F12 medium. Then, the three media were supplemented with 10% fetal bovine serum, 100 units/mL penicillin and 100 μg/mL streptomycin. The cultures were maintained in a humidified incubator containing 5% (v/v) CO_2 at 37°C.

Cytotoxicity Experiment

The cytotoxic effects of the *P. igniarius* extracts were detected using the MTT calorimetric method. Briefly, cells (3×10^3 cells/well) were seeded in 96-well plates and incubated for 24 h. The supernatant was subsequently aspirated, and the cells were exposed to various concentrations of extracts and 0.05% DMSO (v/v). After 72 h of incubation, MTT solution (0.5 mg/mL) was added to each well and incubated for 4 h. Thereafter, the medium containing MTT was removed and replaced with 120 μL of DMSO to dissolve the formazan crystals. Next, the plates were shaken for 20 min, and the absorbance at 570 nm was recorded using an enzyme-linked immunosorbent assay reader (TECAN, Switzerland).

In addition, HT-29 cells (5×10^5 cells/well) were seeded into a six-well plate and incubated for 24 h. Then, the medium was replaced with RPMI-1640 medium containing different concentrations of dichloromethane extract of *P. igniarius* (DCMPI). After incubation for 72 h, the cytomorphology of the cells was observed and digitally photographed using a phase contrast microscope (Olympus, Japan).

Chemical Profile Analysis by UPLC-ESI-Q/TOF-MS

The UPLC-ESI-Q/TOF-MS system consisted of an Acquity™ ultra performance liquid chromatography (UPLC) system (Waters Corporation, Milford, MA, United States) and a Synapt G2 mass spectrometer (MS) (Waters MS-Technologies, Manchester, United Kingdom) equipped with an electrospray ion (ESI) source. The system and data were controlled by MassLynx (V4.1) software. Chromatography was performed on an Acquity UPLC BEH C_{18} column (2.1 × 150 mm, 1.7 μm, Waters Corporation, Milford, MA, United States) at a flow rate of 0.3 mL/min and a 40°C column temperature. The optimal mobile phases consisted of A (HCOOH: CH_3CN = 0.1: 100, v/v) and B (HCOOH: H_2O = 0.1: 100, v/v): 0–1 min, 1–8% A; 1–2.5 min, 8–15% A; 2.5–4.5 min, 15–20% A; 4.5–5.5 min, maintained at 20% A; 5.5–7.5 min, 20–30% A; 7.5–13 min, 30–60%; 13–14 min, 60–99% A; and 14–15 min, maintained at 99% A. The extracts were dissolved in methanol to a concentration of 1 mg/mL and filtered through a 0.22 μm membrane. A 2 μL aliquot of sample solution was injected for analysis.

The full-scan LC-MS data were acquired in both positive and negative ion modes from 50 to 1500 Da with a 0.3 s scan time. The optimal Q/TOF-MS conditions were as follows: capillary voltage 3.0 kV, sampling cone voltage 40.0 V and extraction cone voltage 5.0 V for positive ion mode; capillary voltage 2.4 kV, sampling cone voltage 35.0 V and extraction cone voltage 3.5 V for negative ion mode. The source temperature and desolvation gas temperature were set to 150 and 350°C, respectively, and the cone gas flow and desolvation gas flow were set to 60 L/h and 550 L/h, respectively. The collision energy was set to 4 eV for positive ion mode and 2 eV for negative ion mode. Sodium formate solution was used to calibrate the mass spectrometer prior to the experiment. Leucine-enkephalin was used as an external reference (Lock-Spray™) to correct the mass during data acquisition via a LockSpray interface, generating reference ions at *m/z* 556.2771 Da ($[M+H]^+$) and *m/z* 554.2615 Da ($[M-H]^-$) in the positive and negative ion modes, respectively.

Constituent Identification

All LC-MS and MS/MS data were processed with MassLynx™ (V4.1) software. Molecular formula speculations of the compounds were determined with Elemental Composition software. Structural identification of the main compounds, which included the chemical structure, accurate molecular mass and potential molecular fragmentation pathways, was determined with Mass Fragment software. Previously published compounds were identified by comprehensively searching databases, such as PubMed[1], Chemspider[2], HMDB[3], and Metlin[4]. Compounds with standard materials were validated using reference standards.

Main Ingredient Quantification for DCMPI

DCMPI was dissolved in methanol to a concentration of 1 mg/mL as a sample solution. Mother stock solutions (approximately 1 mg/mL) of protocatechuic aldehyde, osmundacetone, eriodictyol, naringenin and sakuranetin were separately prepared in MeOH. Further, combined spiking stock solutions of the five reference substances were prepared in MeOH from the mother stock solutions by stepwise dilution in the ranges of 4.61–73.15 μg/mL for protocatechuic aldehyde, 3.97–63.44 μg/mL for osmundacetone, 3.91–62.50 μg/mL for eriodictyol, 4.20–67.19 μg/mL for naringenin and 4.04–64.69 μg/mL for sakuranetin. The sample solution and each combined spiking stock solution were filtered through a 0.22 μm membrane, and a 2 μL volume was injected into the UPLC-ESI-Q/TOF-MS system for analysis. The LC-MS conditions were the same as those previously described.

Prediction of Drug Targets for DCMPI

Eight major DCMPI components, including five validated components (protocatechuic aldehyde, osmundacetone,

[1] http://www.ncbi.nlm.nih.gov/pubmed

[2] http://www.chemspider.com/

[3] http://www.hmdb.ca/

[4] http://metlin.scripps.edu

eriodictyol, naringenin and sakuranetin) and three identified components (inoscavin A, phelligrin A and phelligrin B) with a peak area greater than 5% were included in the network pharmacology study. By searching for the relevant predictive genes of the 8 main components at the websites PharmMapper Server[5], SEA Search Server[6], STITCH[7] and TCMSP[8], the DCMPI prediction genes were obtained.

Collection of Predicted Targets Related to Colon Cancer

Two main methods were used to identify colon cancer-related targets. To identify the main DEGs between normal human colon samples and colon cancer samples, GDS4382 microarray data were downloaded from the GEO[9]. The data set consisted of 34 human samples; GEO analysis was performed using 17 normal colon samples and 17 colon cancer samples. DEGs were defined by the Bioconductor/R limma package. $P < 0.05$ and a fold change ≥ 2 were applied. The known targets associated with colon cancer were derived from five databases, GAD, OMIM[10], TTD[11], DrugBank[12] and CoolGen[13], using 'colon cancer' as the key word.

Construction of the PPI Network

Protein–protein interaction data from the six currently available PPI databases, the Human Protein Reference Database, the Biomolecular Interaction Network Database, the Biological General Repository for Interaction Datasets, the Database of Interacting Proteins and the Molecular INTeraction Database, were searched using the Cytoscape plugin BisoGenet. An interactive network of DCMPI drug targets and colon cancer-related targets was constructed based on interaction data, and the network was visualized utilizing Cytoscape software (version 3.2.1).

Definition of Network Topology Feature Set

By calculating the 'betweenness centrality,' 'degree centrality,' 'eigenvector centrality,' 'closeness centrality,' 'network centrality' and 'local average connectivity' using CytoNCA, the topological nature of each node in the interactive network was analyzed. The definitions and calculation formulas of these six parameters represent the topological importance of the nodes in the network, with more important nodes yielding higher quantitative values in the network.

[5]https://omictools.com/pharmmapper-tool
[6]http://sea.bkslab.org/
[7]http://stitch.embl.de/
[8]http://lsp.nwu.edu.cn/tcmspsearch.php
[9]http://www.ncbi.nlm.nih.gov/geo/
[10]http://www.omim.org/
[11]https://db.idrblab.org/ttd/
[12]http://www.drugbank.ca/
[13]http://ci.smu.edu.cn/CooLGeN/Home.php

GO Enrichment and Pathway Analysis

DAVID Bioinformatics Resources 6.8[14] was used to perform GO enrichment analysis of the differentially expressed targets to explore their roles in many BPs. Twenty significantly enriched terms in the CC, BP, and MF categories are shown. ClueGO is a Cytoscape plugin for visualizing the non-redundant features of a large number of gene clusters in a functional grouping network to assess the enrichment of DCMPI candidate targets. The ClueGO network was created using kappa statistics, reflecting the relationship between terms based on the similarity of related genes. The significances of terms and groups are automatically calculated.

Nuclear Staining With DAPI

HT-29 colon cancer cells were seeded into 24-well plates (5×10^4 cells/well) and treated with 30 and 60 μg/mL DCMPI for 24 h. Then, the cells were rinsed with PBS, stained with DAPI (0.5 μg/mL) and further incubated for 20 min in the dark. The slides were observed under a fluorescence microscope (Nikon, Japan), and the cells with nucleus condensation or fragmentation were considered apoptotic.

Apoptosis Assay With Annexin V-FITC/PI Staining

HT-29 colon cancer cells were seeded into 6-well plates (5×10^5 cells/well) and cultured overnight prior to exposure to different concentrations of DCMPI (30 μg/mL, 60 μg/mL) for 24 h. Then, the percentage of apoptotic cells was determined by an Annexin V-FITC/PI staining kit following the manufacturer's protocol. Cells were then analyzed with the Guava Easy cytometer (Merck Millipore Co. Ltd., Darmstadt, Germany) within 1 h.

Mitochondrial Membrane Potential (Δψm) Measurements

Mitochondrial membrane potential (Δψm) was monitored utilizing the JC-1 cationic dye (Molecular Probes) as recommended by the manufacturer. HT-29 cells were seeded into 6-well plates (5×10^5 cells/well) and cultured overnight prior to exposure to different concentrations of DCMPI (30 μg/mL, 60 μg/mL) for 24 h and then resuspended in a buffer solution containing 10 μg/mL JC-1 cationic dye. After 20 min of incubation in the dark at 37°C, the samples were rinsed with PBS to remove unreacted dye. The fluorescence intensity was read with the Guava Easy cytometer within 1 h.

Intracellular ROS Measurement

The cell-permeable dye DCFH-DA (Molecular Probes) was used to assay intracellular ROS levels. This dye diffuses into cells and becomes trapped inside by de-esterification. After a reaction with peroxides, the fluorescent product, 5-chloromethyl-2′-7′-dichlorofluorescein (DCF), is formed. HT-29 cells were seeded into 6-well plates (5×10^5 cells/well) and cultured overnight prior to exposure to different concentrations of DCMPI (30 μg/mL, 60 μg/mL) for 24 h and then

[14]https://david.ncifcrf.gov/

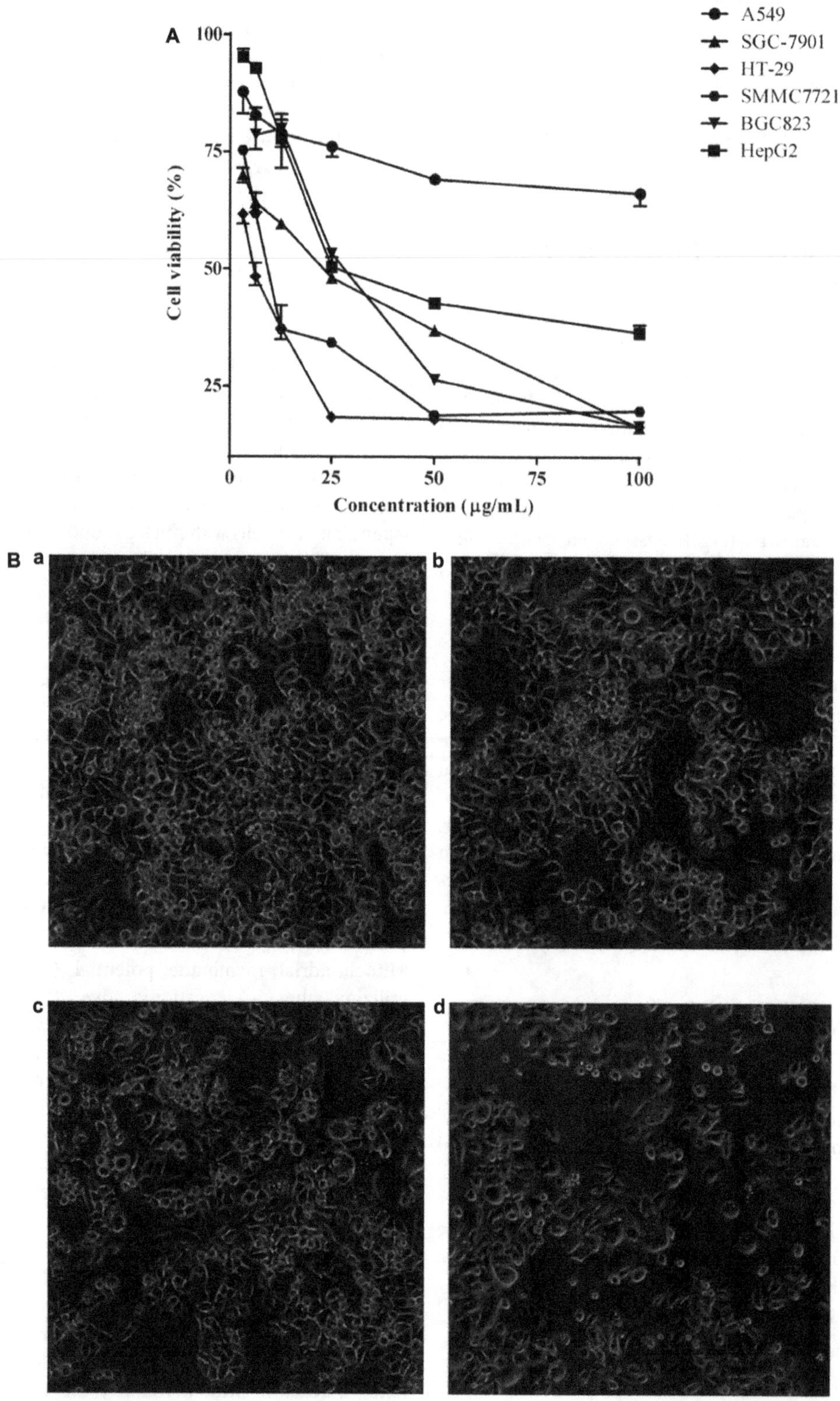

FIGURE 1 | (A) Cytotoxic effects of DCMPI on the A549, SGC-7901, HT-29, SMMC7721, BGC-823 and HepG2 cell lines as determined by the MTT assay for 72 h. **(B)** Microscopic observation of HT-29 cells after administrating DCMPI for 72 h **(a)**: untreated; **(b)**: treated with 12.5 μg/mL DCMPI; **(c)**: treated with 25 μg/mL DCMPI; **(d)**: treated with 50 μg/mL DCMPI).

resuspended in DMEM/F-12 medium containing 10 μM DCFH-DA. Thereafter, the samples were incubated in the dark at 37°C for 20 min and then rinsed with PBS to remove unreacted dye. The fluorescence intensity was read with the Guava Easy cytometer within 1 h.

Apoptosis-Related Protein Assay

Protein extraction was performed as follows: after treatment with DCMPI (30 μg/mL, 60 μg/mL) for 24 h, HT-29 cells were cultured, collected, rinsed twice with ice-cold PBS, lysed, incubated in RIPA buffer containing a 1% protease inhibitor cocktail for 30 min on ice, and then centrifuged at 12,000 × *g* for 15 min. The supernatants were harvested and prepared by mixing with 5× sample buffer for subsequent Western blot analysis. The protein samples were then separated by 10% SDS-PAGE and transferred onto 0.22 μm polyvinylidene fluoride membranes (Millipore, Bedford, MA, United States). The membranes were blocked with 5% non-fat skim milk for 1 h at room temperature and then incubated with the appropriate primary antibodies overnight at 4°C. The membranes were incubated with a horseradish peroxidase-conjugated secondary antibody at room temperature for 2 h, followed by rinsing three times with 1× TBST. The protein bands were visualized utilizing ECL detection reagents (Bio-Rad, United States).

Statistical Analysis

All data were analyzed with GraphPad Prism 5.0 software (GraphPad Software, Inc., La Jolla, CA, United States) and SPSS 20.0 Software (SPSS, Inc., Chicago, IL, United States). Furthermore, all statistical comparisons were performed using one-way analysis of variance followed by a *post hoc* Dunnett's test. Values of $P < 0.01$ were considered statistically significant.

RESULTS

Cell Cytotoxicity Assay of *P. igniarius* Extracts

The cell viability inhibition induced by *P. igniarius* extracts, including the petroleum ether fraction, dichloromethane fraction, ethyl acetate fraction, *n*-butanol fraction and ethanol extract of *P. igniarius*, was evaluated *in vitro* with an MTT assay. Moreover, each cancer cell line was incubated with different concentrations of *P. igniarius* extracts for 72 h to compare their cytotoxicities. Notably, DCMPI as the strongest inhibitor decreased the viabilities of all the tested cell lines in a concentration-dependent manner, and especially significant cytotoxicity was observed in HT-29 cells (**Figure 1A**). Normal HT-29 cells appeared whole, healthy, and polygonal in shape under a microscope; however, after administering DCMPI, the HT-29 cells exhibited a number of morphological alterations, including cell shrinkage, condensed chromatin, membrane blebbing, and an increased density of apoptotic cells (**Figure 1B**).

Characterization of DCMPI Chemical Constituents

The chemical profiles of DCMPI were analyzed by UPLC-ESI-Q/TOF-MS. All LC-MS data, including retention times, accurate molecular masses, and MS/MS data, are necessary for the structural analysis of compounds. The element compositions were calculated and clearly confirmed by combining with a mass accuracy (ppm) less than 5.0 using MarkerLynx (4.1) software. The majority of the components detected in the positive ion mode were also detected in the negative ion mode; therefore, data analysis was performed in only the negative ion mode. Using the optimal UPLC and Q/TOF-MS conditions described

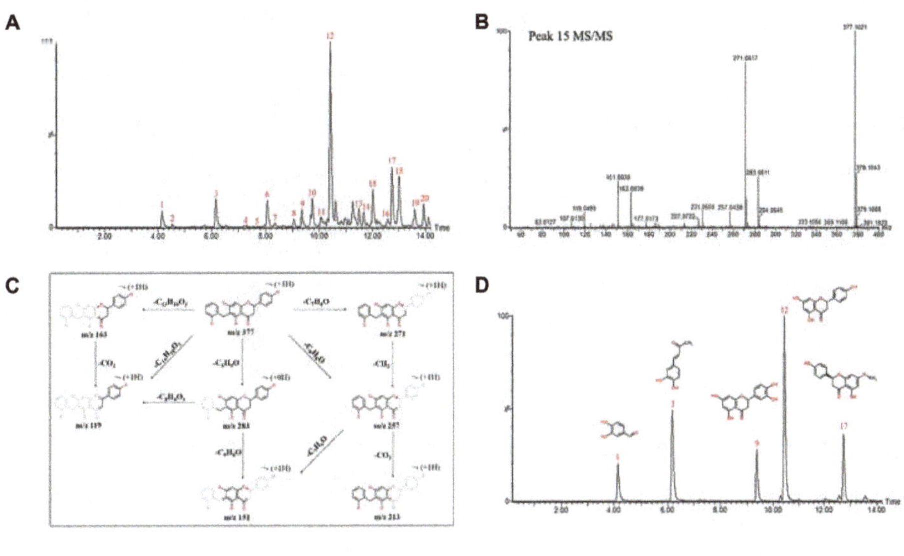

FIGURE 2 | (A) UPLC-ESI-Q/TOF-MS BPI chromatogram of DCMPI. **(B)** Mass fragment spectrum of Phelligrin A in the negative ion mode. **(C)** Possible fragmentation mechanistic pathway of Phelligrin A. **(D)** Typical mixed standard substance chromatograms of protocatechuic aldehyde, osmundacetone, eriodictyol, naringenin, and sakuranetin.

TABLE 1 | Characterization of chemical constituents of DCMPI by UPLC-ESI-Q/TOF-MS.

No.	RT (min)	Formula	Measured mass (m/z)	Theoretical mass (m/z)	Error (ppm)	Fragment ions	Identify
1	4.17	$C_7H_6O_3$	137.0233	137.0239	−4.4	137[M-H]$^-$, 108[M-H-CHO]$^-$, 92[M-H-COOH]$^-$	Protocatechuic aldehyde
2	4.55	$C_9H_6O_4$	177.0182	177.0188	−4.5	177[M-H]$^-$, 161[M-H-O]$^-$, 135[M-H-COCH$_2$]$^-$	Esculetin
3	6.18	$C_{10}H_{10}O_3$	177.0552	177.0552	0	177[M-H]$^-$, 162[M-H-CH$_3$]$^-$, 134[M-H-COCH$_3$]$^-$	Osmundacetone
4	7.29	$C_{12}H_{10}O_4$	217.0499	217.0511	−0.9	217[M-H]$^-$, 177[M-H-C$_3$H$_4$]$^-$, 161[M-H-C$_3$H$_4$O]$^-$	Inotilone
5	7.53	$C_{41}H_{72}O_{10}$	723.5004	723.4989	2.1	723[M-H]$^-$, 677[M-H-COH-OH]$^-$	Not identified
6	8.09	$C_{15}H_{12}O_6$	287.0453	287.0556	−4.5	287[M-H]$^-$, 259[M-H-CO]$^-$, 243[M-H-COCH$_3$]$^-$, 152[M-H-C$_8$H$_7$O$_2$]$^-$, 125[M-H-C$_9$H$_6$O$_3$]$^-$	Dihydrokaempferol
7	8.39	$C_{25}H_{20}O_9$	463.1023	463.1029	−1.3	463[M-H]$^-$, 407[M-H-CH$_3$-CO-CH]$^-$, 379[M-H-CH$_3$-CO-CH-CO]$^-$, 243[M-H-C$_6$H$_5$O$_2$-C$_6$H$_7$O$_2$]$^-$, 217[M-H-C$_6$H$_5$O$_2$-C$_7$H$_5$O$_3$]$^-$, 159[M-H-C$_6$H$_5$O$_2$-C$_6$H$_7$O$_2$-COOH-CO]$^-$, 135[M-H-C$_6$H$_5$O$_2$-C$_7$H$_5$O$_3$-C$_5$H$_6$O]$^-$	Davallialactone
8	9.05	$C_{26}H_{18}O_{10}$	489.0821	489.0822	−0.2	489[M-H]$^-$, 445[M-H-CO$_2$]$^-$, 403[M-H-C$_3$H$_2$O$_3$]$^-$, 335[M-H-C$_8$H$_9$O$_2$-OH]$^-$, 241[M-H-C$_8$H$_9$O$_2$-C$_5$H$_3$O$_3$]$^-$, 159[M-H-C$_{16}$H$_{10}$O$_8$]$^-$, 135[M-H-C$_{19}$H$_{14}$O$_7$]$^-$	Hypholomine B
9	9.37	$C_{15}H_{12}O_6$	287.0554	287.0556	−0.7	287[M-H]$^-$, 151[M-H-C$_8$H$_8$O$_2$]$^-$, 135[M-H-C$_7$H$_4$O$_4$]$^-$, 107[M-H-C$_9$H$_8$O$_4$-]$^-$	Eriodictyol
10	9.74	$C_{25}H_{18}O_9$	461.0872	461.0873	−0.2	461[M-H]$^-$, 377[M-H-C$_4$H$_4$O$_2$]$^-$, 333[M-H-C$_5$H$_4$O$_4$]$^-$, 257[M-H-C$_{11}$H$_8$O$_4$]$^-$, 241[M-H-C$_{11}$H$_8$O$_5$]$^-$, 159[M-H-C$_{15}$H$_{10}$O$_7$]$^-$, 134[M-H-C$_{17}$H$_{11}$O$_7$]$^-$	Epi-inoscavin A
11	10.12	$C_{25}H_{18}O_9$	461.0869	461.0873	−0.9	461[M-H]$^-$, 377[M-H-C$_4$H$_4$O$_2$]$^-$, 333[M-H-C$_5$H$_4$O$_4$]$^-$, 257[M-H-C$_{11}$H$_8$O$_4$]$^-$, 241[M-H-C$_{11}$H$_8$O$_5$]$^-$, 159[M-H-C$_{15}$H$_{10}$O$_7$]$^-$, 145[M-C$_{16}$H$_{12}$O$_7$]$^-$	Inoscavin A
12	10.42	$C_{15}H_{12}O_5$	271.0607	271.0606	0.4	271[M-H]$^-$, 177[M-H-C$_6$H$_6$O]$^-$, 151[M-H-C$_8$H$_8$O]$^-$, 119[M-H-C$_7$H$_4$O$_4$]$^-$, 107[M-H-C$_9$H$_8$O$_3$]$^-$	Naringenin
13	11.46	$C_{22}H_{18}O_7$	393.0969	393.0974	−1.3	393[M-H]$^-$, 365[M-H-CO]$^-$, 299[M-H-C$_6$H$_6$O]$^-$, 287[M-H-C$_7$H$_6$O]$^-$, 259[M-H-C$_8$H$_6$O$_2$]$^-$, 243[M-H-C$_8$H$_6$O$_3$]$^-$, 231[M-C$_9$H$_6$O$_3$]$^-$	Oxyphelligrin A
14	11.65	$C_{16}H_{14}O_6$	301.0704	301.0712	−2.7	301[M-H]$^-$, 165[M-H-C$_8$H$_8$O$_2$]$^-$, 135[M-H-C$_8$H$_6$O$_4$]$^-$	Folerogenin
15	12.00	$C_{22}H_{18}O_6$	377.1011	377.1025	−3.7	377[M-H]$^-$, 283[M-H-C$_6$H$_6$O]$^-$, 271[M-H-C$_7$H$_6$O]$^-$, 257[M-H-C$_8$H$_8$O]$^-$, 231[M-H-C$_9$H$_6$O$_2$]$^-$, 213[M-H-C$_9$H$_8$O$_3$]$^-$, 163[M-C$_{13}$H$_{10}$O$_3$]$^-$, 119[M-C$_{14}$H$_{10}$O$_5$]$^-$	Phelligrin A
16	12.53	$C_{13}H_{18}O_3$	221.1174	221.1178	−1.8	221[M-H]$^-$, 205[M-H-O]$^-$, 177[M-H-C$_2$H$_4$O]$^-$, 149[M-H-C$_3$H$_4$O$_2$]$^-$	Dehydrovomifoliol
17	12.7	$C_{16}H_{14}O_5$	285.0751	285.0763	−4.2	285[M-H]$^-$, 169[M-H-C$_8$H$_8$O]$^-$, 119[M-H-C$_9$H$_{10}$O$_3$]$^-$	Sakuranetin
18	12.98	$C_{22}H_{18}O_6$	377.1019	377.1025	−1.6	377[M-H]$^-$, 283[M-H-C$_6$H$_6$O]$^-$, 271[M-H-C$_7$H$_6$O]$^-$, 257[M-H-C$_8$H$_8$O]$^-$, 231[M-H-C$_9$H$_6$O$_2$]$^-$, 213[M-H-C$_9$H$_8$O$_3$]$^-$, 163[M-C$_{13}$H$_{10}$O$_3$]$^-$, 119[M-C$_{14}$H$_{10}$O$_5$]$^-$	Phelligrin B
19	13.56	$C_{23}H_{20}O_6$	391.1174	391.1182	−2.0	391[M-H]$^-$, 297[M-H-C$_6$H$_6$O]$^-$, 285[M-H-C$_7$H$_6$O]$^-$, 271[M-H-C$_8$H$_8$O]$^-$, 245[M-H-C$_9$H$_6$O$_2$]$^-$, 165[M-H-C$_{15}$H$_{14}$O$_2$]$^-$, 119[M-C$_{15}$H$_{12}$O$_5$]$^-$, 93[M-C$_{17}$H$_{14}$O$_5$]$^-$	Methylphelligrin A
20	13.88	$C_{23}H_{20}O_6$	391.1174	391.1182	−2.0	391[M-H]$^-$, 297[M-H-C$_6$H$_6$O]$^-$, 285[M-H-C$_7$H$_6$O]$^-$, 271[M-H-C$_8$H$_8$O]$^-$, 245[M-H-C$_9$H$_6$O$_2$]$^-$, 165[M-H-C$_{15}$H$_{14}$O$_2$]$^-$, 119[M-C$_{15}$H$_{12}$O$_5$]$^-$, 93[M-C$_{17}$H$_{14}$O$_5$]$^-$	Methylphelligrin B

above, the BPI chromatogram was obtained in the negative ion mode (**Figure 2A**). A total of 20 peaks were obtained from the BPI chromatogram, and 19 of these peaks were identified or characterized (**Table 1**). Peak 15 was tentatively characterized as phelligrin A based on the mass spectrum and fragmentation pathway illustrated in **Figures 2B,C**.

Quantification of Five Main DCMPI Ingredients

The established quantitative method was applied to determine the contents of protocatechuic aldehyde, osmundacetone, eriodictyol, naringenin, and sakuranetin in DCMPI. The linear parameters of the five ingredients are listed in **Table 2**. Typical chromatograms of the five ingredients are shown in **Figure 2D**. DCMPI contained approximately 1.17% protocatechuic aldehyde, 0.62% osmundacetone, 1.10% eriodictyol, 3.59% naringenin, and 3.71% sakuranetin.

Putative DCMPI Target Prediction

By screening the eight main components of DCMPI (the structures are shown in **Figure 3A**) in the PharmMapper Server, SEA Search Server, STITCH and TCMSP databases, potential targets of DCMPI were obtained. A total of 1727 potential targets were predicted for the 8 main compounds (196 for protocatechuic aldehyde, 149 for osmundacetone, 284 for eriodictyol, 293 for naringenin, 285 for sakuranetin, 250 for inoscavin A, 270 for phelligrin A, and 264 for phelligrin B), and 473 targets remained after deleting duplicates.

Compound-Target Network Construction and Analysis

Traditional Chinese medicine always exhibit versatile biological and pharmacological activities with complex chemical compositions by acting on multiple targets. Studying the complicated interactions between compounds and their targets at the system level may help comprehensively understand the mechanisms underlying TCM effects. We constructed a compound-target network based on the 8 candidate DCMPI compounds and their 473 potential targets. In total, 480 nodes and 1988 compound-target interactions are embodied in this network (**Figure 3B**).

GO Enrichment and Pathway Analysis

GO analysis of the putative DCMPI targets was employed based on DAVID software for the visualization, annotation, and integrated discovery described by the BP, CC, and MF terms. In total, 671 BPs, 73 CCs, and 192 MFs that were enriched for this dataset were identified, of which 140 BPs, 55 CCs, and 140 MFs had P-values < 0.05. **Figure 3C** exhibits an overview of the GO analysis, and 20 remarkably enriched terms in the BP, CC, and MF categories are shown.

Collection of Colon Cancer-Related Targets

We herein collected colon cancer-related targets from two main sources: DEGs obtained from publicly available microarray data and disease-related databases. As shown **Figure 4**, 200 DEGs were identified from the GEO repository microarray data, while other targets were obtained from five databases: 163 from GAD, 54 from OMIM, 25 from TTD, 66 from DrugBank, and 246 from CoolGen. After removing redundant genes, 349 colon cancer-related targets were collected. Of these, 84 genes were also the targets of DCMPI, which suggests an obvious therapeutic potential for *P. igniarius*.

Identification of Candidate DCMPI Targets for Colon Cancer Treatment

Numerous evidence in network biology has shown that genes and proteins exert their functions via interactions. Thus, we selected proteins as nodes for constructing the network. To elaborate the pharmacological mechanism by which DCMPI ameliorates colon cancer, we established PPI networks that may reflect the behavior and properties of biological molecules. First, a putative target PPI network of DCMPI-related genes was obtained using Cytoscape 3.2.1 software with the plugin BisoGenet (8933 nodes and 195,493 edges) and database retrieval of the PPI network of colon cancer-related targets (4615 nodes and 113,727 edges). We then merged these two networks to obtain a core PPI (CPPI) network that consisted of 4614 nodes and 113,727 edges. Subsequently, colon cancer targets of DCMPI were screened using the topological features of CPPI. Then, utilizing a Cytoscape plugin (CytoNCA), the main hubs of the network were screened by calculating the topological features for each hub, which were identified when their degree exceeded twice the median degree of all nodes in the network. A flow chart depicting the core target screening is presented in **Figures 5A–C**.

Pathway Enrichment Analysis of DCMPI Targets

A Cytoscape plugin (ClueGO) was applied to further define the pathways involved in the biological networks identified

TABLE 2 | Linearity for the five ingredients using UPLC-ESI-Q/TOF-MS.

Compound name	RT (min)	Traces (m/z)	Calibration curves	Linear range (μg/mL)	R^2
Protocatechuic aldehyde	4.14	137.02	$y = 67.8718x + 451.627$	4.61–73.15	0.9963
Osmundacetone	6.17	177.05	$y = 188.218x + 930.296$	3.97–63.44	0.9944
Eriodictyol	9.37	287.05	$y = 84.2368x – 79.8782$	3.91–62.50	0.9998
Naringenin	10.42	271.05	$y = 353.18x + 1012.13$	4.20–67.19	0.9961
Sakuranetin	12.73	285.07	$y = 127.728–263.059$	4.04–64.69	0.9985

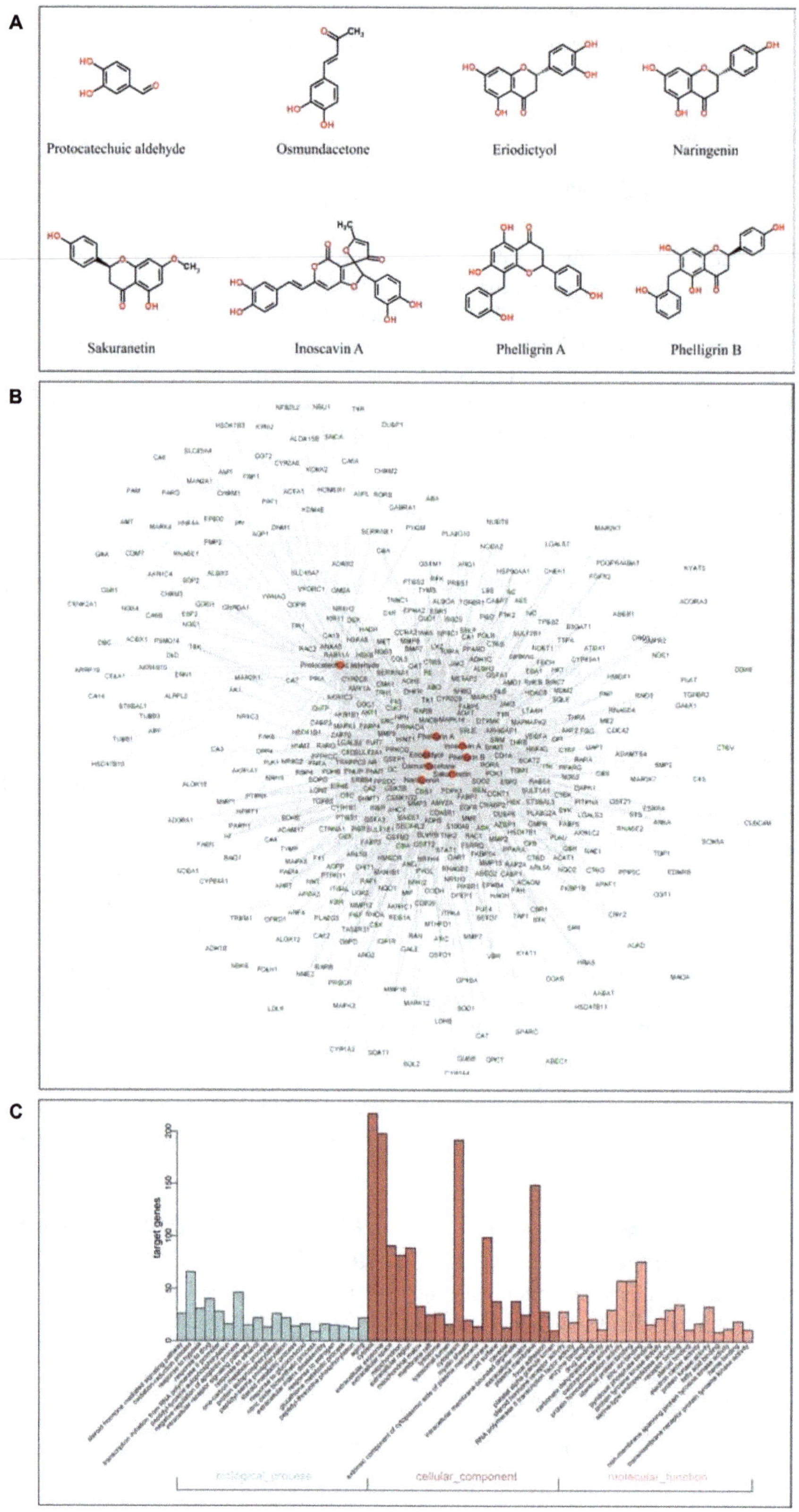

FIGURE 3 | GO analysis of putative DCMPI targets and compound-target network construction. **(A)** Chemical structures of the eight main ingredients. **(B)** GO analysis of BP, cell component, and MF terms was performed on putative DCMPI targets, and the top 20 terms with $P < 0.05$ are shown. **(C)** The compound-target network was constructed by linking the 8 main compounds (red dots) and their potential targets (green dots).

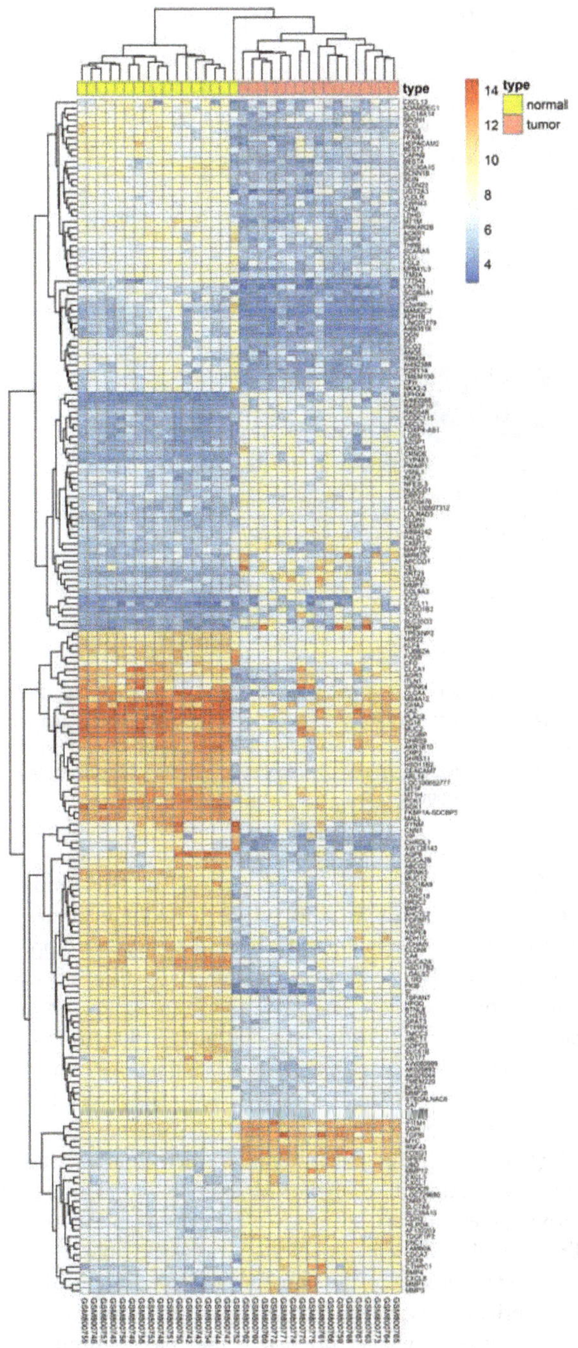

FIGURE 4 | Identification of colon cancer-related targets using pre-existing microarray data. Two hundred DEGs identified by the limma package were highly related to colon cancer. $P < 0.05$ and FC > 2 were considered cut-off values.

above. As shown in **Figures 5D,E**, the biological networks consisted of 189 nodes and 1503 edges, and the potential targets were mainly assigned to positive regulation of ROS metabolic processes, intrinsic apoptotic pathways and mammary gland development. Of these, the first two pathways have well-established roles in cell apoptosis, and the results suggested that DCMPI is highly likely to exert its antitumor effect via the apoptotic pathway.

Nuclear Staining With DAPI

In this study, HT-29 cells were monitored by DAPI staining to determine the pro-apoptotic effect of DCMPI. The administration of DCMPI at doses of 30 and 60 μg/mL for 24 h dramatically induced nuclear morphological changes, such as apoptotic bodies and nuclear fragmentation, compared with the control group (**Figure 6A**).

Apoptosis Assay With Annexin V-FITC/PI Staining

Next, the percentage of apoptotic cells induced by DCMPI treatment was detected by Annexin V-FITC/PI staining. As shown in **Figure 6B**, the numbers of HT-29 cells in both early- and late-stage apoptotic populations were remarkably increased in response to DCMPI (30 and 60 μg/mL). Therefore, this finding was consistent with the DAPI staining results and confirmed that DCMPI induced HT-29 cell apoptosis in a concentration-dependent manner.

Mitochondrial Membrane Potential (MMP, Δψm) Assessment

The loss of Δψm, which occurs prior to caspase activation, is regarded as a hallmark of apoptosis. To determine whether DCMPI treatment activated the mitochondria-mediated apoptotic pathway, we utilized the JC-1 fluorescent probe to evaluate alterations in Δψm by flow cytometry. In apoptotic cells with low Δψm, JC-1 remains in the monomeric form, and the loss of Δψm is followed by a red-to-green shift. The percentage of green JC-1 was significantly elevated by treatment with DCMPI (**Figure 6C**), and DCMPI thus markedly increased the mitochondrial membrane permeability and induced Δψm collapse.

Intracellular ROS Detection

Reactive oxygen species generation was closely associated with the cancer cell death caused by mitochondrial dysfunction and subsequent mitochondria-induced apoptosis. To identify the roles of ROS in DCMPI-induced colon cancer cell death, we measured intracellular ROS production by DCFH-DA staining with flow cytometry. DCMPI significantly increased the accumulation of fluorescent dye in HT-29 cells in a concentration-dependent manner (**Figure 6D**).

Apoptosis-Related Protein Assay

DCMPI not only significantly up-regulated the protein expression of Bax and Bad but also simultaneously attenuated the protein levels of Bcl-2 and Bcl-xl. These results revealed that DCMPI alters the Bax/Bcl-2 ratio in HT-29 cells, which subsequently stimulates the mitochondrial-mediated apoptosis pathway. Furthermore, DCMPI (30 and 60 μg/mL) induced both PARP and caspase-3/9 cleavage to aggravate HT-29 cell apoptosis (**Figure 7**).

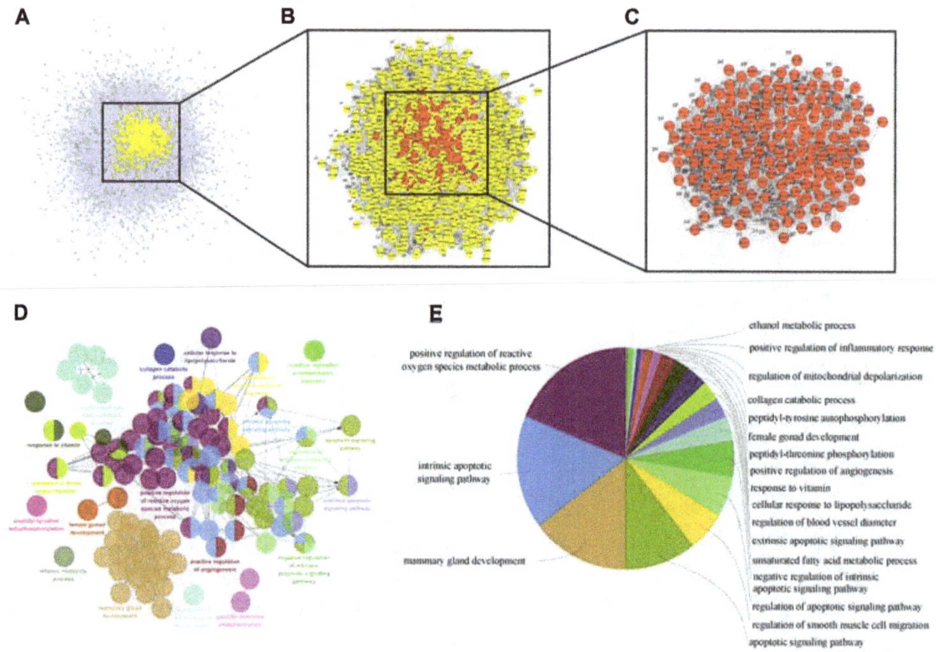

FIGURE 5 | Candidate target identification and ClueGO pathway analysis. **(A)** Core CPPI network of DCMPI targets. **(B)** Large hubs of the DCMPI CPPI network extracted from **(A)** whose degrees were more than twice the median degree of all nodes in the network. **(C)** PPI network of the main DCMPI targets extracted from **(B)** constructed by calculating 6 topological features. **(D,E)** A functionally grouped network of enriched categories was generated for the target genes. GO terms are represented as nodes, and the node size represents the term's enrichment significance. Functionally related groups partially overlap. Only the most significant term in the group is labeled. Representative enriched pathway ($P < 0.05$) interactions among the main DCMPI targets.

To clarify whether apoptosis is initiated by caspase cascade activation, we adopted the caspase inhibitor Z-VAD-FMK. Western blot analysis revealed that the cleavage of PARP and caspase 3/9 caused by DCMPI was dramatically inhibited by Z-VAD-FMK (50 μM) pretreatment (**Figure 8**). Together, these results clearly support that DCMPI induces HT-29 cell apoptosis via the mitochondrial apoptosis pathway.

DISCUSSION

Recently, medicinal fungi were shown to be ubiquitously present in nature, recognized as a promising source of food and medicine with multi-targeted effects and to have low toxicity (Gargano et al., 2017). Intriguingly, numerous preclinical and clinical trials have demonstrated that medicinal fungi contain a variety of structurally unique metabolites, which most likely possess significant activities like anti-inflammatory and antitumor (Piska et al., 2017). For instance, *P. igniarius* has been proposed as a prevalent type of edible and medicinal mushroom that has multiple highly effective protective properties (Dong et al., 2016). More importantly, *P. igniarius* attracts overwhelming attention as a potential candidate for anticancer therapeutics (De Silva et al., 2012). Cancer is a complex disease and tumorigenesis is related to inflammation (Guo et al., 2017). *P. igniarius* has potential anti-inflammatory and antitumor activities, hopeful to be developed a functional food for the prevention and control of inflammation-induced tumorigenesis in the future. Previous studies had established that the ethanol extract of *P. igniarius* suppresses SK-Hep-1 and RHE cell proliferation in a dose-dependent manner (Song et al., 2008). Furthermore, the hot water extract of *P. igniarius* directly inhibits S180 tumors and simultaneously exhibits an immune-regulatory effect on S180-bearing mice (Yang et al., 2006). However, to date, these studies largely emphasize the pharmacological effects of *P. igniarius* extracts, and no studies have characterized the chemical composition *P. igniarius* extracts or clarified their underlying mechanisms.

Traditional Chinese medicine network pharmacology was a new research strategy for translating TCM from an experience-based medicine to an evidence-based medicine system, which predicted the target profiles and pharmacological actions of herbal compounds, and revealed drug-gene-disease co-module associations to interpret the combinatorial rules and network regulation effects of herbal formulae (Liang et al., 2014; Li and Zhang, 2013). It provided a new paradigm for revealing the pharmacodynamics substance basis and mechanisms of TCM and revealing the problem of the effectiveness of TCM (Wang et al., 2017).

Therefore, we herein utilized a combination method that included a cytotoxicity test, phytochemical analysis, TCM network pharmacology, and cell and molecular biology experiments to elucidate the antitumor substances and

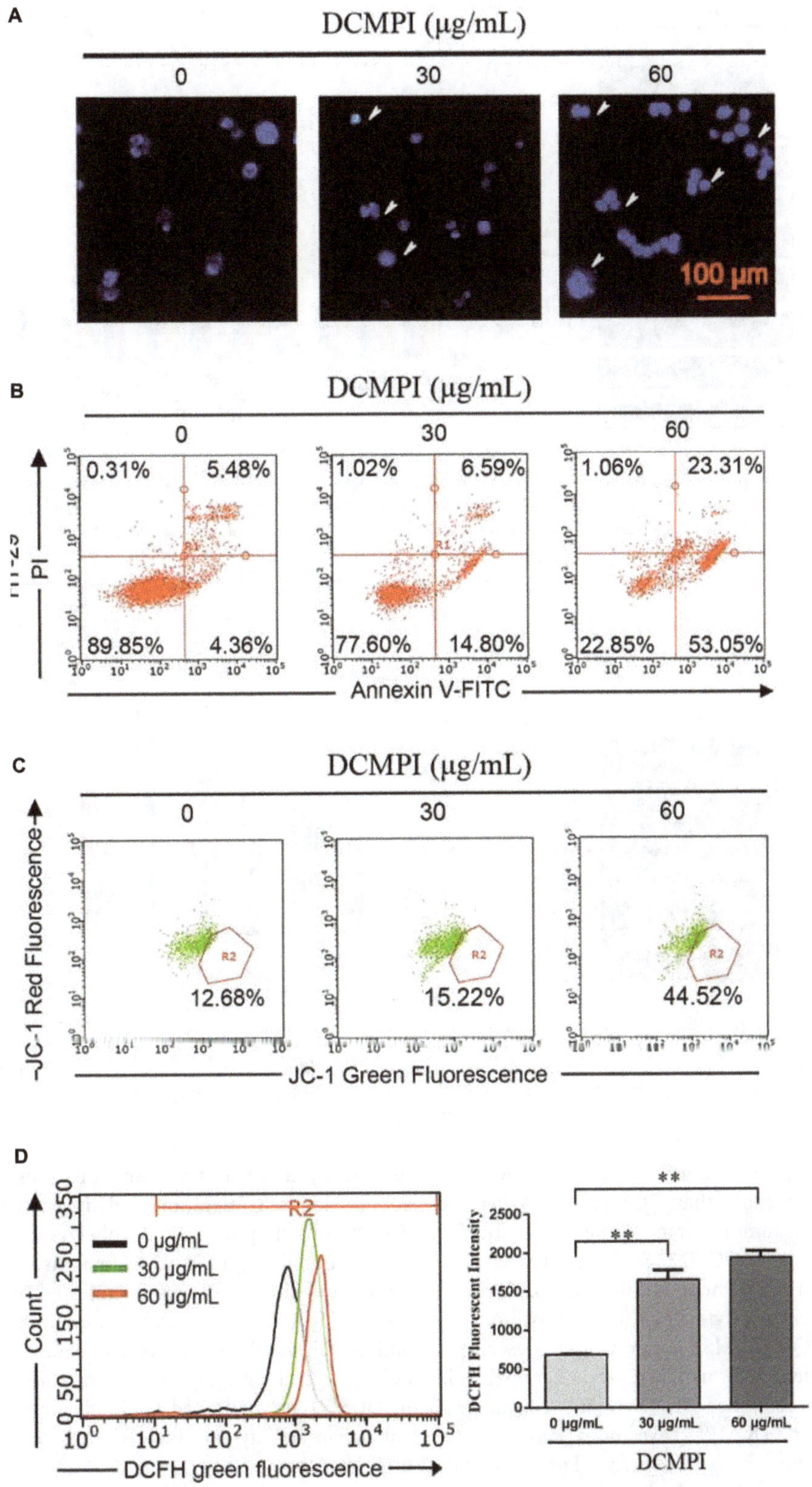

FIGURE 6 | DCMPI induced apoptosis in HT-29 colon cancer cells. **(A)** Nuclear morphological changes were observed in DCMPI-exposed HT-29 cells by DAPI staining. **(B)** The percentage of apoptotic cells induced by DCMPI treatment was detected by Annexin V/PI double-staining analysis. **(C)** The effect of DCMPI on the mitochondrial membrane potential, which was determined using a JC-1 staining assay and flow cytometry. **(D)** The effect of DCMPI on the intracellular ROS, which was detected using DCFH-DA probes and flow cytometry. $^{**}P < 0.01$. The data are presented as the mean ± SD from at least three independent experiments.

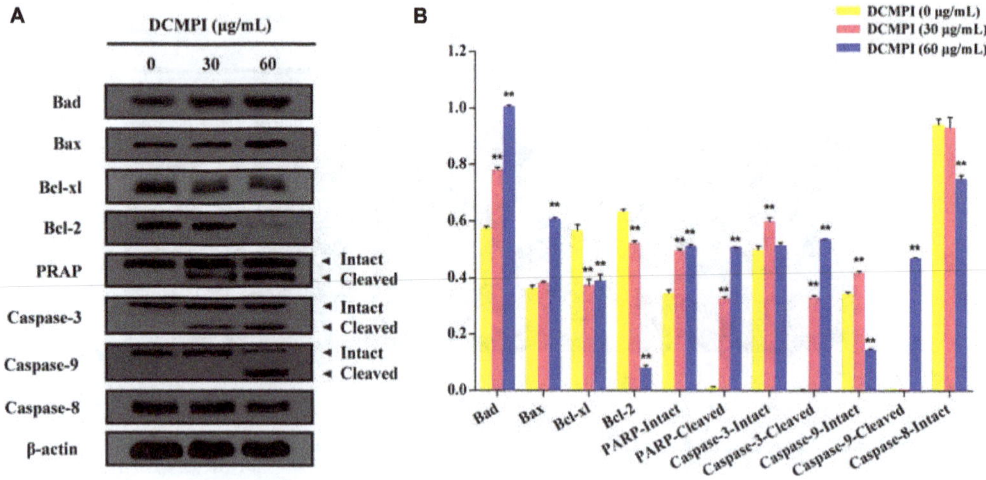

FIGURE 7 | Western blot analysis of apoptosis-related protein expression. **(A)** Bad, Bax, Bcl-xl, Bcl-2, PARP, caspase-3, caspase-9, and caspase-8 protein expression in HT-29 cells after DCMPI treatment (30 and 60 μg/mL) for 24 h. **(B)** Densitometric analysis of Bad, Bax, Bcl-xl, Bcl-2, PARP, caspase-3, caspase-9, and caspase-8 expression. $^{**}P < 0.01$. The data are presented as the mean ± SD from at least three independent experiments.

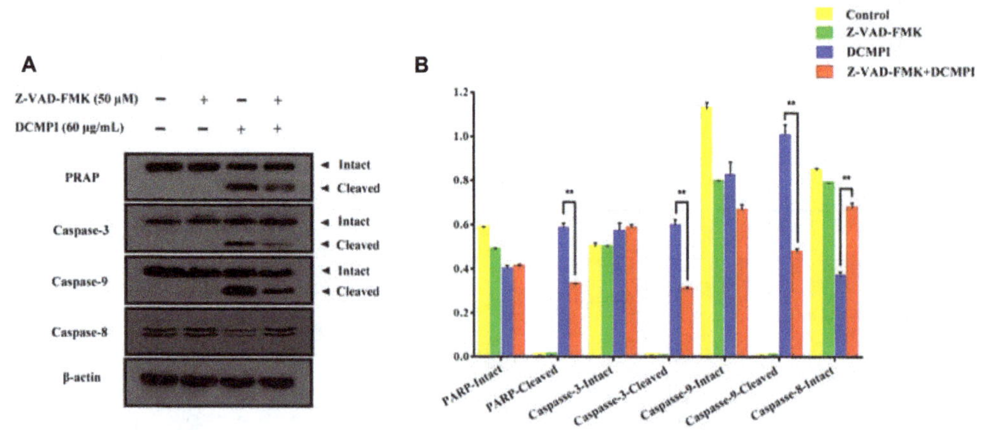

FIGURE 8 | The effect of Z-VAD-FMK (50 μM) pretreatment and DCMPI (60 μg/mL) treatment on the cleavage of PARP and caspase-3/9 in HT-29 cells. **(A)** PARP, caspase-3, caspase-9, and caspase-8 protein expression in HT-29 cells after treatment for 24 h. **(B)** Densitometric analysis of PARP, caspase-3, caspase-9, and caspase-8 expression. $^{**}P < 0.01$. The data are presented as the mean ± SD from at least three independent experiments.

potential mechanisms of *P. igniarius*. First, cytotoxicity experiments were used to show that DCMPI had a certain inhibitory effect on each tumor strain. Among the strains, the inhibitory effects on the BGC-823, SMMC7721 and HT-29 cell lines were higher than those on the others. Second, we elucidated the systemic phytochemical composition of DCMPI via UPLC-ESI-Q/TOF-MS. As previously described, 19 constituents were identified or tentatively characterized, and 5 of them were quantified by standard substances. Numerous ingredients in DCMPI have been reported to possess antitumor activity or cytotoxicity. For example, naringenin, a flavanone compound, has highly effective, diverse bioactivities, including anticancer activity (Chang et al., 2017). Eriodictyol also exerts multiple bioactive effects, and it especially inhibits cell proliferation and transformation (Zhu et al., 2015). Dihydrokaempferol serves as a flavonol extensively in citrus fruits and provides anticancer effects via suppressing cell migration and invasion (Liu X. et al., 2017). The flavonoids phelligrin A, phelligrin B, methylphelligrin A and methylphelligrin B were first discovered in the *Phellinus* family and shown to possess multiple bioactivities (Wu et al., 2011). Furthermore, several studies revealed that phelligrin A and phelligrin B provide selective cytotoxicity against cancer cells (Lee and Yun, 2011). In summary, the main compounds in DCMPI are attributed to the flavone family, and most have anticancer activity and likely account for the antitumor activity of *P. igniarius*.

Because of their complex compositions and mechanisms of action, investigating the pharmacology of TCM is a daunting task. Here, to explore the antitumor mechanism of DCMPI, we selected eight major components of DCMPI and utilized TCM network pharmacology approach to clarify their potential mechanisms. The network pharmacological analysis showed that DCMPI exerted its anticolon cancer function mainly via the positive regulation of ROS metabolic processes and intrinsic apoptotic pathways.

Apoptosis induction has been recognized as an essential mechanism in antitumor therapeutics (Janssen, 2001). Notably, numerous studies have demonstrated that anticancer agents exert their anti-proliferative effects mainly via two different apoptosis pathways involving mitochondria or death receptors (Liu B. et al., 2017). In particular, the mitochondria-associated pathway is a classic intrinsic pathway that is initiated by ROS overproduction, resulting in the depletion of $\Delta\psi m$ (Kuranaga, 2012). In general, a variety of protein molecules are involved in regulating the mitochondrial apoptotic pathway, including pro-apoptotic members (e.g., Bax and Bad) and anti-apoptotic members (e.g., Bcl-2 and Bcl-xl) (Czabotar et al., 2014). Furthermore, the pathway activates the specific pivotal proteinases as initiator caspase-9 and effector caspase-3, which subsequently leads to DNA fragmentation and nuclear PARP degradation during apoptosis (Kuranaga, 2012).

To verify the network pharmacology prediction results, *in vitro* cell experiments were carried out. DAPI and Annexin V-FITC/PI staining were performed to determine the apoptotic alterations associated with the cytotoxicity of HT-29 cells. Apoptotic bodies, nuclear fragmentation and early- and late-stage apoptotic populations were increased by DCMPI. Therefore, the cytotoxic effect of DCMPI on HT-29 cells appeared to be mediated by apoptosis. Apoptosis is considered to be a regulated form of cell death, and dysregulated apoptosis leads to a variety of aberrant pathological conditions and subsequent diseases, especially cancer (Sankari et al., 2012; Goldar et al., 2015). Remarkably, two main signaling pathways involving caspase-mediated apoptosis have been identified: the mitochondrial-mediated intrinsic pathway and the death receptor-mediated extrinsic pathway (Khan et al., 2014). Compelling evidence has indicated that increased levels of intracellular ROS result in mitochondrial swelling and MMP loss, which, in turn, activates the intrinsic apoptotic pathway. Because ROS overproduction not only causes severe DNA damage but also suppresses tumor growth, aggravated cell structures break down, and cancer cells die (Renschler, 2004). In this study, DCMPI stimulated the generation of intracellular ROS in a dose-dependent manner, induced MMP collapse and ultimately contributed to mitochondria-mediated apoptosis.

Bcl-2 family members, including Bcl-2, Bcl-xl, Bax, and Bad, are major regulators located in the mitochondria (Borkan, 2016). As anti-apoptotic proteins, Bcl-2 and Bcl-xl intervene in various apoptotic signals, whereas Bax and Bad serve as pro-apoptotic proteins and trigger the activation of caspases by mitochondrial dysfunction. In the present study, DCMPI down-regulated anti-apoptotic Bcl-xl and Bcl-2 expression and simultaneously enhanced the translocation of the activated pro-apoptotic proteins Bax and Bad. More importantly, subsequent activation of the caspase-dependent pathway was recognized as a pivotal step in the apoptotic process, and a series of initiator

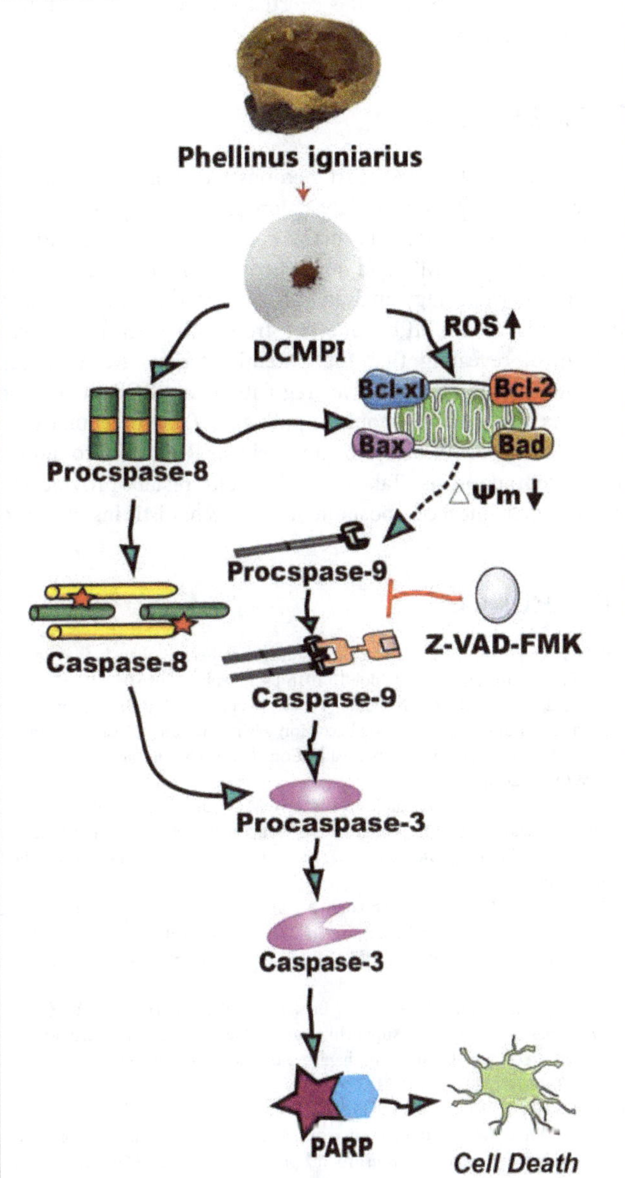

FIGURE 9 | Molecular mechanisms underlying the antitumor activity of DCMPI. DCMPI increased intracellular ROS levels and induced HT-29 cell apoptosis mainly mediated via the mitochondrial apoptosis pathway.

caspases was involved in the progression. Briefly, activation of the initiator caspase as caspase-9 activates downstream or executioner caspases undergoing apoptosis, such as caspase-3 (Nuñez et al., 1998; Kim and Hong, 2011). Furthermore, executioner caspase activation was responsible for a series of apoptotic biochemical characteristics, especially the cleavage of PARP, which facilitated cellular disassembly and resulted in DNA fragmentation. Herein, our findings demonstrated that DCMPI induced apoptosis in HT-29 cells by up-regulating cleaved caspase-3/9 and PARP. In addition, pretreatment with the pan-caspase inhibitor Z-VAD-FMK inhibited caspase and PARP cleavage, which confirmed that the pro-apoptotic effect of DCMPI in HT-29 cells was exerted via a caspase-dependent pathway (**Figure 9**).

CONCLUSION

In the current study, we first demonstrated that the DCMPI dramatically suppressed HT-29 colon cancer cell proliferation. Then, we characterized 19 main constituents of DCMPI by UPLC-ESI-Q/TOF-MS, and quantified 5 of them. Furthermore, network pharmacology analysis focusing on the 8 high content compounds of DCMPI (different from other fractions) was performed, revealing that the potential targets were mainly associated with the positive regulation of ROS metabolic processes and intrinsic apoptotic pathways. Finally, cellular tests verified that DCMPI increased intracellular ROS levels to induce HT-29 cell apoptosis. Taken together, our results provide the antitumor chemical composition of and mechanistic insights into *P. igniarius*, which may be exploited as a promising therapeutic option for colon cancer.

AUTHOR CONTRIBUTIONS

YD and PQ wrote the manuscript. YD, PQ, RZ, LZ, PZ, and YW conducted the research and analyzed the data. CL, KC, DS, and HZ conceived or designed the studies. All authors read and approved the final manuscript.

FUNDING

This research was funded by National Natural Science Foundation of China (Nos. 81603349 and 81673809) and Key Research and Development Plan of Zhejiang Province (No. 2015C03033).

REFERENCES

Borkan, S. C. (2016). The role of BCL-2 family members in acute kidney injury. *Semin. Nephrol.* 36, 237–250. doi: 10.1016/j.semnephrol.2016.04.001

Cao, H., Li, S., Xie, R., Xu, N., Qian, Y., Chen, H., et al. (2018). Exploring the mechanism of dangguiliuhuang decoction against hepatic fibrosis by network pharmacology and experimental validation. *Front. Pharmacol.* 9:187. doi: 10.3389/fphar.2018.00187

Chang, H. L., Chang, Y. M., Lai, S. C., Chen, K. M., Wang, K. C., Chiu, T. T., et al. (2017). Naringenin inhibits migration of lung cancer cells via the inhibition of matrix metalloproteinases-2 and -9. *Exp. Ther. Med.* 13, 739–744. doi: 10.3892/etm.2016.3994

Czabotar, P. E., Lessene, G., Strasser, A., and Adams, J. M. (2014). Control of apoptosis by the BCL-2 protein family: implications for physiology and therapy. *Nat. Rev. Mol. Cell Biol.* 15, 49–63. doi: 10.1038/nrm3722

De Silva, D. D., Rapior, S., Fons, F., Bahkali, A. H., and Hyde, K. D. (2012). Medicinal mushrooms in supportive cancer therapies: an approach to anti-cancer effects and putative mechanisms of action. *Fungal Divers.* 55, 1–35. doi: 10.1007/s13225-012-0151-3

Dong, Y., He, Y., Yu, Z. M., Zhang, Y., Wang, N. N., Shou, D., et al. (2016). Metabolomic investigation of rat serum following oral administration of the willow bracket medicinal mushroom, phellinus igniarius (Agaricomycetes), by UPLC-HDMS. *Int. J. Med. Mushrooms* 18, 699–711. doi: 10.1615/IntJMedMushrooms.v18.i8.60

Dong, Y., Wang, H., Zhang, Y., An, N., Zhang, Y., and Shou, D. (2015). Ultra high performance liquid chromatography with synapt high-definition mass spectrometry and a pattern recognition approach to characterize chemical constituents and rat metabolites after the oral administration of *Phellinus igniarius*. *J. Sep. Sci.* 38, 1137–1148. doi: 10.1002/jssc.201401293

Gargano, M. L., van Griensven, L. J. L. D., Isikhuemhen, O. S., Lindequist, U., Venturella, G., Wasser, S. P., et al. (2017). Medicinal mushrooms: valuable biological resources of high exploitation potential. *Plant Biosyst.* 151, 548–565. doi: 10.1080/11263504.2017.1301590

Goldar, S., Khaniani, M. S., Derakhshan, S. M., and Baradaran, B. (2015). Molecular mechanisms of apoptosis and roles in cancer development and treatment. *Asian Pac. J. Cancer Prev.* 16, 2129–2144. doi: 10.7314/APJCP.2015.16.6.2129

Guo, Y., Nie, Q., Maclean, A. L., Li, Y., Lei, J., and Li, S. (2017). Multiscale modeling of inflammation-induced tumorigenesis reveals competing oncogenic and oncoprotective roles for inflammation. *Cancer Res.* 77, 6429–6441. doi: 10.1158/0008-5472.CAN-17-1662

Hare, J. I., Lammers, T., Ashford, M. B., Puri, S., Storm, G., and Barry, S. T. (2017). Challenges and strategies in anti-cancer nanomedicine development: an industry perspective. *Adv. Drug Deliver. Rev.* 108, 25–38. doi: 10.1016/j.addr.2016.04.025

Huang, T., Ning, Z., Hu, D., Zhang, M., Zhao, L., Lin, C., et al. (2018). Uncovering the mechanisms of chinese herbal medicine (mazirenwan) for functional constipation by focused network pharmacology approach. *Front. Pharmacol.* 9:270. doi: 10.3389/fphar.2018.00270

Janssen, O. (2001). Staurosporine and conventional anticancer drugs induce overlapping, yet distinct pathways of apoptosis and caspase activation. *Oncogene* 20, 1193–1202. doi: 10.1038/sj.onc.1204221

Jeon, T. I., Jung, C. H., Cho, J. Y., Park, D. K., and Moon, J. H. (2013). Identification of an anticancer compound against HT-29 cells from *Phellinus linteus* grown on germinated brown rice. *Asian Pac. J. Trop. Biomed.* 3, 785–789. doi: 10.1016/S2221-1691(13)60156-2

Khan, K. H., Blancocodesido, M., and Molife, L. R. (2014). Cancer therapeutics: targeting the apoptotic pathway. *Crit. Rev. Oncol. Hemat.* 90, 200–219. doi: 10.1016/j.critrevonc.2013.12.012

Kim, B. M., and Hong, S. H. (2011). Sequential caspase-2 and caspase-8 activation is essential for saikosaponin a-induced apoptosis of human colon carcinoma cell lines. *Apoptosis* 16, 184–197. doi: 10.1007/s10495-010-0557-x

Kim, B. Y., Song, K. H., Lim, C. Y., and Cho, S. I. (2017). Therapeutic properties of scutellaria baicalensis in db/db mice evaluated using connectivity map and network pharmacology. *Sci. Rep.* 7:41711. doi: 10.1038/srep41711

Kuranaga, E. (2012). Beyond apoptosis: caspase regulatory mechanisms and functions in vivo. *Genes Cells* 17, 83–97. doi: 10.1111/j.1365-2443.2011.01579.x

Lee, I. K., and Yun, B. S. (2011). Styrylpyrone-class compounds from medicinal fungi phellinus and inonotus spp. and their medicinal importance. *J. Antibiot.* 64, 349–359. doi: 10.1038/ja.2011.2

Li, S., and Zhang, B. (2013). Traditional chinese medicine network pharmacology: theory, methodology and application. *Chin. J. Nat. Med.* 11, 110–120. doi: 10.3724/SP.J.1009.2013.00110

Li, X., Wu, Q., Xie, Y., Ding, Y. R., Du, W. W., Sdiri, M., et al. (2015). Ergosterol purified from medicinal mushroom *Amauroderma rude* inhibits cancer growth in vitro and in vivo by up-regulating multiple tumor suppressors. *Oncotarget* 6, 17832–17846. doi: 10.18632/oncotarget.4026

Liang, X., Li, H., and Li, S. (2014). A novel network pharmacology approach to analyse traditional herbal formulae: the Liu-Wei-Di-Huang pill as a case study. *Mol. BioSyst.* 10, 1014–1022. doi: 10.1039/c3mb70507b

Liu, B., Sun, R., Luo, H., Liu, X., Jiang, M., Yuan, C., et al. (2017). Both intrinsic and extrinsic apoptotic pathways are involved in Toll-like receptor 4 (TLR4)-induced cell death in monocytic THP-1 cells. *Immunobiology* 222, 198–205. doi: 10.1016/j.imbio.2016.10.002

Liu, X., Xiang, M., Fan, Y., Yang, C., Zeng, L., Zhang, Q., et al. (2017). A root-preferential DFR-Like gene encoding dihydrokaempferol reductase involved in anthocyanin biosynthesis of purple-fleshed sweet potato. *Front. Plant Sci.* 8:279. doi: 10.3389/fpls.2017.00279

Ma, X., dan Guo, D., Peterson, E. C., Dun, Y., and Li, D. Y. (2016). Structural characterization and anti-aging activity of a novel extracellular polysaccharide from fungus Phellinus sp. in a mammalian system. *Food Funct.* 7, 3468–3479. doi: 10.1039/c6fo00422a

Nuñez, G., Benedict, M. A., Hu, Y., and Inohara, N. (1998). Caspases: the proteases of the apoptotic pathway. *Oncogene* 17, 3237–3245. doi: 10.1038/sj.onc.1202581

Piska, K., Sułkowska-Ziaja, K., and Muszyńska, B. (2017). Edible mushroom pleurotus ostreatus (Oyster mushroom)-Its dietary significance and biological activity. *Acta Sci. Pol Hortoru.* 16, 151–161.

Renschler, M. F. (2004). The emerging role of reactive oxygen species in cancer therapy. *Eur. J. Cancer* 40, 1934–1940. doi: 10.1016/j.ejca.2004.02.031

Sangdee, K., Buranrat, B., Naksuwankul, K., Jaihan, P., and Sangdee, A. (2017). Antibacterial and anti-breast cancer cell line activities of Sanghuangporus sp. 1 extracts. *Trop. J. Pharm. Res.* 16, 613–620. doi: 10.4314/tjpr.v16i3.16

Sankari, S. L., Masthan, K. M., Babu, N. A., Bhattacharjee, T., and Elumalai, M. (2012). Apoptosis in cancer–an update. *Asian Pac. J. Cancer Prev.* 13, 4873–4878. doi: 10.7314/APJCP.2012.13.10.4873

Shou, D., Dong, Y., Wang, N. N., Li, H. Y., Zhang, Y., and Zhu, Y. (2016). Simultaneous quantification of antioxidant compounds in phellinus igniarius using ultra performance liquid chromatography-photodiode array detection-electrospray ionization tandem mass spectrometry. *PLoS One* 11:e0163797. doi: 10.1371/journal.pone.0163797

Siegel, R. L., Miller, K. D., and Jemal, A. (2016). Cancer statistics, 2016. *CA Cancer J. Clin.* 66, 7–30. doi: 10.3322/caac.21332

Song, T. Y., Lin, H. C., Yang, N. C., and Hu, M. L. (2008). Antiproliferative and antimetastatic effects of the ethanolic extract of *Phellinus igniarius* (Linnearus: Fries) quelet. *J. Ethnopharmacol.* 115, 50–56. doi: 10.1016/j.jep.2007.09.001

Wang, X., Yu, S., Jia, Q., Chen, L., Zhong, J., Pan, Y., et al. (2017). Niaoduqing granules relieve chronic kidney disease symptoms by decreasing renal fibrosis and anemia. *Oncotarget* 8, 55920–55937. doi: 10.18632/oncotarget.18473

Wu, C. S., Lin, Z. M., Wang, L. N., Guo, D. X., Wang, S. Q., Liu, Y. Q., et al. (2011). Phenolic compounds with NF-κB inhibitory effects from the fungus phellinus baumii. *Bioorg. Med. Chem. Lett.* 21, 3261–3267. doi: 10.1016/j.bmcl.2011.04.025

Yang, Q., Hu, X. G., Wan, Q., and Wang, W. Q. (2006). Study on anti-tumor effect of medicinal fungi Phellinus igniarius extracts. *Chin. J. Chinese Mater. Med.* 31, 1713–1715.

Zhang, Q., Yu, H., Qi, J., Tang, D., Chen, X., Wan, J. B., et al. (2017). Natural formulas and the nature of formulas: exploring potential therapeutic targets based on traditional Chinese herbal formulas. *PLoS One* 12:e0171628. doi: 10.1371/journal.pone.0171628

Zhou, C., Jiang, S. S., Wang, C. Y., Li, R., and Che, H. L. (2014). Different immunology mechanisms of *Phellinus igniarius* in inhibiting growth of liver cancer and melanoma cells. *Asian Pac. J. Cancer Prev.* 15, 3659–3665. doi: 10.7314/APJCP.2014.15.8.3659

Zhu, G., Guo, H., Huang, Y., Wu, C. T., and Zhang, X. F. (2015). Eriodictyol, a plant flavonoid, attenuates LPS-induced acute lung injury through its antioxidative and anti-inflammatory activity. *Exp. Ther. Med.* 10, 2259–2266. doi: 10.3892/etm.2015.2827

6

An Integrated Pharmacology-Based Analysis for Antidepressant Mechanism of Chinese Herbal Formula Xiao-Yao-San

Naijun Yuan [1†], Lian Gong [1†], Kairui Tang [1], Liangliang He [1,2], Wenzhi Hao [1], Xiaojuan Li [1], Qingyu Ma [1] and Jiaxu Chen [1]*

[1] *Formula-Pattern Research Center, School of Traditional Chinese Medicine, Jinan University, Guangzhou, China,* [2] *College of Pharmacy, Jinan University, Guangzhou, China*

***Correspondence:**
Jiaxu Chen
chenjiaxu@hotmail.com*

† These authors share first authorship

Clinical studies and basic science experiments have widely demonstrated the antidepressant and anxiolytic effects of the herbal formula Xiao-Yao-San (XYS). However, the system mechanism of these effects has not been fully characterized. The present study conducted a comprehensive network pharmacological analysis of XYS and sorted all pharmacologically active components (149) through the TCMSP webserver. Then, all potential molecular targets (449) were predicted, of which there were 99 genes clearly related to depression. To further investigate the mechanism of antidepressant effects of XYS, a compound-depression targets (C-DTs) network was constructed, and Gene Ontology (GO) functional and KEGG pathway enrichment analyses were performed for the 99 targets. Enrichment results revealed that XYS could regulate multiple aspects of depression through these targets, related to metabolism, neuroendocrine function, and neuroimmunity. Prediction and analysis of protein–protein interactions resulted in selection of three hub genes (AKT1, TP53, and VEGFA). In addition, a total of seven ingredients from XYS could act on these hub genes and they were identified through ultra-high-performance liquid chromatography-quadrupole time-of-flight mass spectrometry (UPLC-Q/TOF-MS), including paeoniflorin, quercetin, luteolin, acacetin, aloe-emodin, Glyasperin C, kaempferol. Hereafter, we investigated the effects of paeoniflorin and its predicted target, the results suggest that it can reverse the neurotoxicity produced by CORT and could be a neuroprotective effect by promoting the phosphorylation of Akt. Overall, our research revealed the complicated antidepressant mechanism of XYS, and also provided a rational strategy for revealing the complex composition and function of Chinese herbal formula.

Keywords: network pharmacology, Xiao-Yao-San, depression, Chinese herb formula, integration analysis methods

INTRODUCTION

Depression is a psychological disorder with widespread prevalence, affecting more than 350 million individuals worldwide, and the prevalence is gradually increasing (Kuo et al., 2015). Because of high morbidity and mortality, depression has received extensive attention. Currently, the main treatment strategy for depression is pharmacotherapy, but antidepressants typically do not completely alleviate depressive symptoms and may lead to drug addiction and adverse side effects for patients (Tom et al., 2014; Solem et al., 2017).

Development of medicines that have antidepressant effects and produce less side effects than current antidepressants is a priority. Therefore, complementary and alternative medicine (CAM) and traditional Chinese medicine (TCM) have received attention as potential strategies for treatment and prevention of depression. Xiao-Yao-San (XYS) has been used in TCM clinics for more than a century to treat various diseases with characteristic features of liver stagnation and spleen deficiency syndrome (LSSDS) (Meng et al., 2013). There are eight Chinese herbs in XYS: *Angelica sinensis* (Oliver) Diels (AS, family: Apiaceae); *Paeonia lactiflora* Pallas (PN, family: Paeoniaceae); *Bupleurum Chinense* De Candolle (BR, family: Apiaceae); *Atractylodes macrocephala* Koidzumi (AMR, family: Compositae); *Poria cocos* (Schweinitz) Wolf (PR, family: Polyporaceae); *Mentha canadensis* Linnaeus (MH; family: Lamiaceae); *Glycyrrhiza uralensis* Fischer (GRH; family: Leguminosea); *Zingiber officinale* Roscoe (ZRR, family: Zingiberaceae).

XYS has been widely prescribed as a safe and effective treatment or adjuvant therapy for depression, because psychological stress syndromes primarily are classified as LSSDS in TCM theory. Clinical studies and basic science experiments have demonstrated the antidepressant and anxiolytic effects of XYS (Dai et al., 2010; Chen and Hou, 2017), but the associated mechanisms have not been characterized.

Systems pharmacology is an emerging field that integrates bioinformatics and experimental methods to advance drug discovery and provides a method for clarification of mechanisms of action of Chinese herbs (Berger and Iyengar, 2009). A drug (active compounds)-targets-diseases (clinical symptoms) network can be constructed and analyzed using a holistic view though this method (Kim et al., 2019; Zhou et al., 2019). It can determine the enrichment of targets, and elucidate complex effects and pharmacological mechanisms of Chinese herbs (Kloft et al., 2016). The present study aimed to identify the bioactive components and mechanisms of action of the TCM formula XYS in the treatment of depression using system network pharmacological analysis.

Abbreviations: CAM, Complementary and alternative medicine; TCM, Traditional Chinese Medicine; XYS, Xiao-Yao-San; LSSDS, Liver stagnation and spleen deficiency syndrome; AS, *Angelica sinensis* (Oliver) Diels; PN, *Paeonia lactiflora* Pallas; BR, *Bupleurum Chinense* De Candolle; AMR, *Atractylodes macrocephala* Koidzumi; PR, *Poria cocos* (Schweinitz) Wolf; MH, *Mentha canadensis* Linnaeus; GRH, *Glycyrrhiza uralensis* Fischer; ZRR, *Zingiber officinale* Roscoe; OB, oral bioavailability; DL, drug-likeness; DEGs, differentially expressed genes; PCA, principal component analysis; GO, Gene Ontology; CC, cellular component; MF, molecular function; KEGG, Kyoto Encyclopedia of Genes and Genomes; MW, molecular weight; ALogP, the value of partition coefficient between octanol and water; nHdon, the number of possible hydrogen-bond donors; nHacc, and the number of hydrogen-bond acceptors; BDNF, brain-derived neurotrophic factor; UPLC–Q/TOF-MS, ultra-high performance liquid chromatography-quadrupole time-of-flight mass spectrometry; CORT, corticosterone; PF, paeoniflorin.

MATERIALS AND METHODS

Data Preparation

Construction of XYS Chemical Constituent Databases

All chemical constituents of each of the herbs in XYS were obtained from the TCMSP data server (Traditional Chinese Medicine Systems Pharmacology Database and Analysis Platform, http://lsp.nwu.edu.cn/tcmsp.php), which is a unique systems-level pharmacology server for TCM (Ru et al., 2014). TCMSP can also provide pharmacology-related properties and predict targets and related diseases for each active ingredient based on critically evaluated pharmacological and clinical knowledge. This ground-breaking data server highlights the role that systems pharmacology can play in the traditional Chinese medicine discipline. Moreover, ADME properties data were also derived from TCMSP, comprising molecular weight (MW), octanol-water coefficient (ALogP), number of possible hydrogen-bond donors (nHdon), and number of hydrogen-bond acceptors (nHacc).

Evaluation the Drug-Likeness

Potential drugs in XYS were mainly identified by integrating oral bioavailability (OB) and drug-likeness (DL) properties. Comprehensive analysis of bioavailability and structural descriptors for predicting OB values for each compound were previously determined *in-silico* (Xue et al., 2012). [OB%]. Data server-dependent DL models were used to determine solubility and chemical stability based on the Tanimoto coefficient, using the following formula: $T(A, B) = (A \times B)/(|A|^2 + |B|^2 - A \times B)$ (Tao et al., 2013). Then, according to recommendations from TCMSP, we selected screening criteria of OB $\geq$ 30% and DL $\geq$ 0.18 for determination of possible bioactive components.

Known Antidepressant Drug/Drug-Like Compounds Database Construction

Known antidepressant drug/drug-like compounds from the cMap database

Gene profiling of depression was performed using GSE12654 from GEO database, which contains frozen brain tissues from 11 depressed individuals and brain tissues from 15 non-depressed individuals (Iwamoto et al., 2004). Differentially expressed genes (DEGs) with the criteria $|\log FC| > 1.2$ and $P < 0.05$ were determined by "limma" package in R studio software. Moreover, the connectivity map (cMap) database is a collection of genome-wide transcriptional expression data from cultured human cells treated with bioactive small molecules that uses simple pattern-matching algorithms allowing for elucidation of functional connections between drugs, genes, and diseases through transitory common gene expression changes (Fang et al., 2003). After determining dysregulated genes, we converted the associated gene symbols to Affymetrix probe IDs, as the cMap database is based on these identifiers. $P < 0.05$ was used as the threshold for statistical significance.

Known antidepressant drug/drug-like compounds from DrugBank database

DrugBank (http://www.drugbank.ca/) is a unique online database used as a bioinformatics and cheminformatics resource that compiles extensive drug-related information (Wishart et al., 2017). Therefore, DrugBank was also searched for antidepressant drugs or drug-like compounds which were approved by the United States Food and Drug Administration (FDA) for clinical trials.

Principal Component Analysis and Correlation Analysis

To evaluate the chemical distribution of antidepressant-related compounds in XYS, we used principal component analysis (PCA) for physicochemical-related parameters (MW, ALogP, nHDon, and nHAcc) though the prcomp function in R studio software. Therefore, known antidepressant drug/drug-like compounds from cMap, DrugBank, and active ingredients from XYS were also analyzed by PCA. Furthermore, the correlation of ADME properties of these compounds was also analyzed. Pearson r coefficients were calculated to evaluate the correlation between the three groups.

Target prediction

Corresponding protein targets of each active ingredient in XYS were predicted using several databases. Predicted targets from TCMSP were extracted and converted to target names using UniProtKB (http://www.uniprot.org) (Emmanuel et al., 2016). Then, PubChem, STITCH (Kuhn et al., 2012), and PharmMapper were used to obtain potential targets. The prediction results from the PharmMapper server (http://lilab.ecust.edu.cn/pharmmapper/) were based on the pharmacophore model, and this server is a large, in-house collection of pharmacophore databases extracted from all targets in TargetBank, DrugBank, BindingDB, and PDTD (Wang et al., 2017). Target information was set to Homo sapiens and aggregated for further analysis.

Network Construction

Construction of an Active Compound-Targets Network for XYS

To clarify the relationship between active compounds in XYS (C) and depression-related targets, depression-related genes were retrieved from the OMIM database (Ada et al., 2005), DisGeNET database (Piñero et al., 2015), TTD database (Zhu et al., 2010), and GSE12654 gene chip. Intersections of disease (depression)-related genes (DGs) with the above predicted targets were determined to create an XYS antidepressant C-DTs network. This network was constructed and visualized using Cytoscape 3.4.0 software.

Comprehensive Analysis

Functional enrichment analysis of XYS related targets

To analyse targets groups of active compounds in XYS, we used enrichment analysis, as this method can effectively increase the reliability of the identification of biological phenomena, resulting in meaningful annotation information. (i) GO annotation: In this study, "clusterProfiler" package in R studio was used for GO (Gene Ontology) enrichment analysis. "ClusterProfiler" is based on multiple resources, and also serves as a user-friendly enrichment tool with integrated gene cluster analysis (Yu et al., 2012). This R package provides for GO gene annotation enrichment analysis, including cellular component (CC), molecular function (MF), and biological process (BP) analyses. $P < 0.05$ were considered statistically significant. (ii) KEGG pathway analysis: To explore potential biological mechanisms of predicted targets, the "clusterProfiler" R package was used to annotate Kyoto Encyclopedia of Genes and Genomes (KEGG) pathways of targets genes potentially regulated by active compounds contained in XYS. In addition, significantly enriched KEGG pathways should contain at least three genes, and have $P < 0.05$.

Interactions between targets in the C-DTs network

Protein–protein interaction data analysis is an important mechanism to characterize the molecular basis of disease. Interactions between each target in the C-DTs network which could be regulated by XYS were searched using the STRING website, which is a comprehensive prediction server (Szklarczyk et al., 2017). Interaction scores should be more than 0.9 to indicate appropriate confidence in identified protein interactions. Using this tool, it is feasible to discover targets related to active components of XYS based on protein network.

Key Active Compounds Screening and Evaluation

Key active compounds screening

To evaluate the antidepressant role of each active compound in XYS, hub DGs were identified using four different analysis methods in "cytoHubba" of cytoscape 3.4.0 software (Chin et al., 2014). The potential key active compounds in XYS for treatment of depression were incorporated into a Sankey diagram to reveal relationships between "hub genes - active compounds."

UPLC–Q/TOF-MS analysis

The test samples of XYS according to the prescription proportion of 'Chinese Pharmacopeia' (AS: PN: BR: AMR: PR: ZRR: GRH: MH = 5: 5: 5: 5: 5: 5: 4: 1) were provided by Jiuzhitang Co., Ltd. (Commission, 2015). And the fine powder was carried out by crushing and mixing all herbs. Next, we accurately weighted 1 g of above powder and added 50% methanol to dissolve, then using ultrasonic treatment at room temperature for 30 min. After centrifuging at 13,000 rpm for 10 min, we injected in supernatant (2 μL) for further UPLC-Q/TOF-MS analysis.

The information of equipment used in the UPLC-Q/TOF-MS analysis was detailed described in our previous research (He et al., 2018). The universal mixed mobile phase composed of water (solvent A) and acetonitrile (solvent B), both of which contain 0.1% formic acid (v/v). Gradient elution system used a flow rate of 0.4 mL/min, and adopted as follow: 5% B, 0–0.5 min; 5–80% B, 0.5–10 min; 80–100% B, 10–12 min; 100% B, 12–13 min; 100–5% B, 13–14 min; 5% B, 14–15 min. The injection volume was set as 2 μL and under 280 nm wavelength to detect. Mass spectral data were collected in Centroided. And the purity of all reference standards was above 98% that analyzed by HPLC (High performance liquid chromatography).

Experiments and Molecular Evaluation

Cell culture

Differentiated PC12 cells were employed in the experiments. RPIM 1640 basic medium supplemented with 5% fetal bovine serum (Gibco, Rockville, MD, USA), 10% Horse serum (Gibco, Rockville, MD, USA), and 1% antibiotic mixture comprising penicillin and streptomycin (Gibco, Rockville, MD, USA). Cells were under the 5% CO_2 in a humidified incubator (Thermo, USA) at 37°C. NGF (nerve growth factor, 50 ng/ml, 48 h) was used for PC12 differentiation.

Cell viability assay

The effect of paeoniflorin reverse neurotoxicity from corticosterone, cell viability was determined by the MTT assay (Fotakis and Timbrell, 2006). Briefly, PC12 cells were seeded into 96-well plate with the concentration of $5 \times 10^3/100$ μl, then incubated the cells under the conventional culture condition overnight. After 24 h treatment that with the mixture of 200μM CORT plus different concentrations of paeoniflorin (10 μM, 20 μM, 40 μM), 10 μl MTT (0.5 mg/ml) was added to each well, followed by 4 h of incubation at 37°C. Then carefully remove the supernatant, and 100 μl DMSO was added to each well to dissolve the formazan crystal. The absorbance was recorded at 570 nm by microtiter plate reader. Cell viability was calculated as a percentage of the untreated or vehicle-treated control and averaged from three independent experiments.

Western blot analysis

Total protein was extracted from the PC-12 cells in different groups. Briefly, the collected were immediately lysed in RIPA lysis buffer containing PMSF and phosphatase protein inhibitor (Beyotime Biotechnology, Jiangsu, China). The protein lysates separated by 10% SDS-PAGE gel were electrophoretically transferred to polyvinylidene difluoride (PVDF) membranes (Millipore, Billerica, MA, USA). The following specific primary antibodies were used for incubate membranes overnight at 4°C: anti-GAPDH (Beijing BioDee Biotechnology Co., Ltd.), anti-AKT (Cell Signaling Technology), anti-Phospho-AKT (Cell Signaling Technology). After probed with a 1:5000 dilution of horseradish peroxidase (HRP) conjugated secondary antibody (Beijing BioDee Biotechnology Co., Ltd.), the labeled proteins were detected by using enhanced chemiluminescence (ECL) detection.

Molecular docking evaluation

Furthermore, AutoDock 4.0 was used to evaluate the hub genes with active compounds, which is widely used for the study of bound conformation and binding free energy of ligand to the protein (Forli et al., 2016).

Statistical Analysis

Data are presented as means ± standard deviation. The standard two-tailed student's t-test was used for analysis and $P < 0.05$ were considered significant.

RESULTS

Bioactive Compounds in Xiaoyao San

Bioactive ingredients in XYS and corresponding ADME information were extracted from the TCMSP data server by filtering by drug-like threshold (OB > 30% and DL > 0.18). Several of the herbal medicines in XYS contain the same active ingredients, such as quercetin, a natural flavonoid, which is present in BR and in GRH. In addition, stigmasterol is present in AS, RB and ZRR. In total, 149 active compounds were identified in XYS, including 12 in PN, 2 in AS, 18 in BR, 15 in PR, 7 in AMR, 91 in GRH, 5 in ZRR, and 10 in MH. Detailed information regarding these molecules is summarized in **Table S1**.

To determine the molecular diversity of the constituents of each herbal medicine, the constituents were evaluated based on four significant physicochemical properties (**Figures 1A–D, Table 1**): MW, ALogP, nHdon, and nHacc. (i) MW index indicated that PR had the highest average MW of bioactive components (467.78 ± 37.66), and RG (348.41 ± 63.69) had the lowest average MW of active components. (ii) Bioactive components in AS had the highest average ALogP value (7.86 ± 0.31), and MHH constituents had the lowest average ALogP value (2.32 ± 2.27). (iii) HM had the highest average number of nHdon (3.60 ± 2.01), and RAM (0.43 ± 0.53) had the lowest average number of nHdon. (iv) The herbal constituents with the highest and lowest average number of hydrogen-bond acceptors were MHH and AS, respectively.

Identified Antidepressant Drugs and PCA

We retrieved the publicly available microarray dataset GSE12654 from GEO, which included frozen brain tissues of 11 humans with depression and 15 individuals without depression (Iwamoto et al., 2004). After applying thresholds log|FC| >1.2 and $P < 0.05$ using "limma" in R studio, a total of 29 significantly differentially expressed genes between depressed and normal patients were identified. Fourteen genes were down-regulated, and 15 genes were up-regulated (**Table S2**).

Furthermore, to evaluate the relationship between ingredients form XYS and other known-compounds, we first identified the known-compounds which contain anti-depression function based on the DEGs results from cMap data server. Finally, 12 significant compounds with adequate relative connection mean scores (absolute value >0.5) were identified. Of the twelve compounds, 2 had high positive connection scores, and the other ten compounds possess negative connectivity scores, indicating they can act with these dysregulated genes in depression. **Figure 2A** and **Table 2** summarize these results. In addition, a search of the DrugBank database resulted in identification of 64 FDA-approved compounds for treatment of depression (**Table 2**).

PCA was performed to characterize the physicochemical parameters (MW, ALogP, nHDon, and nHAcc) of these antidepressant drugs/compounds. PC1 and PC2, as shown in **Figure 2B** and **Table S3**, showed a distribution of different color nodes that flocked together, indicating extensive overlap among the three groups of ingredients in XYS, and the antidepressant compounds determined by cMap and Drugbank. Furthermore,

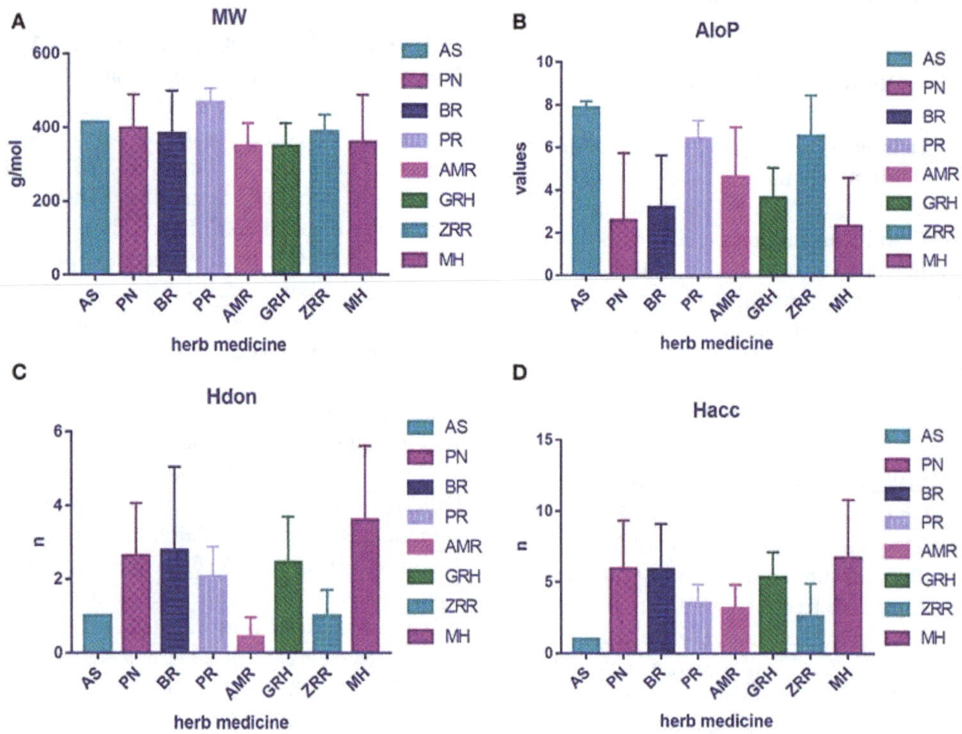

FIGURE 1 | The physicochemical property of bioactive compounds from each herb in XYS. **(A)** physicochemical diversity including molecular weight (MW); **(B)** the value of partition coefficient between octanol and water (ALogP); **(C)** number of possible hydrogen-bond donors (Hdon); **(D)** number of hydrogen-bond acceptors (Hacc).

TABLE 1 | The average physicochemical value of each herb.

	MW	AloP	Hdon	Hacc
AS	413.78 ± 1.43	7.86 ± 0.31	1.00 ± 0	1.00 ± 0
PN	398.06 ± 91.19	2.58 ± 3.15	2.62 ± 1.45	5.92 ± 3.43
BR	382.10 ± 117.32	3.20 ± 2.43	2.78 ± 2.26	5.89 ± 3.33
PR	467.78 ± 37.66	6.43 ± 0.85	2.07 ± 0.79	3.53 ± 1.30
AMR	347.24 ± 64.13	4.60 ± 2.34	0.43 ± 0.53	3.14 ± 1.68
GRH	348.41 ± 63.69	3.66 ± 1.40	2.45 ± 1.25	5.33 ± 1.78
ZRR	388.88 ± 4.29	6.53 ± 1.92	1.00 ± 0.71	2.60 ± 2.30
MH	358.59 ± 130.19	2.32 ± 2.27	3.60 ± 2.01	6.70 ± 4.11

the significant positive correlation between these compounds of three groups (**Figure 2C, Table S3**). In ADME properties, Pearson r value is 0.3404 ($P < 0.0001$) for MW, AlogP ($r = 01969$, $P = 0.003$), Hdon ($r = 0.3018$, $P < 0.0001$), Hacc ($r = 0.351$, $P < 0.0001$). These results indicated that bioactive compounds from XYS are highly correlated with known antidepressant compounds in molecular properties, and could as potential drug therapies for depression treatment.

Targets of Xiaoyao San

An *in silico* target screening approach was performed to identify the putative targets of each bioactive component of XYS. Predictive tools were used, including the TCMSP server, STITCH, and PharmMapper data servers. In total, 446 targets were identified for 149 bioactive compounds (9 compounds did not receive predictions), and many compounds were predicted to target the same proteins, such as Monoamine Oxidase B (gene symbol: MAOB). Depression-related putative targets were obtained from Therapeutic Target, DrugBank, OMIM, and DisGeNET databases, and DEGs resulting from analysis of GSE12654. Finally, 121 bioactive compounds in XYS which associated with 99 depression-related targets were identified. Multiple therapeutic targets were mediated by active ingredients of XYS, such as IL2, IL4, IL6, IL10, and STAT3, which are involved in immune and inflammatory responses closely associated with depression. For example, STAT3 (Signal transducer and activator of transcription 3), a component of the JAK/STAT signaling pathway, influences the fate and function of brain cells.

Construction of a Compound-Depression Target Network (C-DT)

A C-DT network was constructed (**Figure 3**) for further biological analysis. This network contained information regarding complex relationships between all bioactive compounds in XYS and their depression-related targets. There were 220 nodes in the C-DT network composed of 121 active ingredients and 99 depression targets, connected by 1583 interactions, the details were listed in **Table S4**. As shown in **Figure 3**, node size indicated the number of connections

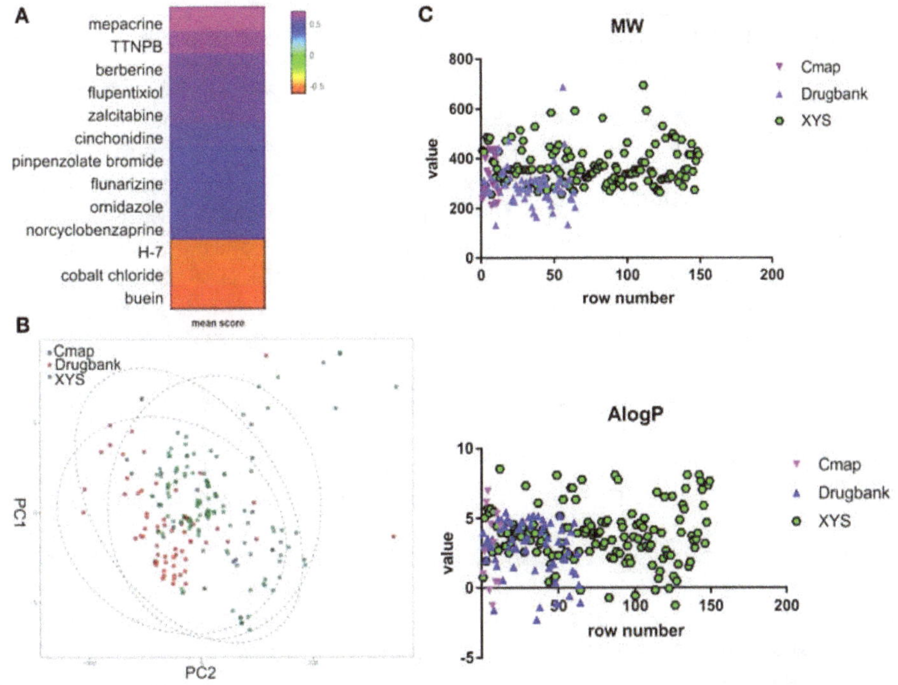

FIGURE 2 | (A) Heatmap for mean scores of cMap antidepressant compounds. The color represents different relative connection mean score. **(B)** PCA analysis for physicochemical properties of antidepressant potential molecules. Each node indicates a compound, cMap (blue), Drugbank (red), XYS (XYS), the circle means 95%. **(C)** the correlation analysis for ADME properties of each group (the property of Hdon and Hacc have not shown).

calculated using "NetworkAnalyzer," an analytical tool in cytoscape 3.7.0.

Enrichment Analysis of the C-DT Network

GO and KEGG Pathway Analysis

To investigate biological functions associated with this interaction network relative to treatment of depression, we performed GO and KEGG pathway enrichment analyses using the "clusterprofile" R package. Three GO categories were analyzed, which included CC, MF, and BP. The top 15 GO enrichment results for each category are listed in **Table 3**. Direct outcomes are shown in **Figure 4A**. These targets were significantly involved in formation of neuronal receptor and cell, which are directly related to generation of brain cells and tissue. Molecular functions involved activity and binding of various molecules, neurotransmitter receptors, cytokines, transmembrane receptor protein kinases, and nuclear receptor, as well as cytokine receptor binding, phoshphatase, and steroid. Moreover, combined BP results indicated that XYS may regulate depression-related biological processes, such as "regulation of cell migration," "reactive oxygen species metabolic process," and "aging" to exert antidepressant effects.

KEGG signaling pathway results are shown in **Figure 4** and **Table 4**. The top enriched terms were related to several critical pathways associated with disease, such as "PI3K-Akt signaling pathway," "MAPK signaling pathway," and "neuroactive ligand-receptor interaction" (**Figure 4B** and **Figure S1**). These findings demonstrated complex pathological features of depression and the potential of XYS as an antidepressant.

PPI Network Analysis and Screening of Key Active Ingredients

To investigate the characteristics of protein targets in the C-DT network, protein–protein interactions were analyzed using the STRING online database, and the related PPI network was constructed and visualized using cytoscape software. Using confidence of 0.9 as the threshold, we found 90 nodes and 288 interactions in the PPI network. In addition, we used four different analysis methods (Stress, Closeness, MNC and EcCentricity) using the "cytoHubba" plugin to identify the top 10 hub nodes in the PPI network. Detailed results are shown in **Figures 5A–D**, and the top hub genes based on these four indices were summarized in a Venn diagram (**Figure 5E**, **Table S5**). Thus, 3 core genes were identified as hubs: AKT1, TP53, and VEGFA. Furthermore, based on GO and KEGG analyses, these three core genes were enriched in multiple biological processes and signaling pathways. For instance, AKT1 is involved in myelination of the peripheral nervous system, peripheral nervous system axon ensheathment, and the neurotrophin signaling pathway, all of which are closely related to depression (Barros et al., 2009; Musashe et al., 2016; Liu et al., 2018). Using these core genes, a Sankey diagram (**Figure 6A**) was used to facilitate shown of bioactive compounds that can act on multiple targets. Nine ingredients of XYS and their hub targets were identified,

TABLE 2 | Antidepressant compounds from cMap and Drugbank.

Name	CAS	MW	AlogP	Hdon	Hacc	Mean score	p-value
cMap						**Mean score**	**p-value**
Cobalt chloride	7791-13-1	237.92	0.95	6	8	−0.825	4E-05
Butein	487-52-5	272.256	2.61	4	5	0.628	0.0002
Mepacrine	83-89-6	399.96	6.13	1	4	0.65	0.0015
TTNPB	71441-28-6	348.49	6.93	1	2	−0.63	0.0036
Berberine	2086-83-1	336.37	−0.2	0	4	0.444	0.0065
Flupentixol	2709-56-0	434.521	4.56	1	7	−0.58	0.0122
Zalcitabine	7481-89-2	211.221	−1.3	2	3	0.586	0.0137
Cinchonidine	485-71-2	294.398	3.2	1	3	−0.47	0.0189
Pipenzolate-bromide	125-51-9	434.37	0.41	4	6	−0.414	0.0192
Flunarizine	40218-96-0	404.51	5.3	0	4	−0.431	0.0204
Ornidazole	16773-42-5	219.625	0.37	1	4	−0.459	0.0208
Norcyclobenzaprine	303-50-4	261.37	4.43	1	1	0.51	0.0221
DRUGBANK							
Setiptiline	57262-94-9	261.368	3.96	0	1		
Reboxetine	71620-89-8	313.4	3.1	1	4		
Minaprine	25905-77-5	298.3828	2.03	1	5		
Mianserin	24219-97-4	264.3648	3.52	0	2		
Demexiptiline	24701-51-7	278.35	3.21	1	3		
Mirtazapine	85650-52-8	265.3529	2.9	0	3		
Escitalopram	128196-01-0	324.3919	3.5	0	3		
Oxitriptan	4350-9-8	220.2246	−1.6	4	4		
Tianeptine	72797-41-2	436.952	2.07	2	5		
Tranylcypromine	155-09-9	133.19	1.58	1	1		
Dimetacrine	4757-55-5	294.4338	4.96	0	2		
Vilazodone	163521-12-8	441.5249	4.21	2	4		
Desipramine	50-47-5	266.38	4.9	1	2		
Sulpiride	15676-16-1	341.43	0.57	2	5		
Adinazolam	37115-32-5	351.83	4.4	0	4		
Butriptyline	35941-65-2	293.45	5.44	0	1		
Dosulepin	113-53-1	295.44	4.98	0	1		
Trazodone	19794-93-5	371.86	2.9	0	4		
Nefazodone	83366-66-9	470	4.7	0	5		
Citalopram	59729-33-8	324.39	3.5	0	3		
Isocarboxazid	59-63-2	231.25	1.49	2	3		
Agomelatine	138112-76-2	243.3	2.83	1	2		
Pirlindole	60762-57-4	226.3	2.8	1	1		
Trimipramine	739-71-9	294.43	4.2	0	2		
Doxepin	1668-19-5	279.38	4.29	0	2		
Protriptyline	438-60-8	263.3767	4.7	1	1		
Imipramine	50-49-7	280.41	4.8	0	2		
Amoxapine	14028-44-5	313.78	3.4	1	3		
Venlafaxine	93413-69-5	277.4	2.69	1	3		
Bupropion	34911-55-2	239.74	3.6	1	2		
Sertraline	79617-96-2	306.23	5.1	1	1		
Nortriptyline	72-69-5	263.3767	4.51	1	1		
Maprotiline	10262-69-8	277.4	5.1	1	1		
Clomipramine	303-49-1	314.852	5.19	0	2		
Toloxatone	29218-27-7	207.229	1.26	1	3		
L-Tyrosine	60-18-4	181.19	−2.3	3	4		
Chlorprothixene	113-59-7	315.86	5.18	0	1		
L-Phenylalanine	63-91-2	165.19	−1.4	2	3		
Fluoxetine	54910-89-3	309.33	4.05	1	2		
Amitriptyline	50-48-6	277.4	4.92	0	1		
Vortioxetine	508233-74-7	298.45	4.51	1	2		
Fluvoxamine	54739-18-3	318.33	3.2	1	4		
Paroxetine	61869-08-7	329.37	3.6	1	4		
Levomilnacipran	96847-54-0	246.35	1.42	1	2		
Pizotifen	15574-96-6	295.44	4.7	0	1		
Milnacipran	92623-85-3	246.348	1.72	1	2		
Viloxazine	46817-91-8	237.3	1.71	1	4		
Pramipexole	104632-26-0	211.33	0.4	2	3		
Acamprosate	77337-76-9	181.21	−1.1	2	4		
Flibanserin	167933-07-5	390.4	3.32	1	3		
Cyclobenzaprine	303-53-7	275.3874	5.2	0	1		
Penbutolol	38363-40-5	291.428	4.15	2	3		
Alprazolam	28981-97-7	308.765	2.12	0	3		
Bromazepam	1812-30-2	316.15	2.05	1	3		
Pipradrol	467-60-7	267.37	3.36	2	2		
Fosnetupitant	1703748-89-3	688.61	2.57	1	6		
Levomefolic acid	31690-09-2	459.4558	−0.6	7	12		
Duloxetine	116539-59-4	297.42	4	1	2		
Phenelzine	51-71-8	135.19	1.2	2	2		
Rotigotine	99755-59-6	315.48	4.7	1	2		
Moxonidine	75438-57-2	241.677	1.01	2	6		
Carbamazepine	298-46-4	236.27	2.45	1	1		
Desvenlafaxine	93413-62-8	263.38	0.21	2	3		
L-Tryptophan	73-22-3	204.2252	−1.1	3	3		

including quercetin, luteolin, acacetin, aloe-emodin, gadelaidic acid, Glyasperin C, kaempferol, naringenin, paeoniflorin.

Identification of the Chemical Characterization of XYS

As shown in **Figure 6B**, the chemical base peak ion (BPI) chromatogram of XYS based on the positive and negative ion modes of UPLC-Q-TOF/MS. According to the above analysis, nine key compounds of XYS were further examined. All of the key compounds from XYS, seven ingredients (paeoniflorin, quercetin, luteolin, acacetin, aloe-emodin, Glyasperin C, kaempferol) were successful identified by UPLC-Q-TOF/MS analysis, the details were listed in **Table 5**. Among them, we found major compounds are flavonoids, only paeoniflorin as monoterpene glycoside, and most importantly it is a principal ingredient of *Paeonia lactiflora* Pallas (**Figure 7A**). Thus, we next performed cellular model and investigated the neuron protected effect of paeoniflorin *in vitro.*

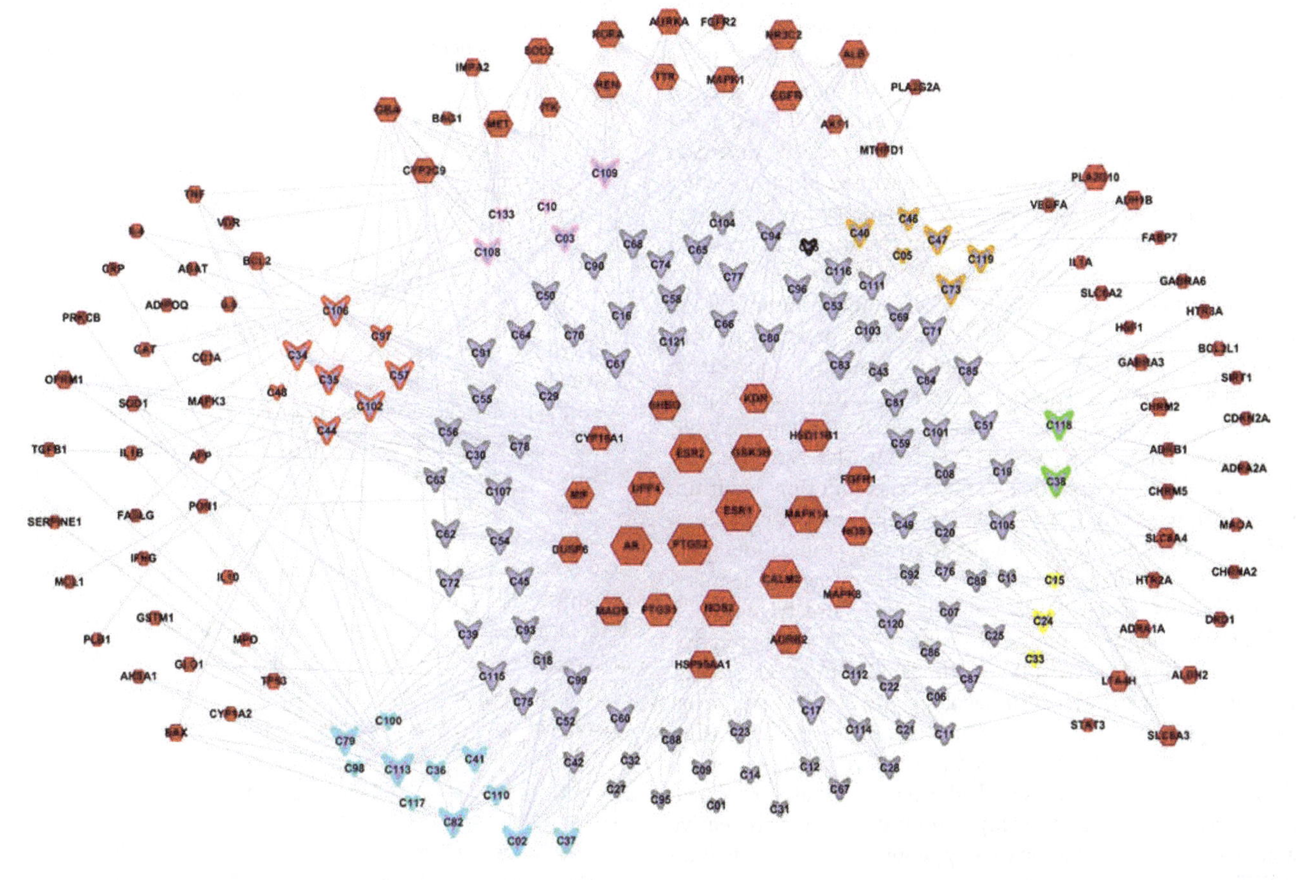

FIGURE 3 | The C-DTs network. Nodes with red means depression related targets. Lavender means bioactive compounds from XYS, border color means different herbal (red: MH; orange: PR; yellow: AMR; green: AS; cyan: BR; gray: GRH; pink: PN; black: ZRR; some compounds exist in many kinds of herbal, they are randomly assigned to the corresponding colors of these herbal). And the size of each node indicate the number of connections.

Evaluations

To determine the protected effect of Paeoniflorin from CORT neurotoxicity, the cell viability assay was examined. The detailed MTT assay results as shown in **Figure 7B**, that 200 μM CORT reduced the cell viability of PC12 cells, whereas treatment 20 and 40 μM paeoniflorin were very significant able to moderate the cell viability ($P < 0.01$). Western blot analysis results showed that compared with the control cells, the expression of p-Akt in CORT stimulated cells was significantly decreased ($P < 0.01$). However, the down-regulated expression of p-Akt was significantly reversed by paeoniflorin treatment (**Figures 7C,D**).

Furthermore, quercetin and luteolin could act on all hub genes, so we further validated their molecular docking to detect and calculate the binding energy between small molecules and proteins. The best bound conformation site of quercetin and luteolin binding to proteins were shown in **Figure 8**, respectively. The binding energy between quercetin with AKT1 is −17.6341 kcal/mol, and luteolin with AKT1 is −12.7977 kcal/mol, that initiated both two compounds had strong binding activity with AKT1. Similarly, these two compounds contain strong binding activity with other hub targets, the binding energy between quercetin with VEGFA and TP53 (−67.4121 kcal/mol), luteolin with VEGFA and TP53 (−53.3754 kcal/mol).

DISCUSSION

Traditional Chinese medicine (TCM) is being more frequently chosen by patients to treat depressive and anxiety disorders. A meta-analysis reported that use of XYS as an adjuvant therapy with antidepressant drugs in 1,837 patients was more effective in improving symptoms than antidepressants alone (Zhang et al., 2011). Furthermore, previous studies indicated that XYS treatment of depression and anxiety involves several biological aspects. For instance, some psychological disorders have been associated with increased cytokine levels resulting from immune activation, known as the "cytokine hypothesis" (Sharma, 2016). Inflammatory cytokines may act as modulators of 5-HT (serotonin) receptors, and upregulate indoleamine 2,3-dioxygenase (IDO), resulting in anxiety-like disorders (Myint and Kim, 2003). The antidepressant-like effects of XYS were associated with downregulation of peripheral IL-1β, IFN-γ, TNF-α, and IL-6, and increased synthesis of tryptophan hydroxylase (TPH) and IDO, which play a role in promoting

5-HT synthesis (Jiao et al., 2019). XYS significantly inhibited TNF-α release in serum and the hippocampus through activation of the TNF-α/JAK2-STAT3 pathway, as shown in our preliminary study (Li et al., 2017). Moreover, the HPA axis and brain-derived neurotrophic factor (BDNF) have also been widely studied in the context of pathogenesis and treatment of depressive disorders (Jiang et al., 2016). Previous studies have demonstrated that XYS could reverse chronic stress-induced anxiety-like symptoms by regulating the apelin-APJ system in the hypothalamus and activity of the HPA axis (Yan et al., 2018).

Many studies have demonstrated the antidepressant effects of XYS, which involves multiple pathways associated with depression. Therefore, the complex bioactive ingredients and targets with potential antidepressant activities require clarification. Previous studies using High Performance Liquid Chromatography coupled with LTQ Orbitrap Mass Spectrometry (HPLC-LTQ-Orbitrap-MS) identified paeoniflorin, liquiritin, glycyrrhizic acid, ferulic acid, saikosaponins A and C, curcumin, and poria cocos alcohol were eight active compounds identified in XYS (Li et al., 2015). Yuzhi Zhou and his colleagues identified 4 components: Z-ligustilide, palmitic acid, atractylenolide I, and atractylenolide II in XYS using gas chromatography–mass spectrometry (GC-MS) methods (Zhou et al., 2012). In addition, network pharmacology methods have been used to predict and analyse 13 components of XYS (Gao et al., 2015). However, no comprehensive analysis of all bioactive compounds in XYS had been previously reported. Therefore, the present study adopted a comprehensive systematic network pharmacology approach for evaluation of XYS.

In this study, we identified 149 compounds in active fractions of XYS. PCA analysis and correlation analysis was used to compare these compounds with antidepressants approved by the FDA and small molecule drugs predicted by the cMap database. This was the first comparative study of drug properties of TCM formula compounds using Drugbank and a gene chip combined with cMap. Our results indicated that these 149 bioactive compounds in XYS possessed potential antidepressant properties. Therefore, we constructed a compound-depression targets (C-DTs) network, and further enriched this network using GO KEGG pathways analyses of 99 depression-related targets. CC enrichment results indicated that a considerable number of genes were involved in formation of nerves and synapses. Synapses are the fundamental structures for information transmission between neurons, and they adapt to stimuli by continuously modifying neural connections and neurological circuits. Therefore, synaptic plasticity is the main manifestation of neuroplasticity, and depression and other psychological disorders are typically associated with decreased synaptic plasticity in the hippocampus (Wainwright and Galea, 2013). Molecular functions associated with components of XYS involved activity and binding of various molecules, such as neurotransmitter receptors, cytokines, transmembrane receptor protein kinases, nuclear receptors, cytokine receptor binding, steroids, and catecholamines. Moreover, a large number of genes were significantly enriched as BP terms in regulation of aging, reactive oxygen species metabolic processes, and inflammatory response, which are associated with pathogenesis of depression. Combined BP results indicated that XYS may act via generation of nerves and synapses, alteration of neurotransmitter receptor function, and regulation of cytokines, resulting in antidepressant effects. The PI3K/Akt signaling pathway was enriched to the greatest degree, resulting in association of 20 genes. It has been wildly regarded to modulate antidepressant-like functions and contributes to synaptic plasticity and neurotransmission formation (Ludka et al., 2016). Furthermore, several metabolic pathways directly related to the nervous system such as "neuroactive ligand-receptor interaction," "GABAergic synapse," and "neurotrophin signaling pathway" were also enriched. Analysis of the PPI network identified hub nodes which were most closely related to other proteins: AKT1, TP53, VEGFA. These proteins were consistent with our enrichment analysis, and have been previously reported to be related to neurotrophic factors and depression.

TABLE 3 | GO enrichment analysis.

ID	Description	Count	q value
BP			
GO:0030335	positive regulation of cell migration	24	3.57E-14
GO:1901615	organic hydroxy compound metabolic process	24	3.70E-14
GO:0032496	response to lipopolysaccharide	23	1.75E-16
GO:0002237	response to molecule of bacterial origin	23	3.87E-16
GO:0031667	response to nutrient levels	23	6.90E-14
GO:0009991	response to extracellular stimulus	23	1.68E-13
GO:0072593	reactive oxygen species metabolic process	22	3.04E-17
GO:0006979	response to oxidative stress	22	1.45E-13
GO:0035690	cellular response to drug	21	3.64E-14
GO:0018108	peptidyl-tyrosine phosphorylation	21	1.39E-13
MF			
GO:0019902	phosphatase binding	11	2.94E-07
GO:0005057	NA	11	2.94E-07
GO:0005125	cytokine activity	12	2.94E-07
GO:0030594	neurotransmitter receptor activity	9	9.10E-07
GO:0019903	protein phosphatase binding	9	1.03E-06
GO:0004702	NA	9	1.03E-06
GO:0008227	G protein-coupled amine receptor activity	7	1.03E-06
GO:0005496	steroid binding	8	1.33E-06
GO:0005126	cytokine receptor binding	12	1.33E-06
GO:1901338	catecholamine binding	5	2.33E-06
CC			
GO:0045121	membrane raft	16	4.00E-10
GO:0098857	membrane microdomain	16	4.00E-10
GO:0098589	membrane region	16	4.57E-10
GO:0043235	receptor complex	15	4.60E-08
GO:0031983	vesicle lumen	14	9.61E-08
GO:0060205	cytoplasmic vesicle lumen	13	7.21E-07
GO:0034774	secretory granule lumen	12	3.03E-06
GO:0005901	caveola	7	3.90E-06
GO:0044853	plasma membrane raft	7	1.67E-05
GO:0031093	platelet alpha granule lumen	5	0.0004881

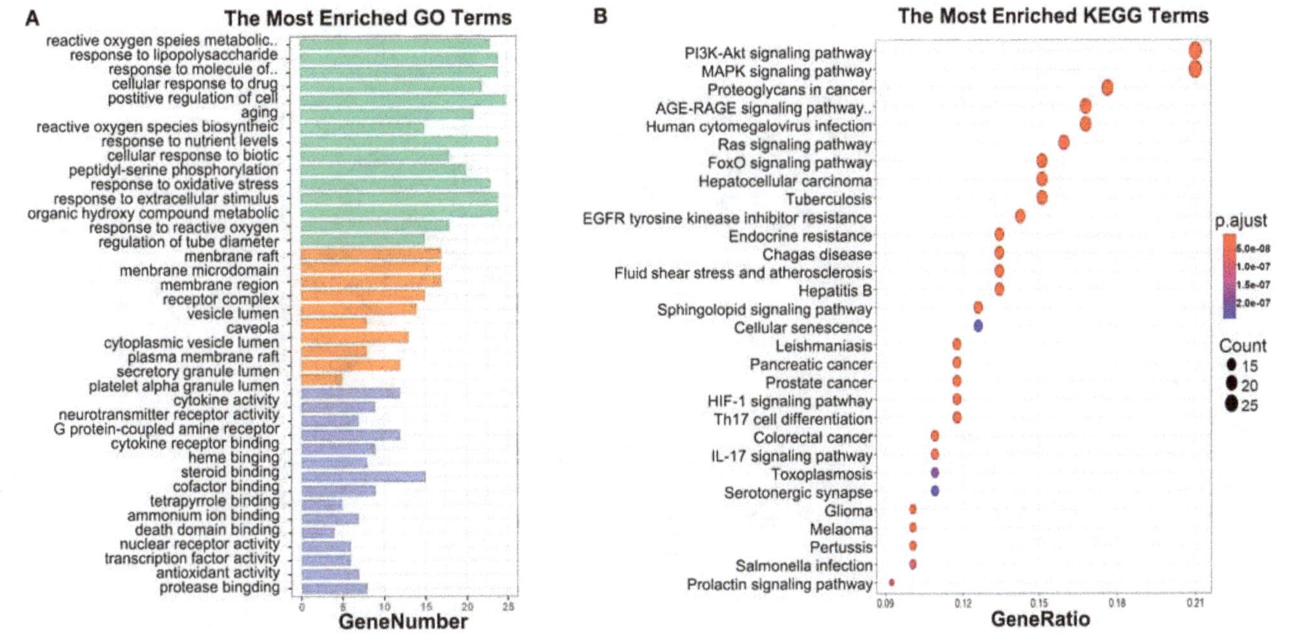

FIGURE 4 | (A) GO enrichment. Each bar indicates a CC/MF/BP term, color means enriched type (green color present CC, orange present MF, light blue present BP), and abscissa represents the number of enriched genes. **(B)** KEGG enrichment. Dotplot for KEGG pathway, the size of each node indicates enriched counts. abscissa represents the enriched gene ratio. Color means enriched adjust *P*-value.

TABLE 4 | KEGG pathway.

ID	Description	p.adjust	Count
hsa04151	PI3K-Akt signaling pathway	6.80E-08	20
hsa04010	MAPK signaling pathway	2.59E-08	19
hsa05163	Human cytomegalovirus infection	4.02E-09	18
hsa04933	AGE-RAGE signaling pathway in diabetic complications	4.07E-13	17
hsa05152	Tuberculosis	1.47E-09	17
hsa05205	Proteoglycans in cancer	2.59E-08	16
hsa04014	Ras signaling pathway	1.44E-07	16
hsa01521	EGFR tyrosine kinase inhibitor resistance	1.90E-12	15
hsa05418	Fluid shear stress and atherosclerosis	2.74E-09	15
hsa05142	Chagas disease (American trypanosomiasis)	9.13E-10	14

Bioactive ingredients in XYS were classified in the following categories: volatile oils, alkaloids, flavonoids, saponins, and polysaccharides. Among these, polysaccharides can regulate intestinal flora to moderate depression though the brain-gut-microbiota axis (Cryan and Dinan, 2012; Schwalm et al., 2016), and flavonoids can cross the blood-brain barrier, directly acting on brain targets (Youdim et al., 2003). We concluded that XYS exerts its effects in many ways through the actions of many compounds and may confer advantages over the compounds by reducing drug resistance.

After identified hub targets, 9 ingredients of XYS could interact with them, and 7 of them were identified by UPLC-Q/TOF-MS analysis. As a result, we found that 3 hub genes predicted by the PPI network could be regulated by quercetin and luteolin, which are both flavonoids. Nevertheless, most of the reports of flavonoids are limited to *in vitro* experiments, and these flavonoids are common constituents in a variety of herbs. It is considered important to clarify their specific role in the treatment (Heinricha et al., 2020). Actually, many studies have verified their neuroprotective effects *in vitro* and *in vivo*. For instance, the genes regulated by luteolin could act as receptors in the central nervous system, resulting in antidepressant effects (Sasaki et al., 2013; Akınrınde and Adebıyı, 2019). Quercetin, a flavonoid, is a component of *Bupleurum Chinense* Dc. This flavonoid confers antioxidant activity and anti-inflammatory effects in the treatment of neurological diseases. A previous study reported that quercetin relieved anxiety and depression of chronic stress rats by protecting neurons from oxidation and inflammation (Mehta et al., 2017). In LPS-induced neuroinflammation of mice, quercetin still exhibited a function of eliminating inflammation through significantly reduced LPS-induced proliferation of astrocytes in the brain and decreased the expression of inflammatory factors (Khan et al., 2018). Additionally, researchers found that quercetin could inhibit neuronal apoptosis to preventing anxiety-like behaviors *in vivo* via regulating the Akt1 and ASK1/JNK3/caspase-3 expression (Pei et al., 2016). Besides, in a previous network pharmacology study, quercetin was found also as a high contribution compound of Huangqi and Huanglian for treating diabetes, participated in polypharmacological and synergistic mechanisms (Yue et al., 2017).

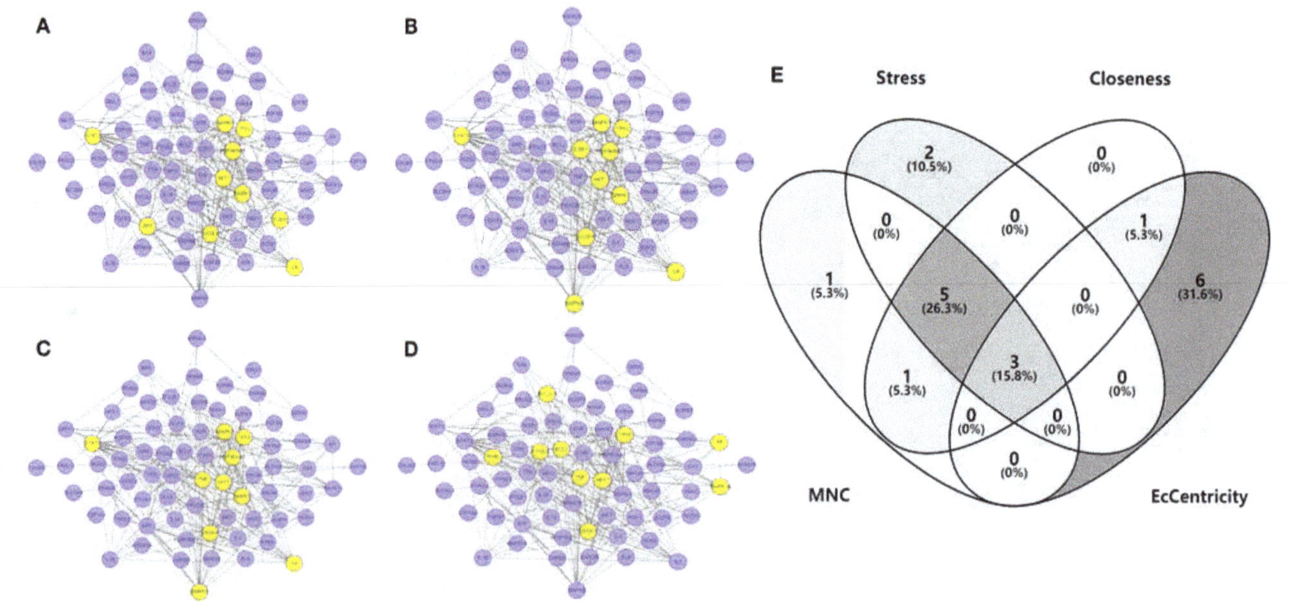

FIGURE 5 | (A–D) PPI network analysis. Networks represent the analysis results of the based different aspect (Stress, Closeness, MNC and EcCentricity), respectively. The highlight yellow nodes are hub targets (top 10). And the light purple nodes are also highest confidence protein targets from C-DTs network. **(E)** Venn diagram. The overlapping genes were selected which as core hub targets for further analysis.

However, among these 7 ingredients, only paeoniflorin, a monoterpene glycoside compound, as main component of herb (*Paeonia lactiflora* Pallas) from XYS. And it is one of the quality identification standards for XYS in the Chinese Pharmacopeia. Thus, it should be a representative compound from this formula, so that the current research further analyzed its neuroprotective effect and validated its potential roles with predicted target Akt. Previous reports by several researchers had provided clues supporting the role for paeoniflorin in the protection of neuron cells and the therapeutic effects in neurological diseases (Mao et al., 2012; Cong et al., 2019). Gu et al. had demonstrated that paeoniflorin via upregulating the p-Akt expression and Bcl-2/Bax ratio to reduce neuron death in Alzheimer's disease mice (Gu et al., 2016). Recent evidence suggests that CUMS rats had improved depressive-like behavior after paeoniflorin treatment, it could be regulated by acting on the ERK-CREB signaling pathway (Zhong et al., 2018). Consist with previous findings, we found paeoniflorin can reverse the neurotoxicity produced through CORT and promote the phosphorylation of Akt. On the one hand, from the perspective of network pharmacology, the representative importance of paeoniflorin in XYS has been clarified for the first time. On the other hand, our results indicated that paeoniflorin as the XYS's representative compound which could modulate the several signaling upstream target AKT's expression, that validate the current network pharmacology prediction.

LIMITATIONS AND CONCLUSIONS

Current research based on network pharmacology which could provide a novel and systematic analysis way for the research of Chinese herbal formula. However, there are still some limitations in our article. Firstly, as we all know, components of Chinese herbal are complicated, it's doubtful whether there are synergistic or side effects caused by the interaction between compounds that is hard to clarified in the prediction and composition identification of this study. Secondly, although CORT is one of the most common methods to simulate depression *in vitro*, the pathogenesis of depression is complicated, which means that it is difficult to simulate whole pathogenic factors *in vitro*. Moreover, western blots suggested that paeoniflorin could regulate the phosphorylation of Akt, but it is only in protein expression level. The direct or indirect regulation between them would need to be further explored. Last but not least, hub genes were selected by PPI network in our study that they are usually as upstream molecules or central molecules in those important signaling pathways. However, there still exist multiple downstream proteins in pathogenesis of depression. And thus, it is important to discover and identify more compounds that interact with these downstream proteins through future works.

Overall, this study systematically summarized key active compounds in XYS and comprehensively analyzed potential mechanisms of its action and pathways. We also evaluated

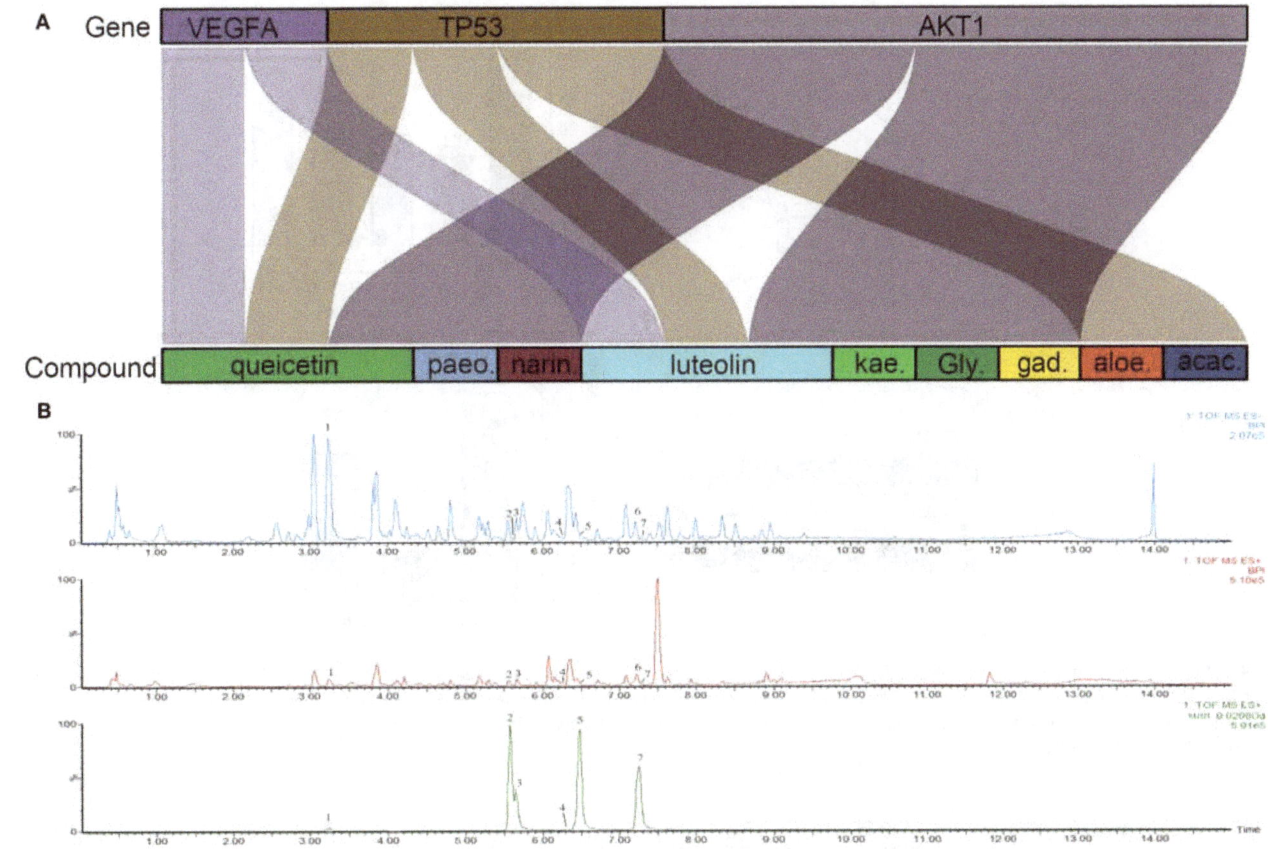

FIGURE 6 | (A) Sankey diagram. Sankey diagram direct shown the relationship between compounds and targets. The blocks on the up represent the hub targets. And the underneath blocks indicate compounds, as follow: quercetin, luteolin, acacetin, aloe-emodin, gadelaidic acid, Glyasperin C, kaempferol, naringenin, paeoniflorin. **(B)** The chemical base peak intensity (BPI) chromatogram of key compounds characterization of XYS in positive ion mode and negative ion mode determined by UPLC-Q-TOF/MS. Identification No.:1. Paeoniflorin; 2. Kaempferol; 3. Quercetin; 4. Aloe emodin; 5. Luteolin; 6. Glyasperin C; 7. Acacetin.

TABLE 5 | Chemical composition of key ingredients from XYS identified by UPLC-Q/TOF-MS.

No.	Time	Selected ion	Elemental composition	Calculated mass	Mass error	(ESI+) MS/MS fragmentation	(ESI-) MS/MS fragmentation	Identification
1*	3.24	[M-H+HCOOH]$^-$	C24H29O13	525.1608	1.7	319.1174, 301.1065, 197.0806, 179.0711, 151.0758, 105.0337	479.1556, 449.1453, 431.1345, 327.1080, 165.0547, 121.0291	Paeoniflorin
2*	5.57	[2M-H]$^-$	C30H19O12	571.0877	3.2	161.0232, 153.0192	285.0414, 151.0039	Kaempferol
3*	5.65	[M+H]$^+$	C15H11O7	303.0505	1.6	229.0497, 179.0344, 153.0188, 109.0290	603.0786, 301.0354, 151.0037, 121.0288	Quercetin
4*	6.29	[M+H]$^+$	C15H11O5	271.0606	−0.7		269.0459	Aloeemodin
5*	6.48	[2M-H]$^-$	C30H19O12	571.0877	−2.6	153.0192, 109.0289	285.0407	Luteolin
6	7.20	[M+H]$^+$	C21H25O5	357.1702	0.6	301.1076, 221.1179, 165.0555	355.1546	Glyasperin C
7*	7.26	[M+H]$^+$	C16H13O5	285.0763	−2.5	270.0524, 242.0575, 153.0183	283.0612, 211.0396	Acacetin

**Accurately identified with reference standards.*

for representative compound paeoniflorin *in vitro*. The current findings provide a basis and new insights for XYS in the treatment of depression. Certainly, we will explore widely experiments of pharmaceutical ingredients to better understand the effects of XYS, such as component analyses, identification of drugs, and metabolic studies in animal models.

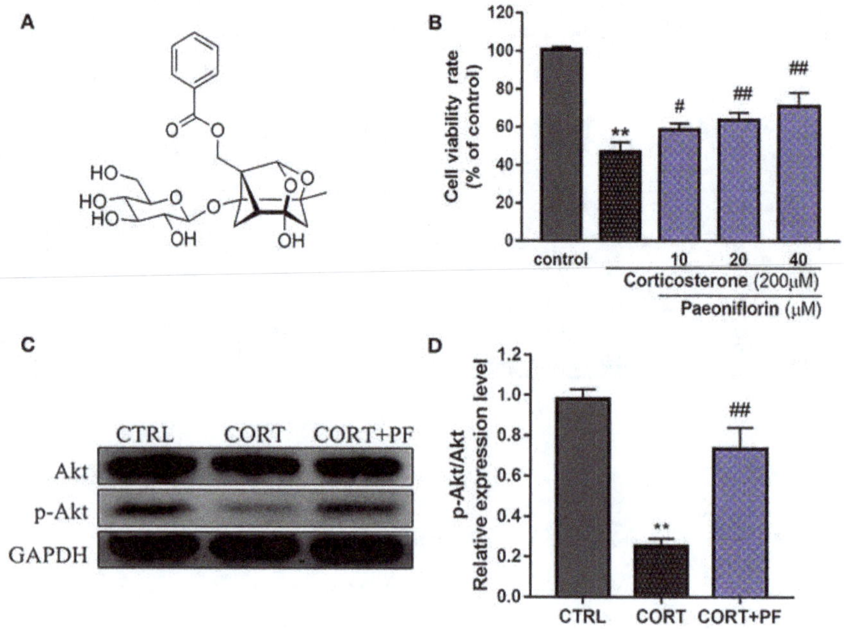

FIGURE 7 | (A) Chemical structure of Paeoniflorin; **(B)** Viability of PC12 cells assessed using MTT assay following culture of 200μM CORT with different dosages of paeoniflorin (10, 20, 40μl/ml) for 24 h. **(C)** Western blots of p-Akt expression in different treated condition PC-12 cells. GAPDH as the loading control. **(D)** Densitometry data analysis were quantified using Image J software. Compare with control group, $^{**}P$ <0.01; compare with CORT group, $^{\#}P$ < 0.05, $^{\#\#}P$<0.01; n = 3. PF, paeoniflorin; CORT, corticosterone.

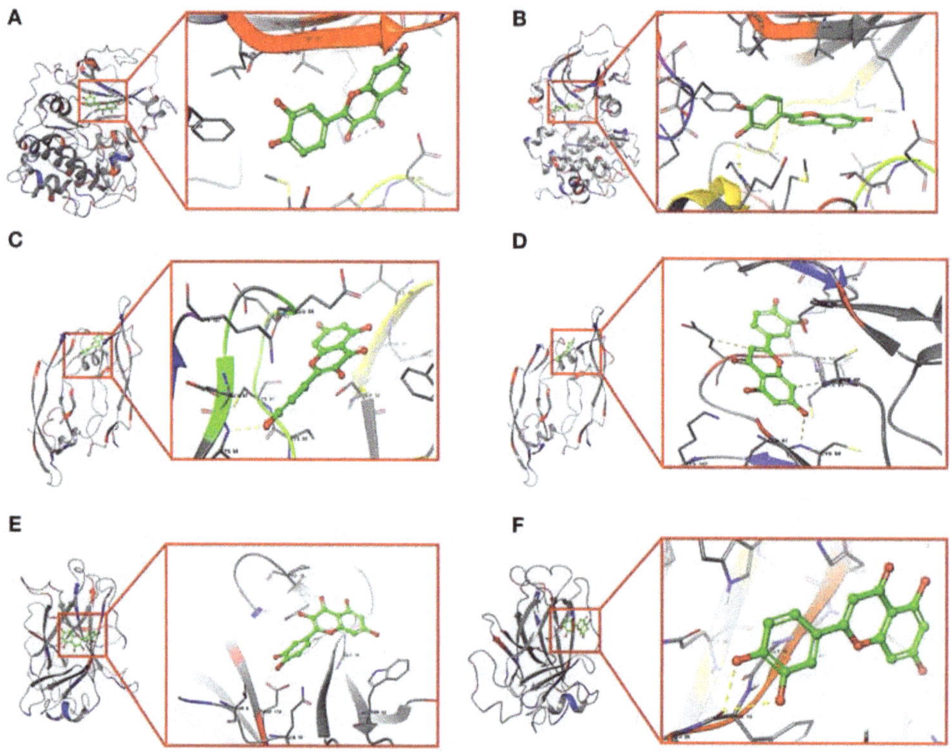

FIGURE 8 | Structural model and binding site of active ingredients with hub targets. **(A)** Docking site between AKT1 with quercetin. **(B)** Docking site between AKT1 with luteolin. **(C)** Docking site between VEGFA with quercetin. **(D)** Docking site between VEGFA with luteolin. **(E)** Docking site between TP53 with quercetin. **(F)** Docking site between TP53 with luteolin.

AUTHOR CONTRIBUTIONS

NY and JC main contributed research conception and design. NY, KT, LH, WH, XL, and QM collected and processed data. NY, LG, and KT wrote sections of the manuscript. All authors contributed to manuscript revision, read, and approved the final submitted version. JC takes primary responsibility for communication with the journal and editorial office during the submission process, throughout peer review, and during publication.

FUNDING

This work was financially supported by the National Natural Science Foundation of China (Nos. 81630104, 81803998, 81973748).

ACKNOWLEDGMENTS

The authors gratefully appreciate the reviewers and editors for their constructive suggestions and kind help. And we sincerely appreciate Dr. Huang Chuiguo for his warm help.

SUPPLEMENTARY MATERIAL

Figure S1 | Distribution of partial targets of XYS on the Neuroactive ligand-receptor interaction signaling pathway. The red nodes are potential targets. The green nodes are relevant targets in the pathway.

Table S1 | Bioactive ingredients of XYS.

Table S2 | The DEmRNAs of GSE12654.

Table S3 | (A) PCA analysis for physicochemical properties of potential antidepressant molecules; **(B)** Correlation analysis for properties between each molecular group.

Table S4 | C-DTs network.

Table S5 | Compounds acting on hub targets.

REFERENCES

Ada, H., Scott, A. F., Amberger, J. S., Bocchini, C. A., and Mckusick, V. A. (2005). Online Mendelian Inheritance in Man (OMIM), a knowledgebase of human genes and genetic disorders. *Nucleic Acids Res.* 33, 514–517. doi: 10.1093/nar/gki033

Akinrinde, A. S., and Adebiyi, O. E. (2019). Neuroprotection by luteolin and gallic acid against cobalt chloride-induced behavioural, morphological and neurochemical alterations in Wistar rats. *Neurotoxicology* 74, 252–263. doi: 10.1016/j.neuro.2019.07.005

Barros, C. S., Nguyen, T., Spencer, K. S., Nishiyama, A., Colognato, H., and Müller, U. (2009). Betal integrins are required for normal CNS myelination and promote AKT-dependent myelin outgrowth. *Development* 136, 2717–2724. doi: 10.1242/dev.038679

Berger, S. I., and Iyengar, R. (2009). Network analyses in systems pharmacology. *Bioinformatics* 25, 2466–2472. doi: 10.1093/bioinformatics/btp465

Chen, Z., and Hou, C. (2017). An effect of Xiaoyao San plus fluoxetine hydrochloride on depression. *Clin. J. Chin. Med.* 10:28.

Chin, C. H., Chen, S. H., Wu, H. H., Ho, C. W., Ko, M. T., and Lin, C. Y. (2014). cytoHubba: identifying hub objects and sub-networks from complex interactome. *BMC Syst. Biol.* 8(Suppl. 4):S11. doi: 10.1186/1752-0509-8-S4-S11

Commission, N. P. (2015). *Pharmacopoeia of the People's Republic of China*. Beijing: China Medical Science and Technology Press.

Cong, C., Kluwe, L., Li, S., Liu, X., Liu, Y., Liu, H., et al. (2019). Paeoniflorin inhibits tributyltin chloride-induced apoptosis in hypothalamic neurons via inhibition of MKK4-JNK signaling pathway. *J. Ethnopharmacol.* 237, 1–8. doi: 10.1016/j.jep.2019.03.030

Cryan, J. F., and Dinan, T. G. (2012). Mind-altering microorganisms: the impact of the gut microbiota on brain and behaviour. *Nat. Rev. Neurosci.* 13, 701–712. doi: 10.1038/nrn3346

Dai, Y., Li, Z., Xue, L., Dou, C., Zhou, Y., Zhang, L., et al. (2010). Metabolomics study on the anti-depression effect of xiaoyaosan on rat model of chronic unpredictable mild stress. *J. Ethnopharmacol.* 128, 482–489. doi: 10.1016/j.jep.2010.01.016

Emmanuel, B., Damien, L., Michael, T., Michel, S., Parit, B., Bridge, A. J., et al. (2016). UniProtKB/Swiss-Prot, the manually annotated section of the UniProt knowledgebase: how to use the entry view. *Methods Mol. Biol.* 1374, 23–54. doi: 10.1007/978-1-4939-3167-5_2

Fang, Z., Polacco, M., Chen, S., Schroeder, S., Hancock, D., Sanchez, H., et al. (2003). cMap: the comparative genetic map viewer. *Bioinformatics* 19, 416–417. doi: 10.1093/bioinformatics/btg012

Forli, S., Huey, R., Pique, M. E., Sanner, M. F., Goodsell, D. S., and Olson, A. J. (2016). Computational protein-ligand docking and virtual drug screening with the AutoDock suite. *Nat. Protoc.* 11, 905–919. doi: 10.1038/nprot.2016.051

Fotakis, G., and Timbrell, J. A. (2006). *In vitro* cytotoxicity assays: comparison of LDH, neutral red, MTT and protein assay in hepatoma cell lines following exposure to cadmium chloride. *Toxicol. Lett.* 160, 171–177. doi: 10.1016/j.toxlet.2005.07.001

Gao, Y., Gao, L., Gao, X. X., Zhou, Y. Z., Qin, X. M., and Tian, J. S. (2015). [An exploration in the action targets for antidepressant bioactive components of Xiaoyaosan based on network pharmacology]. *Acta Pharm. Sin.* 50, 1589–1595. doi: 10.16438/j.0513-4870.2017-0914

Gu, X., Cai, Z., Cai, M., Liu, K., Liu, D., Zhang, Q., et al. (2016). Protective effect of paeoniflorin on inflammation and apoptosis in the cerebral cortex of a transgenic mouse model of Alzheimer's disease. *Mol. Med. Rep.* 13, 2247–2252. doi: 10.3892/mmr.2016.4805

He, L., Qin, Z., Li, M., Chen, Z., Zeng, C., Yao, Z., et al. (2018). Metabolic profiles of ginger, a functional food, and its representative pungent compounds in rats by ultraperformance liquid chromatography coupled with quadrupole time-of-flight tandem mass spectrometry. *J Agric Food Chem.* 66, 9010–9033. doi: 10.1021/acs.jafc.8b03600

Heinricha, M., Appendinob, G., Efferthc, T., Fürstd, R., Izzoe, A. A., Kayserf, O., et al. (2020). Best practice in research - overcoming common challenges in phytopharmacological research. *J. Ethnopharmacol.* 246:112230. doi: 10.1016/j.jep.2019.112230

Iwamoto, K., Kakiuchi, C., Bundo, M., Ikeda, K., and Kato, T. (2004). Molecular characterization of bipolar disorder by comparing gene expression profiles of postmortem brains of major mental disorders. *Mol. Psychiat.* 9, 406–416. doi: 10.1038/sj.mp.4001437

Jiang, Y. M., Li, X. J., Meng, Z. Z., Liu, Y. Y., Zhao, H. B., Na, L., et al. (2016). Effects of Xiaoyaosan on stress-induced anxiety-like behavior in rats: involvement of CRF1 receptor. *Evid. Based Complement Alternat Med.* 2016:1238426. doi: 10.1155/2016/1238426

Jiao, H., Yan, Z., Ma, Q., Li, X., Jiang, Y., Liu, Y., et al. (2019). Influence of Xiaoyaosan on depressive-like behaviors in chronic stress-depressed rats through regulating tryptophan metabolism in hippocampus. *Neuropsychiatr. Dis. Treat.* 15, 21–31. doi: 10.2147/NDT.S185295

Khan, A., Ali, T., Rehman, S. U., Khan, M. S., Alam, S. I., Ikram, M., et al. (2018). Neuroprotective Effect of Quercetin Against the Detrimental Effects of LPS in the Adult Mouse Brain. *Front. Pharmacol.* 9:1383. doi: 10.3389/fphar.2018.01383

Kim, S., Lee, S., Lee, M., and ethnopharmacology, S.L.J.J.o. (2019). A systems pharmacology approach to investigate the mechanism of Oryeong-san formula for the treatment of hypertension. *J Ethnopharmacol.* 244:112129. doi: 10.1016/j.jep.2019.112129

Kloft, C., Trame, M. N., and Ritter, C. A. (2016). Systems pharmacology in drug development and therapeutic use - a forthcoming paradigm shift. 94, 1–3. doi: 10.1016/j.ejps.2016.07.014

Kuhn, M., Szklarczyk, D., Franceschini, A., Mering, C. V., Jensen, L. J., and Bork, P. (2012). STITCH 3: zooming in on protein–chemical interactions. *Nucleic Acids Res.* 40, 876–880. doi: 10.1093/nar/gkr1011

Kuo, D. C., Mina, T., Shah, A. A., and Anu, M. (2015). Depression and the suicidal patient. *Emerg. Med. Clin. North Am.* 33, 765–778. doi: 10.1016/j.emc.2015.07.005

Li, N., Liu, Q., Li, X. J., Bai, X. H., Liu, Y. Y., Zhao, H. B., et al. (2015). TCM formula xiaoyaosan decoction improves depressive-like behaviors in rats with type 2 diabetes. *Evid Based Complem. Alternat. Med.* 2015:415243. doi: 10.1155/2015/415243

Li, X. J., Ma, Q. Y., Jiang, Y. M., Bai, X. H., Yan, Z. Y., Liu, Q., et al. (2017). Xiaoyaosan exerts anxiolytic-like effects by down-regulating the TNF-α/JAK2-STAT3 pathway in the rat hippocampus. *Sci. Rep.* 7:353. doi: 10.1038/s41598-017-00496-y

Liu, W., Xue, X., Xia, J., Liu, J., and Qi, Z. (2018). Swimming exercise reverses CUMS-induced changes in depression-like behaviors and hippocampal plasticity-related proteins. *J Affect Disord.* 227, 126–135. doi: 10.1016/j.jad.2017.10.019

Ludka, F. K., Constantino, L. C., Dal-Cim, T., Binder, L. B., Zomkowski, A., Rodrigues, A. L., et al. (2016). Involvement of PI3K/Akt/GSK-3β and mTOR in the antidepressant-like effect of atorvastatin in mice. *J. Psychiatr. Res.* 82, 50–57. doi: 10.1016/j.jpsychires.2016.07.004

Mao, Q., Zhong, X., Qiu, F., Li, Z., and Huang, Z. (2012). Protective effects of paeoniflorin against corticosterone-induced neurotoxicity in PC12 cells. *Phytother Res.* 26, 969–973. doi: 10.1002/ptr.3673

Mehta, V., Parashar, A., and Udayabanu, M. (2017). Quercetin prevents chronic unpredictable stress induced behavioral dysfunction in mice by alleviating hippocampal oxidative and inflammatory stress. *Physiol. Behav.* 171, 69–78. doi: 10.1016/j.physbeh.2017.01.006

Meng, Z. Z., Chen, J. X., Jiang, Y. M., and Zhang, H. T. (2013). Effect of xiaoyaosan decoction on learning and memory deficit in rats induced by chronic immobilization stress. *Evid. Based Complement. Alternat. Med.* 2013L:297154. doi: 10.1155/2013/297154

Musashe, D. T., Purice, M. D., Speese, S. D., Doherty, J., and Logan, M. A. (2016). Insulin-like signaling promotes glial phagocytic clearance of degenerating axons through regulation of draper. *Cell Rep.* 16, 1838–1850. doi: 10.1016/j.celrep.2016.07.022

Myint, A. M., and Kim, Y. K. (2003). Cytokine–serotonin interaction through IDO: a neurodegeneration hypothesis of depression. *Med. Hypothes.* 61, 519–525. doi: 10.1016/S0306-9877(03)00207-X

Pei, B., Yang, M., Qi, X., Shen, X., Chen, X., Biochemical, F. Z. J., et al. (2016). Quercetin ameliorates ischemia/reperfusion-induced cognitive deficits by inhibiting ASK1/JNK3/caspase-3 by enhancing the Akt signaling pathway. *Biochem. Biophys. Res. Commun.* 478, 199–205. doi: 10.1016/j.bbrc.2016.07.068

Piñero, J., Queraltrosinach, N., Bravo, À., Deupons, J., Bauermehren, A., Baron, M., et al. (2015). DisGeNET: a discovery platform for the dynamical exploration of human diseases and their genes. *Database* 2015:bav028. doi: 10.1093/database/bav028

Ru, J., Li, P., Wang, J., Zhou, W., Li, B., Huang, C., et al. (2014). TCMSP: a database of systems pharmacology for drug discovery from herbal medicines. *J. Cheminform.* 6:13. doi: 10.1186/1758-2946-6-13

Sasaki, K., El Omri, A., Kondo, S., Han, J., and Isoda, H. (2013). Rosmarinus officinalis polyphenols produce anti-depressant like effect through monoaminergic and cholinergic functions modulation. *Behav. Brain Res.* 238, 86–94. doi: 10.1016/j.bbr.2012.10.010

Schwalm, N. D., Townsend, G. E., and Groismana, E. A. (2016). Multiple signals govern utilization of a polysaccharide in the gut bacterium bacteroides thetaiotaomicron. *mBio* 7:e01342-16. doi: 10.1128/mBio.01342-16

Sharma, A. (2016). Systems genomics support for immune and inflammation hypothesis of depression. *Curr. Neuropharmacol.* 14, 749–758. doi: 10.2174/1570159X.14666160106155331

Solem, S., Hagen, R., Wang, C. E., Hjemdal, O., Waterloo, K., Eisemann, M., et al. (2017). Metacognitions and mindful attention awareness in depression: a comparison of currently depressed, previously depressed and never depressed individuals. *Clin. Psychol. Psychother.* 24, 94–102. doi: 10.1002/cpp.1983

Szklarczyk, D., Morris, J. H., Cook, H., Kuhn, M., Wyder, S., Simonovic, M., et al. (2017). The STRING database in 2017: quality-controlled protein–protein association networks, made broadly accessible. *Nucleic Acids Res.* 45, D362–D368. doi: 10.1093/nar/gkw937

Tao, W., Xu, X., Wang, X., Li, B., Wang, Y., Li, Y., et al. (2013). Network pharmacology-based prediction of the active ingredients and potential targets of Chinese herbal Radix Curcumae formula for application to cardiovascular disease. *J. Ethnopharmacol.* 145, 1–10. doi: 10.1016/j.jep.2012.09.051

Tom, B., Michael, B., and Mazda, A. (2014). Chronic and treatment resistant depression: diagnosis and stepwise therapy. *Dtsch. Arztebl. Int.* 111, 766–775. doi: 10.3238/arztebl.2014.0766

Wainwright, S. R., and Galea, L. A. M. (2013). The neural plasticity theory of depression: assessing the roles of adult neurogenesis and PSA-NCAM within the Hippocampus. *Neural Plast.* 2013:805497. doi: 10.1155/2013/805497

Wang, X., Shen, Y., Wang, S., Li, S., Zhang, W., Liu, X., et al. (2017). PharmMapper 2017 update: a web server for potential drug target identification with a comprehensive target pharmacophore database. *Nucleic Acids Res.* 45, W356–W360. doi: 10.1093/nar/gkx374

Wishart, D. S., Feunang, Y. D., Guo, A. C., Lo, E. J., Marcu, A., Grant, J. R., et al. (2017). DrugBank 5.0: a major update to the DrugBank database for 2018. *Nucleic Acids Research* 46, D1074–D1082. doi: 10.1093/nar/gkx1037

Xue, X., Wuxia, Z., Chao, H., Yan, L., Hua, Y., Yonghua, W., et al. (2012). A novel chemometric method for the prediction of human oral bioavailability. *Int. J. Mol. Sci.* 13, 6964–6982. doi: 10.3390/ijms13066964

Yan, Z., Jiao, H., Ding, X., Ma, Q., Li, X., Pan, Q., et al. (2018). Xiaoyaosan improves depressive-like behaviors in mice through regulating apelin-APJ system in hypothalamus. *Molecules* 23:1073. doi: 10.3390/molecules23051073

Youdim, K. A., Dobbie, M. S., Gunter, K., Proteggente, A. R., Abbott, N. J., and Rice-Evans, C. (2003). Interaction between flavonoids and the blood-brain barrier: *in vitro* studies. *J. Neurochem.* 85, 180–192. doi: 10.1046/j.1471-4159.2003.01652.x

Yu, G., Wang, L., Han, Y., and He, Q. (2012). clusterProfiler: an R Package for comparing biological themes among gene clusters. *Omics J. Integr. Biol.* 16, 284–287. doi: 10.1089/omi.2011.0118

Yue, S-J., Liu, J., Feng, W.-W., Zhang, F.-L., Chen, J.-X., Xin, L-T et al. (2017). System pharmacology-based dissection of the synergistic mechanism of Huangqi and Huanglian for diabetes mellitus. *Front. Pharmacol.* 8:694. doi: 10.3389/fphar.2017.00694

Zhang, Y., Han, M., Liu, Z., Wang, J., He, Q., and Liu, J. (2011). Chinese herbal formula xiao yao san for treatment of depression: a systematic review of randomized controlled trials. *Evidence Based Complement. Altern. Med.* 2012:931636. doi: 10.1155/2012/931636

Zhong, X., Li, G., Qiu, F., and Huang, Z. (2018). Paeoniflorin ameliorates chronic stress-induced depression-like behaviors and neuronal damages in rats via activation of the ERK-CREB pathway. *Front. Psychiatry* 9:772. doi: 10.3389/fpsyt.2018.00772

Zhou, W., Chen, Z., Wang, Y., Li, X., Lu, A., Sun, X., et al. (2019). Systems pharmacology-based method to assess the mechanism of action of weight-loss herbal intervention therapy for obesity. *Front. Pharmacol.* 10:1165. doi: 10.3389/fphar.2019.01165

Zhou, Y., Ren, Y., Ma, Z., Jia, G., Gao, X., Zhang, L., et al. (2012). Identification and quantification of the major volatile constituents in antidepressant active fraction of xiaoyaosan by gas chromatography–mass spectrometry. *J. Ethnopharmacol.* 141, 187–192. doi: 10.1016/j.jep.2012.02.018

Zhu, F., Han, B. C., Kumar, P., Liu, X. H., Ma, X. H., Wei, X. N., et al. (2010). Update of TTD: therapeutic target database. *Nucleic Acids Res.* 38, D787–D791. doi: 10.1093/nar/gkp1014

7

Salvia miltiorrhiza Bge. (Danshen) for Inflammatory Bowel Disease: Clinical Evidence and Network Pharmacology-Based Strategy for Developing Supplementary Medical Application

Siyuan Zhang[1], *Hua Luo*[1], *Shiyi Sun*[2], *Yating Zhang*[2], *Jiaqi Ma*[2], *Yuting Lin*[2], *Lin Yang*[1], *Dechao Tan*[1], *Chaomei Fu*[2], *Zhangfeng Zhong*[1]* *and Yitao Wang*[1]*

[1]*Macau Centre for Research and Development in Chinese Medicine, Institute of Chinese Medical Sciences, University of Macau, Taipa, Macao, China,* [2]*School of Pharmacy, Chengdu University of Traditional Chinese Medicine, Chengdu, China*

Correspondence:
Zhangfeng Zhong
zhangfengzhong@um.edu.mo
Yitao Wang
ytwang@um.edu.mo

Inflammatory bowel disease (IBD) is a non-specific colorectal disease caused by multifaceted triggers. Although conventional treatments are effective in the management of IBD, high cost and frequent side effects limit their applications and have turned sufferers toward alternative and complementary approaches. *Salvia miltiorrhiza* Bge (Danshen) is an herbal medicine that reportedly alleviates the symptoms of IBD. A large body of research, including clinical trials in which Danshen-based products or botanical compounds were used, has unmasked its multiple mechanisms of action, but no review has focused on its efficacy as a treatment for IBD. Here, we discussed triggers of IBD, collected relevant clinical trials and analyzed experimental reports, in which bioactive compounds of Danshen attenuated rodent colitis in the management of intestinal integrity, gut microflora, cell death, immune conditions, cytokines, and free radicals. A network pharmacology approach was applied to describe sophisticated mechanisms in a holistic view. The safety of Danshen was also discussed. This review of evidence will help to better understand the potential benefits of Danshen for IBD treatment and provide insights for the development of innovative applications of Danshen.

Keywords: inflammatory bowel disease, *Salvia miltiorrhiza* bge, danshen, clinical trial, network pharmacology

INTRODUCTION

Inflammatory bowel disease (IBD), including ulcerative colitis (UC) and Crohn's disease (CD), is a non-specific intestinal disease characterized by chronic inflammation (Olsen et al., 2009). The prevalence rates of UC and CD have risen to 294 and 213 per 100,000 respectively in Europe while the incidence rate of IBD in Hong Kong has tripled to 3.1 per 100,000, illustrating the scale of the disease as a public health issue (Burisch et al., 2013; Mak et al., 2020). Patients with IBD suffer from abdominal pain, diarrhea, hematochezia and weight loss related to pathological changes including ulcerative activation, mucosal damage, and autoimmune disturbance (Petryszyn and Paradowski, 2018). Multi-faceted extrinsic and intrinsic triggers (the latter including microorganisms, genetic susceptibility, and immunological overreaction) are thought to contribute to the initiation and aggravation of IBD. Dyshomeostasis in gut microflora may lead to bacterial invasion through the intestinal barrier and an abnormal immune response with overexpression of inflammatory factors, causing IBD-like symptoms (Lee, 2015). However, the precise etiology is not yet fully understood. Anti-inflammatory agents, such as sulfasalazine and mesalazine, with a long history of utilization, are conventional treatments while biological immunosuppressants, steroids, and even microbiome-inspired therapeutics are effective (Plichta et al., 2019). Although therapeutics of this kind can bring rapid alleviation of symptoms, a limited recovery, high recurrence rates, heavy economic burden, and severe adverse events are major drawbacks and have encouraged sufferers to seek alternative methods for better management of IBD.

Complementary and alternative approaches provide significant benefits for IBD treatment. As a critical part of global supplementary medicine, herbal medicine has attracted much attention due to the unique therapeutic effects of natural material. An abundant body of medical herbs, such as *Coptis chinensis* Franch (Huanglian), *Zingiber officinale* Rosc (Ganjiang), and *Paeonia lactiflora* Pall (Shaoyao), have shown the potentials in the management of colitis (Cao et al., 2019). Among these anti-IBD phytotherapies, Danshen exhibited multilevel efficacies and Danshen-containing products have been utilized in clinic as satisfying treatments. Danshen (*Salvia miltiorrhiza* Bge.) was first recorded in Shennong's herbal classic of materia medica, Shennong Bencao Jing, a botanical monograph written in the Eastern Han dynasty (AD25-AD220) in China. Danshen is widely applied in the treatment of systemic, especially cardiovascular diseases (Wang L. et al., 2017). More recently, research has shown that natural compounds isolated from Danshen have anti-inflammatory, anti-oxidative and anti-bacterial properties, and are effective in immune regulation and intestinal epithelium protection (Ma et al., 2016; Cao et al., 2017). Danshen extract or molecule compounds could improve colitis symptoms, such as gastro-intestinal bleed, weight loss, and lethal rate in rodent colitis models. In addition, Danshen-based products have shown therapeutic efficacy in clinical trials with attenuation of symptoms and protection from disease recurrence (Deng et al., 2016; Zhu, 2018; Zhu, 2019). Danshen product has been approved by College ter Beoordeling van Geneesmiddelen-Medicines Evaluation Board (CBG-MEB) and used in Europe since 2016.

While these findings imply that Danshen can have a significant impact on IBD, the related molecular mechanisms have not been clearly identified due to methodological limitations related to the "multi-compounds-multi-targets" approach of modeling a sophisticated regulatory network of signal transduction (Luo et al., 2020). Interdisciplinary research has led to the development of identification tools, establishment of a holistic index-assessment system, crosstalk with decussate subjects, and improved statistical analysis methods (Liu et al., 2017; Bai et al., 2018).

This review is a systematic evaluation of the efficacy and safety of Danshen in the treatment of IBD evidenced by experimental studies and clinical trials. Bioactive compounds existing in Danshen were identified, relevant clinical trials were sourced and experimental reports were analyzed to unmask potential mechanisms of Danshen in IBD. To minimize the limitations of the "one-compound-single-target" approach, which does not include the multiple targets in disease, a network pharmacology approach was utilized to estimate and visualize potential actions of Danshen. The safety of Danshen and Danshen-containing products was also discussed. The review provides new ideas about novel applications of Danshen in IBD.

THE PATHOLOGY OF IBD

IBD is a chronic inflammatory disease induced by multi-faceted triggers including epigenetic factors and genetic susceptibility (Olsen et al., 2009). Smoking is a significant environmental risk factor for exacerbating IBD at any age, including infancy (Shouval and Rufo, 2017), but does not have the same impact in UC patients (Blackwell et al., 2019). Mental stress, health status, infectious diseases, vitamin D deficiency, unhealthy diets characterized by high fat (especially saturated acid), high sugar, high cholesterol, and low fiber, all contribute to the pathogenesis of IBD (Mouli and Ananthakrishnan, 2014; Lewis and Abreu, 2017; Khalili et al., 2018). Antigens and dietary nutrients have an important role in maintaining homeostasis between intestinal bacteria and commensal microflora. For instance, breast-feeding helps to decrease the risks of IBD by improving the homeostatic ecosystem in the infant gut (Andrew R. Barclay et al., 2009). Differences in intestinal microflora structure between patients with IBD and healthy volunteers demonstrated that gut microorganisms are an important factor in the disease, consistent with evidence that animal colitis could be induced in healthy mice by inoculating intestinal microflora from those with UC (Plichta et al., 2019). In addition to the type of gut bacteria, their distribution, abundance, and mobility are important factors in the initiation of IBD (Guo et al., 2020). Fungi, viruses, and parasites also influence gut homeostasis. Interestingly, certain parasites have a beneficial effect on the host immune response, and therefore on colitis (Harris, 2016; Pickard et al., 2017). However, this effect needs to be explored further to provide more compelling evidence on the roles of primary and secondary metabolites in the patho-physiological course of IBD (Segal et al., 2019).

It is well known that invasive pathological bacteria and toxins lead to dysfunction of intestinal epithelial cells and damage in intestinal integrity, which consequently disturbs the host immune response and aggravates inflammatory cascades in mucosal tissues (Katsanos and Papadakis, 2017). The intestinal barrier is a defensive structure composed of host cells, mucosal matrix, synergic bacteria, and immune triggers such as antibodies, antimicrobial peptides, cytokines, and chemokines (Lee, 2015). With the ability to regenerate rapidly in damaged tissues, intestinal epithelial and mesenchymal stem cells have important roles in maintaining mucosal structure and protective functions (Chami et al., 2018). Tight junctions (TJs) between epithelial cells are fundamental to intestinal barrier integrity, and their condition is indicative of the degree of inflammatory damage in IBD. Consequently, mucosal healing is a significant feature of remission in IBD.

IBD involves dysfunction of the innate and adaptive immune systems, with overexpression of inflammatory mediators followed by excessive immune responses inducing chronic or acute inflammatory damage to the colon (Soufli et al., 2016). Macrophages and monocytes play a part in this damage and a range of dysregulated immune cells have been found to disrupt cellular homeostasis (Park et al., 2017). Another notable feature is the abnormal presence of adaptive immune cells including Th1, Th2, Th17, and Treg lymphocytes, which are important to the hosts' recognition and neutralization of gut antigens (Friedrich et al., 2019). Aberrant expression of pro-inflammatory cytokines such as tumor necrosis factor-α (TNF-α), IL-6, IL-1β, and Interferon-γ (IFN-γ), reflects a persistent disturbed immune response which initiates and aggravates intestinal inflammation (Katsanos and Papadakis, 2017). In patients with UC, the lamina propria and mucosa are infiltrated by Th1 and Th17-profile cells, and a similar process occurs in patients with CD *via* IL-23/IL-17 axis (Feagan et al., 2016; Friedrich et al., 2019). Therapeutic management of intractable IBD requires monoclonal antibodies with high intensity and specific targeting of representative cytokines, and research in this area has increased understanding of chronic inflammatory diseases and their etiologies.

Risk factors for IBD include economic status, lifestyle, diet, society stress, and genetic factors, the latter consistent with evidence of higher risk in certain ethnic or genetic groups (Ng et al., 2013; Eka et al., 2014). Genome-wide gene expression studies have unmasked the existence of a set of IBD-related genes, which participate in different locations and stages of IBD, in parallel with distinctions between UC and CD phenotypes (Noble et al., 2008; Olsen et al., 2009). Mutation of nucleotide binding oligomerization domain-containing protein 2 (NOD2), associated with toll-like receptors (TLRs) and NOD-like receptors (NLRs), is followed by dysfunction of autophagy and inflammatory responses while deletion of mucin 1 (MUC1) and MUC4 disturbs the mucosal homeostasis (Ramanan et al., 2014; Vancamelbeke et al., 2017). Genetic abnormality associated with the host's immune response, intestinal barrier protection, or inflammatory signal transduction may contribute to the manifestation of IBD-associated symptoms (Eka et al., 2014). However, knowledge of candidate sites is not yet sufficient to evaluate the pathology and to form the basis of diagnostic tests for IBD. Further research is needed to investigate the mechanisms involved. Since holistic outcomes result from sophisticated triggers and interactions at a molecular level, a detailed understanding of molecular mechanisms is important to shed light on prognosis, protection, and amelioration of IBD.

PHYTOCHEMICAL CHARACTERS OF DANSHEN

Phytochemical profiling of Danshen began in the 1930s (Zhou et al., 2005) and enhances understanding of Danshen's role in disease treatment. With novel extraction, separation, and identification techniques applied in plant research, ingredients have been retrieved from Danshen and their structure are described (Guo et al., 2014). The principal bioactive compounds of Danshen are divided into two parts according to structural characteristics (Zhang XZ. et al., 2016). One is the hydrophilic phenolic acids. The core phenolic structure, in a C_6C_3 cluster, exists in both polyphenolic salvianolic compounds like Salvianolic acid B (SAB) and non-polyphenolic compounds such as Salvianic acid A (SA), Caffeic acid (CA), and Protocatechuic aldehyde (PA). The second group, most termed tanshinones, consist of lipophilic phenanthraquinones and their derivatives, is classified into diterpenoids, tricyclic diterpenoids and royleanone tanshinones (Wang L. et al., 2017). Diterpenoid tanshinone, which is represented by Tanshinone IIA (TIIA), Tanshinone IIB (TIIB), and Cryptotanshinone, is constructed according to the basic phenanthraquinone cluster with 1,2-o-quinones core and furan-like units (Hatfield et al., 2013). In addition, the furan or dihydrofuran ring is displaced by isopropyl cluster in tricyclic diterpenoids while royleanone tanshinones are characterized by 1,4-p-quinones, with Miltirone and Isotanshinone respectively.

Despite differences in structure, compounds of Danshen display common therapeutic effects on IBD, including anti-inflammatory properties of tanshinones and anti-oxidative properties of salvianolic acids (Wang L. et al., 2017; Gao et al., 2017). Other compounds were reported such as triterpenoids and flavones, and including physiological constituents (amino acids and metallic elements) (Guo et al., 2014). In addition, many species of essential oils were discovered in the flower of Danshen rather than the root and rhizome, indicating that novel applications may be found by exploiting all parts of the plant (Liang et al., 2009). However, few reports about non-tanshinone or non-salvianolic acid compounds of Danshen have focused on the management of colitis. For more details on the structure of compounds of Danshen, supplementary reviews are available (Zhou et al., 2005; Zhang XZ. et al., 2016; Wang L. et al., 2017). The compounds outlined above are included in the present review and are depicted in **Figure 1**.

PHARMACOLOGICAL ACTIONS AND MECHANISMS OF DANSHEN FOR IBD TREATMENT

Attenuation of Animal Symptoms in IBD Models With Utilization of Danshen

Since IBD is associated with abnormal immune response caused by multifactorial triggers, it is important to establish experimental models to mimic and investigate this abnormality. Dextran sulfate sodium (DSS) and 2,4,6-trinitrobenzene sulfonic acid (TNBS) disturb the intestinal epithelial barrier and render colonic proteins immunogenic, resulting in a comprehensively dysfunctional immune response including excessive Th1/Th17 activation, cytokine release, and infiltration by immune cells (Kiesler et al., 2015). Compounds of Danshen may protect against DSS and TNBS and thus attenuate animal colitis-indications including weight loss, diarrhea, undereating, shortening colon length, colon weight change, rectal bleeding, diminished health status, alternation in

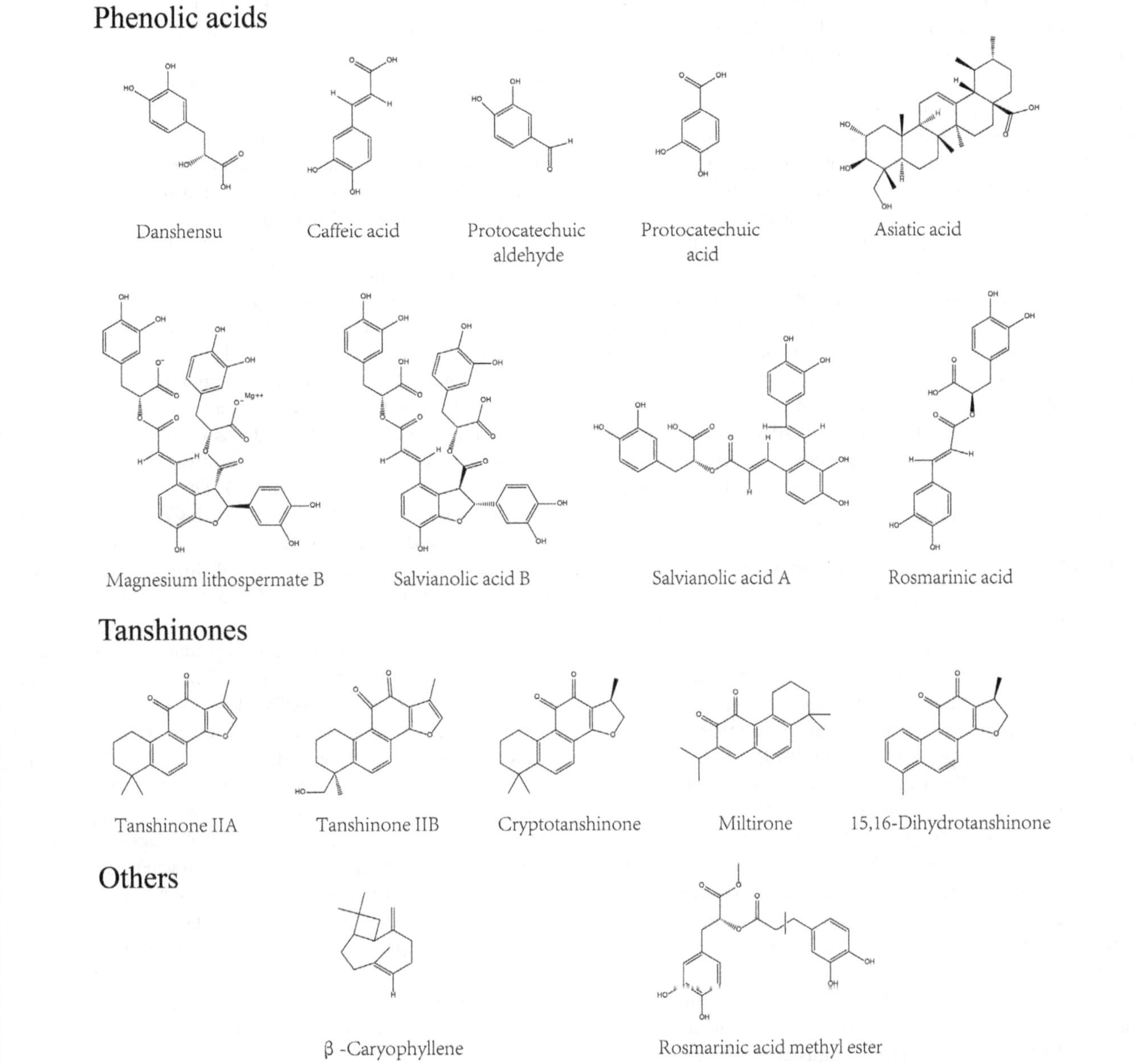

FIGURE 1 | Characteristic compounds of Danshen. Compounds derived from Danshen were divided into phenolic acids, tanshinones and others by their structural characters and pharmacological effects.

spleen scale, or liver weight change. In addition to these benefits, Danshen was associated with histological changes related to epithelial integrity, the infiltration of neutrophils (marked by CD177) and macrophages (marked by F4/80), T cells and B cell function, and reduction in crypts (Jeong et al., 2015; Jin et al., 2017; Wang et al., 2018).

Intestinal Epithelial Barrier and Gut Microflora Regulated by Danshen

A feature of IBD is irreversibly degraded integrity of the intestinal epithelial barrier, including TJs classified into Zonula occludens (ZO), Occludins, and claudins (Lee, 2015). Myosin light chain kinase (MLCK), which monitors permeability of the epithelial barrier, interacts with TJs by contraction of the perijunctional actomyosin ring (Feng et al., 2020). Therefore, research has focused on the roles of MLCK in colonic epithelium dysfunction. SAB, the major water-soluble compound of Danshen with anti-inflammatory and anti-oxidative properties, might attenuate abnormality of MLCK after TNBS exposure in rats. Similar to the results *in vivo*, SAB induced microRNA-1 to suppress MLCK detected by dual luciferase reporter assay in IL-1β-stimulated Caco2 intestinal monolayer, consequently ameliorating loss of epithelial ZO-1 and claudin-2 (Xiong et al., 2016; Feng et al., 2020). Similarly, Salvianolic acid A (SAA) attenuated disruption of ZO-1 and Occludin mRNA triggered by DSS (Wang et al., 2018).

Homeostasis of gut microflora is another important factor associated with IBD. While it remains unclear whether bioactive ingredients reverse microbial dysbiosis in the treatment of IBD or ameliorate the inflammatory status to balance microflora distribution, these interactions and their implications for treatment of disease have attracted considerable research interest. For example, SAB and SAA might restore acid balance and promote healthy gut microbiota, with a significant decrease in *Bacteroides* and an increase in *S24-7* (Wu et al., 2018). Consistent with this, enriched microflora populations, particularly *Akkermansia spp*, and improved microbiota balance had been round in DSS-exposed rats treated with SAA and CA (Zhang Z. et al., 2016; Wang et al., 2018). It was of interest that the gut-kidney axis may contribute to regulation of gut microbiota by Magnesium lithospermate B (MLB), suggesting holistic interactions among diverse organs (Zhao et al., 2019b).

Cell Death Controlled by Danshen

Apoptosis, programmed cell death, acts as a regulatory system in response to extrinsic signals. Morphological and physiological changes during apoptosis can be observed while DNA fragments can be detected by TUNEL assay. The measurement of caspase protein expression, activity, and cleavage-associated maturity, in which B-cell lymphoma 2 (Bcl-2) family members take part, reflects the process of apoptosis (Nagata, 2018). Of note, Caspase-3 is an important mediator in this process. B cells interact closely with cleaved Caspase-3 and Ki-67 while the peroxisome proliferators-activated receptors γ (PPAR-γ) signaling pathway was influenced by the molecular binding of β-Caryophyllene (BC) to Cannabinoid receptor 2 (CB2). In DSS-induced and lipopolysaccharide (LPS)-stimulated experimental models, treatment with BC suppressed expression of macrophage inflammatory protein 2 (MIP2), C-X-C motif chemokine ligand 1 (CINC-1/CXCL1), TNF-α and IL-4 by inhibiting the Nuclear factor kappa B (NF-κB)- extracellular regulated protein kinases (ERK1/2) axis, and attenuated damage due to inflammation (Bento et al., 2011). As cell proliferation and survival are both disturbed in IBD pathogenesis, Rosmarinic acid (RA) was shown to regulate apoptosis-associated mediators including Bcl-XL, Bcl-2, and X-linked inhibitor of apoptosis (XIAP) with its mutually anti-inflammatory performance to obtain remission of DSS-induced colitis. In addition, levels of Cyclin D1 and cyclin dependent kinase 4 (Cdk4), two direct biomarkers for the cell cycle, were also restored to normal after treatment of RA, which protected cellular status when exposed to deleterious factors (Jin et al., 2017). Meanwhile, Tanshinol could protect normal colorectal mucosal cell from apoptosis *via* improvement of low density lipoprotein receptor (VLDR) (Zhu et al., 2021).

Necroptosis is another form of cell death triggered by inflammation and found in the intestinal epithelium of UC patients. When the apoptosis trigger Caspase-8 is blocked, necroptosis regulated by kinases receptor-interacting protein 1 (RIP1)/RIP3/mixed lineage kinase domain-like protein (MLKL) axis is initiated (Tkachenko, 2019). Necroptosis and pyroptosis (an inflammatory programmed cell death) both protect the host from invasive bacteria and feature cell swelling, membrane rupture and cellular content expulsion. NLR family pyrin domain containing 3 (NLRP3) is the most well-studied NLR member to oligomerize apoptosis-associated speck-like protein (ASC), activate Caspase-1 and bring pro-IL-18 and pro-IL-1β to maturation, resulting in Gasdermin-mediated pyroptosis (Kovacs and Miao, 2017). Dihydrotanshinone I (DT) might attenuate DSS-induced damage in the colon and overexpression of pro-inflammatory cytokines through the RIPs-MLKL-Caspase-8 axis, independently of necroptosis (Guo et al., 2018), a property also found in Cryptotanshinone (Min et al., 2020). Asiatic acid (AA) had been found to attenuate colitis symptoms more effectively than sulfasalazine, the therapeutic agent conventionally used in IBD for many years. AA achieved this by scavenging ROS and sustaining mitochondrion membrane integrity, as identified by Mitosox staining and JC-1 staining. Following this attenuation, NLRP3, Caspase-1, and IL-1β were suppressed, as demonstrated both *in vivo* and *in vitro* (Guo et al., 2015). In addition, MLB decreased TNF-α both in DSS-induced chronic and acute colitis with significant suppression of NLPR3/ASC/Caspase-1 pathway (Jiang et al., 2016).

Autophagy is a conserved process in mammals whereby cellular components are degraded and recycled. The ratio of microtubule-associated light chain 3–II (LC3-II) to LC3-I is an important biomarker for this process while other relevant proteins including beclin-1 and Sequestosome 1 (SQSTM1)/p62 play significant roles. It is unclear whether autophagy reduces or increases inflammation, and the interactions of autophagy with the immune response, cell stress, and cellular signal transduction with respect to the etiology of IBD have attracted much attention (Kabat et al., 2016). For example, Tanshinone IIA Sodium Sulfonate (TSS) had shown regulatory effects on LC3-II/LC3-I, beclin-1, and autophagosome, which might contribute to its role in the protection of intestinal epithelium integrity and in downregulation of inflammatory factors including IL-1β, TNF-α, and IL-6 in LPS-induced model (Yang et al., 2018).

Immunology and Cytokines Induced by Danshen

Although the etiology of IBD is not yet fully understood, evidence increasingly points to a critical role of immunity dysfunction in bacterial penetration of the intestine. Cytokines, which are released by immune cells and a small proportion of non-immune cells, participate in mucosal responsiveness and aggravate inflammatory cascades during the pathological process of IBD (Friedrich et al., 2019). Therefore, anti-inflammatory compounds isolated from Danshen have been tested for their impacts on cytokine-profile etiology characterized by TNF-α, IL-6, IL-1β, IFN-γ and other cytokines. Most of the research on the therapeutic effects of Danshen constituents had focused on pro-inflammatory cytokines as an indicator of disease severity (Zhang Z. et al., 2016; Crespo et al., 2017; Wang et al., 2018).

Cyclooxygenase-2 (COX-2), an immediate-early pro-inflammatory mediator, is induced in response to inflammatory stress with crosstalk of cytokines including TNF-α, IL-1α and IFN-α/β (Jin et al., 2017). After treatment with various Danshen-sourced compounds, the high level of COX-2 was reduced, indicating anti-inflammatory properties of Danshen (Crespo et al., 2017; Jin et al., 2017; Zhao et al., 2018). Similarly, Danshen had protective effects on the multifaceted agents including transcriptional factors and pro- and anti-inflammatory cytokines which trigger the differentiation of T helper cells. Th1 is induced by T-bet and triggers a strong immune response damaging cellular homeostasis, which is suppressed by Th2 and similar cytokines including IL-4 and IL-10. A Danshen patent drug consisting of SA (8%) and PA (16%) might restore dysregulation of T-bet in TNBS-induced murine colitis (Xu Dekui et al., 2012). Certain cytokines have unique properties, such as IL-12 which is essential to activate the development of Th1 cells and release of IFN-γ (Soufli et al., 2016). IL-12 was reduced in DSS-induced mice serum and restored to normal by treatment with CA (Zhang Z. et al., 2016). IL-22 has positive and negative effects, participating both in intestinal mucosal repair and in the inflammation process (Friedrich et al., 2019). Incidentally, RA was manifested to decreased levels of IL-22 in DSS-induced model (Jin et al., 2017). The transcriptional factor forkhead box P3 (Foxp3) is the most reliable biomarker of regulatory T cells (Tregs), responsible for regulating the autoimmune system. The injection of Danshen powder had been found to increase Foxp3 and mRNA in TNBS-induced mouse spleen, enhancing its anti-inflammatory function, specifically its attenuation of MPO (Xu et al., 2014). Of interest, transforming growth factor β (TGF-β) had been found to participate in the management of Foxp3+ Treg cell dynamics, supported by SAA's regulatory role in inflamed colonic mucosa (Wang et al., 2018). As highlighted by research on the immune regulatory ability of Miltirone, a receptor agonist derived from Danshen (Wang H. et al., 2017), IL-8, an important biomarker of IBD, is overexpressed in damaged intestinal tissues and consequently recruits neutrophils (Liu et al., 2016). Similarly, IL-17, along with chemokines, growth factors, and adhesion molecules form an interactive network which enhances the infiltration of immune cells. The DSS-induced release of pro-inflammatory mediator monocyte chemoattractant protein-1 (MCP-1) or overexpression of IL-17 mRNA might be ameliorated by TIIA (Zhang et al., 2015), and CA respectively, the latter closely correlated with colonic histopathological scores (Ye et al., 2009).

Free Radicals and Oxidative Stress Balanced by Danshen

In hypoxic conditions, stable hypoxia-inducible factor (HIF)-1α dimerizes with HIF-1β to translocate into cell nuclei and regulate relevant genes for oxidative sensitive mediators and associated proteins such as VEGF which triggers angiogenesis to increase oxygen supply (Perrotta et al., 2015). Rosmarinic acid methyl ester (RAME), a less hydrophilic derivative of RA, suppressed hypoxia inducible factor-prolyl hydroxylase-2 (HPH) and enhanced the release of stable HIF-1α to produce VEGF. This effect formed the basis of RAME treatment to attenuate experimental colitis characterized by pro-inflammatory indicators including MPO, CINC3, COX-2 and inducible nitric oxide synthase (iNOS) (Jeong et al., 2015).

The Nuclear factor E2-related factor 2 (Nrf2) signaling pathway plays an important protective role against inflammation-related oxidative harm marked by reactive oxygen species (ROS), the imbalance of which is regarded as a significant etiological factor for IBD. In this pathway, external stimuli trigger the production of superoxide anion which is transformed into hydrogen peroxide and catalyzed by the catalase/myeloperoxidase (CAT/MPO) enzymatic complex to induce an increase in neutrophils (Balmus et al., 2016). Research had shown that SAB (Xiong et al., 2016), DT (Guo et al., 2018), AA (Guo et al., 2015), RA (Zhao et al., 2018), CA (Ye et al., 2009), and Protocatechuic acid (PAC) (Crespo et al., 2017), suppressed MPO in inflamed colonic tissues, indicating anti-inflammatory and anti-oxidative abilities of Danshen.

Of interest, iNOS and its product nitric oxide (NO), are abundant in inflamed tissues of patients with IBD and in experimental colitis tissue, having alternative impacts which depend on the quantities of NO, stimuli, duration of disease, and even anatomical sites (Soufli et al., 2016). These effects of NO may derive from the reaction with free radical superoxide anion (O2-) to form peroxynitrite (ONOO-) (Kolios et al., 2004). As might be expected, RA, with attenuating effects on colitis syndromes, correlated negatively with NO and iNOS mRNA. In addition, in DSS-induced mice the anti-inflammatory effect of RA, suppressing TNF-α, IL-6 and IL-1β, was enhanced when in combination with black rice anthocyanin-rich extract (Zhao et al., 2018). Other compounds isolated from Danshen including TIIA (Zhao et al., 2018) and PAC (Farombi et al., 2016) also exhibited beneficial impacts on the expression of NO and iNOS. Levels of oxidized-glutathione (GSH), along with relevant enzymes for glutathione metabolism including glutathione peroxidase (GPx) and glutathione-S-transferase (GST), directly reflect cellular oxidative stress. In the DSS-triggered ulcerative colitis model, PAC significantly restored decreased GPx, GST, and Superoxide dismutase (SOD) with resulting reduction in colorectal inflammation. Similar effects also occurred in hepatic tissues indicating that PAC might achieve this outcome *via* complex mechanisms (Farombi et al., 2016). Another report sustained the semblable observation, in which GSSG/GSH ratio, SOD-1, Nrf2, and CAT were reserved (Crespo et al., 2017). In addition, antioxidant properties of SAB might offer protection from TNBS and LPS induced damage, which was noted by NADPH oxidase 4 (NOX4), iNOS, malondialdehyde (MDA), GSH, SOD, and ROS (Xiong et al., 2016).

Multiple Signaling of IBD Mediated by Danshen

In addition to the aforementioned indicators of IBD severity, cellular transducers form a sophisticated network of signaling pathways in response to extrinsic stress in disease. Research on multiple signaling mediators has the potential to reveal key factors in progression of this disease.

TLRs on the cell membrane surface could recognize stimuli like bacteria and mismatched mediators. When TLR4, one typical kind of TLRs recognizing lipopolysaccharide, is activated, NF-κB would be the fundamental mediator to the initiation and progression of inflammatory diseases like IBD (Mitchell et al., 2016). NF-κB is released after phosphorylation of IκB by IκB kinase (IKK) and then translocates into nuclei to activate promoters of inflammation. Research has shown that compounds of Danshen prevent this release and therefore have a major role to play in limiting inflammation (Nennig and Schank, 2017). Kim et al. reported that, with treatment of 70% ethanol extraction of Danshen, EGFP fluorescence was inhibited in small intestinal segments from *cis*- NF-κB^{EGFP} transgenic mice stressed by LPS, indicating blockage of NF-κB. The inhibitory mechanism was multifactorial and more research was needed to define which bioactive compounds are key to limiting inflammation (Kim et al., 2005). Consistent with the above findings, compared with a DSS-induced model without any treatment, CA suppressed the NF-κB signaling pathway, with decreased levels of nuclear p-p65 and p65, and a decline in IL-6, TNF-α, and IFN-γ. In addition to suppression, balance of gut microflora including *Firmicute*, *Bacteroidetes*, and *Akkermansia* was restored, facilitating intestinal damage remission (Zhang Z. et al., 2016). PAC, the metabolite of Cyanidin-3 β -D-Glycoside (CG), had also been found to inhibit hyperactive NF-κB in a mouse model. With better anti-inflammatory ability than CG, PAC attenuated colitis-associated parameters, including excessive pro-inflammatory triggers (Jang et al., 2016).

As well as hydrophilic components of Danshen, anti-inflammatory properties have also been demonstrated in the lipophilic components, *via* management of NF-κB signaling. Miltirone, an element of tanshinones, downregulated TLR4/NF-κB/IQGAP2 to attenuate colonic inflammation in TNBS-treated mice (Wang H. et al., 2017). Meanwhile, cryptotanshione could inhibit TLR4/p38 MAPK/NF-κB p65 pathway in the colitis (Min et al., 2020).

After phosphorylation at tyrosine residues or serine residues by JAKs, signal transducers and activators of transcription (STATs) accelerate dimerization and consequently translocate into nuclei and activate relevant genes of cytokines and pro-inflammatory enzymes. This contributes to initiating IBD and other chronic inflammatory diseases (Crespo et al., 2017). Synergistically, interactive modification of crosstalk with STATs assists responses to extrinsic and intrinsic factors. RA's amelioration of DSS-induced colitis derived from decussate suppression of NF-κB and STAT3 signaling transduction characterized by diminished phosphorylation at tyrosine 705 residue rather than serine 727 residue. Following the management of cellular signals, inflammatory mediators including MPO, IL-22, Cdk4, and Cyclin D1 were simultaneously controlled (Jin et al., 2017). As the upstream trigger in STAT3 signaling pathway, Sphingosine-1-phosphate (S1P) and its catalytic synthase, sphingosine kinase (SphK), remain in excess in chronic IBD. PAC had been shown to attenuate excessive SphK1 and S1P receptor (S1P1R) in TNBS-treated mice with impact on S1P-related genes SGPP2 and S1PL. Along with management of the SphK/S1P axis, PAC ameliorated colitis severity depending on antioxidant profile indicated by GSH, CAT, SOD-1, and Nrf2 and intersections with synergistic pathways including AKT, ERK, STAT3, and NF-κB (Crespo et al., 2017).

Intestinal pregnane x receptor (PXR) is inactive in IBD patients, which reflects the necessary role of PXR in maintaining intestinal barrier integrity (Zhang et al., 2015). CYP3A4, CYP4B1, and other xenobiotic-metabolizing genes encoding cytochrome P450 monooxygenases are considered metabolically important in IBD. A compound isolated from Danshen, TIIA, acts as an efficacious PXR agonist. Research on experimental colitis found that levels of metabolic enzymes including CYP3A11, CYP3A13, MDR1, and Gsta1 were restored during disease remission (Zhang et al., 2015). CA restored normal weight in DSS-exposed mice with attenuation of MPO and CYP4B1 expression (Ye et al., 2009; Ye et al., 2011). Other research showing similar regulatory effects suggested CA as a mediator of both pro-inflammatory IL-17 and anti-inflammatory IL-4, indicating multiple functions of CA (Ye et al., 2009). In addition to colonic damage, various organs including liver, kidney, spleen, immune units, and functional systems such as blood coagulation characterized by Plasminogen activator inhibitor-1 (PAI-1) might be adversely affected by pathological changes in IBD. It is therefore of note that PAC ameliorated Aspertate aminotransferase (AST), Alanine transaminase (ALT), and Alkaline phosphatase (ALP), factors indicative of liver toxicity, and restored normal levels of hepatic antioxidant biomarkers including lipid peroxidation, GSH, and H_2O_2, resulting in reduced colitis symptoms. However, more evidence is needed to understand the relationship between liver disruption and colitis (Farombi et al., 2016). MLB was found to significantly attenuate symptomatic indices including serum PAI-1, gross bleeding, and damaged mucus and crypt, particularly at a high dose (Jiang et al., 2013). Relevant research is described in **Table 1**, **Table 2**, and **Figure 2**.

CLINICAL TRIALS OF DANSHEN AS A TREATMENT OF UC

Danshen is traditionally used for menstrual disorder, traumatic injury, anxiety, depression, and cardiovascular diseases. Recent investigations have reported that Danshen and its constituents may have potential for protection against cancer, inflammation, allergy, oxidation and harmful microorganisms, and may have a role in immune regulation (Gao et al., 2017; Gu et al., 2017; Li et al., 2018). Evidence-based therapeutic effects on diabetes, autoimmune disease, alcohol dependence, and nervous system disorders such as Parkinson's disease and Alzheimer's disease suggest the scope for a range of clinical applications, which sustain the Danshen-based pharmaceutic industry (Yin et al., 2009; Su et al., 2015).

Two or more participant herbs with different therapeutic functions are combined to create a formula with the potential to treat complex clinical disorders. In Chinese herbal medicine, a core characteristic herb within this combination determines the

TABLE 1 | Pharmacological details of action of Danshen compounds in experimental colitis.

Compound/ Product	Animal model	Colitis symptoms	Immunology and cytokines	Free radicals and oxidative stress	Cell death	Multiple signaling pathways	Intestinal barrier	Microenvironment	Cites
Danshen powder for injection	BALB/C mice (TNBS(100 mg/kg)); BALB/C mice (TNBS(1%))	DAI↓ Colorectal damage↓	TNF-α↓ T-bet↓ T-bet (mRNA)↓ MPO activity↓ Foxp3 (mRNA)↑ Foxp3↑						Xu Dekui et al. (2012) Xu et al. (2014)
Total phenolic acids + Tanshinones	C57BL/6 mice (DSS (2%))	DAI↓ Colon length↑ Colorectal damage↓	TNF-α↓ IL-6↓ IL-1β↓ COX-2↓			NF-κB↓ TLR4↓ p-PI3K↓ p-AKT↓ mTOR↓			Peng et al. (2020)
Salvianolic acid A	Sprague Dawley rats (DSS (3%))	Body wight↑ Liver weight↓ DAI↓ Colorectal damage↓	TNF-α(mRNA)↓ IL-1β(mRNA)↓ IL-6 (mRNA)↓ TGF-β(mRNA)↓				ZO-1 (mRNA) ↑ Occuldin (mRNA)↑	Gut microbial diversity↑ *Akkermansia* spp.↑	Wang et al. (2018)
Salvianolic acid B	C57BL/6 mice (DSS(2.2%)) Sprague-Dawley rats (TNBS/IL-1β); C57BL/6 mice (DSS(4%)) (IL-1β; 200 mg/kg)	DAI↓ Colon length↑ Body weight↑ Colorectal damage↓ Food intake↑	Infiltration: CD3+↓ CD177+↓ F4/80+↓ TNF-α↓ IL-6↓ IL-1β↓ MPO↓	iNOS↓ MDA↓ GSH↑ SOD↑ ROS↓	Apoptosis↓ Bax↓ Bcl-2↑	Production of acetic acid, propionic acid and miRNA-1↑ NOX4↓	ZO-1↑ Claudin-2↓ Monolayer integrity↑ Occludin↑	*S24-7*↑ *Bacteroides*↓	Xiong et al. (2016), Wu et al. (2018), Feng et al. (2020)
Tanshinol	C57BL/6J mice (5% DSS)	Colon length↑ Colorectal damage↓ Percent survival↑	TNF-α↓ IL-6↓ IL-1β↓			VLDLR↑			Zhu et al. (2021)
Tanshinone IIA sodium sulfonate	C57BL/6J mice (LPS(30 mg/kg))	Colorectal damage↓ Length of jejunum and ileum villus↑	TNF-α↓ IL-6↓ IL-1β↓ TNF-α(mRNA)↓ IL-6 (mRNA)↓ IL-1β(mRNA)↓		LC3-II/LC3-I ↑ Beclin-1↑ Beclin-1 (mRNA)↑ LC3 (mRNA)↑ Autophagosome formation↑				Yang et al. (2018)
Tanshinone IIA	BALB/C mice (DSS(4%)); BALB/c mice (TNBS); BC57BL/6 mice (DSS(3%))	Diarrhea↓ Bleeding↓ Body weight↑ Colorectal damage↓ Colon length↑ DAI↓	TNF-α(mRNA)↓ IL-6 (mRNA)↓ MCP(mRNA)↓ TNF-α↓ IL-1β↓ MPO↓ Ly6G positive lymphocyte infiltrates↓ MMP-8↓ IL-6↓ IL-10↓	iNOS (mRNA)↓ GSH↑ ROS↓		PXR transactivation↑ DNA-binding by PXR↑ PXR↑ PXR (mRNA)↑ CYP3A4↑ CYP3A4 (mRNA)↑ CYP3A11 (mRNA)↑ CYP3A13 (mRNA)↑ MDR1α(mRNA)↑ GSTα1 (mRNA)↑ NF-κB p65↓	Intestinal permeability↓		Zhang et al. (2015), Bai et al. (2008), Liu et al. (2016)
15,16-Dihycrotanshinone I	C57BL/6 mice (DSS(5%))	DAI↓Colon length↑ Body weight↑ Colorectal damage↓	TNF-α↓ MPO↓ IL-6↓ COX-2↓ IL-1β↓	iNOS↓	RIP1↓ RIP3↓ caspase-8↑ MLKL↓	HMGB1↓			Guo et al. (2018)
Cryptotanshinone	C57BL/6 mice (DSS(4.5%))	DAI↓ Colon length↑ Body weight↑	TNF-α↓ MPO↓ IL-6↓ IL 1β↓ COX-2↓	iNOS↓					Min et al. (2020)

(Continued on following page)

TABLE 1 | *(Continued)* Pharmacological details of action of Danshen compounds in experimental colitis.

Compound/ Product	Animal model	Colitis symptoms	Immunology and cytokines	Free radicals and oxidative stress	Cell death	Multiple signaling pathways	Intestinal barrier	Microenvironment	Cites
		Colorectal damage↓							
Miltirone	C57BL/6 mice (TNBS (100 mg/kg))	DAI↓ Colon length↑ Body weight↑ Colorectal damage↓	TNF-α↓ IL-6↓ IL-1β↓ IL-8↓			TLR4↓ MyD88↓ NF-κB p65↓ TLR4 (mRNA)↓ MyD88 (mRNA)↓ IQGAP2↑ IQGAP2 (mRNA)↑			Wang et al. (2017a)
Rosmarinic acid	ICR mice (DSS(5%)); C57BL/6 mice (DSS(3%))	Body weight↑ DAI↓ Spleen weight↓ Colorectal damage↓	MPO↓ IL-6↓ IL-1β↓ IL-22↓ COX-2↓ TNF-α↓ COX-2 (mRNA)↓ TNF-α(mRNA)↓ IL-6 (mRNA)↓ L-1β(mRNA)↓	iNOS↓ NO↓ iNOS(mRNA)↓	Survivin↓ Bcl-2 ↓ Bcl-xL↓ XIAP↓ Cdk4↓ Cyclin D1↓	NF-κB p65↓ p65 translocation↓ p-IκBα↓ IκBα↑ p-STAT3↓ p-STAT3 translocation↓			Jin et al. (2017), Zhao et al. (2018)
Rosmarinic acid methyl ester	Rats (TNBS)	Colorectal damage↓	MPO↓ CINC-3↓ iNOS↓ COX-2↓	HIF-1α↑ Stabilization of HIF-1α↑ Inhibition of HPH↑ VEGF↑					Jeong et al. (2015)
Asiatic acid	C57BL/6 mice (DSS(2.5%))	DAI↓ Colon length↑ Body weight↑ Colorectal damage↓	TNF-α↓ IL-6↓ IL-1β↓ MPO↓ IFN-γ↓ TNF-α(mRNA)↓ IL-6 (mRNA)↓ IL-1β(mRNA)↓ IFN-γ(mRNA)↓		Caspase-1 activation↓ Caspase-1 p10↓				Guo et al. (2015)
β-Caryophyllene	CD1 mice (DSS(3%))	DAI↓ Colon length↑ Body weight↑ Colorectal damage↓	TNF-α(mRNA)↓ IL-1β(mRNA)↓ CXCL1/KC(mRNA)↓ IFN-γ(mRNA)↓ IL-4↑ MPO activity↓ Foxp3 (mRNA)↑ TNF-α↓ IL-1β↓ CXCL1/KC↓ IFN-γ↓ MIP-2↓			CB2(mRNA)↓ CINC-1 (mRNA)↓ PPARγ(mRNA)↑ NF-κB p65↓ p-CREB↓ p-ERK↓ p-IKKα/β↓ Cleaved caspase-3↓			Bento et al. (2011)
Protocatechuic acid	BALB/C mice (TNBS); Wistar rat (DSS(5%)); ICR mice (TNBS(2.5%))	Body weight↑ Colorectal damage↓DAI↓ Colon length↑	MPO↓ TNF-α↓ IL-6↓ IL-1β↓ COX-2↓ TNF-α(mRNA)↓ IL-6 (mRNA)↓ IL-1β(mRNA)↓ COX-2 (mRNA)↓	Nrf2↑ MDA ↓ GSH↑ SOD↑ CAT↑ GST↑ GPx↑ H_2O_2↓ iNOS↓ NO↓		SphK1↓ S1PR1↓ SphK1 (mRNA)↓ S1PR1(mRNA)↓ S1PL (mRNA)↑ SGPP2(mRNA)↓ S1P↓ p-STAT3↓ p-AKT↓ p-ERK1/2↓ NF-κB p65↓ AST↓ ALT↓ ALP↓			Crespo et al. (2017); Farombi et al. (2016); Jang et al. (2016)
Magnesium lithospermate B	BALB/C mice (DSS(5%))	Body weight↑ Colorectal damage↓	CD40/CD40L↓ IL-6↓ CD40 (mRNA)↓ CD40L (mRNA)↓		ASC↓ NLRP3↓ Caspase-1↓	PAI-1↓			Jiang et al. (2013),

(Continued on following page)

TABLE 1 | *(Continued)* Pharmacological details of action of Danshen compounds in experimental colitis.

Compound/ Product	Animal model	Colitis symptoms	Immunology and cytokines	Free radicals and oxidative stress	Cell death	Multiple signaling pathways	Intestinal barrier	Microenvironment	Cites
		Microvilli integrity ↑	TNF-α↓						Jiang et al. (2016)
Caffeic acid	C3H/HeOuJ mice (DSS(1.25%)); C57BL/6 mice (DSS(2.5%))	Food intake↓ Colon length↑ Body weight↑ Colorectal damage↓ DAI↓	MPO↓ IL-17 (mRNA)↓ IL-4 (mRNA)↑ IL-6↓ TNF-α↓ IFN-γ↓ IL-12↑ Infiltration of $CD3^+$ T cells↓ CD177 + neutrophils↓ F4/80 + macrophage↓	iNOS(mRNA)↓		Cyp4b1 (mRNA)↑ Cytoplasmic IκBα↑ p65 translocation↓		*Akkermansia*↑	Ye et al. (2009), Zhang et al. (2016b)

PAI-1, Plasminogen activator inhibitor type-1; AST, aspertate aminotransferase; ALT, alanine transaminase; ALP, alkaline phosphatase; Cebpb, CCAAT/enhancer-binding protein and beta; Hp, haptoglobin; S100a8, S100 calcium binding protein a8; Saa3 = serum amyloid A3; DAI, disease activity index.

therapeutic direction of the formula. Danshen is introduced in Chinese herbal medicine theory as a medicine to treat blood-associated diseases (Liao et al., 2019), and reports of its effectiveness as a treatment for IBD and related syndromes are rare. However, medicinal formulae in which Danshen is the main constituent are increasingly applied to the management of IBD. In addition, many clinical trials using Chinese patent drugs mostly consisting of Danshen such as Danshen Injection have been reported.

In this review, papers describing clinical trials on the effectiveness of Danshen for the treatment of UC, the most frequently occurring phenotype of IBD, were sought from the following databases: China National Knowledge Infrastructure (CNKI), Chinese Science and Technology Periodical database (VIP), Wanfang, Chinese biomedical literature service system (SinoMed), and other resources in Chinese or in English based on Pubmed, MEDLINE, embase, and the Cochrane Central Register of Controlled Trials. To build a complete figure, "Danshen", "*Salvia miltiorrhiza* Bge.", and "ulcerative colitis" were regarded as search terms without limitations. Then, only randomized controlled trials (RCTs) till Dec. 2020 without significant bias assessed by Cochrane criteria and in which patients were diagnosed with UC were included in the review.

Overall, 19 clinical trials with a total of 1,440 patients were included in **Figure 3**. Although diagnostic criteria varied between these trials, patients who were eligible generally exhibited typical symptoms of UC characterized by hematochezia, abdominal pain, and consistent diarrhea. Only two trials used the Mayo Score to assess the disease course (Deng et al., 2016; Liu et al., 2019) while 5 trials recorded the precise location of ulcers, such as descending colon, sigmoid colon and rectum (Dong, 2004; Zhu, 2018; Zhu, 2019) and at least eight trials described the pathological course of UC including severity and remission phases (Han et al., 2005; Yang and Zhang, 2005). No significant heterogeneity in age, treatment course, disease course, gender, or ethnicity was found among the trials. Danshen-based interventions consisted of Compound Danshen injection (Li and Luo, 2011; Zheng et al., 2013), Danshen injection (Zheng et al., 2013), Danshen powder for injection (Li, 2019), Tanshinone capsule (Xiong and Wang, 2016; He, 2018), Danshen Chuanxiong injection (Sheng et al., 2014; Xu, 2015). Characteristics of these products including pharmaceutical forms, dose, frequency, and mode of administration were shown in **Tables 3, 4, 5**. All interventions in experimental groups were combinations of Danshen products and conventional treatments for UC including sulfasalazine, mesalazine, probiotics, antibiotics, or dexamethasone and these were compared with only the conventional treatments in the control groups.

The rate of clinical efficacy attributed to Danshen plus conventional treatment of UC ranged from 83.3 to 96.9%, suggesting that either aqueous or lipophilic constituents of Danshen exhibited therapeutic effects. Although 11 trials reported adverse events including rash, headache, diarrhea, nausea, abdominal pain, and dizziness (Han et al., 2005; Sheng

TABLE 2 | Pharmacological details of action of Danshen compounds *in vitro* or *ex vivo*

Compound/Product	Cell types	Stimulus	Doses of danshen compound/ product	Mediated biomarkers	Cites
Danshen water-soluble extract	IEC-18 Small intestinal segments Primary intestinal epithelial cells	LPS, 10 μg/ml	100, 250, 500 μg/ml	ICAM-1 (mRNA)↓, NF-κB↓ p-IκBa↓ IκBa↑ p-p38↑ IKK activity (directly)↓ NF-κB transcriptional activity↓ RELA nuclear translocation↓ NF-κB recruitment to the ICAM-1↓	Kim et al. (2005)
Salvianolic acid B	Caco-2 intestinal monolayer Raw264.7	IL-1β, 10 ng/ml	20, 40, 80 μM	ROS↓MLCK↓ miRNA-1↑ZO-1↑ Claudin-2↓ Monolayer integrity↑	Xiong et al. (2016)
Tanshinol	Normal colorectal mucosal cell	LPS, 8 μg/ml	25, 50, 100 μM	IL-8↓ IL-1β↓ IL-6↓ IL-8 (mRNA)↓ IL-1β(mRNA)↓ IL-6 (mRNA)↓ cell apoptosis↓ Bax↓ Bcl-2↑ Cleaved-Caspase 9↓ Cleaved-Caspase 3↓ VLDLR↑ VLDLR (mRNA)↑	Zhu et al. (2021)
Tanshinone IIA	LS174T Peripheral blood neutrophils	LPS, 1 μg/ml	2.5, 5, 10, 20 μM; 50 μM	TNF-α↓ IL-1β↓ MPO↓ IL-6↓ IL-10↓ neutrophil migration↓ ROS↓ PXR transactivation↑ DNA-binding by PXR↑ PXR↑ PXR (mRNA)↑ CYP3A4↑ CYP3A4 (mRNA)↑ CYP3A11 (mRNA)↑	(Zhang et al., 2015); Liu et al. (2016)
15,16-Dihydrotanshinone I	RAW 264.7 HT-29	LPS, 1 μg/ml TNF, 20 ng/ml + BV6, 0.5μM + ZVAD 20 μM	0.1, 0.2, 0.5 μM	TNF-α↓ IL-6↓ COX-2↓ iNOS↓ Nitrite↓p-RIP1↓ p-RIP3↓ caspase-8↑ p-MLKL↓	Guo et al. (2018)
Cryptotanshinone	RAW 264.7 HT-29	LPS, 1 μg/ml TNF, 20 ng/ml + BV6, 0.5μM + ZVAD 20 μM	2, 5, 10 μM	TNF-α↓ IL-6↓ COX-2↓ iNOS↓ RIP3↓ TLR4↓ p-p65↓ p-p38↓ p-ERK1/2↓ p-SAPK/JNK↓	Min et al. (2020)
Miltirone	IEC-6	LPS, 0.5 mg/L	5, 15, 50 μM	TLR4↓ MyD88↓ NF-κB p65↓ TLR4 (mRNA)↓ MyD88 (mRNA)↓ IQGAP2↑ IQGAP2 (mRNA)↑	Wang et al. (2017a)
Asiatic acid	THP-1 Peritoneal macrophages	LPS, 100 ng/ml + ATP, 5 mM	15, 30, 60 μM	IL-1β↓Mitochondrial ROS generation↓Caspase-1 activation↓ Caspase-1 p10↓ NLRP3 inflammasome formation ↓	Guo et al. (2015)
β-Caryophyllene	IEC-6 Lymph Node Macrophage Marrow-Derived Macrophage	LPS, 10 μg	10 μM	TNF-α↓ IL-1β↓ CXCL1/KC↓	Bento et al. (2011)
Protocatechuic acid	Peritoneal macrophage	LPS, 100 ng/ml	10 μM	TNF-α↓ NF-κB p65↓	Jang et al. (2016)

et al., 2014; Liu et al., 2019), these side effects were ameliorated after cessation of treatment. Similar rates of adverse events between experimental groups and control groups suggested that Danshen is a safe treatment.

In the patients taking Danshen products, both duration and severity of clinical symptoms including abdominal pain, blood stool, diarrhea, and tenesmus were ameliorated. Endoscopic evaluation of mucosal condition showed improvement with less erosion, better healing in ulcers, and improvement in microenvironment ecosystem, and the recurrence of UC was decreased. The following biomarkers representing inflammation and microcirculation were also at healthy levels: IL-6, IL-8, IL-10, TNF-α (Zhu, 2018; Li, 2019), C-reactive protein (CRP), D-Lactate (DL), D-dimer (D-D), blood sedimentation, serum levels of platelet (PLT), plasma fibrinogen (FIB), and mean platelet volume (MPV) (Xiong and Wang, 2016; He, 2018). Based on the collective clinical evidence, Danshen was considered as a potential auxiliary treatment for UC.

The clinical evidence summarized above suggests that Danshen may be considered as a potential auxiliary treatment for UC. However, while the included studies were randomized and controlled, they were found to be of low quality due to methodological flaws including small samples, and potentially biased selection processes. Hence, more standardized clinical trials of randomized, double-blind, and multi-centered design are needed to further test the safety and efficacy of Danshen products.

NETWORK PHARMACOLOGY APPROACH UNMASKING THE HOLISTIC MECHANISM OF DANSHEN

In contrast to conventional medicine, the holistic nature of Chinese herbal medicine is characterized by multi-compounds, multi-targets, multi-functions, and multi-systems, acting co-operatively toward a desired outcome. This network model challenges researchers to explain its precise mechanisms of action. Network pharmacology, rooted in systems biology, is a flexible approach combining the disciplines of bioinformatics, computational analysis, and polypharmacology, which can be used to investigate the complex interactions inherent in Chinese herbal medicine (Zhang et al., 2019). Network pharmacology therefore offers the possibility of a solution to multiple element profile complexity, in which intersections and interactions of physiological proteins and other biological factors are important (Hu et al., 2019). The paradigm of network pharmacology also accelerates drug discoveries featuring as combinatorial rules and compound-gene associations (Shao Li and Zhang., 2013). In recent years, network pharmacology has been wildly employed

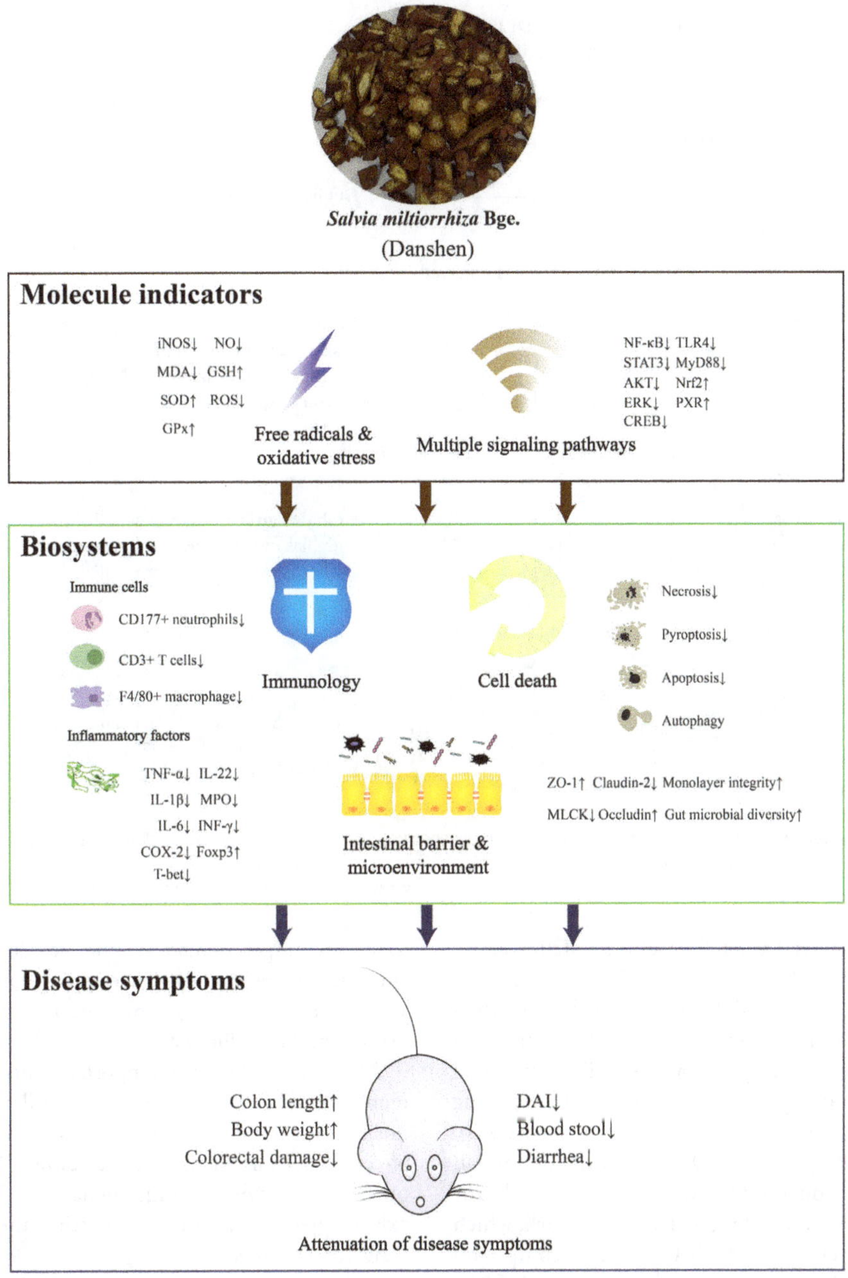

FIGURE 2 | The mechanisms of action of Danshen as a treatment of inflammatory bowel disease (IBD). Danshen exhibited ameliorative effects on IBD among molecular indicators, biosystems and symptoms. The up or down arrows indicated promoting or inhibitory effects of Danshen on the disease indicators.

in Chinese medicine research, including pharmacology, phytochemistry, and pharmacokinetics, providing a holistic view on the complex relationships between herbal medicine and the host (Zhao et al., 2019a; Yuan et al., 2020).

Hence, we applied this approach in an attempt to explain the mechanisms by which Danshen acts as a treatment for IBD. Compounds with oral bioavailability (OB) $\geq$ 30% and drug-likeness (DL) $\geq$ 0.18 were selected based on the Traditional Chinese Medicine System Pharmacology database and Analysis Platform (TCMSP) evaluation criteria (Jiang et al., 2019). Other supplementary compounds with potentiality, bioactivity, and experimental manipulation of which was described in "Pharmacological actions and mechanisms of Danshen for IBD treatment", were included to construct and enrich the compound library of Danshen (**Supplementary Material S1**). The Traditional Chinese Medicine Integrated database (TCMID) (Huang et al., 2018) and PubChem were consulted to find and remove duplications and mismatched compounds and then all eligible compounds were validated to exist in Danshen. MOL2, SMILES, and SDF formats of each compound were captured

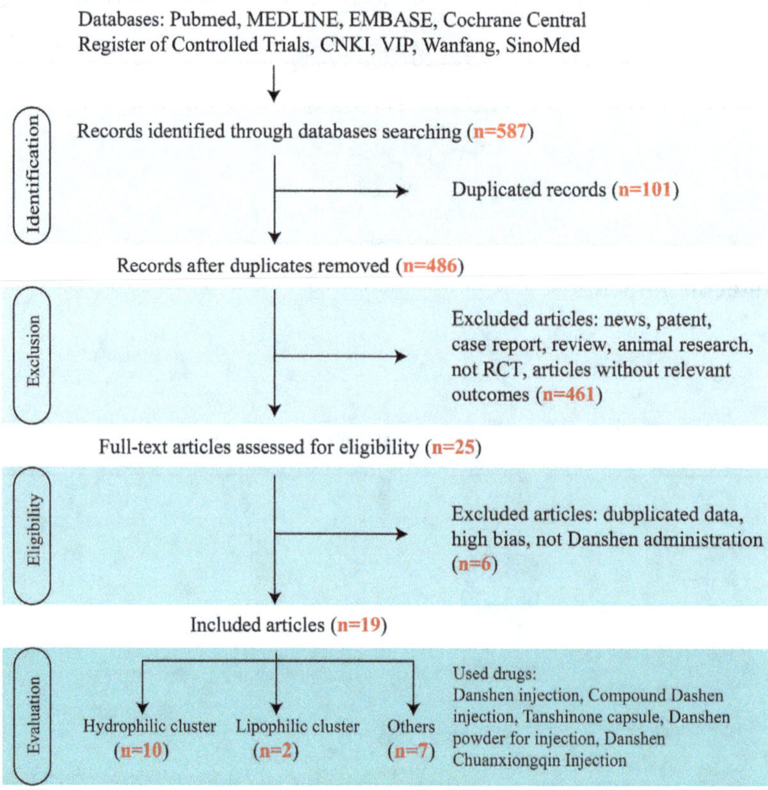

FIGURE 3 | Flow diagram of study selection of clinical trials. Clinial records on Danshen products for inflammatory bowel disease (IBD) were screened through the steps of identification, exclusion, eligibility, and evaluation.

and then uploaded to Swiss Target Prediction (Gfeller et al., 2014), STITCH (Kuhn et al., 2008), and TCMSP to retrieve predictive targets. The following databases were also searched to construct a disease library: Online Mendelian Inheritance in Man (OMIM), Therapeutic Target database (TTD), National Center for Biotechnology Information (NCBI), the Pharmacogenomics Knowledge base (PharmGKB), Malacards, and Drugbank. The entry identifiers of all targets were manually converted into Uniprot symbols for uniformity. An herb-compound-target-disease network, which was formed by intersected targets between the compound library and the disease library (**Supplementary Material S2**), was created using Cytoscape 3.5.1 to explore the multi-level Danshen treatment. The intrinsic protein-protein interactions (PPIs) of IBD and Danshen were visualized using STRING (Szklarczyk et al., 2019). In addition, all eligible targets were input to DAVID Bioinformatics Resources for Kyoto Encyclopedia of Genes and Genomes (KEGG) pathways and ClueGO plugin for Gene Ontology (GO) (Bindea et al., 2009).

In total, 64 compounds were identified for 66 IBD-Danshen overlapping targets, reflecting a range of possible functions of Danshen in the treatment of IBD. The resulting "herb-compound-target-disease" network, which included 130 hub nodes and 124 literature-supported lines of 346 intersectional ones, represented potential targets for botanical compounds in the treatment of IBD. Each objective compound could have more than one target, which in turn could interact with various compounds (**Figure 4**). Overlapping targets were uploaded to yield PPIs featuring 66 hubs and 404 interactions (**Supplementary Figure S1**).

Meanwhile, evidence-supported functions including positive regulation of cytokine production, inflammatory response, and positive regulation of programmed cell death appeared to be affected by Danshen in **Supplementary Figure S2**. In addition, other processes of cell component and cell activity cooperated to exhibit pleiotropic effects, reflecting the holistic principles of Danshen treatment.

As putative targets of compounds of Danshen were included in the integrated network of multiple regulatory systems responding to extrinsic and endogenous irritants, KEGG was used to imply direct and indirect signaling transduction of Danshen's potential action (**Supplementary Material S3**). The results were concentrated on TNF signaling pathway, JAK/STAT signaling pathway, TLR/NLR signaling pathway, NF-κB signaling pathway, HIF signaling pathway, PI3K/AKT/PTEN signaling pathway, and MAPK signaling pathway, all playing irreplaceable roles in the process of IBD multiply regulated by Danshen. When comparing positions of Tanshinones with Salvianolic acids in the network, some common targets, such as NF-κB, IL-6, and TNF, which were enriched in inflammatory-associated signaling pathways, were correlated with these two clusters of Danshen compounds. Meanwhile, certain specific targets, such as PPAR-γ to

TABLE 3 | Clinical trials of Danshen products as supplementary interference in the regulation of ulcerative colitis (UC) (Hydrophilic cluster).

Study design	Interventions	Approach, duration, dose, frequence of danshen treatment	Participants	Amount	Information of patients *m*, f, age (year), course (year)	Clinical efficacy (C/T)	Adverse events	Outcome measurements	References
RCT	C:mesalazine T:mesalazine, Danshen powder for injection	i.v.gtt, 8w, 0.4 g, qd	C:51 T:51	102	C: N, N, N, N T: N, N, N, N	78.43%/ 94.12%	C: 4, abdominal pain, nausea, diarrea T: 7, abdominal pain, nausea, diarrea	TNF-α, IL-6, IL-8, Hcy	Li, (2019)
RCT	C:mesalazine T:mesalazine + Danshen injection	i.v.gtt, 4w, 10ml, qd	C:27 T:27	54	C: 16, 11, 39.84 ± 9.68, 2.75 ± 1.28 T: 15, 12, 38.53 ± 10.37, 2.51 ± 1.74	70.37%/ 96.30%	C: 4, hash, nausea, diarrea T: 3, hash, diarrea	TNF-α, IL-6, IL-8	Zhu, (2018)
RCT (random number table)	C:probiotics + mesalazine T:probiotics + mesalazine + Danshen injection	i.v.gtt, 6m, 20ml, qd	C:46 T:47	93	C: 25, 21, 33.17 ± 6.50, 4.88 ± 3.12 T: 24, 23, 34.2 ± 6.46, 4.90 ± 3.09	73.91%/ 93.62%	C: 3, nausea, dizziness T: 5, nausea, localized edema, hypotension	D-lactate, DAO, QOL score	Yang, (2017)
RCT	C:probiotics + mesalazine T:probiotics + mesalazine + Danshen injection	i.v.gtt, 4w, 20 ml,qd	C:32 T:32	64	C: 18, 14, 39.9 ± 6.5, N T: 17, 15, 40.4 ± 8.5, N	N	C: 6 T: 8	defecating frequency, haemorrhoids blood in stool, Mayo Score, Blood sendimentation, PLT	Liu et al. (2019)
RCT	C:ornidazole + sulfasalazine T:ornidazole + sulfasalazine + Danshen injection	i.v.gtt, 4w,20ml, qd	C:30 T:30	60	C: 22, 8, 47.9 ± 8.1, 3.2 ± 0.7 T: 20, 10, 48.1 ± 7.9, 3.1 ± 0.6	53.30%/ 83.30%	C: 1, headache T: 1, headache	DAI, CRP, Blood sendimentation	Yao et al. (2016)
RCT	C:mesalazine T:mesalazine + Danshen injection	i.v.gtt, 4w,20ml, qd	C:49 T:49	98	C: 29, 20, 37.6 ± 5.8, 4.2 ± 0.8 T: 28, 21, 37.4 ± 5.7, 4.2 ± 0.9	77.55%/ 93.88%	C: N T: N	TNF-α, IL-8, PLT, FIB	Zhu, (2019)
RCT (random number table)	C:mesalazine T:mesalazine + Danshen injection	i.v.gtt, 4w,20 ml+	C:55 T:55	110	C: 23, 32, 57.6 ± 7.5, 4.5 ± 1.3 T: 25, 30, 58.3 ± 8.2, 4.8 ± 1.4	80.00%/ 94.50%	C: N T: N	TNF-α, IL-6, IL-8, FIB, PLT, MPV, Recurrence rate	Deng et al. (2016)
RCT (random number table)	C:mesalazine T:mesalazine + Danshen injection	i.v.gtt, 4w,20ml, qd	C:43 T:43	86	C: 25, 18, 45.4 ± 1.3, 2.4 ± 0.3 T: 23, 20, 45.6 ± 1.2, 2.3 ± 0.4	81.40%/ 95.40%	C: 5, nausea, fever, hash T: 3, nausea, fever, disturbance in respiration	CRP, Blood sendimentation, D-lactate	Sun, (2019)
RCT	C:mesalazine T:mesalazine + Danshen injection	i.v.gtt, 4w, 4ml, qd	C:36 T:36	72	C: 19, 17, 44.6 ± 2.5, 3.2 ± 1.2 T: 20, 16, 44.2 ± 2.7, 3.3 ± 1.4	77.78%/ 94.44%	C: 4, nausea, diarrhea, hash T: 2, diarrhea, hash	IL-8, IL-10, TNF-α, FIB, PLT, MPV	Du, (2019)
RCT	C: sulfasalazine T:mesalazine + Danshen injection	i.v.gtt, 4w, 4ml, qd	C:50 T:50	100	C: 26, 24, 36.6 ± 12.7, 2.1 T: 27, 23, 36.8 ± 11.3, 2.3	62.00%/ 84.00%	C: N T: N	D-dimer, FIB, blood viscosity	Huang, (2005)

RCT, random control trial; i.v.gtt, intravenously guttae; qd, quaque die; Hcy, homocysteine; DAO, diamine oxidase; DAI, disease activity index; CRP, C-reactive protein; PLT, serum levels of platelet; FIB, plasma fibrinogen; MPV, mean platelet volume; N, not available; T, dansheh treatment; C, conventional treatment.

TABLE 4 | Clinical trials of Danshen products as supplementary interference in the regulation of ulcerative colitis (UC) (Lipophilic cluster).

Study design	Interventions	Approach, duration, dose, frequence of danshen treatment	Participants (T/C)	Amount	Information of patients n, m/f, age (year), course (year)	Clinical efficacy	Adverse events	Outcome measurements	References
RCT (random number table)	C:mesalazine T:mesalazine + Tanshinone capsule	p.o., 4w, 1g, tid	C:44< T:44	88	C: 26, 18, 45.88 ± 9.22, 7.21 ± 5.30 T: 24, 20, 44.56 ± 10.11, 8.06 ± 4.83	N	N	PLT, MPV, APTT, FIB, D-D, CRP, TF, TFPI	He, (2018)
RCT (random number table)	C:mesalazine T:mesalazine + Tanshinone capsule	p.o., 8w,1g, tid	C:35 T:35	70	C: 15, 20, 46.8 ± 7.1, 5.2 ± 2.1 T: 16, 19, 47.4 ± 6.2, 5.1 ± 2.3	N	N	CRP, TNF-α, IL-6, APTT, FIB, PLT, MPV, PAG, D-D	Xiong and Wang, (2016)

N, no information; RCT, random control trial; CRP, C-reactive protein; PLT, serum levels of platelet; FIB, plasma fibrinogen; MPV, mean platelet volume; p.o, per os; tid, three times daily; PAG, platelet aggregation; APTT, activation partial prothrombin time; FIB, fibrinogen; D-D, D-dimer; CRP, C-reactive protein.; m: male; f:female; T: danshen treatment; C:conventional treatment.

Salvianolic acid B, and estrogen receptors to Tanshinones, achieving in dynamic regulated functions, improved multilevel management of Danshen's therapies of IBD.

Network Pharmacology Evaluation Method Guidance-Draft, the recent guidance for network pharmacology research, provided a systematic evaluation method (Li, 2021). Therefore, we employed this criterion to assess the network object of Danshen-IBD, especially from aspects of data retrieving, network analysis, and outcome evaluation. We performed our work to meet fundamental requirements of the Network Pharmacology Evaluation Method Guidance-Draft but need validated data, such as existing compounds, functional proteins, and further experimental verification.

SAFETY OF DANSHEN PRODUCTS FOR IBD

Danshen and its phytochemical constituents possess multiple therapeutic efficacies and have the potential in transformation of novel drugs. During the development of pharmaceutical industry, drug safety is necessary for further research. Danshen and Danshen-containing products can be tolerated for clinical usage (Jia et al., 2019). With safety tested by a set of toxicity research on various mammals including Sprague-Dawley rats, Beagle dogs, and mice, Danshen and Danshen-containing products, offer an optional treatment of IBD with acceptable tolerance (Gao et al., 2009; Li et al., 2009; Wang et al., 2012). In 2017, a real world study, employing data of 30180 consecutive inpatients from 36 hospitals, stated that a Danshen-containing product called *Salvia Miltiorrhiza* Depside Salt for Infusion was of good tolerance by the general population (Yan et al., 2017). In the included trials in "CLINICAL TRIALS OF DANSHEN AS A TREATMENT OF UC", side events, which best reflect safety of Danshen products on human being, had no significant difference between control groups and Danshen-intervention groups. Meanwhile, the treatment course ranged from 4 to 8 weeks, covering the general treatment course in clinic. Although Tanshione IIA exhibited potential cardiotoxicity and other severe toxicity in zebrafish embryos at high concentrations, as Danshen-containing products are mostly made by hydrophilic constituents of Danshen, there remains the declaration of safety of Danshen-containing products for IBD treatments (Wang T. et al., 2017).

CONCLUSION

IBD is a chronic inflammatory disease, which induces heavy burden and lacks satisfying treatments. Although innovative drugs like monoclonal antibodies and specific agents achieve in better management and less side events, the high cost asks for economical and practical agents that are specific to IBD. Danshen is a classical herbal material frequently prescribed in Chinese medicine with a long history of over 2000 years. This herb possesses multiple therapeutic effects with low toxicity and is attracting more attention as a potential IBD treatment.

Clinical trials in which Danshen products were used supplementarily with conventional treatments indicated the efficacy of Danshen on symptoms and disease biomarkers. The Danshen products of hydrophilic cluster is used more often in clinical trials and these products like Danshen injection have shown ensured efficacy. However, as quality control of Chinese medicine injection is in challenge because of the sophistication of compounds directly entering blood, the side events can not be neglected, which asks for further evaluation on the safety of Danshen products used for IBD. Meanwhile, methodological issues including small sample sizes and flawed outcome measurements limit believability of the conclusion on Danshen's capacity.

The compounds of Danshen are fundamentally classified by their solubility as phenolic acids and tanshinone derivatives. The development of instruments of high resolution, accuracy, and sensitivity, makes it possible to discover novel compounds

TABLE 5 | Clinical trials of Danshen products combined with other Chinese herbal products as supplementary interference in the regulation of ulcerative colitis (UC).

Study design	Interventions (T/C)	Approach, duration, dose, frequence of danshen treatment	Mayor constituents of danshen products	Treatment course (day)	Amount	Participant amount (T/C) T: M, F, age, duration of disease; C: M, F, age(y), duration of disease(y)	Clinical efficacy (T/C)	Outcome measurements	Adverse events	References
RCT	Fufang Danshen Injection + Sulfasalazine/Sulfasalazine	en, 40ml, bid	Salvianic acid A, Protocatechuic aldehydrate, Salvianolic acid B	28	63	32/31; T: 14, 18, 43.5 ± 2.7,N/C: 15, 16, 42.3 ± 2.5, N	96.9%/ 61.3%	N	N	Li and Luo, (2011)
RCT (registration order)	Fufang Danshen Injection + Sulfasalazine + Tinidazole + Dexamethasone/ Sulfasalazine + Tinidazole + Dexamethasone	i.v.gtt, 24ml, qd	Salvianic acid A, Protocatechuic aldehydrate, Salvianolic acid B	28	48	23/25; T: N, N, N, N/C: N, N, N, N	86.9%/ 84.0%	Relapse rate	T: N/C: 32% (8) nausea, burning sensation, liver dysfunction	Dong, (2004)
RCT (random number table)	Fufang Danshen Injection + Sulfasalazine/Sulfasalazine	ivqtt, 20ml, qd	Salvianic acid A, Protocatechuic aldehydrate, Salvianolic acid B	20	60	30/30; T: 17, 13, 34.5 ± 4.8, 20.8 ± 7.4m/ C: 15, 15, 35.9 ± 5.3, 27.6 ± 6.9m	90%/ 76.67%	Endoscopic remission; Relapse rate	N	Zheng et al. (2013)
RCT	Danshen Injection + Huangqi Injection + Dexamethasone/ Dexamethasone	i.v.gtt, 40–70ml, qd	Salvianic acid A, Protocatechuic aldehydrate, Salvianolic acid B, Astragaloside IV, Astragaloside III, Astragaloside I	28	56	26/30; T: 15, 11, 39,N/C: 16, 14, 40, N	N	Duration of symptoms; Minimum dose of glucocorticoid	N	Yang and Zhang, (2005)
RCT	Danshen Injection + Huangqi Injection + Dexamethasone + Conventional treatments/ Dexamethasone + Conventional treatments	i.v.gtt, 0.8–1.2 ml/kg, qd	Salvianic acid A, Protocatechuic aldehydrate, Salvianolic acid B, Astragaloside IV, Astragaloside III, AstragalosideI	28	84	46/38; T: N, N, N/C: N, N, N	N	Duration of symptoms; Minimum dose of glucocorticoid	T: N/C: 13.2% (5) interstinal perforation, worsen condition	Han et al. (2005)
RCT (random number table)	Danshen Chuanxiongqin Injection + Sulfasalazine/ Sulfasalazine	i.v.gtt, 5ml, qd	Salvianic acid A, Protocatechuic aldehydrate, Isoferulic acid, Rosmarinic acid, Salvianolic acid A, Ligustrazine hydrochloride	28	86	43/43; T: 27, 16, 45.9 ± 9.2, 3.6 ± 0.7 years/C: 26, 17, 46.3 ± 9.6, 3.2 ± 0.6 y	95.3%/ 74.4%	Symptom scores	T: 16.3% (7)/C: 18.6% (8) gastrointestinal response, rash, headache gastrointestinal response, rash, headache	Xu, (2015)
RCT (registration order)	Danshen Chuanxiongqin Injection + Clostridium Butyricum Capsule + Methalazine/Clostridium Butyricum Capsule + Methalazine	i.v.gtt, 10ml, qd	Salvianic acid A, Protocatechuic aldehydrate, Isoferulic acid, Rosmarinic acid, Salvianolic acid A, Ligustrazine hydrochloride	28	46	28/18; T: 17, 11, 43.2, 1.8 years/C: 10, 8, 42.6, 2.1 y	89.3%/ 83.3%	Duration of symptoms; Blood sendimentation; CRP	T: 17.9% (5)/C: 16.7% (3) abdominal distension, nausea, rash abdominal distension, nausea, rash	Sheng et al. (2014)

N, no information; RCT, random control trial; CRP, C-reactive protein; en, enema; i.v.gtt, intravenously guttae; qd, quaque die; bid, bis in die; T, danshen treatment; C, conventional treatment.

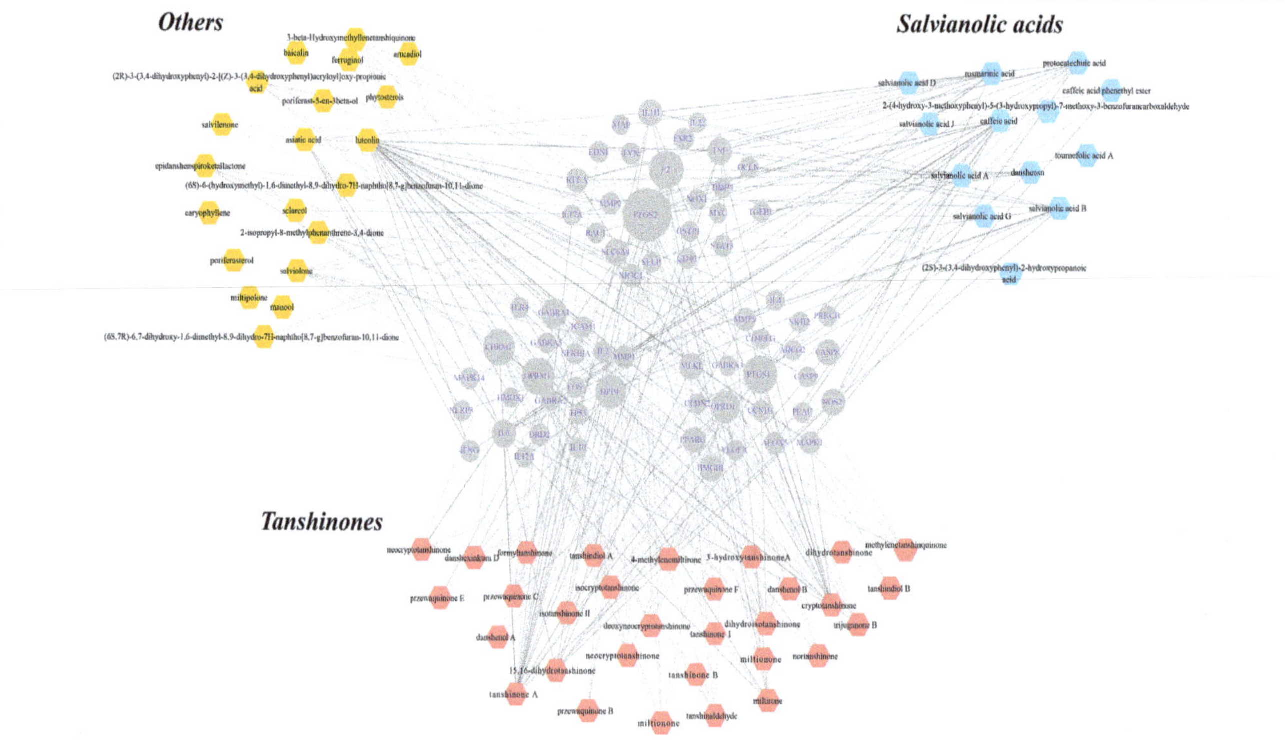

FIGURE 4 | Construction of "herb-compound-target-disease" network for unmasking underlying mechanisms of Danshen for inflammatory bowel disease (IBD). Eligible compounds of Danshen were characterized within three kinds of colors while the round shapes in the center represented intersected targets both of Danshen and IBD. The scale of hubs indicated degree of targets. Solid lines indicated interactions between certain compounds and targets that were supported in the literature.

of Danshen, which might have the potential to manage colitis. For instance, Savianolic acid C, one of the derivates of Savianolic acid B, has significant anti-inflammatory and anti-oxidative effects but has not been tested for colitis (Song et al., 2018). The individual compounds of Danshen with different structural features are reported to possess multiple pharmacological functions in colitis model. With deeper understand in the pathology of IBD, the anti-colitis capacity of compounds of Danshen can be explained clearly in another way. For instance, ferroptosis, which could be controlled by Tanshinone IIA, is recently reported to play an important role in IBD and will be the future field in which Danshen possesses anti-colitis capacity (Guan et al., 2020; Xu et al., 2020). Meanwhile, as a mixture of numerous compounds, Danshen exhibits its effects through multiple reactions among various compounds, different targets, and alternative biosystems. To give concise descriptions, system pharmacology approaches like network pharmacology are applied to visualize molecular mechanisms of Danshen. Although it has been developed for about 10 years, network pharmacology in Chinese medicine is still in infant to mimic the actual bio-reactions. Hence, more methods like omics are encouraged to use together to make a systematic figure of Danshen as a treatment of IBD.

With the case of Danshen in the management of IBD, the usage of medicinal herbs for complex disease shines a light on drug discovery, in which multipotent responses and uniqueness of the individuals are considered. Discovery of innovative compounds and exploring their applications are pivotal aims in the field of herbal medicine, and will contribute to the development of marketable botanical products such as Danshen injection in the future.

AUTHOR CONTRIBUTIONS

SZ designed and drafted the manuscript. ZZ and YW organized and supervised the study. SS, HL, QQ, JM, YL, YZ, and CF analyzed the literature. LY and DT revised the eligible version. All authors read and approved the final manuscript.

FUNDING

This study was supported by the Macao Science and Technology Development Fund (FDCT007/2020/ALC) and the Research Fund of University of Macau (CPG2022-00005-ICMS).

REFERENCES

Bai, A., Lu, N., Guo, Y., and Fan, X. (2008). Tanshinone IIA Ameliorates Trinitrobenzene Sulfonic Acid (TNBS)-induced Murine Colitis. *Dig. Dis. Sci.* 53, 421–428. doi:10.1007/s10620-007-9863-8

Bai, G., Zhang, T., Hou, Y., Ding, G., Jiang, M., and Luo, G. (2018). From Quality Markers to Data Mining and Intelligence Assessment: A Smart Quality-Evaluation Strategy for Traditional Chinese Medicine Based on Quality Markers. *Phytomedicine* 44, 109–116. doi:10.1016/j.phymed.2018.01.017

Balmus, I. M., Ciobica, A., Trifan, A., and Stanciu, C. (2016). The Implications of Oxidative Stress and Antioxidant Therapies in Inflammatory Bowel Disease: Clinical Aspects and Animal Models. *Saudi J. Gastroenterol.* 22, 3–17. doi:10.4103/1319-3767.173753

Barclay, A. R., Russell, R. K., Wilson, M. L., Gilmour, W. H., Satsangi, J., and Wilson, D. C. (2009). Systematic Review: The Role of Breastfeeding in the Development of Pediatric Inflammatory Bowel Disease. *J. Pediatr.* 155, 421–426. doi:10.1016/j.jpeds.2009.03.017

Bento, A. F., Marcon, R., Dutra, R. C., Claudino, R. F., Cola, M., Leite, D. F., et al. (2011). β-Caryophyllene Inhibits Dextran Sulfate Sodium-Induced Colitis in Mice through CB2 Receptor Activation and PPARγ Pathway. *Am. J. Pathol.* 178, 1153–1166. doi:10.1016/j.ajpath.2010.11.052

Bindea, G., Mlecnik, B., Hackl, H., Charoentong, P., Tosolini, M., Kirilovsky, A., et al. (2009). ClueGO: a Cytoscape Plug-In to Decipher Functionally Grouped Gene Ontology and Pathway Annotation Networks. *Bioinformatics* 25, 1091–1093. doi:10.1093/bioinformatics/btp101

Blackwell, J., Saxena, S., Alexakis, C., Bottle, A., Cecil, E., Majeed, A., et al. (2019). The Impact of Smoking and Smoking Cessation on Disease Outcomes in Ulcerative Colitis: a Nationwide Population-Based Study. *Aliment. Pharmacol. Ther.* 50, 556–567. doi:10.1111/apt.15390

Burisch, J., Jess, T., Martinato, M., Lakatos, P. L., and EpiCom, E. (2013). The burden of Inflammatory Bowel Disease in Europe. *J. Crohns Colitis* 7, 322–337. doi:10.1016/j.crohns.2013.01.010

Cao, S. Y., Ye, S. J., Wang, W. W., Wang, B., Zhang, T., and Pu, Y. Q. (2019). Progress in Active Compounds Effective on Ulcerative Colitis from Chinese Medicines. *Chin. J. Nat. Med.* 17, 81–102. doi:10.1016/s1875-5364(19)30012-3

Chami, B., Martin, N. J. J., Dennis, J. M., and Witting, P. K. (2018). Myeloperoxidase in the Inflamed colon: A Novel Target for Treating Inflammatory Bowel Disease. *Arch. Biochem. Biophys.* 645, 61–71. doi:10.1016/j.abb.2018.03.012

Crespo, I., San-Miguel, B., Mauriz, J. L., Ortiz de Urbina, J. J., Almar, M., Tuñón, M. J., et al. (2017). Protective Effect of Protocatechuic Acid on TNBS-Induced Colitis in Mice Is Associated with Modulation of the SphK/S1P Signaling Pathway. *Nutrients* 9. doi:10.3390/nu9030288

Deng, W.-J., Ma, Y., and Ma, L. (2016). Mesalazine in Combination with Danshen Injection for Treatment of Ulcerative Colitis: Curative Efficacy and Effect on Inflammatory Factors and Coagulation Parameters. *Wcjd* 24, 462–466. doi:10.11569/wcjd.v24.i3.462

Dong, X. (2004). Treatment of Ulcerative Colitis by Compound Danshen Intravenous Drip Combined with Drug Enema. *Shandong Med.* 44, 24–25. doi:10.3969/j.issn.1002-266X.2004.10.010

Du, X. (2019). Clinical Analysis of Mesalazine Combined with Salvia Miltiorrhiza Injection on Ulcerative Colitis. *Health Nutr. Chin.* 33, 218.

Ek, W. E., D'Amato, M., and Halfvarson, J. (2014). The History of Genetics in Inflammatory Bowel Disease. *Ann. Gastroenterol.* 27, 294–303.

Farombi, E. O., Adedara, I. A., Awoyemi, O. V., Njoku, C. R., Micah, G. O., Esogwa, C. U., et al. (2016). Dietary Protocatechuic Acid Ameliorates Dextran Sulphate Sodium-Induced Ulcerative Colitis and Hepatotoxicity in Rats. *Food Funct.* 7, 913–921. doi:10.1039/c5fo01228g

Feagan, B. G., Sandborn, W. J., Gasink, C., Jacobstein, D., Lang, Y., Friedman, J. R., et al. (2016). Ustekinumab as Induction and Maintenance Therapy for Crohn's Disease. *N. Engl. J. Med.* 375, 1946–1960. doi:10.1056/NEJMoa1602773

Feng, P. P., Fang, X. S., Zhao, S. H., Fu, J. Y., Zhang, H. T., Yi, Y. L., et al. (2020). Salvianolic Acid B Decreases Interleukin-1β-Induced Colitis Recurrence in Mice. *Chin. Med. J. (Engl)* 133, 1436–1444. doi:10.1097/CM9.0000000000000773

Friedrich, M., Pohin, M., and Powrie, F. (2019). Cytokine Networks in the Pathophysiology of Inflammatory Bowel Disease. *Immunity* 50, 992 1006. doi:10.1016/j.immuni.2019.03.017

Gao, H., Liu, X., Sun, W., Kang, N., Liu, Y., Yang, S., et al. (2017). Total Tanshinones Exhibits Anti-inflammatory Effects through Blocking TLR4 Dimerization via the MyD88 Pathway. *Cell Death Dis* 8, e3004. doi:10.1038/cddis.2017.389

Gao, Y., Liu, Z., Li, G., Li, C., Li, M., and Li, B. (2009). Acute and Subchronic Toxicity of Danshensu in Mice and Rats. *Toxicol. Mech. Methods* 19, 363–368. doi:10.1080/15376510902810672

Gfeller, D., Grosdidier, A., Wirth, M., Daina, A., Michielin, O., and Zoete, V. (2014). SwissTargetPrediction: a Web Server for Target Prediction of Bioactive Small Molecules. *Nucleic Acids Res.* 42, W32–W38. doi:10.1093/nar/gku293

Gu, J.-F., Su, S.-L., Guo, J.-M., Zhu, Y., Zhao, M., and Duan, J.-A. (2017). The Aerial Parts of Salvia Miltiorrhiza Bge. Strengthen Intestinal Barrier and Modulate Gut Microbiota Imbalance in Streptozocin-Induced Diabetic Mice. *J. Funct. Foods* 36, 362–374. doi:10.1016/j.jff.2017.06.010

Guan, Z., Chen, J., Li, X., and Dong, N. (2020). Tanshinone IIA Induces Ferroptosis in Gastric Cancer Cells through P53-Mediated SLC7A11 Down-Regulation. *Biosci. Rep.* 40. doi:10.1042/BSR20201807

Guo, W., Liu, W., Jin, B., Geng, J., Li, J., Ding, H., et al. (2015). Asiatic Acid Ameliorates Dextran Sulfate Sodium-Induced Murine Experimental Colitis via Suppressing Mitochondria-Mediated NLRP3 Inflammasome Activation. *Int. Immunopharmacol* 24, 232–238. doi:10.1016/j.intimp.2014.12.009

Guo, X. Y., Liu, X. J., and Hao, J. Y. (2020). Gut Microbiota in Ulcerative Colitis: Insights on Pathogenesis and Treatment. *J. Dig. Dis.* 21, 147–159. doi:10.1111/1751-2980.12849

Guo, Y., Li, Y., Xue, L., Severino, R. P., Gao, S., Niu, J., et al. (2014). Salvia Miltiorrhiza: an Ancient Chinese Herbal Medicine as a Source for Anti-osteoporotic Drugs. *J. Ethnopharmacol* 155, 1401–1416. doi:10.1016/j.jep.2014.07.058

Guo, Y., Wu, X., Wu, Q., Lu, Y., Shi, J., and Chen, X. (2018). Dihydrotanshinone I, a Natural Product, Ameliorates DSS-Induced Experimental Ulcerative Colitis in Mice. *Toxicol. Appl. Pharmacol.* 344, 35–45. doi:10.1016/j.taap.2018.02.018

Han, W., Liu, Y., and Sun, L. (2005). Clinical Study of Danshen and Huangqi Injection on Ulcerative Colitis. *Aced Per Changchun Coll. Trad Chin. Med.* 21, 7. doi:10.3969/j.issn.1007-4813.2005.04.006

Harris, N. L. (2016). Intimate Gut Interactions: Helminths and the Microbiota. *Cell Res* 26, 861–862. doi:10.1038/cr.2016.72

Hatfield, M. J., Tsurkan, L. G., Hyatt, J. L., Edwards, C. C., Lemoff, A., Jeffries, C., et al. (2013). Modulation of Esterified Drug Metabolism by Tanshinones from Salvia Miltiorrhiza ("Danshen"). *J. Nat. Prod.* 76, 36–44. doi:10.1021/np300628a

He, H. (2018). Effects of Tanshinone Combined with Mesalazineon Coagulation Functionand Tissue TF and TFPI Expressionin Patients with Ulcerative Colitis. *Res. Int. Trad Chin. West. Med.* 10, 225–228. doi:10.3969/j.issn.1674-4616.2018.05.001

Hu, S., Zuo, H., Qi, J., Hu, Y., and Yu, B. (2019). Analysis of Effect of Schisandra in the Treatment of Myocardial Infarction Based on Three-Mode Gene Ontology Network. *Front. Pharmacol.* 10, 232. doi:10.3389/fphar.2019.00232

Huang, L., Xie, D., Yu, Y., Liu, H., Shi, Y., Shi, T., et al. (2018). TCMID 2.0: a Comprehensive Resource for TCM. *Nucleic Acids Res.* 46, D1117–D1120. doi:10.1093/nar/gkx1028

Huang, L. (2005). The Effect on Hypercoagulable State of Ulcerative Colitis Patients by Intervening Treatment of Danshen Injection. *Chin. Archi Trad Chin. Med.* 23, 1901–1902. doi:10.13193/j.archtcm.2005.10.167.huanglx.090

Jang, S.-E., Choi, J.-R., Han, M. J., and Kim, D.-H. (2016). The Preventive and Curative Effect of Cyanidin-3β-D-Glycoside and its Metabolite Protocatechuic Acid against TNBS-Induced Colitis in Mice. *Nat. Prod. Sci.* 22, 282–286. doi:10.20307/nps.2016.22.4.282

Jeong, S., Park, H., Hong, S., Yum, S., Kim, W., and Jung, Y. (2015). Lipophilic Modification Enhances Anti-colitic Properties of Rosmarinic Acid by Potentiating its HIF-Prolyl Hydroxylases Inhibitory Activity. *Eur. J. Pharmacol.* 747, 114–122. doi:10.1016/j.ejphar.2014.11.030

Jia, Q., Zhu, R., Tian, Y., Chen, B., Li, R., Li, L., et al. (2019). Salvia Miltiorrhiza in Diabetes: A Review of its Pharmacology, Phytochemistry, and Safety. *Phytomedicine* 58, 152871. doi:10.1016/j.phymed.2019.152871

Jiang, X., Jiang, Y., Sun, D., and Rong, L. (2013). Protective Effect of Magnesium Lithospermate B against Dextran Sodiumsulfate Induced Ulcerative Colitis in Mice. *Environ. Toxicol. Pharmacol.* 36, 97–102. doi:10.1016/j.etap.2013.03.010

Jiang, X., Zhong, L., Sun, D., and Rong, L. (2016). Magnesium Lithospermate B Acts against Dextran Sodiumsulfate-Induced Ulcerative Colitis by Inhibiting Activation of the NRLP3/ASC/Caspase-1 Pathway. *Environ. Toxicol. Pharmacol.* 41, 72–77. doi:10.1016/j.etap.2015.10.009

Jiang, Y., Liu, N., Zhu, S., Hu, X., Chang, D., and Liu, J. (2019). Elucidation of the Mechanisms and Molecular Targets of Yiqi Shexue Formula for Treatment of Primary Immune Thrombocytopenia Based on Network Pharmacology. *Front. Pharmacol.* 10, 1136. doi:10.3389/fphar.2019.01136

Jin, B. R., Chung, K. S., Cheon, S. Y., Lee, M., Hwang, S., Noh Hwang, S., et al. (2017). Rosmarinic Acid Suppresses Colonic Inflammation in Dextran Sulphate Sodium (DSS)-induced Mice via Dual Inhibition of NF-Kb and STAT3 Activation. *Sci. Rep.* 7, 46252. doi:10.1038/srep46252

Kabat, A. M., Pott, J., and Maloy, K. J. (2016). The Mucosal Immune System and its Regulation by Autophagy. *Front. Immunol.* 7, 240. doi:10.3389/fimmu.2016.00240

Katsanos, K. H., and Papadakis, K. A. (2017). Inflammatory Bowel Disease: Updates on Molecular Targets for Biologics. *Gut Liver* 11, 455–463. doi:10.5009/gnl16308

Khalili, H., Chan, S. S. M., Lochhead, P., Ananthakrishnan, A. N., Hart, A. R., and Chan, A. T. (2018). The Role of Diet in the Aetiopathogenesis of Inflammatory Bowel Disease. *Nat. Rev. Gastroenterol. Hepatol.* 15, 525–535. doi:10.1038/s41575-018-0022-9

Kiesler, P., Fuss, I. J., and Strober, W. (2015). Experimental Models of Inflammatory Bowel Diseases. *Cell Mol Gastroenterol Hepatol* 1, 154–170. doi:10.1016/j.jcmgh.2015.01.006

Kim, J. S., Narula, A. S., and Jobin, C. (2005). Salvia Miltiorrhiza Water-Soluble Extract, but Not its Constituent Salvianolic Acid B, Abrogates LPS-Induced NF-kappaB Signalling in Intestinal Epithelial Cells. *Clin. Exp. Immunol.* 141, 288–297. doi:10.1111/j.1365-2249.2005.02844.x

Kolios, G., Valatas, V., and Ward, S. G. (2004). Nitric Oxide in Inflammatory Bowel Disease: a Universal Messenger in an Unsolved Puzzle. *Immunology* 113, 427–437. doi:10.1111/j.1365-2567.2004.01984.x

Kovacs, S. B., and Miao, E. A. (2017). Gasdermins: Effectors of Pyroptosis. *Trends Cel Biol* 27, 673–684. doi:10.1016/j.tcb.2017.05.005

Kuhn, M., von Mering, C., Campillos, M., Jensen, L. J., and Bork, P. (2008). STITCH: Interaction Networks of Chemicals and Proteins. *Nucleic Acids Res.* 36, D684–D688. doi:10.1093/nar/gkm795

Lee, S. H. (2015). Intestinal Permeability Regulation by Tight junction: Implication on Inflammatory Bowel Diseases. *Intest Res.* 13, 11–18. doi:10.5217/ir.2015.13.1.11

Lewis, J. D., and Abreu, M. T. (2017). Diet as a Trigger or Therapy for Inflammatory Bowel Diseases. *Gastroenterology* 152, 398–e6. doi:10.1053/j.gastro.2016.10.019

Li, G., Gao, Y., Li, S., Li, C., Zhu, X., Li, M., et al. (2009). Study on Toxicity of Danshensu in Beagle Dogs after 3-month Continuous Intravenous Infusion. *Toxicol. Mech. Methods* 19, 441–446. doi:10.1080/15376510903150623

Li, G. H., Li, Y. R., Jiao, P., Zhao, Y., Hu, H. X., Lou, H. X., et al. (2018). Therapeutic Potential of Salviae Miltiorrhizae Radix et Rhizoma against Human Diseases Based on Activation of Nrf2-Mediated Antioxidant Defense System: Bioactive Constituents and Mechanism of Action. *Oxid Med. Cel Longev* 2018, 7309073. doi:10.1155/2018/7309073

Li, L., and Luo, X. (2011). Treatment of Ulcerative Colitis by Compound Danshen Needle Retention Enema Combined with Sal Treatment of Ulcerative Colitis. *Chin. J. Misdiagn* 11, 301–302. CNKI:SUN:ZWZX.0.2011-02-037.

Li, S., and Zhang, B. (2013). Traditional Chinese Medicine Network Pharmacology: Theory, Methodology and Application. *Chin. J. Nat. Med.* 11, 110–120. doi:10.1016/s1875-5364(13)60037-0

Li, S. (2021). Network Pharmacology Evaluation Method Guidance - Draft. *World J. Tradit Chin. Med.* 7, 148–154. doi:10.4103/wjtcm.wjtcm_11_21

Li, X. (2019). Effect of Danshen Powder Injection in the Treatment of Ulcerative Colitis and its Effect on the Levels of Hcy and Inflammatory Factors of Patients. *Clin. Med. Res. Pract.* 2, 26–27. doi:10.19347/j.cnki.2096-1413.201902012

Liang, Q., Liang, Z.-S., Wang, J.-R., and Xu, W.-H. (2009). Essential Oil Composition of Salvia Miltiorrhiza Flower. *Food Chem.* 113, 592–594. doi:10.1016/j.foodchem.2008.08.035

Liao, W., Ma, X., Li, J., Li, X., Guo, Z., Zhou, S., et al. (2019). A Review of the Mechanism of Action of Dantonic® for the Treatment of Chronic Stable Angina. *Biomed. Pharmacother.* 109, 690–700. doi:10.1016/j.biopha.2018.10.013

Liu, C., Yang, J., Zhu, F., Li, X., and Ma, J. (2019). Evaluation of Curative Effects of Danshen Injection Combined with Lactic Acid Bacteria Capsule in Treatment of Ulcerative Colitis. *Heibei Med. J.* 41, 2012–2018. doi:10.3969/j.issn.1002-7386.2019.13.022

Liu, X., He, H., Huang, T., Lei, Z., Liu, F., An, G., et al. (2016). Tanshinone IIA Protects against Dextran Sulfate Sodium- (DSS-) Induced Colitis in Mice by Modulation of Neutrophil Infiltration and Activation. *Oxid Med. Cel Longev* 2016, 7916763. doi:10.1155/2016/7916763

Liu, Z.-j., Shi, Z.-l., Tu, C., Zhang, H.-z., Gao, D., Li, C.-y., et al. (2017). An Activity-Calibrated Chemical Standardization Approach for Quality Evaluation of Salvia Miltiorrhiza Bge. *RSC Adv.* 7, 5331–5339. doi:10.1039/c6ra26281c

Luo, T. T., Lu, Y., Yan, S. K., Xiao, X., Rong, X. L., and Guo, J. (2020). Network Pharmacology in Research of Chinese Medicine Formula: Methodology, Application and Prospective. *Chin. J. Integr. Med.* 26, 72–80. doi:10.1007/s11655-019-3064-0

Ma, S., Zhang, D., Lou, H., Sun, L., and Ji, J. (2016). Evaluation of the Anti-inflammatory Activities of Tanshinones Isolated from Salvia Miltiorrhiza Var. alba Roots in THP-1 Macrophages. *J. Ethnopharmacol* 188, 193–199. doi:10.1016/j.jep.2016.05.018

Mak, W. Y., Zhao, M., Ng, S. C., and Burisch, J. (2020). The Epidemiology of Inflammatory Bowel Disease: East Meets West. *J. Gastroenterol. Hepatol.* 35, 380–389. doi:10.1111/jgh.14872

Min, X., Zeng, X., Zhao, W., Han, Z., Wang, Y., Han, Y., et al. (2020). Cryptotanshinone Protects Dextran Sulfate Sodium-Induced Experimental Ulcerative Colitis in Mice by Inhibiting Intestinal Inflammation. *Phytother Res.* 34, 2639–2648. doi:10.1002/ptr.6693

Mitchell, S., Vargas, J., and Hoffmann, A. (2016). Signaling via the NFκB System. *Wires Syst. Biol. Med.*, 8, 227–241. doi:10.1002/wsbm.1331

Mouli, V. P., and Ananthakrishnan, A. N. (2014). Review Article: Vitamin D and Inflammatory Bowel Diseases. *Aliment. Pharmacol. Ther.* 39, 125–136. doi:10.1111/apt.12553

Nagata, S. (2018). Apoptosis and Clearance of Apoptotic Cells. *Annu. Rev. Immunol.* 36, 489–517. doi:10.1146/annurev-immunol-042617-053010

Nennig, S. E., and Schank, J. R. (2017). The Role of NFkB in Drug Addiction: Beyond Inflammation. *Alcohol Alcohol* 52, 172–179. doi:10.1093/alcalc/agw098

Ng, S. C., Bernstein, C. N., Vatn, M. H., Lakatos, P. L., Loftus, E. V., Jr., Tysk, C., et al. (2013). Epidemiology, Natural History Task Force of the International Organization of Inflammatory Bowel, DGeographical Variability and Environmental Risk Factors in Inflammatory Bowel Disease. *Gut* 62, 630–649. doi:10.1136/gutjnl-2012-303661

Noble, C. L., Abbas, A. R., Cornelius, J., Lees, C. W., Ho, G. T., Toy, K., et al. (2008). Regional Variation in Gene Expression in the Healthy colon Is Dysregulated in Ulcerative Colitis. *Gut* 57, 1398–1405. doi:10.1136/gut.2008.148395

Olsen, J., Gerds, T. A., Seidelin, J. B., Csillag, C., Bjerrum, J. T., Troelsen, J. T., et al. (2009). Diagnosis of Ulcerative Colitis before Onset of Inflammation by Multivariate Modeling of Genome-wide Gene Expression Data. *Inflamm. Bowel Dis.* 15, 1032–1038. doi:10.1002/ibd.20879

Park, J. H., Peyrin-Biroulet, L., Eisenhut, M., and Shin, J. I. (2017). IBD Immunopathogenesis: A Comprehensive Review of Inflammatory Molecules. *Autoimmun. Rev.* 16, 416–426. doi:10.1016/j.autrev.2017.02.013

Peng, K.-Y., Gu, J.-F., Su, S.-L., Zhu, Y., Guo, J.-M., Qian, D.-W., et al. (2021). Salvia Miltiorrhiza Stems and Leaves Total Phenolic Acids Combination with Tanshinone Protect against DSS-Induced Ulcerative Colitis through Inhibiting TLR4/PI3K/AKT/mTOR Signaling Pathway in Mice. *J. Ethnopharmacology* 264, 113052. doi:10.1016/j.jep.2020.113052

Perrotta, I., Moraca, F. M., Sciangula, A., Aquila, S., and Mazzulla, S. (2015). HIF-1α and VEGF: Immunohistochemical Profile and Possible Function in Human Aortic Valve Stenosis. *Ultrastruct. Pathol.* 39, 198–206. doi:10.3109/01913123.2014.991884

Petryszyn, P. W., and Paradowski, L. (2018). Stool Patterns and Symptoms of Disordered Anorectal Function in Patients with Inflammatory Bowel Diseases. *Adv. Clin. Exp. Med.* 27, 813–818. doi:10.17219/acem/68986

Pickard, J. M., Zeng, M. Y., Caruso, R., and Núñez, G. (2017). Gut Microbiota: Role in Pathogen Colonization, Immune Responses, and Inflammatory Disease. *Immunol. Rev.* 279, 70–89. doi:10.1111/imr.12567

Plichta, D. R., Graham, D. B., Subramanian, S., and Xavier, R. J. (2019). Therapeutic Opportunities in Inflammatory Bowel Disease: Mechanistic Dissection of Host-Microbiome Relationships. *Cell* 178, 1041–1056. doi:10.1016/j.cell.2019.07.045

Ramanan, D., Tang, M. S., Bowcutt, R., Loke, P., and Cadwell, K. (2014). Bacterial Sensor Nod2 Prevents Inflammation of the Small Intestine by Restricting the Expansion of the Commensal Bacteroides Vulgatus. *Immunity* 41, 311–324. doi:10.1016/j.immuni.2014.06.015

Segal, J. P., Mullish, B. H., Quraishi, M. N., Acharjee, A., Williams, H. R. T., Iqbal, T., et al. (2019). The Application of Omics Techniques to Understand the Role of the Gut Microbiota in Inflammatory Bowel Disease. *Therap Adv. Gastroenterol.* 12, 1756284818822250–13. doi:10.1177/1756284818822250

Sheng, B., Wu, F., and Yao, A. (2014). Treatment of Salviae Miltiorrhizae and Ligustrazine Hydrochloride Injection, Clostridium Butyricum Live Bacteria Capsules and Salad Diazoxide on Ulcerative Colitis Patients. *West. Med.* 26, 1340–1342. doi:10.3969/j.issn.1672-3511.2014.10.028

Shouval, D. S., and Rufo, P. A. (2017). The Role of Environmental Factors in the Pathogenesis of Inflammatory Bowel Diseases: A Review. *JAMA Pediatr.* 171, 999–1005. doi:10.1001/jamapediatrics.2017.2571

Song, J., Zhang, W., Wang, J., Yang, H., Zhao, X., Zhou, Q., et al. (2018). Activation of Nrf2 Signaling by Salvianolic Acid C Attenuates NF-κB M-ediated I-nflammatory R-esponse B-oth In V-ivo and In V-itro. *Int. Immunopharmacol* 63, 299–310. doi:10.1016/j.intimp.2018.08.004

Soufli, I., Toumi, R., Rafa, H., and Touil-Boukoffa, C. (2016). Overview of Cytokines and Nitric Oxide Involvement in Immuno-Pathogenesis of Inflammatory Bowel Diseases. *World J. Gastrointest. Pharmacol. Ther.* 7, 353–60. doi:10.4292/wjgpt.v7.i3.353

Su, C. Y., Ming, Q. L., Rahman, K., Han, T., and Qin, L. P. (2015). Salvia Miltiorrhiza: Traditional Medicinal Uses, Chemistry, and Pharmacology. *Chin. J. Nat. Med.* 13, 163–82. doi:10.1016/s1875-5364(15)30002-9

Sun, S. (2019). Clinical Analysis of Mesalazine Combined with Salvia Miltiorrhiza Injection on Ulcerative Colitis. *Guid Chin. Med.* 17, 60. doi:10.15912/j.cnki.gocm.2019.04.051

Szklarczyk, D., Gable, A. L., Lyon, D., Junge, A., Wyder, S., Huerta-Cepas, J., et al. (2019). STRING V11: Protein-Protein Association Networks with Increased Coverage, Supporting Functional Discovery in Genome-wide Experimental Datasets. *Nucleic Acids Res.* 47, D607–D613. doi:10.1093/nar/gky1131

Tkachenko, A. S. (2019). Effectiveness of Breast-Conserving Surgery in Patients with Breast Cancer. *J. Clin. Med. Kaz* 1, 12–15. doi:10.23950/1812-2892-jcmk-00658

Vancamelbeke, M., Vanuytsel, T., Farré, R., Verstockt, S., Ferrante, M., Van Assche, G., et al. (2017). Genetic and Transcriptomic Bases of Intestinal Epithelial Barrier Dysfunction in Inflammatory Bowel Disease. *Inflamm. Bowel Dis.* 23, 1718–1729. doi:10.1097/MIB.0000000000001246

Wang, H., Gu, J., Hou, X., Chen, J., Yang, N., Liu, Y., et al. (2017a). Anti-inflammatory Effect of Miltirone on Inflammatory Bowel Disease via TLR4/NF-Kb/iqgap2 Signaling Pathway. *Biomed. Pharmacother.* 85, 531–540. doi:10.1016/j.biopha.2016.11.061

Wang, K., Yang, Q., Ma, Q., Wang, B., Wan, Z., Chen, M., et al. (2018). Protective Effects of Salvianolic Acid A against Dextran Sodium Sulfate-Induced Acute Colitis in Rats. *Nutrients* 10. doi:10.3390/nu10060791

Wang, L., Ma, R., Liu, C., Liu, H., Zhu, R., Guo, S., et al. (2017b). Salvia Miltiorrhiza: A Potential Red Light to the Development of Cardiovascular Diseases. *Curr. Pharm. Des.* 23, 1077–1097. doi:10.2174/1381612822666161010105242

Wang, M., Liu, J., Zhou, B., Xu, R., Tao, L., Ji, M., et al. (2012). Acute and Sub-chronic Toxicity Studies of Danshen Injection in Sprague-Dawley Rats. *J. Ethnopharmacol* 141, 96–103. doi:10.1016/j.jep.2012.02.005

Wang, T., Wang, C., Wu, Q., Zheng, K., Chen, J., Lan, Y., et al. (2017c). Evaluation of Tanshinone IIA Developmental Toxicity in Zebrafish Embryos. *Molecules* 22. doi:10.3390/molecules22040660

Wu, X., Wang, L., Tang, L., Wang, L., Cao, S., Wu, Q., et al. (2018). Salvianolic Acid B Alters the Gut Microbiota and Mitigates Colitis Severity and Associated Inflammation. *J. Funct. Foods* 46, 312–319. doi:10.1016/j.jff.2018.04.068

Xiong, D., and Wang, Y. (2016). Effect of Melalazine Combined with Tanshinone on Inflammatory Factors and Hypercoagulability in Ulcerative Colitis. *J. Hainan Med. Coll.* 22, 2718–2720. doi:10.13210/j.cnki.jhmu.20160814.017

Xiong, Y., Wang, J., Chu, H., Chen, D., and Guo, H. (2016). Salvianolic Acid B Restored Impaired Barrier Function via Downregulation of MLCK by microRNA-1 in Rat Colitis Model. *Front. Pharmacol.* 7, 134. doi:10.3389/fphar.2016.00134

Xu, D., Yu, H., Yu, Q., Wu, S., Liu, D., Lin, Y., et al. (2014). Salvia Miltiorrhiza Increases the Expression of Transcription Factor Foxp3 in Experimental Murine Colitis. *Mol. Med. Rep.* 9, 1947–51. doi:10.3892/mmr.2014.1986

Xu Dekui, X., Simeng, W., Hongbo, Y., Changqing, Z., Dongmei, L., and yan, L. (2012). Salvia Miltiorrhiza Inhibits the Expressions of Transcription Factor T-Bet (T-Bet) and Tumor Necrosis Factor α (TNFα) in the Experimental Colitis in Mice. *Afr. J. Biotechnol.* 11. doi:10.5897/ajb11.1796

Xu, M., Tao, J., Yang, Y., Tan, S., Liu, H., Jiang, J., et al. (2020). Ferroptosis Involves in Intestinal Epithelial Cell Death in Ulcerative Colitis. *Cel Death Dis* 11, 86. doi:10.1038/s41419-020-2299-1

Xu, S. (2015). Clinical Observation of Sulfasalazine Enteric-Coated Tablets Combined with Chuanxiong Danshen Injection for Treatment of Active Ulcerative Colitis. *J. New Chin. Med.* 47, 56–58. doi:10.13457/j.cnki.jncm.2015.06.027

Yan, Y. Y., Yang, Y. H., Wang, W. W., Pan, Y. T., Zhan, S. Y., Sun, M. Y., et al. (2017). Post-marketing Safety Surveillance of the Salvia Miltiorrhiza Depside Salt for Infusion: A Real World Study. *PLoS One* 12, e0170182. doi:10.1371/journal.pone.0170182

Yang, J., and Zhang, Y. (2005). Treatment of 26 Cases of Ulcerative Colitis by Danshen and Huangqi Injection. *Chin. J. Coal Ind. Med.* 8, 600. doi:10.3969/j.issn.1007-9564.2005.06.039

Yang, L. (2017). Effect of Danshen Injection Combined with Bacillus Subtilis Double-Linked Enteric Capsule on Intestinal Mucosal Function of Ulcerative Colitis Patients. *Heilongjiang Med. Pharm.* 40, 149–150. doi:10.3969/j.issn.1008-0104.2017.06.070

Yang, X. J., Qian, J. X., Wei, Y., Guo, Q., Jin, J., Sun, X., et al. (2018). Tanshinone IIA Sodium Sulfonate Attenuates LPS-Induced Intestinal Injury in Mice. *Gastroenterol. Res. Pract.* 2018, 9867150. doi:10.1155/2018/9867150

Yao, J., Wang, J., Sun, R., and Yang, Z. (2016). Effect of Danshen Injection Combined with Ornidazole on Ulcerative Colitis. *Mod. J. Int. Trad Chin. West. Med.* 25, 3864–3865. doi:10.3969/j.issn.1008-8849.2016.34

Ye, Z., Hong, C. O., Lee, K., Hostetter, J., Wannemuehler, M., and Hendrich, S. (2011). Plasma Caffeic Acid Is Associated with Statistical Clustering of the Anticolitic Efficacy of Caffeic Acid in Dextran Sulfate Sodium-Treated Mice. *J. Nutr.* 141, 1989–95. doi:10.3945/jn.111.142208

Ye, Z., Liu, Z., Henderson, A., Lee, K., Hostetter, J., Wannemuehler, M., et al. (2009). Increased CYP4B1 mRNA Is Associated with the Inhibition of Dextran Sulfate Sodium-Induced Colitis by Caffeic Acid in Mice. *Exp. Biol. Med. (Maywood)* 234, 605–16. doi:10.3181/0901-RM-1

Yin, H. Q., Choi, Y. J., Kim, Y. C., Sohn, D. H., Ryu, S. Y., and Lee, B. H. (2009). Salvia Miltiorrhiza Bunge and its Active Component Cryptotanshinone Protects Primary Cultured Rat Hepatocytes from Acute Ethanol-Induced Cytotoxicity and Fatty Infiltration. *Food Chem. Toxicol.* 47, 98–103. doi:10.1016/j.fct.2008.10.018

Yuan, N., Gong, L., Tang, K., He, L., Hao, W., Li, X., et al. (2020). An Integrated Pharmacology-Based Analysis for Antidepressant Mechanism of Chinese Herbal Formula Xiao-Yao-San. *Front. Pharmacol.* 11, 284. doi:10.3389/fphar.2020.00284

Zhang, R., Zhu, X., Bai, H., and Ning, K. (2019). Network Pharmacology Databases for Traditional Chinese Medicine: Review and Assessment. *Front. Pharmacol.* 10, 123. doi:10.3389/fphar.2019.00123

Zhang, X., Wang, Y., Ma, Z., Liang, Q., Tang, X., Hu, D., et al. (2015). Tanshinone IIA Ameliorates Dextran Sulfate Sodium-Induced Inflammatory Bowel Disease via the Pregnane X Receptor. *Drug Des. Devel Ther.* 9, 6343–62. doi:10.2147/DDDT.S79388

Zhang, X. Z., Qian, S. S., Zhang, Y. J., and Wang, R. Q. (2016a). Salvia Miltiorrhiza: A Source for Anti-alzheimer's Disease Drugs. *Pharm. Biol.* 54, 18–24. doi:10.3109/13880209.2015.1027408

Zhang, Z., Wu, X., Cao, S., Wang, L., Wang, D., Yang, H., et al. (2016b). Caffeic Acid Ameliorates Colitis in Association with Increased Akkermansia Population in the Gut Microbiota of Mice. *Oncotarget* 7, 31790–9. doi:10.18632/oncotarget.9306

Zhao, J., Lv, C., Wu, Q., Zeng, H., Guo, X., Yang, J., et al. (2019a). Computational Systems Pharmacology Reveals an Antiplatelet and Neuroprotective Mechanism of Deng-Zhan-Xi-Xin Injection in the Treatment of Ischemic Stroke. *Pharmacol. Res.* 147, 104365. doi:10.1016/j.phrs.2019.104365

Zhao, J., Zhang, Q. L., Shen, J. H., Wang, K., and Liu, J. (2019b). Magnesium Lithospermate B Improves the Gut Microbiome and Bile Acid Metabolic Profiles in a Mouse Model of Diabetic Nephropathy. *Acta Pharmacol. Sin* 40, 507–513. doi:10.1038/s41401-018-0029-3

Zhao, L., Zhang, Y., Liu, G., Hao, S., Wang, C., and Wang, Y. (2018). Black rice Anthocyanin-Rich Extract and Rosmarinic Acid, Alone and in Combination, Protect against DSS-Induced Colitis in Mice. *Food Funct.* 9, 2796–2808. doi:10.1039/c7fo01490b

Zheng, S., Du, G., Lin, X., and Zhang, N. (2013). A Randomized Controlled Study of Compound Danshen Injection Combined with Oxygen Inhalation Combined with Western Medicine in the Treatment of Ulcerative Colitis. *J. Pract. Trad Chin. Intern. Med.* 27, 58–60. doi:10.3969/j.issn.1671-7813.2013.09(s).29

Zhou, L., Zuo, Z., and Chow, M. S. (2005). Danshen: an Overview of its Chemistry, Pharmacology, Pharmacokinetics, and Clinical Use. *J. Clin. Pharmacol.* 45, 1345–59. doi:10.1177/0091270005282630

Zhu, H. (2018). Effect of Melalazine Combined with Danshen Injection on Inflammatory Factors in Patients with Ulcerative Colitis. *Cont Med.* 24, 100–101. doi:10.3969/j.issn.1009-4393.2018.01.051

Zhu, H., Tong, S., Cui, Y., Wang, X., and Wang, M. (2021). Tanshinol Alleviates Ulcerative Colitis by Promoting the Expression of VLDLR. *Drug Dev. Res.* 82, 1258–1268. doi:10.1002/ddr.21840

Zhu, Y. (2019). Effect of Danshen Injection Combined with Mesalazine on Ulcerative Colitis. *Heilongjiang J. Trad Chin. Med.* 2, 249–250. CNKI:SUN: HLZY.0.2019-02-137.

8

Network Pharmacology Based Research on the Combination Mechanism Between Escin and Low Dose Glucocorticoids in Anti-Rheumatoid Arthritis

Leiming Zhang[1†], Yanan Huang[1†], Chuanhong Wu[2†], Yuan Du[1†], Peng Li[3], Meiling Wang[1], Xinlin Wang[1], Yanfang Wang[1], Yanfei Hao[1], Tian Wang[1], Baofeng Fan[4], Zhuye Gao[5*] and Fenghua Fu[1*]*

[1] *Key Laboratory of Molecular Pharmacology and Drug Evaluation, Ministry of Education, School of Pharmacy, Yantai University, Yantai, China,* [2] *The Biomedical Sciences Institute of Qingdao University (Qingdao Branch of SJTU Bio-X Institutes), Qingdao University, Qingdao, China,* [3] *College of Arts and Sciences, Shanxi Agricultural University, Taigu, China,* [4] *Air Force General Hospital, PLA, Beijing, China,* [5] *Xiyuan Hospital, China Academy of Chinese Medical Sciences, Beijing, China*

***Correspondence:**
Baofeng Fan
baofengfan2018@126.com
Zhuye Gao
zhuyegao@126.com
Fenghua Fu
fufenghua@sohu.com

†These authors have contributed equally to this work

Rheumatoid arthritis (RA) is characterized by chronic progressive symmetrical synovitis and destruction of multiple joints. Glucocorticoids (GCs) are widely used in the treatment of RA. However, their adverse effects can be serious. Escin, which is isolated from *Aesculus hippocastanum* L., has been reported to have anti-inflammatory effects. We investigated the anti-RA effect of Escin combined with low dose GCs (dexamethasone, Dex) and the underlying mechanism. Adjuvant-induced RA rats and lipopolysaccharides (LPS)-injured RAW264.7 cells were used to investigate the anti-RA effects of Escin combined with low dose Dex *in vivo* and *in vitro*. The results showed that Escin combined with low-dose Dex significantly decreased arthritic index, serum IL-6 and TNF-α levels, reduced paw swelling, and ameliorated the joint pathology and immune organ pathology. Gene chip results revealed that *Nr3c1* (GR) expression was significantly altered, and that GR was activated by Escin and low dose Dex *in vivo* and *in vitro*. Additionally, Escin combined with low dose Dex also significantly increased GR mRNA expression. However, when GR expression was suppressed by its specific inhibitor, the anti-RA effect of Escin combined with low-dose Dex was abolished. The data in this study demonstrated that Escin combined with Dex reduced the dose of Dex, and exerted significant anti-RA effects, which could also reduce the adverse effects of Dex. This combination might result from GR activation. This study might provide a new combination of drugs for the treatment of RA.

Keywords: rheumatoid arthritis, glucocorticoids, glucocorticoid receptor, Escin, dexamethasone

INTRODUCTION

Rheumatoid arthritis (RA) is a chronic autoimmune disease that causes progressive articular damage, functional loss, and comorbidity. RA affects about 1% of the population, and it can present at any age (McInnes and Schett, 2017). Its physiopathology includes synovial inflammation with pro-inflammatory cytokine overexpression (Courbon et al., 2018).

Glucocorticoids (GCs) are widely used in the treatment of RA. However, long-term and high dose GC use can lead to serious adverse effects, such as immunosuppression, osteoporosis and metabolic disorders (Gossye et al., 2009). One of the methods to minimize the undesirable adverse effects is through administering them with other pharmaceuticals, aiming at synergistic effects to reduce the dose and duration of cortical therapy.

Escin (polyhydroxyolean-12-ene 3-*O*-monodesmosides) is a natural mixture of triterpene saponins isolated from *Aesculus hippocastanum* L. (Xin et al., 2011a). Several studies have reported that it has anti-inflammatory (Wang et al., 2013), anti-edematous (Wang et al., 2011), and anti-cancer properties (Cheong et al., 2018). It was also reported that Escin could synergize with GCs to enhance their anti-inflammatory effect (Xin et al., 2011b).

Recent years, network-based approaches offer the potential to explore, in a systematic way (Hopkins, 2008), the effect of a drug candidate in a global physiological environment (Xiong et al., 2019), and was commonly used to decipher new drug-target relationships in drug discovery (Boezio et al., 2017). And this method was also used in this study to give a constructive result of the Escin effect on RA. Based on the network pharmacology, we investigated whether the combination of Escin and GCs would improve the anti-RA effects and the underlying mechanism.

MATERIALS AND METHODS

Materials

Escin, including sodium aescinate tablets (batch no: 201509321) and sodium aescinate for injection (batch no: 2017110103), were purchased from Shandong Luye Pharmaceutical Co., Ltd. (Yantai, China). Dexamethasone tablets (Dex, batch no: 160601201) were purchased from Chen Xin Pharmaceutical Co., Ltd. (Jining, China). Dexamethasone powder (D4902, purity $\geq$ 97%), lipopolysaccharides (LPS) and 3-(4,5-dimethyl-2-thiazolyl)-2,5-diphenyl-2-H-tetrazolium bromide (MTT) were purchased from Sigma-Aldrich (St. Louis, MO, United States). Complete Freund's adjuvant (CFA) (containing 10 mg/ml of dry, heat-killed Mycobacterium tuberculosis) was purchased from Chondrex Co., Ltd. (Redmond, WA, United States, batch no: 170334). RPMI medium 1640 was purchased from Gibco (Carlsbad, CA, United States, batch no: 1960297). Fetal bovine serum (FBS) was purchase from Zhejiang Tianhang Biological Technology Co., Ltd. (Hangzhou, China, batch no: 11011-8611). Griess reagent kit (S0023) was purchased from Beyotime Institute of Biotechnology (Haimen, China). Primary antibody for IκBα (K2017), and GR (A2518) were purchased from Santa Cruz Biotechnology (Santa Cruz, CA, United States). Primary antibody for *p*-IκBα (S32) and *p*-p65 (S536) were purchased from Cell signaling Technology (Danvers, MA, United States). P65 (ab16502) was purchased from Abcam company (Burlingame, CA, United States). Second antibodies for anti-rabbit IgG HRP-linked antibody and anti-mouse IgG HRP-linked antibody were purchased from Beyotime Institute of Biotechnology (Haimen, China). RU486 (m8046) were purchased from Sigma-Aldrich (United States). qPCR reagents: UltraSYBR Mixture (CW2602M) were purchased from Kang Wei century Biotechnology Co., Ltd. (Beijing, China).

Animals

Animal experimental procedures were performed in strict accordance with the National Institutes of Health Regulations on the use and care of animals for scientific purposes. Male Sprague-Dawley rats (weight, 180–220 g) were purchased from Shandong Jinan PengYue Experimental Animal Breeding Co., Ltd. (Jinan, China). All the rats were housed in diurnal lighting conditions (12 h/12 h) and allowed free access to food and water. All experimental procedures in this study were performed in accordance with the Guidelines for the Care and Use of Laboratory Animals of Yantai University, and were approved by the ethics committee.

Induction of Adjuvant-Induced Rheumatoid Arthritis

Adjuvant-induced RA (AIA) was induced in the rats according to the method described by Pearson (Pearson, 1963). Briefly, the animals were inoculated with a subplantar injection of 0.1 mL CFA into the right hind paw at day 0 and were randomly allocated to 6 groups of eight rats each (n = 10) as follows: the control group; AIA group; AIA + Dex (0.2 $mg \cdot kg^{-1}$) group; AIA + Dex (0.05 $mg \cdot kg^{-1}$) group; AIA + Escin (10 $mg \cdot kg^{-1}$) group; AIA + Escin (10 $mg \cdot kg^{-1}$) + Dex (0.05 $mg \cdot kg^{-1}$) group. Dex and Escin were administered orally 15 days after inoculation, and once daily for a period of 2 weeks (from day 15 to day 28). Body weight was determined on Day 0, 3, 6, 9, 12, 15, 18, 21, 24, and 27.

Measurement of Paw Volume

Paw volume was measured using a Plethysmometer (YLS-7B, Shandong Academy of Medical Sciences, Jinan, China) on Day 0 before CFA injections and thereafter on Day 3, 7, 11, 15, 18, 22, 25, and 28. The change in paw volume was calculated as the difference between the final (28 days) and initial (0 day) paw volume (Lee et al., 2009).

Measurement of Arthritic Index

The morphological features of arthritis such as redness, swelling and erythema were determined using a five-point ordinal scale (0–4) scoring system as follows: 0, narrow paw; 1, mild swelling and erythema of the digits; 2, swelling and erythema of the digits; 3, severe swelling and erythema; 4, gross deformity and inability to use the limb (Paval et al., 2009). Thus, the maximum score for both the paws was 8.

Histopathological Examination

After 2 weeks of Dex/Escin administration, the speen, thymus, right leg joint, and left leg joint tissues with pathologic changes were stained with haematoxylin-eosin (HE) to evaluate the effect of Dex and Escin. The tissues were removed and fixed in 10% buffered formalin (pH = 7.0) for 3 days. Samples were then trimmed, decalcified in 10% EDTA at room temperature for 60 days, embedded in paraffin and cut into slices. Sections (4 μm) were stained with HE. The histopathological changes and severity were observed with a light microscope (Pan et al., 2017).

Immune Organ Index

After Dex/Escin administration for 2 weeks, the spleen and thymus weights were determined and the organ-to-body weight ratio was calculated.

Glucocorticoid Signaling RT2 Profiler OCR Array

The GC signaling gene changes (including 84 genes) in synovial tissue of the joints were detected by Shanghai Bo Hao Biotechnology Co., Ltd. (Shanghai, China) using a RT2 Profiler PCR Array. Briefly, the procedure started with conversion of experimental RNA samples into first-strand cDNA using the RT2 First Strand Kit. Then, the cDNA was mixed with an appropriate RT2 SYBR Green Mastermix. This mixture was aliquoted into the wells of the RT2 Profiler PCR Array. PCR was performed and the relative expression was determined using data from the real-time cycler and the ΔΔCT method.

Cell Culture

Murine RAW264.7 macrophages obtained from the American Type Culture Collection (ATCC, VA, United States), were cultured in complete RPMI 1640 containing 10% heated-inactivated FBS, 100 U/ml penicillin, and 100 μg/ml streptomycin. Cells were incubated at 37°C in a humidified atmosphere of 5% CO_2 in air.

MTT Assay

RAW264.7 cells (5 × 10^4 cells/well) were cultured in 96-well plates for 24 h after Dex/Escin treatment with or without LPS (1 μg/mL). MTT solution (10 μL; 5 mg/ml) was added, and the cells were incubated at 37°C for an additional 4 h. After washing out the supernatant, the insoluble formazan product was dissolved in DMSO. Then, the optical density was measured at 570 nm using a microplate reader.

CCK-8 Assay

RAW264.7 cells (5 × 10^3 cells/well) were cultured in 96-well plates for 24 h after Dex/Escin treatment with or without LPS (1 μg/ml). CCK-8 solution (10 μL) was added to each well of the plate, and the cells were then incubated for 2 h in an incubator. The absorbance was measured at 450 nm using a 96-well plate reader.

Determination of Nitrite

RAW264.7 cells (1 × 10^5 cells/well) were cultured in 96-well plates with Dex/Escin pretreatment for 2 h and incubated with LPS for 24 h. Supernatant (50 μl) was collected and mixed with equal volumes of Griess reagent for 10 min at room temperature. Optical density was measured at 540 nm (Wu et al., 2015b).

Determination of IL-6 and TNF-α

RAW264.7 cells (1 × 10^5 cells/well) were cultured in 96-well plates with Dex/Escin pretreatment for 2 h and then incubated with LPS for 6 h. The concentrations of IL-6 and TNF-α in the culture medium were determined using ELISA kits, in accordance with the manufactures' instructions.

After 2 weeks of Dex/Escin administration, rat serum was obtained. The IL-6 and TNF-α serum concentrations were determined using ELISA kits in accordance with the manufactures' instructions.

RT-PCR Assay

RAW264.7 cells were seeded in six-well plates treated with Dex/Escin and 1 μg/ml LPS for 30 min. Total RNA was isolated and the RNA concentration was detected using a spectrophotometer. Total RNA (1 μg) was converted to cDNA and real-time PCR (RT-PCR) was performed using a PrimeScript^{TM} RT reagent kit. The PCR primers were as follows: GR, sense 5′-GTTGCGCAGCCTGAATGGCG-3′, antisense 5′-GCCGTCACTCCAACGCAGCA-3′; GAPDH, sense 5′-CGA CTTCAACAGCAACTCCCACTCTTCC-3′, antisense 5′-TGG GTGGTCCAGGGTTTCTTACTCCTT-3′. The amplification sequence protocol was conducted using three steps: 1 step: Cycle 1, 95°C 10 min; 2 step: Cycle 40, 95°C 15 s, 60°C 60 s; 3 step: Cycle 1, 95°C 15 s, 60°C 60 s, 95°C 15 s, 60°C 15 s.

Western Blotting

The expression of *p*-p65, p65, *p*-IκBα, IκBα, and GR in rat tissue and RAW264.7 cells was determined by western blot. The rat lysate and RAW264.7 lysates were incubated on ice for 30 min and then centrifuged at 12,000 rpm for 20 min at 4°C. The supernatant was collected, and the protein concentrations contained in the supernatant were measured using the BCA assay. The protein samples with loading buffer added were boiled for 5 min before loading onto SDS-polyacrylamide gel. After electrophoresis, the gel was electroblotted onto PVDF membranes. Membranes were blocked in Tris-buffered saline (TBS) with 1% Tween-20 (TBST) and 5% non-fat dry milk, and incubated with primary antibody overnight at 4°C. Then, the membranes were washed several times with TBST before incubation with horseradish peroxidase-conjugated secondary antibody for 60 min at room temperature. After subsequent washes in TBST, the protein bands were visualized using the ECL detection kit. The relative intensities of the bands were quantified by densitometric analysis. The densitometric plots of the results were normalized to the intensity of the actin band (Wu et al., 2015a).

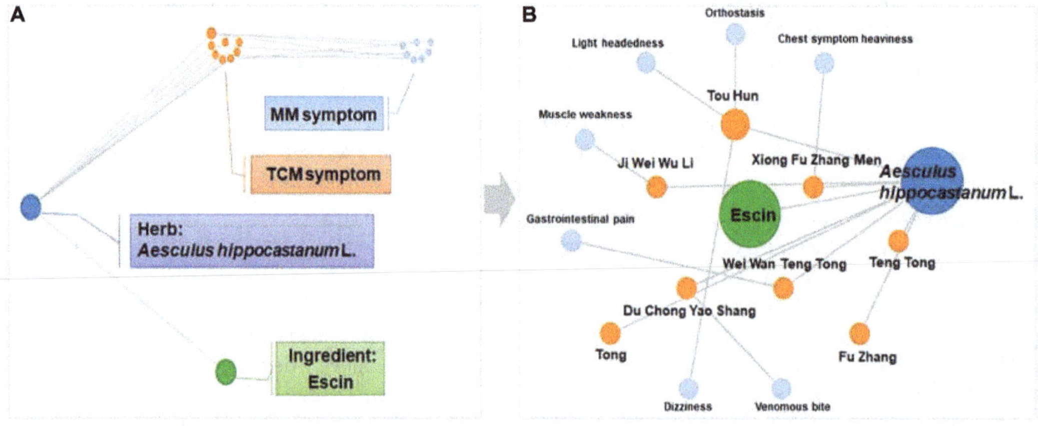

FIGURE 1 | Symptom network of Escin constructed with SymMap. **(A)** Description of network composition. **(B)** The detailed component of Escin network. This network was formed using SymMap (http://www.symmap.org).

Statistics

Data were expressed as the mean ± standard deviation (SD) of at least three independent experiments. The protective effects were assessed using the GraphPad Prism 6 software (GraphPad, San Diego, CA, United States). Relative protein semi-quantification was performed using the QUANTITY ONE software (Bio-Rad, Hercules, CA, United States). Differences between groups were assessed by ANOVA. A *P*-value less 0.05 was considered statistically significant.

RESULTS

Symptom Network of Escin Constructed Using SymMap

Symptom network of Escin was constructed with SymMap[1] (Wu et al., 2019) to predict the disease that Escin might be intervened. As displayed in **Figure 1A**, this network including Herb, Ingredient, Traditional Chinese Medicine symptom (TCM symptom), Modern Medicine symptom (MM symptom). The detailed component of Escin network was displayed in **Figure 1B**. Escin was isolated from *Aesculus hippocastanum* L. TCM symptom related to *Aesculus hippocastanum* L. were Teng Tong, Tong, Du Chong Yao Shang, Ji Wei Wu Li, Xiong Fu Zhang Men, Tou Hun and Wei Wan Teng Tong. Meanwhile, MM symptom correspondent to TCM symptom were Chest symptom heaviness (Xiong Fu Zhang Men), Light headedness, Orthostasis and Dizziness (Tou Hun), Muscle weakness (Ji Wei Wu Li), Gastrointestinal pain (Wei Wan Teng Tong), Venomous bite (Du Chong Yao Shang). Among the symptoms, muscle weakness also occurred in RA. In addition, TCM symptom, Tong, Teng Tong had no related MM symptom until now. However, these symptoms also occurred in RA. This network provide a trace for Escin in anti-RA.

[1]http://www.symmap.org

Effect of Escin Combined With Dex on Arthritic Index and Serum Inflammatory Factor Secretion in AIA Rats

The rats gradually developed multiple-joint RA beginning on day 15 after CFA injection. The arthritic index peaked on day 21 (**Figure 2A**). Dex at daily dose of 0.2 mg/kg and Escin (10 mg/kg) combined with Dex (0.05 mg/kg) significantly reduced the arthritic index compared with the AIA-treated group between days 18 and 27 post-CFA ($P < 0.05$). As illustrated in the representative day 28 paw graphs in **Figure 1B**, the AIA-treated rats displayed a swelling paw compared with the control rats. After administration of Dex (0.2 mg/kg), Dex (0.05 mg/kg), Escin (10 mg/kg) or Escin (10 mg/kg) combined with Dex (0.05 mg/kg), this swelling was ameliorated (**Figure 2B**). Moreover, the serum TNF-α and IL-6 concentrations in AIA rats were significantly higher compared with the control group ($P < 0.05$). The serum TNF-α and IL-6 concentrations in the Dex (0.2 mg/kg), Dex (0.05 mg/kg), Escin (10 mg/kg) and Escin (10 mg/kg) combined with Dex (0.05 mg/kg) groups were significantly lower compared with that the AIA-treated group (**Figures 2C,D**; $P < 0.05$).

Effect of Escin Combined With Dex on Histopathological Changes and Paw Swelling in AIA Rats

Haematoxylin-eosin staining was used to evaluate inflammation and bone lesion induced by AIA. As illustrated in **Figure 3**, no pathological findings of arthritis were observed in normal joints in the control group. However, the AIA-treated group exhibited severe synovitis, with synovial hyperplasia, inflammatory cells infiltration into the joint cavity, and bone and cartilage erosion on the primary and secondary sides. Treatment with Dex (0.2 mg/kg), Escin (10 mg/kg) combined with Dex (0.05 mg/kg), significantly decreased synovial hyperplasia, cartilage surface erosion, and joints degradation ($P < 0.05$), and substantially reduced the amount of infiltrated inflammatory cells. However, low dose Dex (0.05 mg/kg) and Escin (10 mg/kg) alone did not

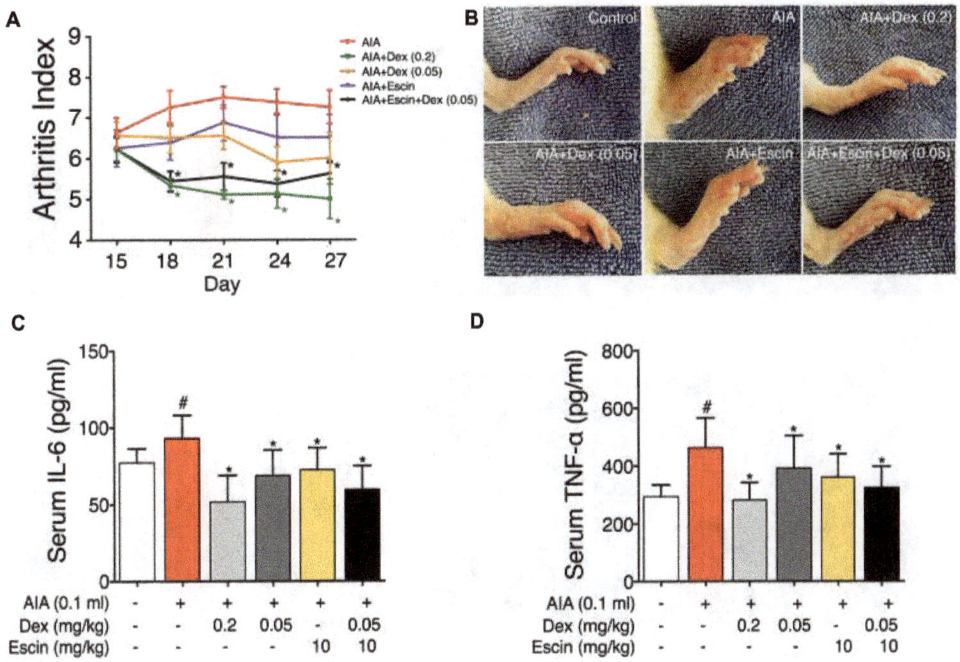

FIGURE 2 | Effect of Escin combined with Dex on arthritic index and serum inflammatory factor secretion in AIA rats. **(A)** Arthritic index was evaluated by 5-point ordinal scale (0–4) scoring system. **(B)** Images for the paws were obtained. **(C,D)** Serum IL-6 and TNF-α were determined with ELISA kits. Data were expressed as the mean ± SD, and were analyzed by ANOVA. $^{\#}P < 0.05$ *versus* the control group; $^{*}P < 0.05$ *versus* the AIA-treated group; Dex, dexamethasone.

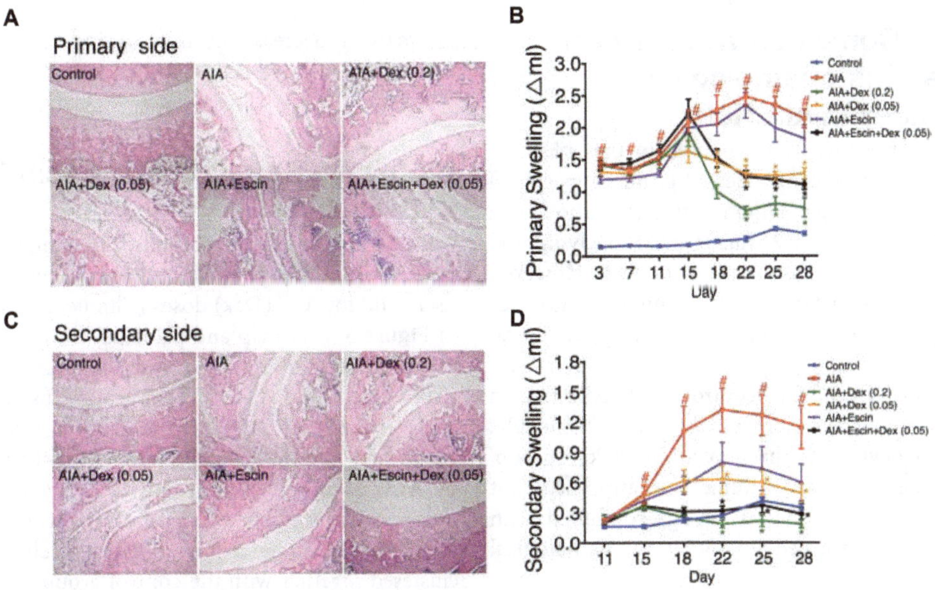

FIGURE 3 | Effect of Escin combined with Dex on histopathological changes and paw swelling in AIA rats. **(A,C)** Histopathological changes of joints in primary side and secondary side were determined with HE staining. **(B,D)** Paw swelling in primary side and secondary side were determined by a Plethysmometer. Data were expressed as the mean ± SD, and were analyzed by ANOVA. $^{\#}P < 0.05$ *versus* the control group; $^{*}P < 0.05$ *versus* the AIA-treated group; Dex, dexamethasone.

reverse these effects. After CFA injection, paw swelling on the primary side significantly increased on day 11 and peaked on day 22 ($P < 0.05$). while paw swelling occurred on the secondary side on day 15 and peaked on day 22. Dex (0.2 mg/kg) and Escin (10 mg/kg) combined with Dex (0.05 mg/kg) significantly decreased paw swelling on the primary and secondary sides beginning on day 22 ($P < 0.05$), and the effect of the combined medication was better than that of low-dose Dex (0.05 mg/kg).

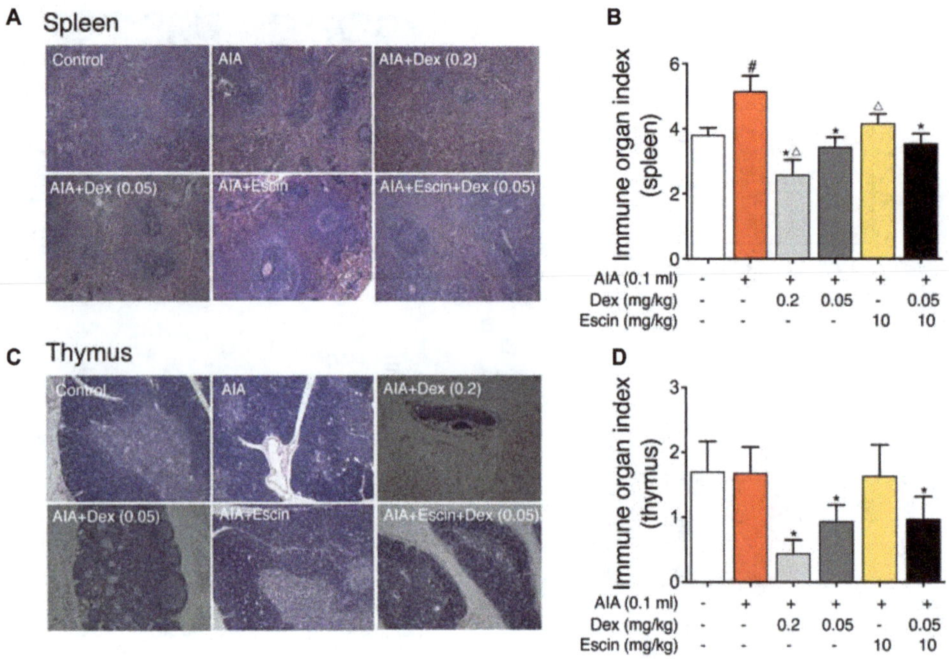

FIGURE 4 | Effect of Escin combined with Dex on immune organ histopathological change and index in AIA rats. **(A,C)** Histopathological changes of spleen and thymus were determined with HE staining. **(B,D)** Immune organ index of spleen and thymus were determined. Data were expressed as the mean ± SD, and were analyzed by ANOVA. $^{\#}P < 0.05$ *versus* the control group; $^{*}P < 0.05$ *versus* the AIA-treated group; $^{\triangle}P < 0.05$ *versus* the Escin (10 mg/kg) combined with Dex (0.05 mg/kg); Dex, dexamethasone.

Effect of Escin Combined With Dex on Immune Organ Histopathological Change and Index in AIA Rats

Red and white pulps were neatly distributed in the spleen of control group. However, in the AIA-treated group, hyperplasia of the white pulp and a larger lymphocyte aggregation area were observed. In the Dex (0.2 mg/kg) group, lymphoid nodules were significantly reduced and atrophied. However, Escin (10 mg/kg) and Escin (10 mg/kg) combined with Dex (0.05 mg/kg) treated groups showed no significant pathological changes (**Figure 4A**).

Rat thymus tissue from the control and AIA-treated groups showed clear demarcation of the dermal medulla and abundant lymphocytes. In the Dex (0.2 mg/kg) group, the rat thymus tissue medullary volume was atrophied, but the Escin (10 mg/kg) and Escin (10 mg/kg) combined with Dex (0.05 mg/kg) groups showed no significant pathological changes (**Figure 4C**).

The AIA-treated group displayed a remarkable increase in spleen index compared with the control rats. However, Dex (0.2 mg/kg) caused a marked decrease in spleen index compared with the AIA-treated rats and control rats. Escin (10 mg/kg) and Escin (10 mg/kg) combined with Dex (0.05 mg/kg) showed no marked decrease, compared with Dex (0.2 mg/kg) (**Figure 4B**). The Dex (0.2 mg/kg) group showed a remarkable decrease in thymus index compared with the AIA-treated rats and control rats ($P < 0.05$). However, Escin (10 mg/kg) and Escin (10 mg/kg) combined with Dex (0.05 mg/kg) showed no marked decrease in thymus index, compared with Dex (0.2 mg/kg) (**Figure 4D**).

Pathways Regulated by Escin Combined With Dex in AIA Rats

Considering that Dex specifically targeting GR, gene chips were further used to explore the combination mechanism between Escin and low GC (Dex) doses (Zhou et al., 2015). As illustrated in **Figure 5**, heat map and principal component analysis results of the gene chip revealed that the AIA group, AIA + Dex (0.05) group, and AIA + Escin group clustered together, which suggested that the AIA + Dex (0.05) group and AIA + Escin group had little influence on the GR pathway that was altered by AIA. AIA + Dex (0.2) clustered together with the control group, which suggested a significant anti-RA effect of Dex (0.2) in AIA-induced rats. However, AIA + Escin + Dex (0.05) group clustered together with the control group and AIA + Dex (0.2) group, which suggested that Escin combined with Dex (0.05) had a similar influence compared with Dex (0.2). Further analysis of specific genes showed that the control group, AIA + Dex (0.2) group and AIA + Escin + Dex (0.05) group shared the same trend in the *Tnf*, *Il-6*, *Nr3c1*, *Sphk1* mRNA expression. Moreover, these three groups improved the expression of *Nr3c1 (GR)* and the key genes, *Sphk1*, in the GR pathway, which suggested that Escin combined with Dex (0.05) might treat the disease by increasing GR expression and further affecting its relevant pathways.

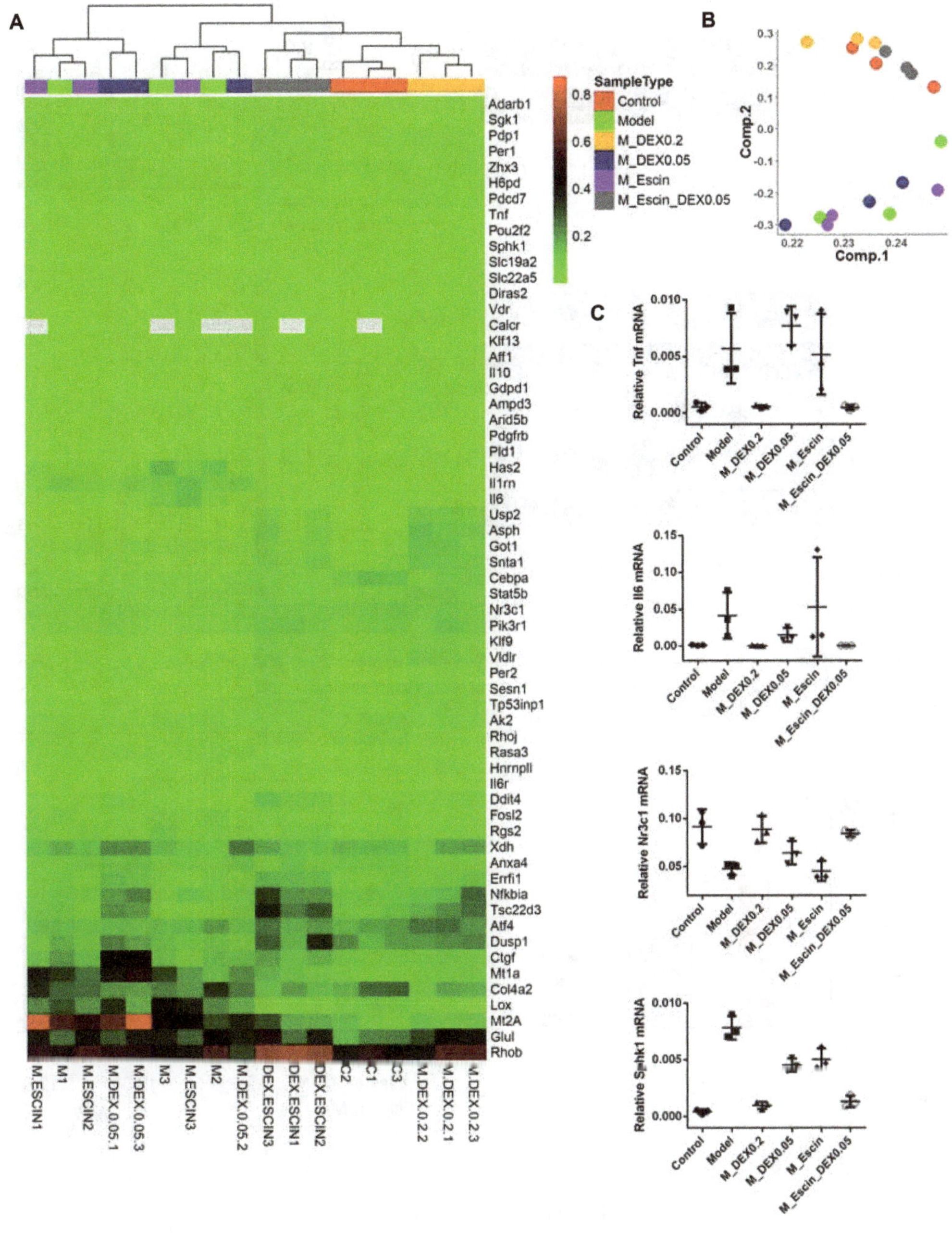

FIGURE 5 | RT[2] profile PCR array rat glucocorticoid signaling. **(A)** Heatmap analysis of the PCR array. Out of all 84 genes in the array, the heatmap includes 61 genes that were significantly changed in Model *versus* Control, M_DEX0.2 *versus* Model, M_DEX0.05 *versus* Model, M_Escin *versus* Model or M_Escin_DEX0.05 *versus* Model. **(B)** Principal component analysis of the PCR array results. The colors of sample points are consistent with the SampleType of **(A)**. **(C)** The relative mRNA expression values of four key genes *Tnf*, *Il6*, *Nr3c1*, and *Sphk1*. Model: AIA; M_DEX0.2: AIA + Dex (0.2); M_DEX0.05: AIA + Dex (0.05); M_Escin: AIA + Escin; M_Escin_DEX0.05: AIA + Escin + Dex (0.05).

Confirmation of the Gene Chip Results in AIA Rats

As illustrated in **Figure 6**, GR expression was significantly down-regulated in the AIA-treated group ($P < 0.05$), and its expression was significantly up-regulated after Dex (0.2 mg/kg) and Escin (10 mg/kg) combined with Dex (0.05 mg/kg) administration ($P < 0.05$). Moreover, the AIA-treated group significantly increased *p*-p65, p65 and *p*-IκBα expression. When administrated with Dex (0.2 mg/kg), Escin (10 mg/kg) combined with Dex (0.05 mg/kg) significantly decreased *p*-p65, p65 and *p*-IκBα expression ($P < 0.05$). Dex (0.05 mg/kg) significantly decreased *p*-p65 and *p*-IκBα expression ($P < 0.05$). Escin (10 m/kg) significantly decreased *p*-p65 expression ($P < 0.05$).

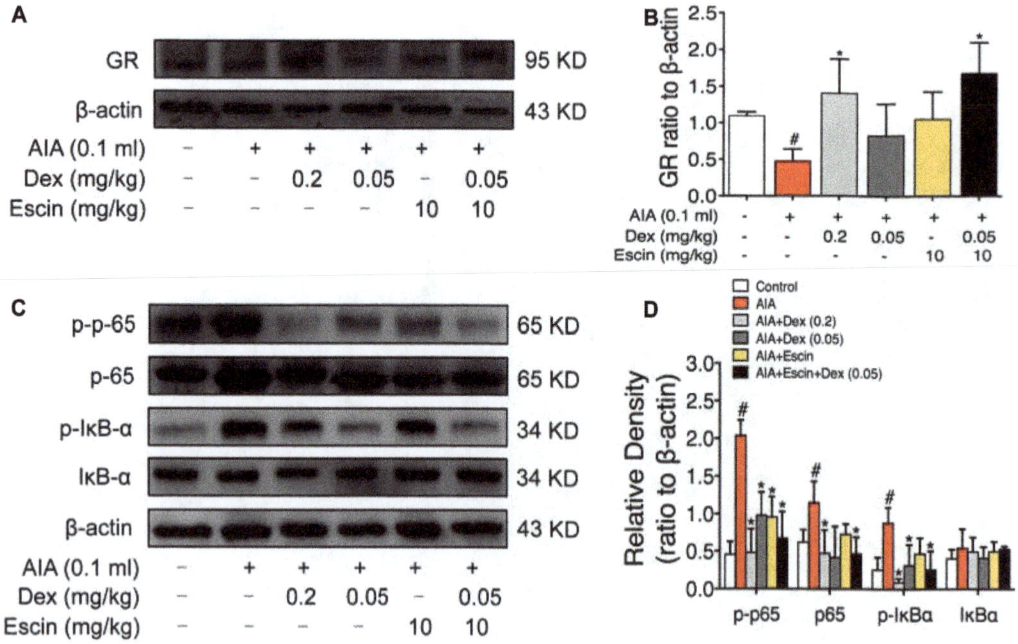

FIGURE 6 | Escin combined with Dex activated GR in AIA rats. **(A,C)** Representative western blots of GR, *p*-p65, p65, *p*-IκBα, IκBα, and β-actin. **(B,D)** The quantified densitometric analysis of GR, *p*-p65, p65, *p*-IκBα, IκBα. Data were expressed as the mean ± SD, and were analyzed by ANOVA. $^{\#}P < 0.05$ *versus* the control group; $^{*}P < 0.05$ *versus* the AIA-treated group; Dex, dexamethasone.

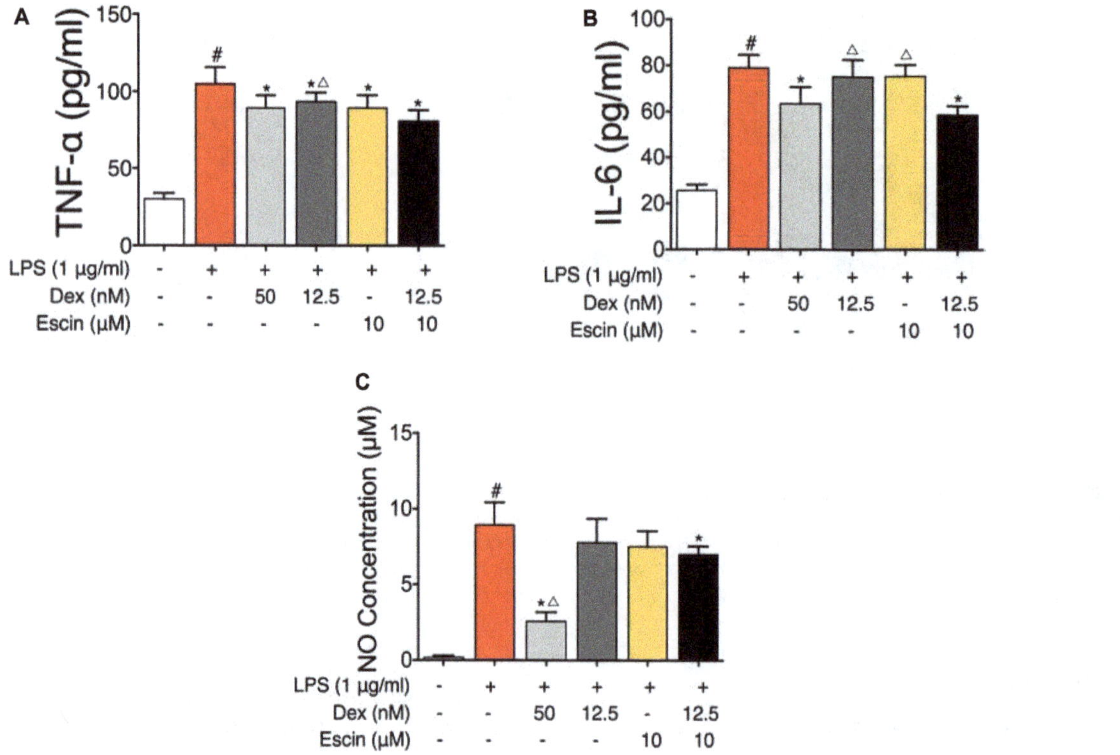

FIGURE 7 | Anti-inflammation effect of Escin combined with Dex in LPS-induced RAW 264.7 cells. **(A,B)** Cell supernatant IL-6 and TNF-α were determined with ELISA kits. **(C)** Cell supernatant NO concentration was determined with Griess reagent kit. Data were expressed as the mean ± SD, and were analyzed by ANOVA. $^{\#}P < 0.05$ *versus* the control group; $^{*}P < 0.05$ *versus* the AIA-treated group; $^{\Delta}P < 0.05$ *versus* the Escin (10 mg/kg) combined with Dex (0.05 mg/kg); Dex, dexamethasone.

Confirmation of the Gene Chip Results in LPS-Induced RAW 264.7 Cells

To further confirm the gene chip results, the LPS-induced RAW264.7 cell model was constructed. As displayed in **Figure 7**, the TNF-α, IL-6 and NO concentrations were significantly increased in the LPS group ($P < 0.05$). Dex (50 nM) and Escin (10 μM) combined with Dex (12.5 nM) significantly decreased the TNF-α, IL-6 and NO concentrations ($P < 0.05$). Moreover, the TNF-α concentration in Escin (10 μM) combined with Dex (12.5 nM) group was significantly lower than the Dex (12.5 nM) group ($P < 0.05$). The IL-6 concentration in the Escin (10 μM) combined with Dex (12.5 nM) group was significantly lower than that in the Dex (12.5 nM) and Escin (10 μM) ($P < 0.05$) group.

We then confirmed GR activation in this cell model *in vitro*. The LPS-treated group significantly decreased GR expression ($P < 0.05$). Escin (10 μM) combined with Dex (12.5 nM) significantly increased GR expression ($P < 0.05$). Moreover, the LPS-treated group significantly increased *p*-p65, *p*-IκBα expression and decreased IκBα expression ($P < 0.05$). Administrated with Escin (10 μM) combined with Dex (12.5 nM) significantly decreased *p*-p65 and *p*-IκBα expression and increased IκBα expression (**Figure 8**) ($P < 0.05$).

Escin Enhances the Effect of Low Dose Glucocorticoids Through GR Activation

GR mRNA expression was also detected. As shown in **Figure 9**, LPS decreased GR mRNA expression significantly. Escin (10 μM) combined with Dex (12.5 nM) significantly increased the GR mRNA. When compared with Dex (50 nM), Dex (12.5 nM) and Escin (10 μM) groups, the Escin (10 μM) combined with Dex (12.5 nM) group displayed a higher GR mRNA expression ($P < 0.05$). Cell supernatant IL-6 concentration in the LPS treated group significantly increased ($P < 0.05$), and the IL-6 concentration in the Dex (50 nM), Dex (12.5 nM), Escin (10 μM), Escin (10 μM) combined with Dex (12.5 nM) groups was significantly decreased compared with LPS ($P < 0.05$). After pre-treatment with the GR specific inhibitor, RU486, the cell supernatant IL-6 concentration was significantly increased in the group treated with Dex (50 nM) and Escin (10 μM) combined with Dex (12.5 nM) ($P < 0.05$). In the LPS-treated group, *p*-p65 expression was increased significantly ($P < 0.05$). Dex (50 nM), Dex (12.5 nM), Escin (10 μM), and Escin (10 μM) combined with Dex (12.5 nM) significantly decreased *p*-p65 expression ($P < 0.05$). After pre-treatment with RU486, *p*-p65expression in Dex (50 nM), Escin (10 μM) and Escin (10 μM) combined with Dex (12.5 nM) group were increased.

DISCUSSION

Rheumatoid arthritis is a chronic systemic disease with clinical manifestations of multi-joints damage, leading to chronic pain, joint deformity and functional disability. There are many types of medications for RA, such as non-steroidal anti-inflammatory drugs (NSAIDs), disease-modifying anti-rheumatic drugs (DMARDs), biological agents and GCs (Scott et al., 2010). GCs are 21-carbon steroid hormones. They are still used in the treatment of RA although a variety of adverse effects exist. Because GCs show strong anti-inflammatory effects and can reduce signs and symptoms of the disease, exert disease-modifying effects, especially in the active stage of RA (Strehl et al., 2017). Indeed the adverse effects of GCs such as infections, immunosuppression and osteoporosis limited their widely clinic use (Dubois-Camacho et al., 2017). So some new treatment strategies for RA with GCs are under development. For example, previous studies reported that transactivation is responsible for most of the adverse reactions of GCs while transrepression is considered to mediate their anti-inflammatory effects (Barnes, 2017). Novel drugs such as selective GR agonists, also called dissociated agonists, are under development (Sundahl et al., 2015). Escin is a natural mixture of triterpene saponins isolated from *Aesculus hippocastanum* L. Based on the network pharmacology, the TCM network related to Escin was constructed. MM symptom muscle weakness was related to RA, and the TCM symptom such as Tong, Teng Tong was also closely related to RA. This was consistent with our previous study. Our previous studies found that Escin exerts synergistic anti-inflammatory effects with GCs (Xin et al., 2011b), shows anti-arthritic effects combined with low dose of GCs with reduced adverse effects (Du et al., 2016). The present study elucidated the possible anti-arthritic mechanism of Escin, which may be another strategy to improve the efficacy and diminish any possible adverse effects of GCs.

The rat AIA model is an easy, reliable, and reproducible experimental model of polyarthritis with a short duration. It has been commonly used for preclinical evaluation of anti-arthritic drugs because of its similar pathology of human RA (Wang et al., 2016). In the present study, we demonstrated that low-dose Dex combined with Escin exerts an enhanced protective effect in a rat model of AIA. After injection of adjuvant, clinical evidence of arthritis occurred and was gradually exacerbated in immunized rats. Escin and Dex were given orally. Rat paw swelling and serum inflammatory factors served as indicators of systemic inflammation. Results revealed that Escin (10 mg/kg) combined with Dex (0.05 mg/kg) and Dex (0.2 mg/kg) significantly decreased the arthritic index, reduced the paw swelling, decreased serum IL-6 and TNF-α levels, and ameliorated the joint pathology. The values of the indexes showed similar trends. However, Escin combined with Dex, improved the effect of the low dose Dex.

It is known to all that high dose and long-term use of glucocorticoids can lead to pleiotropic side effects, including immunosuppression. In the present study, we investigated the effect of Escin combined with Dex on immune organ histopathological change and index in AIA rats. The results demonstrate that Escin combined with low dose of Dex shows good anti-arthritic effects but not induces apoptosis of immune cells or cause damage to immune organs compared to high dose of Dex.

To explore the underlying combination mechanism, a GC signaling RT2 Profiler OCR Array was used. The results revealed that *Nr3c1*, *Asph*, *Got1*, *Il-6*, *Tnf*, and *Sphk1* were altered significantly, especially *Nr3c1*, which showed high expression

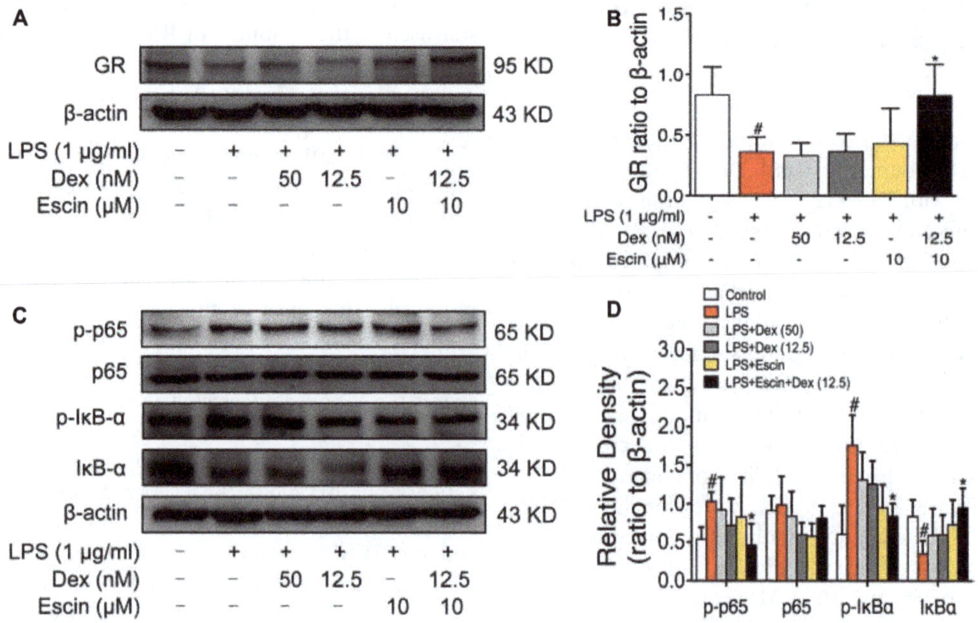

FIGURE 8 | Escin combined with Dex activated GR in LPS-induced RAW 264.7 cells. **(A,C)** Representative western blots of GR, *p*-p65, p65, *p*-IκBα, IκBα and β-actin. **(B,D)** The quantified densitometric analysis of GR, *p*-p65, p65, *p*-IκBα, IκBα. Data were expressed as the mean ± SD, and were analyzed by ANOVA. $^{\#}P < 0.05$ *versus* the control group; $^{*}P < 0.05$ *versus* the AIA-treated group; Dex, dexamethasone.

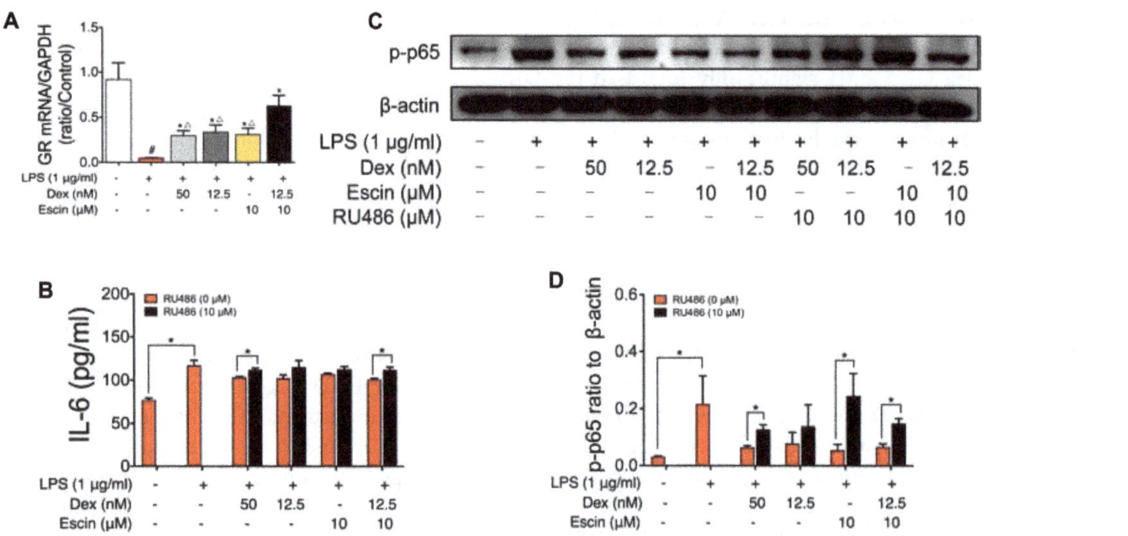

FIGURE 9 | Escin enhances the effect of low dose glucocorticoids through GR activation. **(A)** GR mRNA expression was determined by RT-PCR assay. Data were expressed as the mean ± SD, and were analyzed by ANOVA. $^{\#}P < 0.05$ *versus* the control group; $^{*}P < 0.05$ *versus* the AIA-treated group; $^{\Delta}P < 0.05$ *versus* the Escin (10 mg/kg) combined with Dex (0.05 mg/kg); Dex, dexamethasone. **(B)** Cell supernatant IL-6 was determined with ELISA kits. Data were expressed as the mean ± SD, and were analyzed by ANOVA. $^{*}P < 0.05$; Dex, dexamethasone. **(C,D)** Expression of *p*-p65 was determined by western blotting. Data were expressed as the mean ± SD, and were analyzed by ANOVA. $^{*}P < 0.05$; Dex, dexamethasone.

in both Dex and Escin combined with Dex groups. This result suggests that activation of GR is key events in the combination mechanism between Escin and low doses Dex.

We further confirmed the activation of GR *in vivo* and *in vitro*. Our results revealed that Dex (0.2 mg/kg) and Escin (10 mg/kg) combined with Dex (0.05 mg/kg) significantly up-regulated GR expression in AIA-induced RA rats *in vivo*. The value of GR expression in Escin (10 mg/kg) combined with Dex (0.05 mg/kg) was higher than that of the Dex (0.2 mg/kg) alone. This result was further confirmed in the LPS-induced RAW 264.7 cells *in vitro*. Escin (10 μM) combined with Dex (12.5 nM) significantly up-regulated GR expression *in vitro*.

Ample amounts of evidence support the idea that GCs exert their beneficial effects, at least in part, via interference with the NF-κB signaling pathway (De Bosscher et al., 2006; Gossye et al., 2008). NF-κB signaling pathway activation was also confirmed in the present study. Dex (0.2 mg/kg) and Escin (10 mg/kg) combined with Dex (0.05 mg/kg) activated *p*-p65, p65 and *p*-IκBα expression in AIA rats *in vivo*, and they activated *p*-p65, *p*-IκBα and IκBα in LPS-induced RAW 264.7 cells *in vitro*. This suggests that GR activation plays an important role in the effects of the combination of Escin and Dex.

Additionally, we evaluated the GR mRNA expression. The results revealed that Escin (10 μM) combined with Dex (12.5 nM) showed a significant high GR mRNA expression, and the levels observed in the combination treatment group were higher than that any of drug used alone. These results suggested that activation of GR pathway might be the underlying anti-RA mechanism in the Escin (10 μM) combined with Dex (12.5 nM) group. Additionally, GR was suppressed by its specific inhibitor, RU486. After GR suppression, the cell supernatant IL-6 and the *p*-p65 expression levels were reversed, which further confirmed the important role of GR pathway underlying the effects in the Escin (10 μM) combined with Dex (12.5 nM) group.

CONCLUSION

This study provided comprehensive evidence supporting the anti-RA effects of Escin combined with Dex and the underlying mechanisms of this combined medication. Escin combined with Dex reduced the dose of Dex, and exerts a significant anti-RA effects, which may also reduce the adverse effects of Dex. This combination might be attributed to GR activation. This study might provide a new combination of drugs for the treatment of RA.

AUTHOR CONTRIBUTIONS

LZ, YHu, CW, YD, MW, XW, YW, YHa, and TW were involved in data acquisition. FF, ZG, and BF conceived and designed the study. LZ, YHu, and PL have made statistical analyses. CW and LZ wrote the manuscript. All authors contributed to analysis and interpretation of the data and approved the final manuscript.

FUNDING

This study was supported by the Taishan Scholar Project. This study was also supported by Natural Science Foundation of Shandong Province (Nos. ZR2017MH068, ZR2017LH043, and ZR2017PH073), the Graduate Science and Technology Innovation Fund Project of Yantai University (No. YDZD1811), and the National Natural Science Foundation of China (No. 81703945).

ACKNOWLEDGMENTS

We thank Jodi Smith, Ph.D., from Liwen Bianz Editing China (www.liwenbianji.cn/ac), for editing the English text of a draft of this manuscript.

REFERENCES

Barnes, P. J. (2017). Glucocorticosteroids. *Handb. Exp. Pharmacol.* 237, 93–115. doi: 10.1007/164_2016_62

Boezio, B., Audouze, K., Ducrot, P., and Taboureau, O. (2017). Network-based approaches in pharmacology. *Mol. Inform.* 36:1700048. doi: 10.1002/minf.201700048

Cheong, D. H. J., Arfuso, F., Sethi, G., Wang, L., Hui, K. M., Kumar, A. P., et al. (2018). Molecular targets and anti-cancer potential of escin. *Cancer Lett* 422, 1–8. doi: 10.1016/j.canlet.2018.02.027

Courbon, G., Lamarque, R., Gerbaix, M., Caire, R., Linossier, M. T., Laroche, N., et al. (2018). Early sclerostin expression explains bone formation inhibition before arthritis onset in the rat adjuvant-induced arthritis model. *Sci. Rep.* 8:3492. doi: 10.1038/s41598-018-21886-w

De Bosscher, K., Vanden Berghe, W., and Haegeman, G. (2006). Cross-talk between nuclear receptors and nuclear factor kappaB. *Oncogene* 25, 6868–6886. doi: 10.1038/sj.onc.1209935

Du, Y., Song, Y., Zhang, L., Zhang, M., and Fu, F. (2016). Combined treatment with low dose prednisone and escin improves the anti-arthritic effect in experimental arthritis. *Int. Immunopharmacol.* 31, 257–265. doi: 10.1016/j.intimp.2016.01.006

Dubois-Camacho, K., Ottum, P. A., Franco-Munoz, D., De la Fuente, M., Torres-Riquelme, A., Diaz-Jimenez, D., et al. (2017). Glucocorticosteroid therapy in inflammatory bowel diseases: from clinical practice to molecular biology. *World J. Gastroenterol.* 23, 6628–6638. doi: 10.3748/wjg.v23.i36.6628

Gossye, V., Elewaut, D., Bougarne, N., Bracke, D., Van Calenbergh, S., Haegeman, G., et al. (2009). Differential mechanism of NF-kappaB inhibition by two glucocorticoid receptor modulators in rheumatoid arthritis synovial fibroblasts. *Arthritis Rheum.* 60, 3241–3250. doi: 10.1002/art.24963

Gossye, V., Haegeman, G., and De Bosscher, K. (2008). Therapeutic implications of the nuclear factor-kappaB/nuclear receptor cross-talk. *Front. Biosci.* 13:4122–4143. doi: 10.2741/2997

Hopkins, A. L. (2008). Network pharmacology: the next paradigm in drug discovery. *Nat. Chem. Biol.* 4, 682–690. doi: 10.1038/nchembio.110

Lee, D. Y., Choo, B. K., Yoon, T., Cheon, M. S., Lee, H. W., Lee, A. Y., et al. (2009). Anti-inflammatory effects of *Asparagus cochinchinensis* extract in acute and chronic cutaneous inflammation. *J. Ethnopharmacol.* 121, 28–34. doi: 10.1016/j.jep.2008.07.006

McInnes, I. B., and Schett, G. (2017). Pathogenetic insights from the treatment of rheumatoid arthritis. *Lancet* 389, 2328–2337. doi: 10.1016/S0140-6736(17)31472-1

Pan, T., Cheng, T. F., Jia, Y. R., Li, P., and Li, F. (2017). Anti-rheumatoid arthritis effects of traditional chinese herb couple in adjuvant-induced arthritis in rats. *J. Ethnopharmacol.* 205, 1–7. doi: 10.1016/j.jep.2017.04.020

Paval, J., Kaitheri, S. K., Potu, B. K., Govindan, S., Kumar, R. S., Narayanan, S. N., et al. (2009). Anti-arthritic potential of the plant Justicia gendarussa Burm F. *Clinics* 64, 357–362. doi: 10.1590/S1807-59322009000400015

Pearson, C. M. (1963). Experimental joint disease observations on adjuvant-induced arthritis. *J. Chronic Dis.* 16, 863–874. doi: 10.1016/0021-9681(63)90136-X

Scott, D. L., Wolfe, F., and Huizinga, T. W. (2010). Rheumatoid arthritis. *Lancet* 376, 1094–1108. doi: 10.1016/S0140-6736(10)60826-4

Strehl, C., van der Goes, M. C., Bijlsma, J. W., Jacobs, J. W., and Buttgereit, F. (2017). Glucocorticoid-targeted therapies for the treatment of rheumatoid arthritis. *Expert Opin. Investig. Drugs* 26, 187–195. doi: 10.1080/13543784.2017.1276562

Sundahl, N., Bridelance, J., Libert, C., De Bosscher, K., and Beck, I. M. (2015). Selective glucocorticoid receptor modulation: new directions with non-steroidal scaffolds. *Pharmacol. Ther.* 152, 28–41. doi: 10.1016/j.pharmthera.2015.05.001

Wang, H., Zhang, L., Jiang, N., Wang, Z., Chong, Y., and Fu, F. (2013). Anti-inflammatory effects of escin are correlated with the glucocorticoid receptor/NF-kappaB signaling pathway, but not the COX/PGF2alpha signaling pathway. *Exp. Ther. Med.* 6, 419–422. doi: 10.3892/etm.2013.1128

Wang, S., Wang, Y., Liu, X., Guan, L., Yu, L., and Zhang, X. (2016). Anti-inflammatory and anti-arthritic effects of taraxasterol on adjuvant-induced arthritis in rats. *J. Ethnopharmacol.* 187, 42–48. doi: 10.1016/j.jep.2016.04.031

Wang, T., Jiang, N., Han, B., Liu, W., Liu, T., Fu, F., et al. (2011). Escin attenuates cerebral edema induced by acute omethoate poisoning. *Toxicol. Mechan. Methods* 21, 400–405. doi: 10.3109/15376516.2010.550337

Wu, C., Chen, J., Chen, C., Wang, W., Wen, L., Gao, K., et al. (2015a). Wnt/beta-catenin coupled with HIF-1alpha/VEGF signaling pathways involved in galangin neurovascular unit protection from focal cerebral ischemia. *Sci. Rep.* 5:16151. doi: 10.1038/srep16151

Wu, C., Zhao, W., Zhang, X., and Chen, X. (2015b). Neocryptotanshinone inhibits lipopolysaccharide-induced inflammation in RAW264.7 macrophages by suppression of NF-kappaB and iNOS signaling pathways. *Acta Pharm. Sin. B* 5, 323–329. doi: 10.1016/j.apsb.2015.01.010

Wu, Y., Zhang, F., Yang, K., Fang, S., Bu, D., Li, H., et al. (2019). SymMap: an integrative database of traditional Chinese medicine enhanced by symptom mapping. *Nucleic Acids Res.* 47, D1110–D1117. doi: 10.1093/nar/gky1021

Xin, W., Zhang, L., Fan, H., Jiang, N., Wang, T., and Fu, F. (2011a). Escin attenuates acute lung injury induced by endotoxin in mice. *Eur. J. Pharm. Sci.* 42, 73–80. doi: 10.1016/j.ejps.2010.10.008

Xin, W., Zhang, L., Sun, F., Jiang, N., Fan, H., Wang, T., et al. (2011b). Escin exerts synergistic anti-inflammatory effects with low doses of glucocorticoids in vivo and in vitro. *Phytomedicine* 18, 272–277. doi: 10.1016/j.phymed.2010.08.013

Xiong, Y., Yang, Y., Xiong, W., Yao, Y., Wu, H., and Zhang, M. (2019). Network pharmacology-based research on the active component and mechanism of the antihepatoma effect of *Rubia cordifolia* L. *J. Cell. Biochem.* doi: 10.1002/jcb.28513 [Epub ahead of print].

Zhou, C., Li, G., Li, Y., Gong, L., Huang, Y., Shi, Z., et al. (2015). A high-throughput metabolomic approach to explore the regulatory effect of mangiferin on metabolic network disturbances of hyperlipidemia rats. *Mol. Biosyst.* 11, 418–433. doi: 10.1039/c4mb00421c

9

Network Pharmacological Analysis and Experimental Validation of the Mechanisms of Action of Si-Ni-San Against Liver Fibrosis

Siliang Wang[1†], Cheng Tang[2†], Heng Zhao[3†], Peiliang Shen[4], Chao Lin[5], Yun Zhu[1] and Dan Han[1*]*

[1]Department of Pharmacy, Nanjing Drum Tower Hospital, The Affiliated Hospital of Nanjing University Medical School, Nanjing, China, [2]Department of Respiratory Medicine, Affiliated Hospital of Integrated Traditional Chinese and Western Medicine, Nanjing University of Chinese Medicine, Nanjing, China, [3]Department of Endocrinology, Jinling Hospital, Medical School of Nanjing University, Nanjing, China, [4]School of Pharmacy, School of Medicine and Holistic Integrative Medicine, Nanjing University of Chinese Medicine, Nanjing, China, [5]School of Medicine and Holistic Integrative Medicine, Nanjing University of Chinese Medicine, Nanjing, China

***Correspondence:**
Siliang Wang
wsl_dth@126.com
Dan Han
handanjelly@126.com

†These authors have contributed equally to this work

Background: Si-Ni-San (SNS), a commonly used traditional Chinese medicine (TCM) formula, has potency against liver diseases, such as hepatitis and non-alcoholic fatty liver disease (NAFLD). However, the therapeutic efficacy and pharmacological mechanisms of action of SNS against liver fibrosis remain largely unclear.

Methods: A carbon tetrachloride (CCl_4)-induced liver fibrosis mouse model was adopted for the first time to investigate the beneficial effects of SNS on liver fibrosis. The potential mechanisms of action of SNS were explored using the network pharmacology-based strategy and validated with the aid of diverse assays.

Results: SNS treatment reduced collagen and ECM deposition, downregulated fibrosis-related factor (hyaluronic acid and laminin) contents in serum, maintained the morphological structure of liver tissue, and improved liver function in the liver fibrosis model. Based on network pharmacology results, apoptosis, inflammation and angiogenesis, together with the associated pathways (including VEGF, TNF, caspase, PPAR-γ and NF-κB), were identified as the mechanisms underlying the effects of SNS on liver fibrosis. Further *in vivo* experiments validated the significant mitigatory effects of SNS on inflammatory infiltration and pro-inflammatory cytokine contents (IFNγ, IL-1β and TGF-β1) in liver tissues of mice with liver fibrosis. SNS suppressed pathologic neovascularization as well as levels of VEGFR1, VEGF and VEGFR2 in liver tissues. SNS treatment additionally inhibited hepatic parenchyma cell apoptosis in liver tissues of mice with liver fibrosis and regulated apoptin expression while protecting L02 cells against apoptosis induced by TNF-α and Act D *in vitro*. Activation of hepatic stellate cells was suppressed and the balance between MMP13 and TIMP1 maintained *in vitro* by SNS. These activities may be associated with SNS-induced NF-κB suppression and PPAR-γ activation.

Conclusion: SNS effectively impedes liver fibrosis progression through alleviating inflammation, ECM accumulation, aberrant angiogenesis and apoptosis of hepatic parenchymal cells along with inhibiting activation of hepatic stellate cells through effects on multiple targets and may thus serve as a novel therapeutic regimen for this condition.

Keywords: network pharmacology, Si-Ni-San, liver fibrosis, inflammation, hepatic stellate cell, angiogenesis

INTRODUCTION

Liver fibrosis refers to histological changes induced by chronic inflammation resulting from multiple acute and chronic liver conditions, including infection with viral hepatitis B or C virus (HBV or HCV), alcoholic steatohepatitis, non-alcoholic steatohepatitis (NASH), non-alcoholic fatty liver disease (NAFLD), cholestatic liver disease and biliary disease (Koyama and Brenner, 2017; Mendez-Sanchez et al., 2020; Sterling et al., 2020). Liver injury can cause hepatic stellate cell (HSC) hyperactivity and promote extracellular matrix (ECM) accumulation (Cai et al., 2020). In this case, collagen fibers accumulate within the hepatocyte extracellular space, causing loss of blood supply to hepatocytes (Kisseleva and Brenner, 2020; Meurer et al., 2020). In the absence of appropriate treatment, liver fibrosis can progress to cirrhosis or even liver failure (He et al., 2015). Due to the reversibility of this condition, interventions can effectively improve clinical outcome, even at an advanced stage of liver fibrosis (Koyama et al., 2016). Recent treatments have mainly aimed to inactivate HSCs, protect against apoptosis of hepatic parenchymal cells (HPC), control inflammation and regulate metabolism of the extracellular matrix (ECM) (Hou et al., 2015; Zhou et al., 2019; Chan et al., 2020; Lambrecht et al., 2020).

Few potent antifibrotic drugs have been extensively validated clinically or applied as therapy to date. The existing antifibrotic drugs are limited in that insufficient quantities are absorbed *via* activated HSCs and significant side-effects are generated including hepatotoxicity or tumor occurrence (Fagone et al., 2015; Ma et al., 2017). Therefore, more research attention should be paid to natural herbs, such as traditional Chinese medicine (TCM) formulae, that may provide greater opportunities to prevent and treat chronic liver diseases without inducing side-effects (Song et al., 2019; Wang T. et al., 2020). TCM formulae generally incorporate complex combinations of natural herbs, animal products and minerals, consequently serving as multifunctional therapeutic agents that exert their effects in a holistic manner (Cheung et al., 2012; Gong, 2012; Liu, 2016). Numerous TCM-based formulae and herbal extracts, such as silymarin, emodin and curcumin, have been shown to protect against liver fibrosis through inhibiting inflammation, promoting ECM decomposition, and suppressing activation of HSCs (Zhao et al., 2017; Cao et al., 2018; Liu et al., 2018; Zhao et al., 2018; Jiang et al., 2020).

Si-Ni-San (SNS), a noted TCM formula used for thousands of years in China for coordinating liver and spleen functions, was initially documented by Zhong-Jing Zhang in the Eastern Han Dynasty (Jiang et al., 2003). SNS comprises four herbal medicines: Bupleuri Radix (*Bupleurum chinense* DC., *Bupleurum scorzonerifolium* Willd., Chaihu, CH), Paeoniae Radix Alba (*Paeonia lactiflora* Pall., Baishao, BS), Aurantii Fructus Immaturus (*Citrus* × *aurantium* L., Zhishi, ZS), and Glycyrrhizae Radix et Rhizoma (*Glycyrrhiza glabra* L., *Glycyrrhiza inflata* Batalin, *Glycyrrhiza uralensis* Fisch. ex DC., Gancao, GC) at a ratio of 1:1:1:1. SNS is reported to be efficient in improving "stagnation of Qi due to depression of the liver" in TCM theory and adopted clinically to alleviate several liver diseases, including NAFLD and hepatitis (Zhu et al., 2019). Accumulating studies suggest that the active herbal components of SNS, such as Paeoniflorin in BS, Saikosaponin A in CH, hesperidin in ZS and Liquiritigenin in GC, exert diverse pharmacological effects, such as anti-inflammation, anti-fibrosis, anti-HSC activation and liver protection activities (Zhao et al., 2014; El-Sisi et al., 2017; Geng et al., 2020; Shiu et al., 2020). However, the specific roles and protective mechanisms of action of SNS against liver fibrosis remain unclear.

The TCM formula is characterized by multiple components and targets. Traditional experimental approaches have been unsuccessful in characterizing the underlying complex pharmacological mechanisms. Moreover, due to the current lack of knowledge on specific activities and mechanisms, TCM is not commonly employed on a global scale (Guo et al., 2020). To ensure effective clinical application, the scientific foundation and mechanisms underlying the beneficial effects of TCM require elucidation. Owing to rapid developments in bioinformatics and systems biology approaches, network pharmacology-based analysis presents novel tools that could aid in clarifying the complex pathways of TCM, such as SymMap (Wu et al., 2019) and TCMSP (Zhang R. et al., 2019). Holism is a critical principle of TCM. Integration of network science with abundant TCM experience may therefore help to transform the research pattern from a single drug target to multi-component network targets, which should provide novel insights into the activities and associated mechanisms of the herbal components of TCM (Pun and Chor, 2020). In the present study, we examined the active components and mechanisms underlying the effects of SNS on liver fibrosis using network pharmacology analysis in combination with experimental validation, which were carried out in accordance with Network Pharmacology Evaluation Method Guidance-Draft (Li, 2021).

METHODS

Preparation of Si-Ni-San Experimental Agents

Crude TCM herbs (dried roots of *Bupleurum scorzonerifolium* Willd., dried roots of *Paeonia lactiflora* Pall., dried immature fruits of *Citrus* × *aurantium* L., dried roots and rhizomes of *Glycyrrhiza uralensis* Fisch. ex DC.) were provided by Beijing Tongrentang. In brief, CH, BS, ZS, and GC (25 g each) were extracted twice for 60 min each using boiling water (1:6 and 1:4,

TABLE 1 | The contents of four major ingredients in the freeze-dried powder.

Ingredients	Contents in mg/g
Glycyrrhizic acid	128.3 ± 0.04
Saikosaponin A	91.5 ± 0.02
Paeoniflorin	389.7 ± 0.03
Naringin	134.7 ± 0.05

w/v), followed by filtering and mixing. Afterward, we concentrated the filtrates by reducing pressure and then on an electric thermostatic water bath at 70°C to thick paste [0.8 kg (crude medicine)/L]. Further, the SNS experimental powders were producted through freeze-drying technology, and the process was shown below: refrigeration at −40°C, cryopreservation for 2 h at −20°C, cryopreservation for 16 h at −10°C, drying at 20°C for 5 h, and secondary drying at 35°C for 2 h. The contents of the four major components of the freeze-dried powder were quantified *via* HPLC (**Table 1** and the HPLC chromatograms were shown in **Supplementary Figure S1**).

Animals and Treatment

Male C57BL/6J mice (7 weeks old, 18–20 g) obtained from Beijing Vital River Laboratory Animal Technology Co. Ltd. (Beijing, China) were subjected to a temperature-, light-, and humidity-controlled environment. All animals had free access to food and water and were allowed to acclimatize to the conditions for one week prior to experiments. Experimental protocols were approved by the Animal Care and Use Committee of Nanjing University of Chinese Medicine (Nanjing, China) and conducted according to the Guidelines for the Care and Use of Laboratory Animals (ACU200905, 29th September 2020). Liver fibrosis was induced through intraperitoneal injection with 4% (v/v) carbon tetrachloride (CCl_4) in olive oil at a dose of 5 ml/kg body weight (BW) twice weekly for eight consecutive weeks (Cao et al., 2018). An appropriate amount of SNS freeze-dried powders was collected, prepared into the 500 g (powder)/L solution with distilled water, and used for intragastric administration of experimental animals. The 32 mice were classified into four groups for 8 weeks of treatments as follows: 1) Control group given gavage of distilled water, 2) Model group with liver fibrosis given gavage of distilled water, 3) SNS low-dose (SNS-L) group with liver fibrosis given gavage of SNS at 5 g (powder)/kg BW, and 4) SNS high-dose (SNS-H) group with liver fibrosis given gavage of SNS at 10 g (powder)/kg BW. The BW of individual mice from each group was recorded once weekly for eight consecutive weeks.

Histomorphology Assay

Liver tissues were processed with 10% formalin fixation followed by paraffin embedding, slicing into 5 μm sections, and hematoxylin-eosin (HE) staining for histopathological analysis or Masson trichrome dye and Sirius red staining to examine collagen formation. An upright microscope was utilized to observe histological sections and obtain photographic images. Subsequently, 10 fields of view (FOV) were selected from each sample from all treatment groups for observation. Areas with positive Sirius red or Masson staining were evaluated using Aperio ImageScope-Pathology Slide Viewing Software. Liver fibrosis was graded using a previously reported fibrosis staging system (Goodman, 2007) (**Supplementary Table S1**).

Network Pharmacology Analysis

Data preparation: Data on each herbal component of SNS were collected using the Traditional Chinese Medicine System Pharmacology Database (TCMSP, http://lsp.nwu.edu.cn/tcmsp) (Ru et al., 2014), Traditional Chinese Medicines Integrated Database (TCMID, http://www.megabionet.org/tcmid/) (Huang et al., 2018), and associated literature. The data acquired were uploaded to the ingredient database.

Oral bioavailability (OB) and drug-likeness screening: OB prescreening indicates the distribution level of an oral drug dose in bloodstream, which is a critical prerequisite for identification and application of oral drugs in the clinic. Drug-likeness is a qualitative concept used for evaluating the structural similarities of compounds with therapeutic efficacy in the Drugbank database, which can be determined immediately following drug discovery. Wang and colleagues reported the calculations for the two above parameters in detail (Xu et al., 2012; Tao et al., 2013). At last, in line with the TCMSP database recommendations, an OB of 30%, together with a drug-likeness index of 0.18, (mean value for all molecules within the DrugBank database) (Wang X. et al., 2012), was adopted as the cut-off value for selecting the potential pharmacodynamic components.

Prediction of putative drug targets for SNS: Identification of targets is suggested to be the critical link during drug discovery. In our study, the systemic drug targeting method of Wang and co-workers was adopted for precise determination of potential targets for the therapeutic components of SNS (Li et al., 2014). As for the present systemic drug targeting method, it is conducted from two levels, and it represents a systemic target predicting approach to integrate several algorithms. 1) The HIT database was applied in collection and retrieval of the drug-target interactions verified in experiments. 2) The SysDT model was used to predict the putative compound targets that have not been validated in experiments, and high sensitivity, specificity, and consistency were attained in the prediction of drug-target interactions.

Collection of known liver fibrosis-related targets: Targets known to be related to liver fibrosis were mainly collected based on five resources: 1) MalaCards human disease database (https://www.malacards.org) (Rappaport et al., 2017), 2) OMIM database (http://www.omim.org) (Amberger et al., 2019), 3) Therapeutic Target Database (TTD, http://bidd.nus.edu.sg/group/cjttd/) (Zhu et al., 2010), 4) DrugBank database (https://www.drugbank.ca) (Wishart et al., 2008), and 5) the Genetic Association Database (GAD, https://geneticassociationdb.nih.gov) (Becker et al., 2004). After the redundant targets were deleted, known targets related to liver fibrosis were screened.

GO-BP and KEGG enrichment analyses: Targets were annotated based on the Omicshare (http://www.omicshare.com/tools) database for further clarification of the corresponding functions. Differences of ≤0.05 indicated statistical significance and the enriched terms of GO and KEGG analyses were subsequently determined *via* hypergeometric examination.

Serum Biochemical and Cytokine Analysis

At 24 h following the final injection, 0.8 ml peripheral blood was obtained from every mouse through eyeball enucleation. After 60 min of incubation at ambient temperature, blood samples were centrifuged for 10 min at 3,000 rpm and 4°C to separate serum. After the addition of protein extraction solution, samples were incubated for 30 min on ice and centrifuged at 15,000 rpm to collect supernatant fractions that were stored at −20°C for quantification of protein contents. ELISA kits were utilized to determine the serum levels of laminin (LN; GeneTex, cat no. GTX37121), hyaluronic acid (HA; Abbexa, cat no. abx156663), albumin (Abcam, cat no. ab179887), AST (Nanjing Jiancheng Bio, cat no. C010-2-1), ALT (Nanjing Jiancheng Bio, cat no. C009-2-1), tumor necrosis factor (TNF)-α (R&D systems, cat no. MTA00B), TGF-β1 (R&D systems, cat no. MB100B), interleukin (IL)-1β (R&D systems, cat no. MLB00C) and interferon (IFN)-γ (R&D systems, cat no. MIF00) according to the manufacturers' protocols. The BioTek Synergy instrument was applied for reading optical density (OD) at specific wavelengths.

Examination of Alanine Aminotransferase, Aspartate Aminotransferase, Tumor Necrosis Factor-Alpha, Hydroxyproline and Vascular Endothelial Growth Factor in Liver

Briefly, 150 μL ice-cold lysis buffer was added to homogenize 15 mg liver tissue. The mixture was centrifuged for 15 min at 10,000 rpm and 4°C to collect the supernatant fractions, which were stored at −20°C for quantification of protein levels. ELISA kits were utilized to determine the tissue contents of ALT, AST, TNF-α, hydroxyproline (Hyp, Nanjing Jiancheng Bio, cat no. A030-2-1) and VEGF-A (Invitrogen, cat no. BMS619-2) according to the manufacturers' protocols.

Immunofluorescence Analysis

Immunofluorescence double staining was performed for determination of CD34 expression. Tissue sections were stained with primary anti-CD34 antibody (Abcam, cat no. ab81289), followed by the appropriate secondary goat anti-rabbit IgG (H + L)-FITC antibody (1:200; Bioworld, cat no. BS10950). Finally, sections were mounted with mounting medium for fluorescence with 4′, 6′-diamidino-2-phenylindole (DAPI; Beyotime, cat no. C1002). Fluorescence images were analyzed using ZEN pro 2012 imaging software on a Zeiss inverted microscope.

Terminal Deoxynucleotidyl Transferase-Mediated dUPT Nick-End Labeling Assay

After deparaffinization and rehydration, sections were subjected to the TUNEL assay to detect apoptotic hepatocytes using an Apoptosis Detection Kit (Beyotime, cat no. C1098). Each section was incubated for 15 min with proteinase K at 37°C and 3% hydrogen peroxide added to block endogenous peroxidase activity. After reaction with deoxynucleotidyl transferase, sections were incubated with the anti-digoxigenin conjugate prior to DAB color development. Next, each section was subjected to 0.5% Methyl Green counterstaining and mounting. Five high-power fields of view (FOV) were selected for each section and examined using Image Pro Plus software (Media Cybernetics, Inc., Rockville, MD, United States). The percentage of positively stained cells (apoptotic index) was determined according to the formula: apoptotic index = positive cell number/total cell number × 100%.

Cell Culture

LX2 and L02 cells purchased from the Type Culture Collection of the Chinese Academy of Sciences (Shanghai, China) were used for experimental validation *in vitro*. The human HSC cell line, LX2, was cultivated in RPMI 1640 (Gibco) containing 10% fetal bovine serum (FBS, Gibco). Normal human hepatic L02 cells were cultivated in DMEM (Gibco) containing 10% FBS. The cell culture media contained 100 mg/L streptomycin and 100,000 U/L penicillin. Both cell lines were cultivated under 37°C and 95% O_2/5% CO_2.

For examination of the roles and mechanisms of action of SNS in activated LX2 cells, 5 ng/ml TGF-β1 was used to stimulate quiescent LX2 cells for 24 h in the presence or absence of SNS (50 mg/L). Cells were subsequently harvested to detect related items.

Cell Viability Assay

After digestion, counting and seeding of L02 cells into 96-well plates at a density of 3×10^3 cells/plate for 12 h, fresh medium containing various concentrations of SNS or distilled water was used to replace the original medium for 18 h, followed by incubation of cells with 200 ng/ml Act D and 20 ng/ml TNF-α for 6 h. The MTT assay was conducted at a wavelength of 490 nm to evaluate cell proliferation.

Cell Apoptosis Assay

In the apoptosis assay, cells (3.0×10^5 cells/well) were inoculated in 6-well plates. After treatment with 50 mg/L and 100 mg/L SNS for 42 h, L02 cells were incubated for 6 h with 20 ng/ml TNF-α (Peprotech, cat no. 300-01A) and 200 ng/ml Act D (Merck, cat no. 50-76-0). The cell apoptosis rate was analyzed with the Muse Annexin V and Dead Cell Assay (Millipore, cat no. MCH100105) in keeping with the manufacturer's instructions. All assays were conducted in triplicate.

RNA Isolation and qRT-PCR Analysis

RT-PCR analysis was performed to determine collagen I, α-SMA, fibronectin, VEGFR1, VEGFR2, VEGF, TNF-α, TGF-β1, IL-1β, IFN-γ, TIMP and MMP13 mRNA levels in liver tissue or LX2 cells. Specifically, TRIzol reagent (Invitrogen, cat no. 15596018) was utilized to isolate total RNA from LX2 cells or liver tissues under RNase-free conditions. The resultant total RNA (1 mg) was used to prepare cDNA *via* reverse transcription using Hiscript® II QRTSuperMix (Vazyme, cat no. R223-01) and gDNA Eraser, as recommended by the manufacturer. Quantitative RT-PCR with the SYBR Green Master kit (Bio-Rad) was utilized to quantify specific transcripts and the ABI 7500 RT-PCR system (Applied Biosystems) employed for detection and analysis. All gene-specific primers were prepared by Sangon Biotech. The primer sequences used are presented in **Supplementary Table S2**.

The mRNA expression levels were normalized to β-actin control. The PCR conditions were as follows: 30 s under 95°C, 40 cycles of 5 s under 95°C, and 30 s under 60°C. The comparative CT approach was used to calculate relative levels of mRNA.

Western Blot

Western blot analysis was performed to determine protein expression of collagen I, α-SMA,VEGF, fibrolectin, KDR, TNF-α, TGF-β1, IFN-γ, IL-1β, TIMP, MMP13, cleaved caspase 3, Bax, Bcl2, and GAPDH in LX2 or L02 cells or liver tissue. Specifically, lysis buffer (Beyotime, cat no. P0013C) containing 1 nM phenylmethanesulfonyl fluoride (PMSF) (Beyotime, cat no. ST505) was used to prepare tissue homogenates. After denaturation, proteins were subjected to 8–12% bis-Tris/polyacrylamide gel electrophoresis (Beyotime, cat no. P0690) and subsequently transferred to polyvinylidene fluoride (PVDF) membranes (Amresco). Membranes were coated with Millipore filter (pore size 0.45 mm) and blocked for 2 h using TBST blocking solution containing 0.1% Tween-20 and 5% skimmed milk powder. Next, membranes was subjected to overnight incubation with the appropriate antibodies (Abcam; anti-collagen I, cat no. ab260043; anti-alpha-SMA, cat no. ab124964; anti-fibronectin, cat no. ab268020; anti-VEGFR2, cat no. ab115805; anti-VEGFR1, cat no. ab32152; anti-TIMP1, cat no. ab211926; anti-MMP13, cat no. ab219620; anti-cleaved caspase 3, cat no. ab32042; anti-Bax, cat no. ab32503; anti-Bcl-2, cat no. ab182858; anti-caspase 8, cat no. ab3239; anti-PPARγ, cat no. ab178866; anti-p65, cat no. ab32536 and anti-GAPDH, cat no. ab181602) diluted in TBST (1:1,000) containing 5% bovine serum albumin (BSA) at 4°C. Each membrane was further incubated for 2 h with horseradish peroxidase (HRP)-conjugated secondary antibody (Abcam, cat no. ab6721) diluted in TBST (1:10,000) containing 5% skimmed milk powder at ambient temperature. An enhanced chemiluminescence kit (Applygen Technologies) was employed to detect immunoreactivity. Image-Pro Plus software (version 6.0) was adopted for blot scanning and analysis of band intensity. Band intensity was determined according to the formula: band intensity = sum of all pixel values in a selected segment—background pixel value in the segment.

Statistical Analysis

Data are presented as means ± SD. Student's test was utilized to assess the differences in related parameters between experimental and control groups. One-way ANOVA was adopted to assess differences among several groups and Tukey's test used to determine significance. *p* values <0.05 indicated significant differences. GraphPad Prism software (version 6.0) was employed for statistical analysis.

RESULTS

Si-Ni-San Attenuates CCl_4-Induced Hepatic Pathological Changes and Dysfunction

The CCl_4-induced liver fibrosis mouse model was used due to its convenient time frame (**Figure 1A**). H&E-stained liver tissue sections were subjected to microscopy analysis. As shown in **Figure 1B**, intact hepatic lobules were evident in liver tissues of the blank group along with normal hepatic sinusoids and orderly arranged hepatic cell cords and no hyperplasia of collagen fibers or infiltration of inflammatory cells. In the model group, liver tissues displayed obscure hepatic lobule structure along with destroyed hepatic cell cords, slight cell swelling, necrosis and fatty degeneration, infiltration of inflammatory cells and fibrocytes, which were partially mitigated after SNS treatment. The regulatory effects of SNS on alanine aminotransferase (ALT) and aspartate aminotransferase (AST) in liver tissues and sera of mice with liver fibrosis were further examined. SNS treatment induced a remarkable decrease in the ALT and AST contents relative to the model group ($p < 0.01$) but had no obvious influence on the ratio of liver weight to body weight (**Figures 1C–E**).

Si-Ni-San Alleviates Liver Fibrosis Induced by CCl_4

We initially examined the serum levels of factors related to liver fibrosis, such as hyaluronic acid (HA) and laminin (LN). As illustrated in **Figure 1F,G**, HA and LN levels were slightly increased in the model group compared to the control group, but markedly declined in the SNS group relative to the model group ($p < 0.01$).

The regulatory effects of SNS on collagen and ECM deposition in the liver were examined by visualization through Sirius red and Masson staining and measured based on Hyp and Col-I levels in liver and fibrosis grading scores. Under conditions of CCl_4 induction, collagen was deposited in Sirius red and Masson-stained sections, particularly the perisinusoidal areas and diverse pseudo lobules. In the presence of SNS, the number of pseudo lobules and collagen deposition was decreased (**Figure 1B**). The Hyp levels in liver tissue and fibrosis grading scores were markedly elevated in CCl_4-stimulated mice relative to the control group and conversely reduced in the SNS-treated group (**Figures 1H,I**). CCl_4 treatment triggered an increase in Col-I mRNA and protein expression while SNS exposure had the opposite effect (**Figures 1J,K**).

We further explored the potential role of SNS in HSC activation. Liver tissues stimulated with CCl_4 showed significantly increased mRNA and protein expression of α-SMA and fibronectin, indicative of activated HSCs. SNS exposure led to significant attenuation of α-SMA and fibronectin expression induced by CCl_4, clearly signifying suppression of HSC activation in fibrotic liver (**Figures 1J,K**).

Network Pharmacological Analysis of Si-Ni-San for Liver Fibrosis

Screening of Potential Pharmacodynamic Components and Targets of Si-Ni-San

Despite several studies on the therapeutic mechanisms of action of TCM, limited progress has been reported to date. Currently, no specific and efficient techniques for identification of the active components of herbal medicines are available. One promising

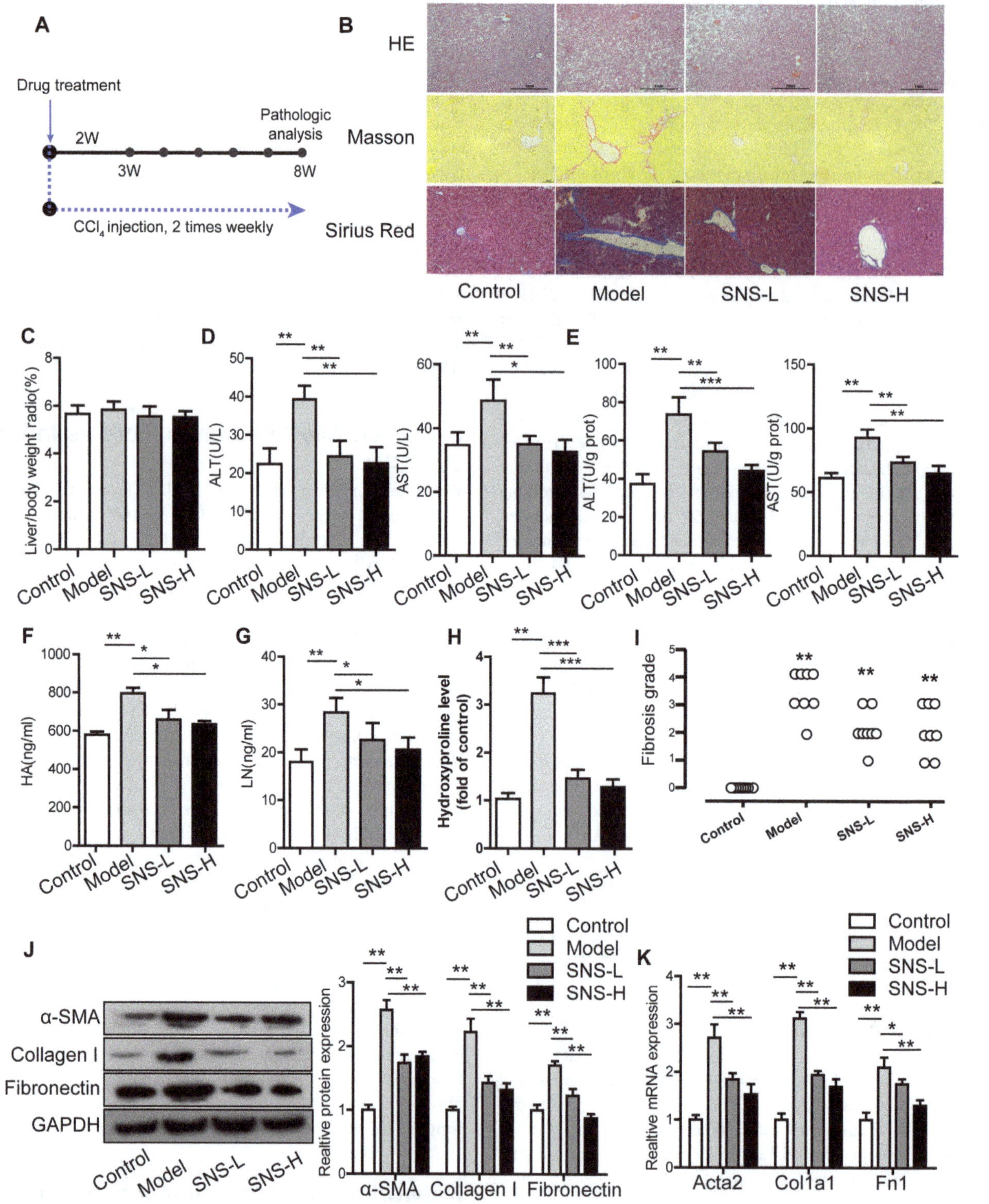

FIGURE 1 | SNS ameliorates hepatic fibrosis in CCl_4-treated mice. **(A)** Flowchart of animal experiments. **(B)** Representative images of liver sections stained with H&E or Masson or Sirius red (magnification, 100×). **(C)** Ratio of liver weight to body weight. **(D)** Concentrations of ALT and AST in serum. **(E)** Concentrations of ALT and AST in liver homogenates. **(F)** Concentrations of HA in serum. **(G)** Concentrations of LN in serum. **(H)** Effect of SNS on liver hydroxyproline. **(I)** Effect of SNS on fibrosis grading score. **(J)** Effects of SNS on protein levels of α-SMA, collagen I and fibronectin in liver tissue. **(K)** Effects of SNS on mRNA levels of Acta2, Col1a1, and Fn1 in liver tissue. Data are presented as mean ± SD (n = 6). $^{*}p < 0.05$, $^{**}p < 0.01$, $^{***}p < 0.001$ compared to control or model group.

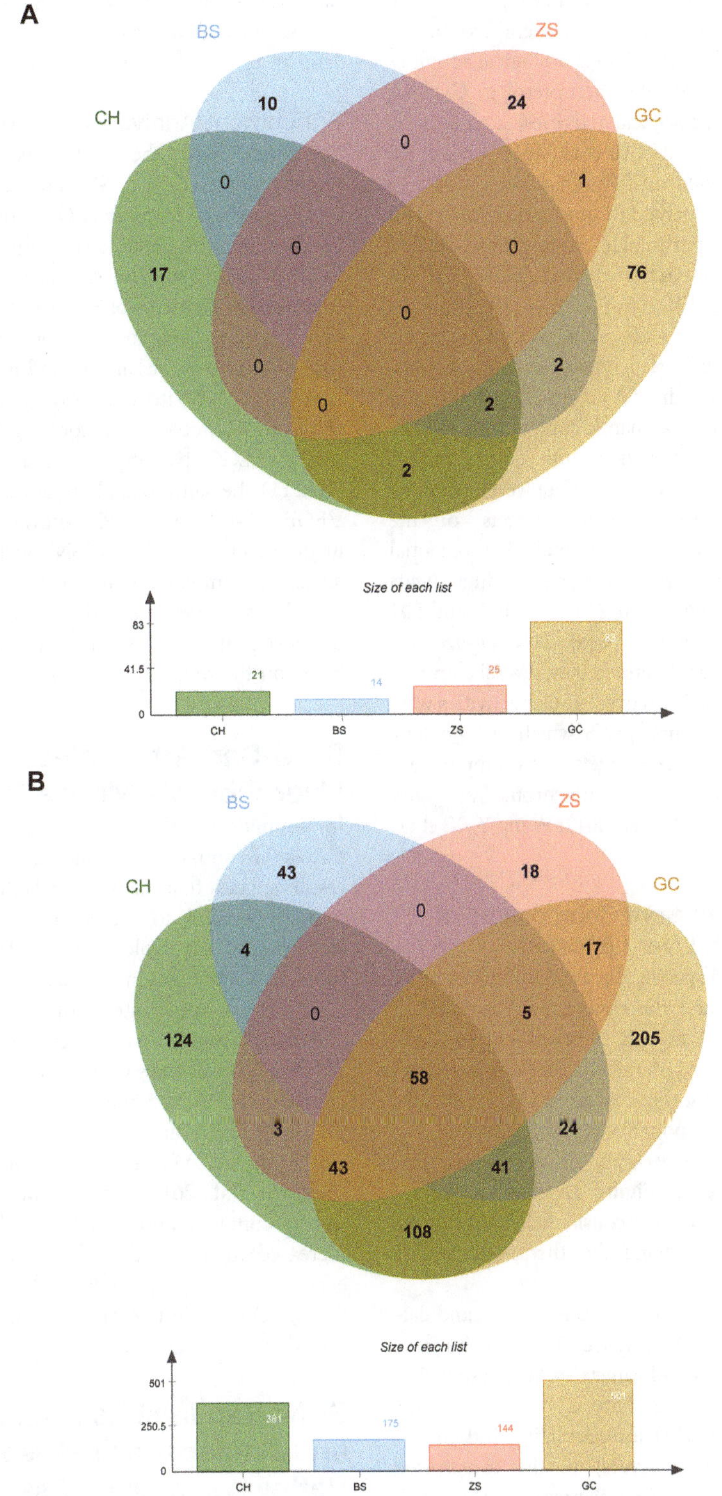

FIGURE 2 | Screening of potential pharmacodynamic components and targets of SNS. **(A)** Venn diagram of potential pharmacodynamic components in each herb of SNS. **(B)** Venn diagram of potential pharmacodynamic targets of each herb of SNS.

approach involves integration of OB screening with drug-likeness evaluation. In the present study, 134 compounds with suitable OB and drug-likeness values were identified as potential pharmacodynamic ingredients of SNS (**Supplementary Table S3**). Specifically, 21, 14, 25, and 83 candidate compounds were detected in CH, BS, ZS, and GC, respectively (**Figure 2A**). Among these, kaempferol, oleanolic acid, isorhamnetin, quercetin, mairin, sitosterol and naringenin have been identified in the different herbal components of SNS and their biological activities extensively characterized. For example, kaempferol in CH, BS, and GC has widespread pharmacological activities, such as anti-fibrosis and anti-inflammation effects (Xu et al., 2019; Bian et al., 2020). Naringenin, widely detected in ZS and GC, exerts diverse pharmacological effects and is involved in modulation of several signaling pathways, such as pathologic angiogenesis-related VEGF/KDR and inflammatory reaction-related NLRP3/NF-κB (Li Q. et al., 2016; Fan et al., 2017).

Overall, TCM prescriptions exert widespread therapeutic effects on complex diseases that are totally dependent on the synergistic actions of multiple compounds on diverse targets. Accordingly, in addition to uncovering the pharmacodynamic components of SNS, it is necessary to explore the potential therapeutic targets. In this study, genomic, chemical and pharmacological data were integrated with a view to predicting the potential targets of the pharmacodynamic components of SNS. In total, 693 potential targets were screened for 134 pharmacodynamic ingredients (**Supplementary Table S4**), among which, 381, 175, 144, and 501 were associated with CH, BS, ZS and GC, respectively (**Figure 2B**). While all four herb components had diverse targets, several common targets were additionally identified. Moreover, similar activities were observed for different herb components of SNS, which were possibly attributable to their regulation of shared targets. For example, both CH and BS have been shown to reverse acute and chronic liver injury induced by various irritants (Wang R. et al., 2012; Wang Y.-X. et al., 2019).

Mining of Core Targets and Core Components of Si-Ni-San Associated With Liver Fibrosis

Liver fibrosis is a polygenic predisposing disease. Determination of the interactions between genes and the environment may aid in illustrating the pathogenesis of liver fibrosis. In our experiments, 834 targets related to liver fibrosis were identified from five resources (**Supplementary Table S5**). Among these, some were also potential targets of pharmacodynamic components of SNS. Overall, 173 candidate targets of SNS for activity against liver fibrosis were predicted (**Supplementary Table S6, Figure 3A**) and the related pharmacodynamic ingredients (n = 119) considered the candidate pharmacological components underlying the therapeutic effects of SNS.

Cytoscape was adopted for constructing the candidate component-target network of SNS (**Figure 3B**). To improve screening of the core components and targets of SNS responsible for therapeutic activity against liver fibrosis, we utilized the Cytohubba plug-in (Chin et al., 2014) for calculating and sorting the node topological parameters (degrees) in the constructed candidate component-target network (**Supplementary Table S7**). Nodes with a degree greater than or equal to two-fold median degree values (=6) for all nodes in the network were selected as the core active ingredients (n = 21, **Supplementary Table S8**) and core targets (n = 19, **Supplementary Table S9**) of SNS and used to establish the core component-target network (**Figure 3C**). Interestingly, all the core active ingredients with the top 5 degree values (quercetin, liquiritigenin, luteolin, puerarin, saikosaponin A) have been shown to reverse the occurrence and development of liver fibrosis through diverse pathways (Li et al., 2015; Chen et al., 2017; Hou et al., 2018; Lee et al., 2019; Zhang Q. et al., 2019).

Enrichment Analysis of Core Targets of Si-Ni-San

For clarification of the multi-target and multi-pathway mechanisms underlying the effects of SNS on liver fibrosis, the Omicshare online tool was utilized to conduct GO biological process (BP) and KEGG pathway analyses for the 19 core targets screened based on their degree values, with the aim of identifying biological processes (BPs) and signal transduction pathways of SNS associated with liver fibrosis ($p < 0.05$, FDR <0.05). Apoptosis, angiogenesis-related proliferation and migration of endothelial cells and immuno-inflammatory responses were the GO-BP items displaying the most significant enrichment (**Figure 4A**). Moreover, the core targets were predominantly related to several KEGG pathways, such as apoptosis-related, liver disease (NAFLD, hepatitis B and hepatocellular carcinoma)-related, TNF, VEGF, NF-κB, and MAPK pathways (**Figure 4B**), implicating their involvement in the effects of SNS on liver fibrosis. Subsequently, tissue and serum samples from the *in vivo* CCl_4-induced liver fibrosis mouse model and a series of experiments *in vitro* were employed to validate the biological processes and signal transduction pathways identified based on the results of network pharmacological analysis.

Si-Ni-San Attenuates Inflammation in the Liver Fibrosis Mouse Model

Inflammation is closely associated with the development of liver fibrosis (Koyama and Brenner, 2017). Our network pharmacology results suggest that the beneficial effects of SNS on liver fibrosis are partially related to regulation of the inflammatory response. Accordingly, we explored the potential involvement of SNS in local and systemic inflammation. Compared with the control group, the serum contents of cytokines (such as TNF-α, IFN-γ, and IL-1β) together with their gene expression patterns in liver tissues of fibrotic mice were remarkably elevated. Interestingly, SNS application reversed the upregulation of these factors (**Figures 5A,B**). TGF-β1 can be excessively produced by various cell types and suggested to serve as the pro-fibrogenic factor in liver fibrosis (Beljaars et al., 2017). Consistently, our findings showed that the serum contents and mRNA levels of TGF-β1 in liver were increased in the model relative to the control group and SNS exposure led to suppression of TGF-β1 upregulation (**Figures 5A,B**). Our collective results suggest that SNS mitigates liver fibrosis through alleviating the proinflammatory milieu.

Si-Ni-San Inhibits Pathological Microvessel and Angiogenesis-Associated Signaling Pathways in Liver Tissue of the Mouse Model

To establish whether SNS affects pathological angiogenesis in liver tissues of the CCl_4-induced liver fibrosis mouse model, CD34 levels were detected using the immunofluorescence assay. The number of fluorescence-stained cells and fluorescence intensity were remarkably increased after CCl_4 stimulation and evidently reduced in the presence of SNS compared with the model

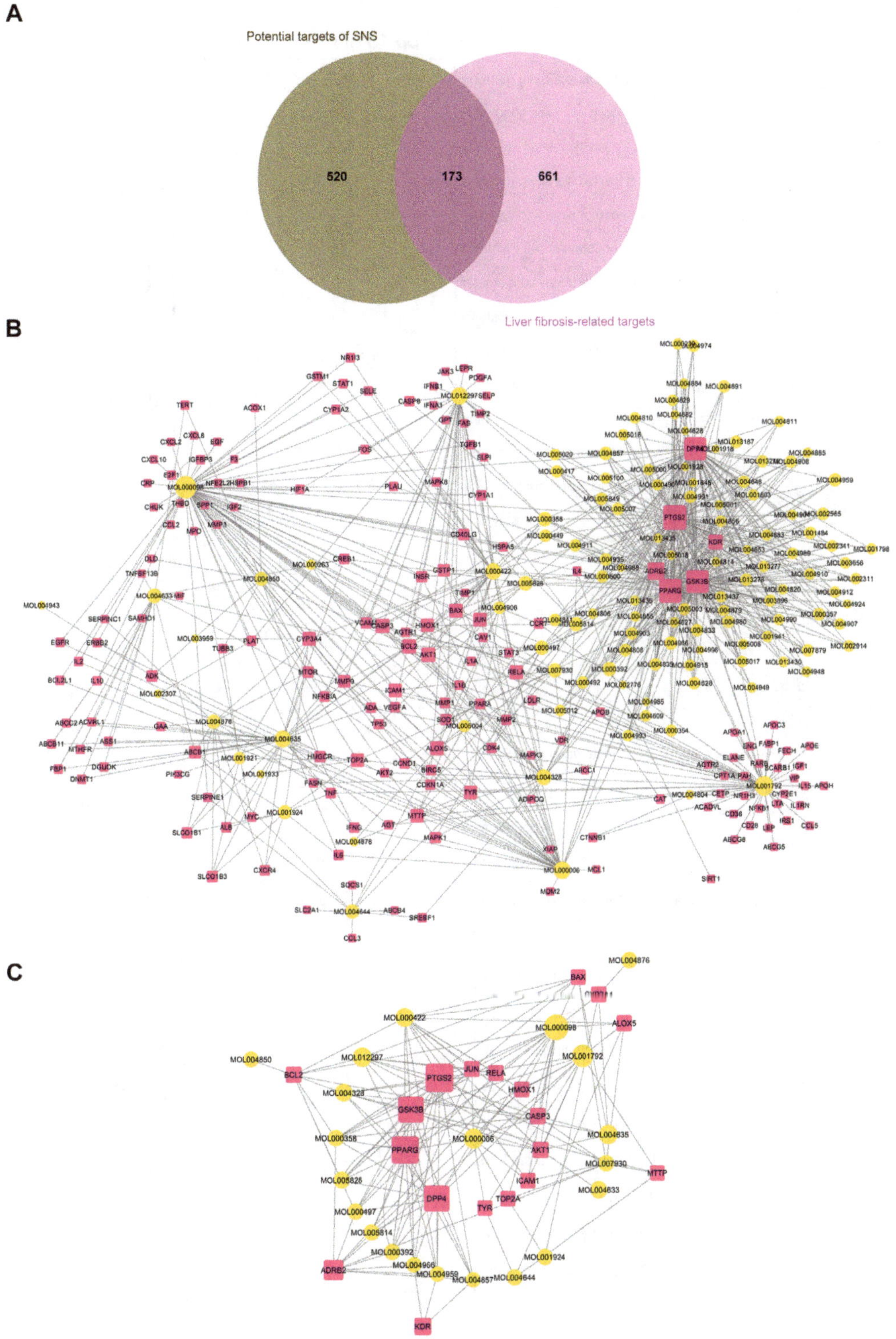

FIGURE 3 | Excavation of the core pharmacodynamic components and targets of SNS with activity against liver fibrosis. **(A)** Venn diagram showing that SNS shares 173 potential targets with known pathological targets of liver fibrosis. **(B)** Candidate active ingredient-target network of SNS. **(C)** Core active ingredient-target network of SNS.

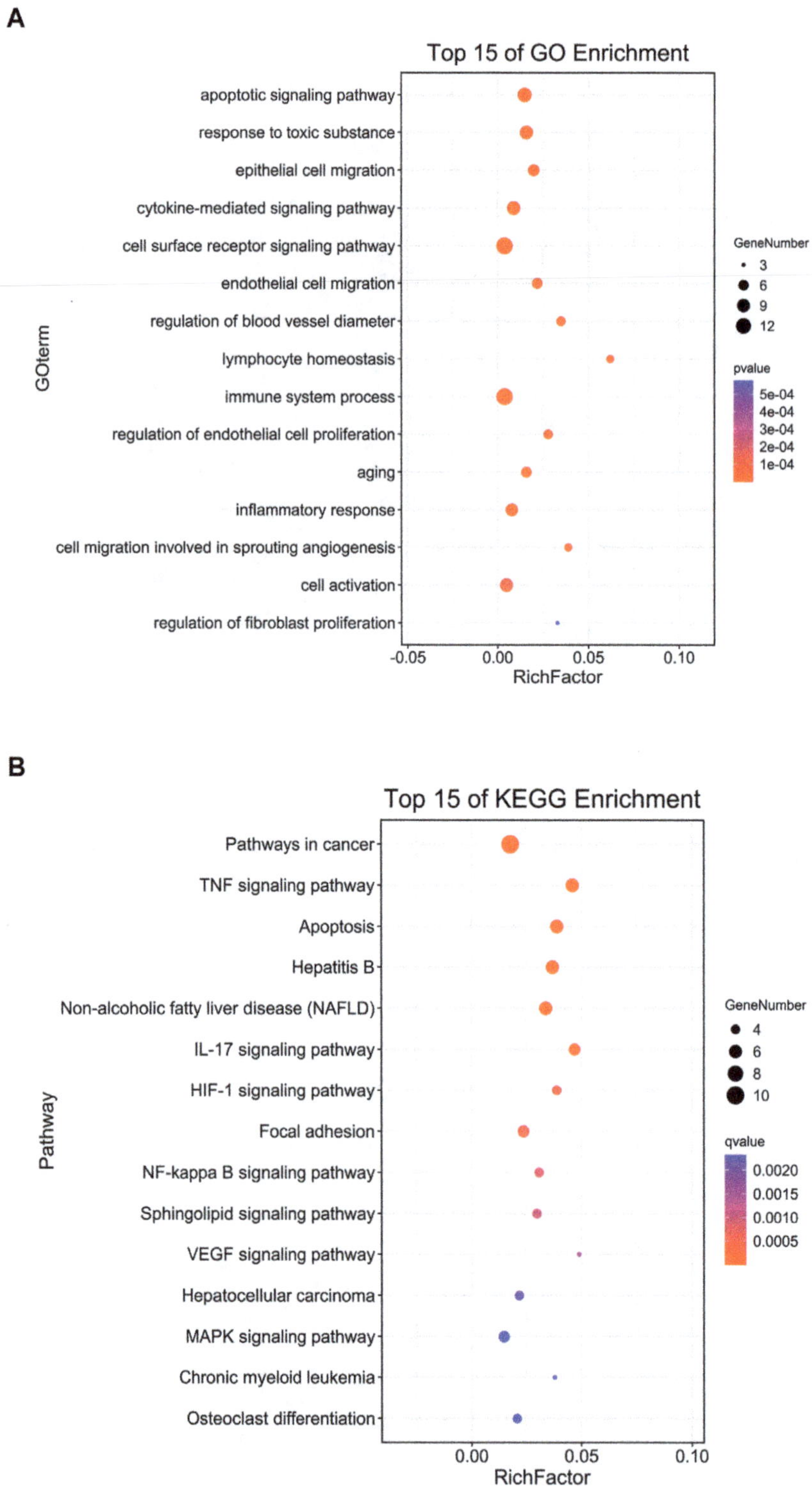

FIGURE 4 | Enrichment analysis of core targets of SNS in treating liver fibrosis based on Omicshare. A *p*-value cut-off of ≤0.05 was considered significant and the hyper-geometric test applied to identify enriched GO-BP terms **(A)** and KEGG pathways **(B)**.

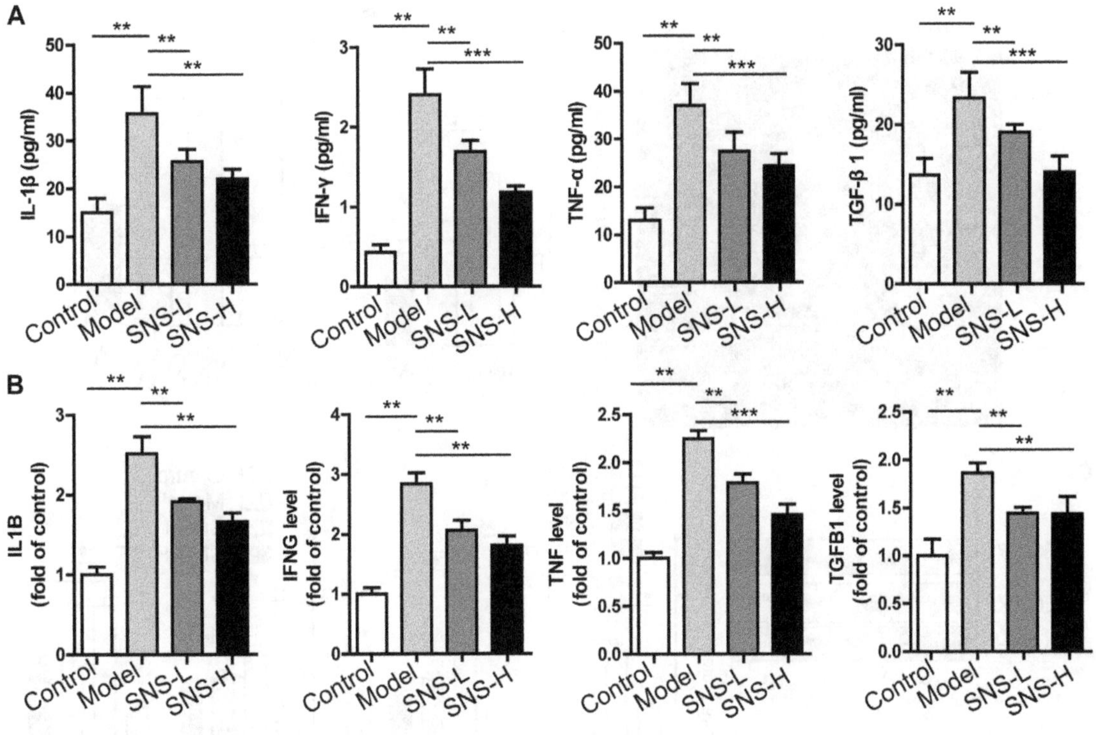

FIGURE 5 | SNS attenuates inflammation in mice with liver fibrosis. Liver and serum samples were obtained from control and fibrotic mice administered water or SNS (5 g/kg and 10 g/kg) at the indicated times. **(A)** Secretion of IL-1β, IFN-γ, TNF-α and TGF-β1 in serum. **(B)** qRT-PCR analysis of f IL-1β, IFN-γ, TNF-α and TGF-β1 mRNA in liver using β-actin as the internal reference. Data are presented as mean ± SD (n = 6). *$p < 0.05$, **$p < 0.01$, ***$p < 0.001$ compared to control or model group.

group ($p < 0.01$; **Figure 6A**). Based on the above findings, we propose that SNS can partially suppress pathological hepatic angiogenesis in the CCl_4-induced liver fibrosis mouse model. VEGF levels in liver tissues were subsequently determined in view of the modulatory effects of SNS on pathological microvessels. According to ELISA findings, CCl_4 elevated the VEGF content in the model relative to the normal group while the VEGF content in SNS treatment groups was markedly reduced compared with the model group ($p < 0.01$) (**Figure 6B**). The results suggest SNS can effectively reduce the production of angiogenesis-related VEGF in mice with CCl_4-induced liver fibrosis after long-term damage. We further determined the mRNA and proteins expression patterns of VEGF receptors (VEGFR1 and VEGFR2). Expression levels of both VEGFR1 and VEGFR2 were markedly decreased following SNS exposure ($p < 0.01$; **Figures 6C,D**).

In summary, SNS suppresses abnormal angiogenesis in tissues of mice with liver fibrosis, which is potentially associated with regulating expression of VEGF and its receptors.

Si-Ni-San Protects Hepatic Parenchymal Cells From Apoptosis *in vivo* and *in vitro*

The TUNEL assay was conducted to examine the involvement of SNS in apoptosis of HPCs in the liver fibrosis mouse model. The proportion of TUNEL-positive HPCs was significantly increased in mice with CCl_4-induced liver fibrosis, which was reversed in the presence of SNS (**Figure 7A**). SNS induced a marked decrease in TNF-α expression upregulated by CCl_4 within liver tissues ($p < 0.05$; **Figure 7B**). Data from western blot analysis showed that SNS reduced the protein levels of cleaved caspase-3, caspase-8 ($p < 0.05$) and Bax ($p < 0.01$) but enhanced the Bcl-2 level ($p < 0.05$) in fibrotic liver tissues of mice, as shown in **Figure 7C**.

We further examined whether SNS plays a similar role in HPC apoptosis *in vitro*. To this end, the MTT assay was conducted to determine the viability of L02 cells after 24 h of SNS treatment. As shown in **Figure 7D**, L02 cell viability was remarkably decreased after TNF-α + Act D treatment ($p < 0.001$) and reversed following SNS exposure. The Muse Annexin V and Dead cell assay was conducted to evaluate apoptosis of L02 cells after 48 h of SNS treatment (**Figure 7E**). Relative to the control group, TNF-α + Act D treatment promoted L02 cell apoptosis ($p < 0.01$), which was suppressed by SNS. Similar results were obtained with the TUNEL assay (**Figure 7F**). In conclusion, SNS suppresses the apoptosis-inducing effects of stimulant on HPCs both *in vivo* and *in vitro*, possibly through regulation of apoptin expression and activation.

Si-Ni-San Reverses Activation of Hepatic Stellate Cells Through Modulating PPAR-γ and NF-κB p65

Activated HSCs have been identified as critical hepatic fibrogenic effector cells, although other cells or processes also contribute significantly to this process. HSCs activated after liver injury proliferate and generate ECM. Our previous

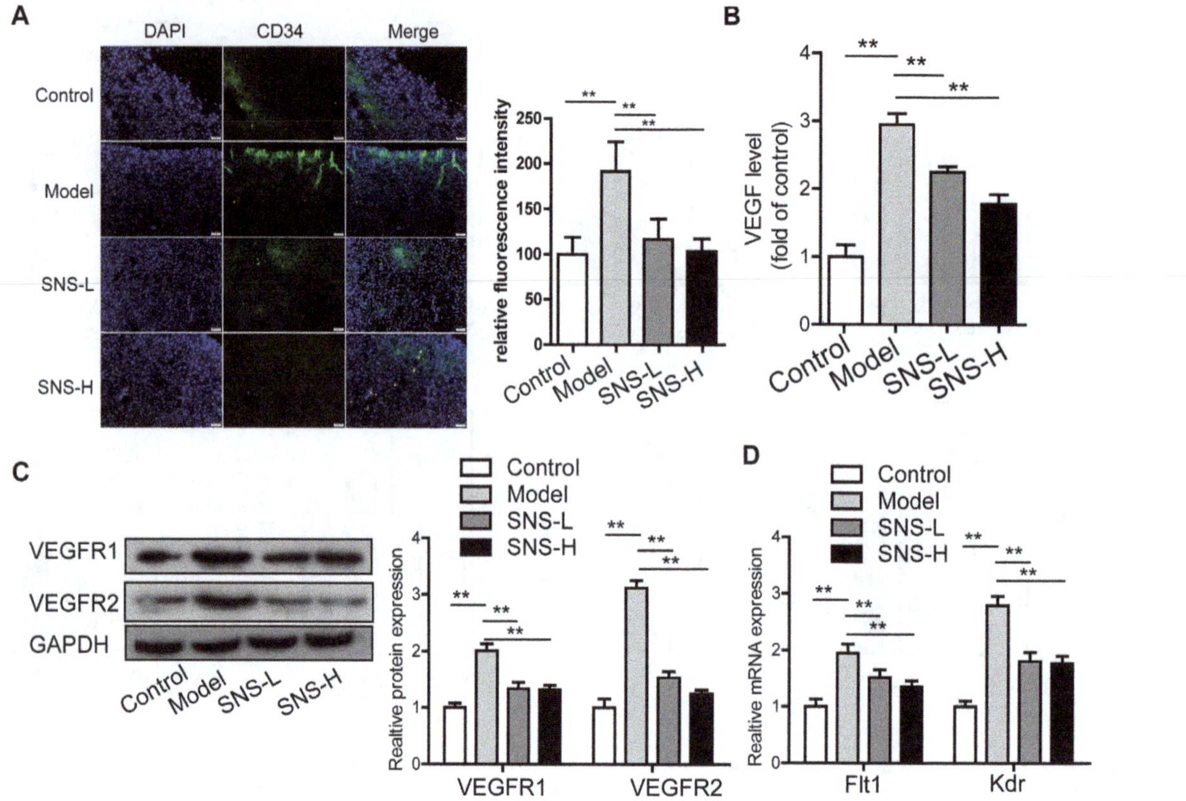

FIGURE 6 | SNS inhibits pathological microvessel and angiogenesis-associated signaling pathways in liver tissue of mice with liver fibrosis. **(A)** Image analysis of fluorescence intensity of CD 34 (pathological microvessels) stained with IF in hepatic tissue of mice with CCl_4-induced liver fibrosis. **(B)** Effect of SNS on VEGF expression in liver tissue. **(C)** Effects of SNS on VEGFR1 and VEGFR2 protein levels in liver tissue. **(D)** Effects of SNS on Flt1 and Kdr mRNA levels in liver tissue. Data are presented as mean ± SD ($n = 6$). $^{*}p < 0.05$, $^{**}p < 0.01$, $^{***}p < 0.001$ compared to control or model group.

experiments demonstrated that SNS suppresses expression of the HSC activation marker α-SMA (**Figure 1**) and activation inducer TGF-β (**Figure 5**) in fibrotic liver tissues of mice in addition to collagen deposition (**Figure 1**). We further examined whether SNS directly acts in suppression of liver fibrosis with the aid of activated LX2 cells. Notably, SNS (50 mg/L) induced a decrease in collagen I, α-SMA and fibronectin mRNA and protein expression in activated LX2 cells (**Figures 8A,B**). Gene analysis data suggest that SNS reduces ECM generation through downregulating TIMP1 mRNA while upregulating MMP13 (**Figure 8C**). These findings indicate that SNS mitigates liver fibrosis by reversing HSC activation and altering the fibrogenesis-fibrolysis balance.

Upregulation of PPAR-γ in activated HSCs is suggested to suppress expression of collagen I, impede TGF-β1 signal transduction, inhibit cell proliferation and increase lipid droplets in the cytoplasm (Hamed et al., 2017). NF-κB p65 functions as a critical inflammation and fibrogenesis regulator in fibrotic liver disease (Wang Y.-H. et al., 2020). According to network pharmacological data, SNS positively affects liver fibrosis and HSC activation potentially through modulation of PPAR-γ and p65. Moreover, our results suggest that SNS promotes PPAR-γ mNRA and protein expression in activated LX2 cells concomitant with downregulation of NF-κB p65 (**Figures 8A,B**). PTGS2 and DPP4 were regulated by 96 and 80 of the 119 candidate compounds of SNS, respectively. No changes in these molecules in activated LX2 cells and liver tissue were observed (data not shown). Accordingly, we propose that SNS suppresses liver fibrosis and HSC activation, at least partly through regulating PPAR-γ and NF-κB p65 expression.

DISCUSSION

Liver fibrosis, a type of progressive disorder, is related to structural destruction of liver tissue, ECM deposition, and new pathological microvessel formation in liver as a result of pathological insult. Liver fibrosis is a pathological process frequently detected in most liver diseases, such as end-stage cirrhosis and hepatocellular carcinoma (HCC) (Sakurai and Kudo, 2013). Numerous therapeutic targets are currently under investigation with a view to identifying antifibrotic agents. Knowledge of these therapeutic targets may aid in: 1)

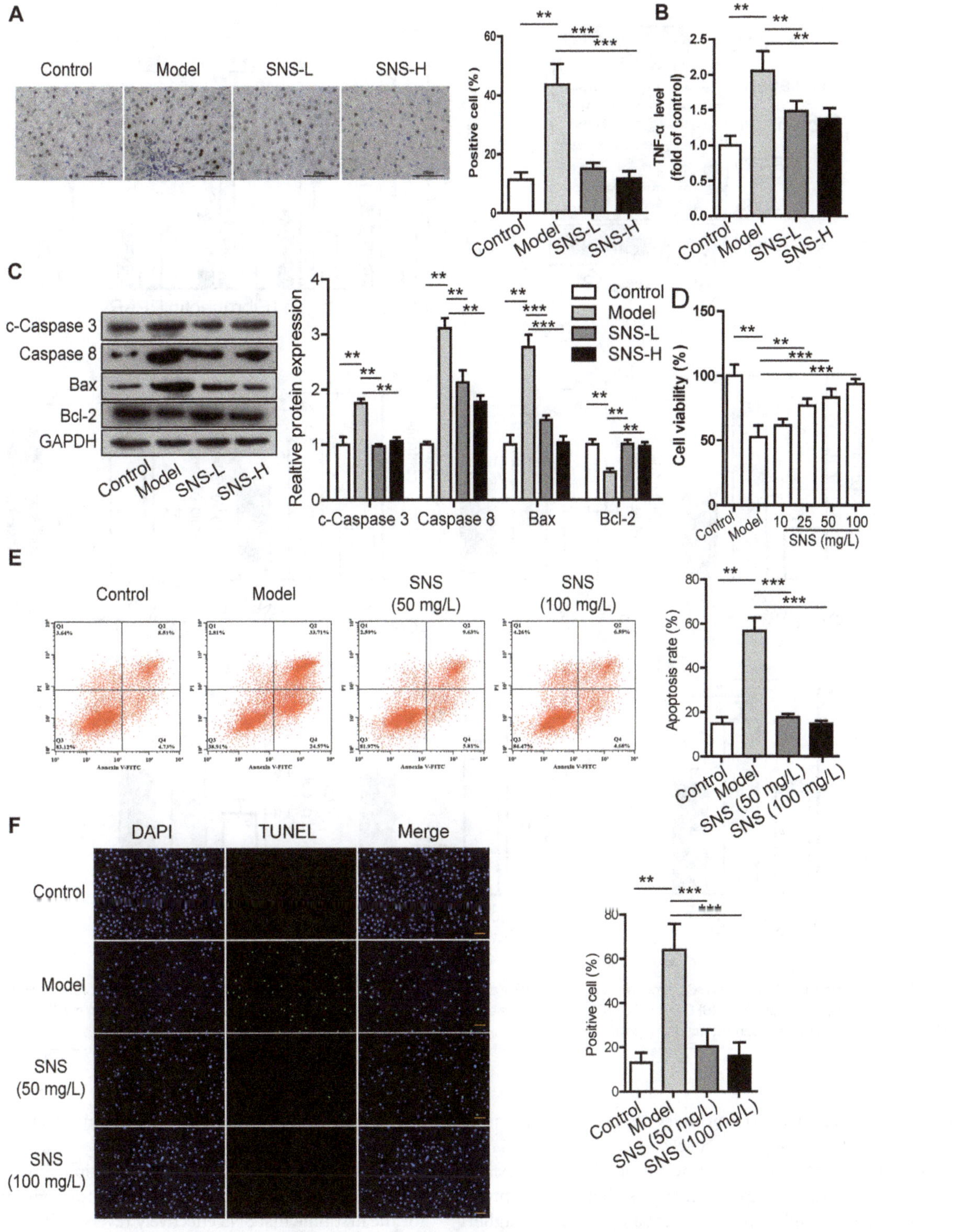

FIGURE 7 | SNS protects hepatic parenchymal cells from apoptosis *in vivo* and *in vitro*. **(A)** TUNEL staining (100×) of liver tissues. **(B)** Effect of SNS on the TNF-α level in liver tissue. **(C)** Effects of SNS on cleaved caspase 3, caspase 8, Bax, and Bcl-2 in liver tissue. **(D)** Effects of SNS on viability of L02 cells stimulated with TNF-α and Act D. **(E)** Evaluation of apoptosis of L02 cells treated with SNS and TNF-α/Act D using the Muse Annexin V and Dead Cell Assay. **(F)** Evaluation of apoptosis of L02 cells treated with SNS and TNF-α/Act D *via* TUNEL staining. Data are presented as mean ± SD (n = 6). $^{*}p < 0.05$, $^{**}p < 0.01$, $^{***}p < 0.001$ compared to control or model group.

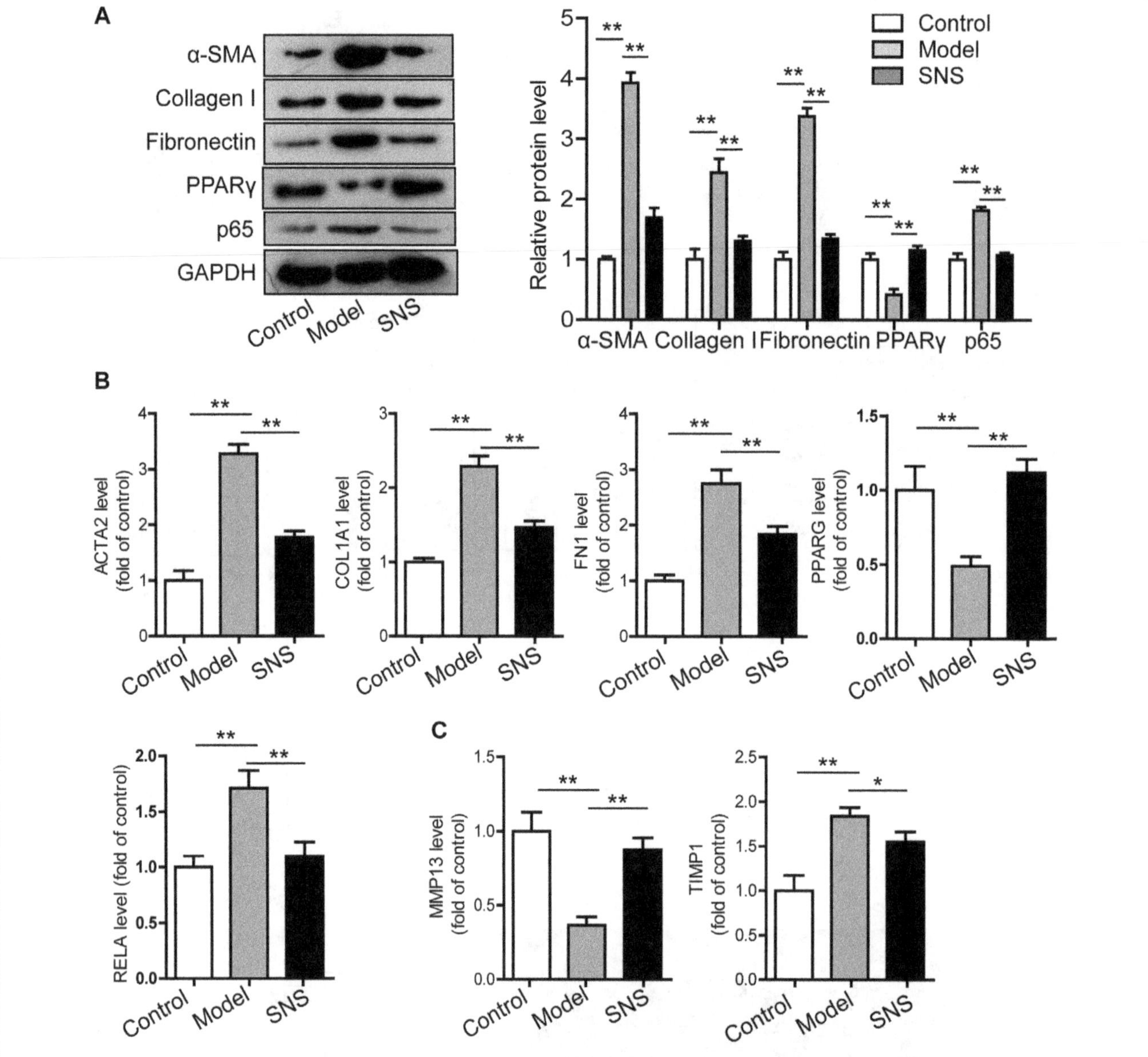

FIGURE 8 | SNS reverses activation of HSCs through modulating PPAR-γ and NF-κB p65. **(A)** Effects of SNS on protein levels of α-SMA, collagen I, fibronectin, p65 and PPARγ in activated LX2 cells. **(B)** Effects of SNS on mRNA levels of ACTA2, COL1A1, FN1, PPARG and RELA in activated LX2 cells. **(C)** Effects of SNS on MMP13 and TIMP1 mRNA levels in activated LX2 cells.

decreasing the incidence of primary disease; 2) mitigating damage to HPCs through the use of hepatoprotectants; 3) suppressing the activation, contractility and fibrogenesis of myofibroblasts; 4) accelerating activated stellate cell apoptosis or reversion; and 5) inhibiting aberrant angiogenesis (Baglieri et al., 2019; Greuter and Shah, 2019; Manka et al., 2019; Chan et al., 2020). To date, the majority of treatments have only focused on a single cell, single cytokine or single signaling molecule without consideration of the overall complex process of liver fibrosis, leading to failure in achieving the expected clinical efficacy. Development of novel antifibrotic treatments involving two or more critical pathogenic targets and/or pathways is thus urgently required (Wang T. et al., 2020).

SNS is a common TCM prescription involving several components and targets. Data from the present study showed for the first time that SNS effectively reverses CCL_4-induced liver fibrosis *in vivo* and facilitates recovery of liver function. We subsequently examined the candidate components and targets in SNS with the aid of network pharmacology analysis. As a result, 119 candidate compounds and 173 corresponding targets were found to be associated with SNS activity against liver fibrosis. Afterwards, the core active ingredients and targets of SNS for inhibiting liver fibrosis were screened through topological analysis. Several core components, such as Glycyrrhizic acid, Saikosaponin A, Paeoniflorin, and Naringin (**Supplementary Table S8**), which have been determined as the quality control substances in the Chinese Pharmacopoeia of the four single medicinal herbs constituting SNS and used for quality control of the experimental medicine in this study, have long been verified to significantly inhibit the diverse stimuli (CCl_4 and dimethylnitrosamine)-induced liver fibrosis *via* multiple pathways. For example, Glycyrrhizic acid was verified to revere the occurrence of liver fibrosis through regulating the TGF-beta pathway and inhibiting parenchymal hepatic cell apoptosis (Liang et al., 2015; Zhou et al., 2016). Paeoniflorin can regulate the local immune-inflammatory responses of liver fibrosis pathology (Chen et al., 2012), while Naringin can suppress the NF-κB signal in hepatic stellate cells to regulate the TIMP-MMP13 pathway-mediated fibrogenesis/fibrolysis balance (Anuja et al., 2018). The core targets were further subjected to functional annotation and pathway enrichment analyses, which revealed that SNS predominantly modulates apoptosis, angiogenesis-related proliferation and migration of endothelial cells and immuno-inflammatory responses *via* TNF, VEGF, NF-κB, and MAPK pathways. Similarly, our experimental results showed that SNS mitigates inflammation in mice with liver fibrosis and protects against apoptosis of HPCs. Moreover, SNS directly suppressed aberrant angiogenesis, HSC activation and ECM accumulation, leading to inhibition of liver fibrosis.

Following induction of liver injury by CCl_4 or other stimulators, a variety of cells generate proinflammatory cytokines, including TNF-α and IL-1β, to promote liver fibrosis (Weiskirchen and Tacke, 2016). In our study, SNS treatment reduced the serum and liver contents of TNF-α, IL-1β as well as IFN-γ in mice with liver fibrosis. The fibrotic pathology may additionally be related to increased expression of TGF-β1 that originally recruits fibroblasts and inflammatory cells at the injury site and subsequently promotes production of ECM and cytokines from these cells (Crosas-Molist et al., 2015). Overexpression of TGF-β1 in transgenic animals is reported to trigger spontaneous liver fibrosis (Kisseleva and Brenner, 2008; Wilson, 2015). Our results showed that SNS induced a decrease in serum and liver levels of TGF-β1 in mice with liver fibrosis, validating our target prediction that the inhibitory effects of SNS on fibrogenesis are related to TGF-β1 modulation. Based on the collective findings, we propose that the beneficial effects of SNS are potentially associated with alleviation of inflammation and ECM deposition with reduced TGF-β1 activity.

Angiogenesis and novel hepatic pathological microvessel formation in chronic liver disease facilitate progression of liver fibrosis (Li, 2020). Activation of HSCs and their conversion to myofibroblasts represent central links in liver fibrosis formation. In addition, activated HSCs produce proangiogenic factors to accelerate hepatic endothelial cell proliferation and migration, leading to promotion of fibrosis (Zadorozhna et al., 2020). In chronic liver disease, many newly formed pathological vessels are immature and useless. As a result, the vascular plexus is formed, which splits around the regenerating hepatocytes and impedes the exchange between hepatocytes and sinusoids. Therefore, regenerating hepatocytes cannot build a normal portal vein branch, thereby aggravating damage to hepatocytes (Kaur and Anita, 2013). In this regard, a vicious cycle is formed between liver fibrosis and pathological angiogenesis in the liver, whereby increased pathological angiogenesis triggers fibrotic progression (Elpek, 2015). VEGF and its receptors, VEGFR1 and VEGFR2, play important roles in this aberrant angiogenesis process (Yan et al., 2015). Our *in vivo* results suggest that SNS not only suppresses angiogenesis in liver tissues of CCl_4-induced mice but also downregulates VEGF and its two receptors. The therapeutic effects of SNS on liver fibrosis may be associated with regulation of aberrant angiogenesis in liver under pathological conditions.

Apoptosis, also known as programmed cell death, is a critical biological process during liver fibrosis (Chakraborty et al., 2012). To date, the majority of studies on treatments for liver fibrosis have focused on inhibition of HPC apoptosis and promotion of HSC apoptosis (Marti-Rodrigo et al., 2020). Typically, HPC apoptosis not only results from liver injury but also serves as a vital inflammatory stimulus for HSC activation (Jaeschke, 2002). Apoptosis is also a self-controlled program that serves to maintain homeostasis. Numerous genes are involved in this process, including the Bcl-2 family, caspase family and TNF (Wei et al., 2018; Wang R. et al., 2019). The induction of fibrotic response may be attributable to persistent HPC apoptosis (Takehara et al., 2004). In addition, apoptotic hepatocyte DNA increases release of collagen, promoting HSC differentiation (Watanabe et al., 2007). Experiments from the current study showed that SNS significantly suppresses the proportion of apoptotic cells in liver tissues induced by CCl_4 and regulates caspase activation and expression of multiple Bcl-2 family proteins. *In vitro*, SNS suppressed apoptosis of L02 cells induced by TNF-α combined with Act D.

MMP13 and TIMP1 are mainly produced by HSC cells and affected by cytokines such as IL-1β, TGF-β1 and TNF-α. Release of MMPs and TIMPs is stringently regulated depending on the HSC activation status (Hernandez-Gea and Friedman, 2011). Under conditions of chronic liver injury, MMP13 and TIMP1 levels are regulated in different ways, resulting in the formation of a positive feedback loop together with subsequent fibrogenesis. In activated HSCs, particularly those with increased TIMP-1 expression, MMP activity is suppressed and matrix proteins accumulate (Hemmann et al., 2007). As evident from our *in vitro* findings, SNS suppressed TIMP1 while upregulating MMP13, leading to recovery of the balance between MMP13 and TIMP1 in activated LX2 cells. SNS induced a significant reduction in the levels of the mesenchymal markers, α-SMA and collagen I, indicating that SNS alleviates liver fibrosis predominantly through mitigating ECM deposition.

NF-κB p65 is a transcription factor and critical inflammation and cell death regulator, which plays a key role in chronic liver disease (Ray, 2012). Activation of p65 in HSCs accelerates fibrogenesis through promoting the activity and survival of HSCs (Luedde and Schwabe, 2011). Interestingly, in our experiments, SNS downregulated NF-κB p65 mRNA and protein expression in activated LX2 cells, confirming data from functional annotation and pathway enrichment analyses supporting significant effects of SNS on the NF-κB p65 signal transduction pathway. In addition, quercetin and puerarin in SNS are reported to exert anti-inflammation and/or antifibrosis effects through suppressing the NF-κB pathway (Li et al., 2013; Li X. et al., 2016). SNS may therefore suppress fibrogenesis progression through regulating activation of NF-κB p65.

PPAR-γ, expressed in HSCs, plays an important role in maintaining cell quiescence (Hazra et al., 2004). PPAR-γ activation blocks TGF-β1/Smad signaling, suppresses HSC proliferation and causes apoptosis, both *in vivo* and *in vitro* (Han et al., 2020). As determined from our network analysis, several candidate components prevent liver injury, inflammation and HSC activation through enhancing PPAR-γ expression. Data from our validation experiments showed that SNS promotes PPAR-γ activity in activated LX2 cells. SNS-induced amelioration of inflammation, promotion of collagen accumulation and regulation of apoptosis may thus be partially achieved through regulation of PPAR-γ activation.

Although this study has explained the material basis and molecular mechanism of SNS against liver fibrosis to a certain extent, there are still some limitations to be futher solved. To begin with, some compounds of herbs in SNS were neglected in consideration of the inadequate data obtained from existing databases and laboratory findings. Secondly, the influence of absolute content of each compound in SNS or the serum and fibrotic liver tissue distribution concentrations on its effect was ignored. Thirdly, this study only illustrated the regulatory effect of SNS on targets, but it did not explain the regulatory effects and patterns of combined actions (synergy, antagonism or additive) of the complex mixture of key active ingredients. As a result, in future research, we aim to extensively examine: 1) the enrichment degrees and contents of screened core active ingredients in the blood or liver tissues of experimental animals or patients through UPLC-MS to further confirm the core active ingredients in SNS against liver fibrosis; 2) the regulatory effect and patterns of combined actions of core active ingredients on the screened core targets and signaling pathways in patients, animal models and *in vitro* experiments using molecular biological technology.

AUTHOR CONTRIBUTIONS

Conceptualization: SW, YZ, and DH; Formal analysis: DH; Funding acquisition: SW and CL; Investigation: CT, HZ, and PS; Resources: CT; Supervision: SW and DH; Validation: PS and CL; Visualization: HZ and PS; Writing—original draft: SW; Writing—review and editing: YZ and DH. All authors have read and agreed to the published version of the manuscript.

FUNDING

This study was financially supported by the National Natural Science Foundation of China (Grant No. 81803916, No. 81903927) and Natural Science Foundation of Jiangsu Province (Grant No. BK20180128).

ACKNOWLEDGMENTS

The authors thank members of their laboratory and their collaborators for their research work.

REFERENCES

Amberger, J. S., Bocchini, C. A., Scott, A. F., and Hamosh, A. (2019). OMIM.org: Leveraging Knowledge across Phenotype-Gene Relationships. *Nucleic Acids Res.* 47 (D1), D1038–D1043. doi:10.1093/nar/gky1151

Anuja, G. I., Shine, V. J., Latha, P. G., and Suja, S. R. (2018). Protective Effect of Ethyl Acetate Fraction of Drynaria Quercifolia against CCl 4 Induced Rat Liver Fibrosis via Nrf2/ARE and NFκB Signalling Pathway. *J. Ethnopharmacology* 216, 79–88. doi:10.1016/j.jep.2017.11.015

Baglieri, J., Brenner, D., and Kisseleva, T. (2019). The Role of Fibrosis and Liver-Associated Fibroblasts in the Pathogenesis of Hepatocellular Carcinoma. *Ijms* 20 (7), 1723. doi:10.3390/ijms20071723

Becker, K. G., Barnes, K. C., Bright, T. J., and Wang, S. A. (2004). The Genetic Association Database. *Nat. Genet.* 36 (5), 431–432. doi:10.1038/ng0504-431

Beljaars, L., Daliri, S., Dijkhuizen, C., Poelstra, K., and Gosens, R. (2017). WNT-5A Regulates TGF-β-Related Activities in Liver Fibrosis. *Am. J. Physiology-Gastrointestinal Liver Physiol.* 312 (3), G219–G227. doi:10.1152/ajpgi.00160.2016

Bian, Y., Dong, Y., Sun, J., Sun, M., Hou, Q., Lai, Y., et al. (2020). Protective Effect of Kaempferol on LPS-Induced Inflammation and Barrier Dysfunction in a Coculture Model of Intestinal Epithelial Cells and Intestinal Microvascular Endothelial Cells. *J. Agric. Food Chem.* 68 (1), 160–167. doi:10.1021/acs.jafc.9b06294

Cai, X., Wang, J., Wang, J., Zhou, Q., Yang, B., He, Q., et al. (2020). Intercellular Crosstalk of Hepatic Stellate Cells in Liver Fibrosis: New Insights into Therapy. *Pharmacol. Res.* 155, 104720. doi:10.1016/j.phrs.2020.104720

Cao, H., Li, S., Xie, R., Xu, N., Qian, Y., Chen, H., et al. (2018). Exploring the Mechanism of Dangguiliuhuang Decoction against Hepatic Fibrosis by Network Pharmacology and Experimental Validation. *Front. Pharmacol.* 9, 187. doi:10.3389/fphar.2018.00187

Chakraborty, J. B., Oakley, F., and Walsh, M. J. (2012). Mechanisms and Biomarkers of Apoptosis in Liver Disease and Fibrosis. *Int. J. Hepatol.* 2012, 1–10. doi:10.1155/2012/6489152012

Chan, Y.-T., Wang, N., Tan, H. Y., Li, S., and Feng, Y. (2020). Targeting Hepatic Stellate Cells for the Treatment of Liver Fibrosis by Natural Products: Is it the Dawning of a New Era? *Front. Pharmacol.* 11, 548. doi:10.3389/fphar.2020.00548

Chen, C.-H., Chen, M.-F., Huang, S. J., Huang, C.-Y., Wang, H.-K., Hsieh, W.-C., et al. (2017). Saikosaponin a Induces Apoptosis through Mitochondria-dependent Pathway in Hepatic Stellate Cells. *Am. J. Chin. Med.* 45 (2), 351–368. doi:10.1142/S0192415X17500227

Chen, X., Liu, C., Lu, Y., Yang, Z., Lv, Z., Xu, Q., et al. (2012). Paeoniflorin Regulates Macrophage Activation in Dimethylnitrosamine-Induced Liver Fibrosis in Rats. *BMC Complement. Altern. Med.* 12, 254. doi:10.1186/1472-6882-12-254

Cheung, F., Feng, Y., Wang, N., Yuen, M.-F., Tong, Y., and Wong, V. (2012). Effectiveness of Chinese Herbal Medicine in Treating Liver Fibrosis: a Systematic Review and Meta-Analysis of Randomized Controlled Trials. *Chin. Med.* 7 (1), 5. doi:10.1186/1749-8546-7-5

Chin, C.-H., Chen, S.-H., Wu, H.-H., Ho, C.-W., Ko, M.-T., and Lin, C.-Y. (2014). cytoHubba: Identifying Hub Objects and Sub-networks from Complex Interactome. *BMC Syst. Biol.* 8 (Suppl. 4), S11. doi:10.1186/1752-0509-8-S4-S11

Crosas-Molist, E., Bertran, E., and Fabregat, I. (2015). Cross-Talk between TGF-β and NADPH Oxidases during Liver Fibrosis and Hepatocarcinogenesis. *Cpd* 21 (41), 5964–5976. doi:10.2174/1381612821666151029112126

El-Sisi, A. E.-D. E. -S., Sokar, S. S., Shebl, A. M., and Mohamed, D. Z. (2017). Antifibrotic Effect of Diethylcarbamazine Combined with Hesperidin against Ethanol Induced Liver Fibrosis in Rats. *Biomed. Pharmacother.* 89, 1196–1206. doi:10.1016/j.biopha.2017.03.013

Elpek, G. Ö. (2015). Angiogenesis and Liver Fibrosis. *Wjh* 7 (3), 377–391. doi:10.4254/wjh.v7.i3.377

Fagone, P., Mangano, K., Mammana, S., Pesce, A., Pesce, A., Caltabiano, R., et al. (2015). Identification of Novel Targets for the Diagnosis and Treatment of Liver Fibrosis. *Int. J. Mol. Med.* 36 (3), 747–752. doi:10.3892/ijmm.2015.2264

Fan, R., Pan, T., Zhu, A.-L., and Zhang, M.-H. (2017). Anti-inflammatory and Anti-arthritic Properties of Naringenin via Attenuation of NF-κB and Activation of the Heme Oxygenase (HO)-1/related Factor 2 Pathway. *Pharmacol. Rep.* 69 (5), 1021–1029. doi:10.1016/j.pharep.2017.03.020

Geng, W., Zhou, G., Zhao, B., Xiao, Q., Li, C., Fan, S., et al. (2020). Liquiritigenin Suppresses the Activation of Hepatic Stellate Cells via Targeting miR-181b/PTEN axis. *Phytomedicine* 66, 153108. doi:10.1016/j.phymed.2019.153108

Gong, Y. (2012). Identifying the Targets for Treatment of Liver Fibrosis and Hepatocellular Carcinoma from Both Western Medicine and Chinese Medicine. *Chin. J. Integr. Med.* 18 (4), 245–249. doi:10.1007/s11655-012-1062-6

Goodman, Z. D. (2007). Grading and Staging Systems for Inflammation and Fibrosis in Chronic Liver Diseases. *J. Hepatol.* 47 (4), 598–607. doi:10.1016/j.jhep.2007.07.006

Greuter, T., and Shah, V. H. (2019). Too Stiff, Too Late . . Timing Is Everything in Antiangiogenic Treatment of Liver Fibrosis. *Hepatology* 69 (1), 449–451. doi:10.1002/hep.30124

Guo, R., Luo, X., Liu, J., Liu, L., Wang, X., and Lu, H. (2020). Omics Strategies Decipher Therapeutic Discoveries of Traditional Chinese Medicine against Different Diseases at Multiple Layers Molecular-Level. *Pharmacol. Res.* 152, 104627. doi:10.1016/j.phrs.2020.104627

Hamed, A. M., El-Kharashi, O. A., Boctor, S. S. A., and Abd-Elaziz, L. F. (2017). Potential Involvement of PPAR α Activation in Diminishing the Hepatoprotective Effect of Fenofibrate in NAFLD. *Biomed. Pharmacother.* 85, 68–78. doi:10.1016/j.biopha.2016.11.114

Han, X., Wu, Y., Yang, Q., and Cao, G. (2021). Peroxisome Proliferator-Activated Receptors in the Pathogenesis and Therapies of Liver Fibrosis. *Pharmacol. Ther.* 222, 107791. doi:10.1016/j.pharmthera.2020.107791

Hazra, S., Xiong, S., Wang, J., Rippe, R. A., Krishna, V., Chatterjee, K., et al. (2004). Peroxisome Proliferator-Activated Receptor γ Induces a Phenotypic Switch from Activated to Quiescent Hepatic Stellate Cells. *J. Biol. Chem.* 279 (12), 11392–11401. doi:10.1074/jbc.M310284200

He, Y., Jin, L., Wang, J., Yan, Z., Chen, T., and Zhao, Y. (2015). Mechanisms of Fibrosis in Acute Liver Failure. *Liver Int.* 35 (7), 1877–1885. doi:10.1111/liv.12731

Hemmann, S., Graf, J., Roderfeld, M., and Roeb, E. (2007). Expression of MMPs and TIMPs in Liver Fibrosis - a Systematic Review with Special Emphasis on Anti-fibrotic Strategies. *J. Hepatol.* 46 (5), 955–975. doi:10.1016/j.jhep.2007.02.003

Hernandez-Gea, V., and Friedman, S. L. (2011). Pathogenesis of Liver Fibrosis. *Annu. Rev. Pathol. Mech. Dis.* 6, 425–456. doi:10.1146/annurev-pathol-011110-130246

Hou, B., Zhao, Y., Qiang, G., Yang, X., Xu, C., Chen, X., et al. (2018). Puerarin Mitigates Diabetic Hepatic Steatosis and Fibrosis by Inhibiting TGF-β Signaling Pathway Activation in Type 2 Diabetic Rats. *Oxidative Med. Cell Longevity* 2018, 1–13. doi:10.1155/2018/45453212018

Hou, J.-L., Xu, D., Shi, G., Wan, M., Goodman, Z., Tan, D., et al. (2015). Long-Term Telbivudine Treatment Results in Resolution of Liver Inflammation and Fibrosis in Patients with Chronic Hepatitis B. *Adv. Ther.* 32 (8), 727–741. doi:10.1007/s12325-015-0232-2

Huang, L., Xie, D., Yu, Y., Liu, H., Shi, Y., Shi, T., et al. (2018). TCMID 2.0: a Comprehensive Resource for TCM. *Nucleic Acids Res.* 46 (D1), D1117–D1120. doi:10.1093/nar/gkx1028

Jaeschke, H. (2002). Inflammation in Response to Hepatocellular Apoptosis. *Hepatology* 35 (4), 964–966. doi:10.1053/jhep.2002.0350964

Jiang, C., Iwaisako, K., Cong, M., Diggle, K., Hassanein, T., Brenner, D. A., et al. (2020). Traditional Chinese Medicine Fuzheng Huayu Prevents Development of Liver Fibrosis in Mice. *Arch. Clin. Biomed. Res.* 04 (5), 561–580. doi:10.26502/acbr.50170125

Jiang, J., Zhou, C., and Xu, Q. (2003). Alleviating Effects of Si-Ni-San, a Traditional Chinese Prescription, on Experimental Liver Injury and its Mechanisms. *Biol. Pharm. Bull.* 26 (8), 1089–1094. doi:10.1248/bpb.26.1089

Kaur, S., and Anita, K. (2013). Angiogenesis in Liver Regeneration and Fibrosis: "a Double-Edged Sword". *Hepatol. Int.* 7 (4), 959–968. doi:10.1007/s12072-013-9483-7

Kisseleva, T., and Brenner, D. A. (2008). Mechanisms of Fibrogenesis. *Exp. Biol. Med. (Maywood)* 233 (2), 109–122. doi:10.3181/0707-MR-190

Kisseleva, T., and Brenner, D. (2020). Molecular and Cellular Mechanisms of Liver Fibrosis and its Regression. *Nat. Rev. Gastroenterol. Hepatol.* 18, 151–166. doi:10.1038/s41575-020-00372-7

Koyama, Y., and Brenner, D. A. (2017). Liver Inflammation and Fibrosis. *J. Clin. Invest.* 127 (1), 55–64. doi:10.1172/JCI88881

Koyama, Y., Xu, J., Liu, X., and Brenner, D. A. (2016). New Developments on the Treatment of Liver Fibrosis. *Dig. Dis.* 34 (5), 589–596. doi:10.1159/000445269

Lambrecht, J., van Grunsven, L. A., and Tacke, F. (2020). Current and Emerging Pharmacotherapeutic Interventions for the Treatment of Liver Fibrosis. *Expert Opin. Pharmacother.* 21 (13), 1637–1650. doi:10.1080/14656566.2020.1774553

Lee, E. H., Park, K.-I., Kim, K.-Y., Lee, J.-H., Jang, E. J., Ku, S. K., et al. (2019). Liquiritigenin Inhibits Hepatic Fibrogenesis and TGF-β1/Smad with Hippo/YAP Signal. *Phytomedicine* 62, 152780. doi:10.1016/j.phymed.2018.12.003

Li, H. (2020). Angiogenesis in the Progression from Liver Fibrosis to Cirrhosis and Hepatocelluar Carcinoma. *Expert Rev. Gastroenterol. Hepatol.* 15, 217–233. doi:10.1080/17474124.2021.1842732

Li, J., Li, X., Xu, W., Wang, S., Hu, Z., Zhang, Q., et al. (2015). Antifibrotic Effects of Luteolin on Hepatic Stellate Cells and Liver Fibrosis by Targeting AKT/mTOR/p70S6K and TGFβ/Smad Signalling Pathways. *Liver Int.* 35 (4), 1222–1233. doi:10.1111/liv.12638

Li, P., Chen, J., Wang, J., Zhou, W., Wang, X., Li, B., et al. (2014). Systems Pharmacology Strategies for Drug Discovery and Combination with Applications to Cardiovascular Diseases. *J. Ethnopharmacology* 151 (1), 93–107. doi:10.1016/j.jep.2013.07.001

Li, Q., Wang, Y., Zhang, L., Chen, L., Du, Y., Ye, T., et al. (2016a). Naringenin Exerts Anti-angiogenic Effects in Human Endothelial Cells: Involvement of ERRα/VEGF/KDR Signaling Pathway. *Fitoterapia* 111, 78–86. doi:10.1016/j.fitote.2016.04.015

Li, R., Xu, L., Liang, T., Li, Y., Zhang, S., and Duan, X. (2013). Puerarin Mediates Hepatoprotection against CCl4-Induced Hepatic Fibrosis Rats through Attenuation of Inflammation Response and Amelioration of Metabolic Function. *Food Chem. Toxicol.* 52, 69–75. doi:10.1016/j.fct.2012.10.059

Li, S. (2021). Network Pharmacology Evaluation Method Guidance-Draft. *World J. Tradit. Chin. Med.* 7 (1), 146–154. doi:10.1093/nar/gky1021

Li, X., Jin, Q., Yao, Q., Xu, B., Li, Z., and Tu, C. (2016b). Quercetin Attenuates the Activation of Hepatic Stellate Cells and Liver Fibrosis in Mice through Modulation of HMGB1-Tlr2/4-NF-Kb Signaling Pathways. *Toxicol. Lett.* 261, 1–12. doi:10.1016/j.toxlet.2016.09.002

Liang, B., Guo, X. L., Jin, J., Ma, Y. C., and Feng, Z. Q. (2015). Glycyrrhizic Acid Inhibits Apoptosis and Fibrosis in Carbon-Tetrachloride-Induced Rat Liver Injury. *Wjg* 21 (17), 5271–5280. doi:10.3748/wjg.v21.i17.5271

Liu, F., Zhang, J., Qian, J., Wu, G., and Ma, Z. (2018). Emodin Alleviates CCl4-induced L-iver F-ibrosis by S-uppressing E-pithelial-mesenchymal T-ransition and T-ransforming G-rowth F-actor-β1 in R-ats. *Mol. Med. Rep.* 18 (3), 3262–3270. doi:10.3892/mmr.2018.9324

Liu, P. (2016). Inhibition of Pathological Angiogenesis of Chinese Medicine against Liver Fibrosis. *Chin. J. Integr. Med.* 22 (8), 569–572. doi:10.1007/s11655-016-2468-3

Luedde, T., and Schwabe, R. F. (2011). NF-κB in the Liver-Linking Injury, Fibrosis and Hepatocellular Carcinoma. *Nat. Rev. Gastroenterol. Hepatol.* 8 (2), 108–118. doi:10.1038/nrgastro.2010.213

Ma, R., Chen, J., Liang, Y., Lin, S., Zhu, L., Liang, X., et al. (2017). Sorafenib: A Potential Therapeutic Drug for Hepatic Fibrosis and its Outcomes. *Biomed. Pharmacother.* 88, 459–468. doi:10.1016/j.biopha.2017.01.107

Manka, P., Zeller, A., and Syn, W.-K. (2019). Fibrosis in Chronic Liver Disease: An Update on Diagnostic and Treatment Modalities. *Drugs* 79 (9), 903–927. doi:10.1007/s40265-019-01126-9

Martí-Rodrigo, A., Alegre, F., Moragrega, Á. B., García-García, F., Martí-Rodrigo, P., Fernández-Iglesias, A., et al. (2020). Rilpivirine Attenuates Liver Fibrosis through Selective STAT1-Mediated Apoptosis in Hepatic Stellate Cells. *Gut* 69 (5), 920–932. doi:10.1136/gutjnl-2019-318372

Méndez-Sánchez, N., Valencia-Rodríguez, A., Coronel-Castillo, C., Vera-Barajas, A., Contreras-Carmona, J., Ponciano-Rodríguez, G., et al. (2020). The Cellular Pathways of Liver Fibrosis in Non-alcoholic Steatohepatitis. *Ann. Transl Med.* 8 (6), 400. doi:10.21037/atm.2020.02.184

Meurer, S. K., Karsdal, M. A., and Weiskirchen, R. (2020). Advances in the Clinical Use of Collagen as Biomarker of Liver Fibrosis. *Expert Rev. Mol. Diagn.* 20 (9), 947–969. doi:10.1080/14737159.2020.1814746

Pun, J., and Chor, W. (2020). Use of Questioning between Traditional Chinese Medicine Practitioners and Patients to Realize TCM Philosophy: Holism, Five Elements and Yin-Yang in the Context of Doctor-Patient Communication. *Health Commun.*, 1–14. doi:10.1080/10410236.2020.1828533

Rappaport, N., Twik, M., Plaschkes, I., Nudel, R., Iny Stein, T., Levitt, J., et al. (2017). MalaCards: an Amalgamated Human Disease Compendium with Diverse Clinical and Genetic Annotation and Structured Search. *Nucleic Acids Res.* 45 (D1), D877–D887. doi:10.1093/nar/gkw1012

Ray, K. (2012). Activation of NF-Kb Signaling in Hepatocytes Induces Liver Fibrosis. *Nat. Rev. Gastroenterol. Hepatol.* 9 (5), 244. doi:10.1038/nrgastro.2012.61

Ru, J., Li, P., Wang, J., Zhou, W., Li, B., Huang, C., et al. (2014). TCMSP: a Database of Systems Pharmacology for Drug Discovery from Herbal Medicines. *J. Cheminform* 6, 13. doi:10.1186/1758-2946-6-13

Sakurai, T., and Kudo, M. (2013). Molecular Link between Liver Fibrosis and Hepatocellular Carcinoma. *Liver Cancer* 2 (3-4), 365–366. doi:10.1159/000343851

Shiu, L.-Y., Huang, H. H., Chen, C. Y., Cheng, H.-Y., Chen, C. I., and Kuo, S. M. (2020). Reparative and Toxicity-Reducing Effects of Liposome-Encapsulated Saikosaponin in Mice with Liver Fibrosis. *Biosci. Rep.* 40 (8). doi:10.1042/BSR20201219

Song, Y., Zhao, J., Wang, S., Huang, H., Hong, J., Zuo, J., et al. (2019). The Efficacy of Chinese Patent Medicine Combined with Entecavir for the Treatment of Chronic HBV-Related Liver Fibrosis or Cirrhosis. *Medicine (Baltimore)* 98 (22), e15732. doi:10.1097/MD.0000000000015732

Sterling, R. K., King, W. C., Wahed, A. S., Kleiner, D. E., Khalili, M., Sulkowski, M., et al. (2020). Evaluating Noninvasive Markers to Identify Advanced Fibrosis by Liver Biopsy in HBV/HIV Co-infected Adults. *Hepatology* 71 (2), 411–421. doi:10.1002/hep.30825

Takehara, T., Tatsumi, T., Suzuki, T., Rucker, E. B., 3rd, Hennighausen, L., Jinushi, M., et al. (2004). Hepatocyte-specific Disruption of Bcl-xL Leads to Continuous Hepatocyte Apoptosis and Liver Fibrotic Responses. *Gastroenterology* 127 (4), 1189–1197. doi:10.1053/j.gastro.2004.07.019

Tao, W., Xu, X., Wang, X., Li, B., Wang, Y., Li, Y., et al. (2013). Network Pharmacology-Based Prediction of the Active Ingredients and Potential Targets of Chinese Herbal Radix Curcumae Formula for Application to Cardiovascular Disease. *J. Ethnopharmacology* 145 (1), 1–10. doi:10.1016/j.jep.2012.09.051

Wang, R., Song, F., Li, S., Wu, B., Gu, Y., and Yuan, Y. (2019a). Salvianolic Acid A Attenuates CCl4-Induced Liver Fibrosis by Regulating the PI3K/AKT/mTOR, Bcl-2/Bax and Caspase-3/cleaved Caspase-3 Signaling Pathways. *Dddt* Vol. 13, 1889–1900. doi:10.2147/DDDT.S194787

Wang, R., Xiong, A.-Z., Teng, Z.-Q., Yang, Q.-W., Shi, Y.-H., and Yang, L. (2012a). Radix Paeoniae Rubra and Radix Paeoniae Alba Attenuate CCl4-Induced Acute Liver Injury: an Ultra-performance Liquid Chromatography-Mass Spectrometry (UPLC-MS) Based Metabolomic Approach for the Pharmacodynamic Study of Traditional Chinese Medicines (TCMs). *Ijms* 13 (11), 14634–14647. doi:10.3390/ijms131114634

Wang, T., Jin, W., Huang, Q., Li, H., Zhu, Y., Liu, H., et al. (2020a). Clinical Efficacy and Safety of Eight Traditional Chinese Medicine Combined with Entecavir in the Treatment of Chronic Hepatitis B Liver Fibrosis in Adults: A Network Meta-Analysis. *Evidence-Based Complement. Altern. Med.* 2020, 1–15. doi:10.1155/2020/7603410

Wang, X., Xu, X., Tao, W., Li, Y., Wang, Y., and Yang, L. (2012b). A Systems Biology Approach to Uncovering Pharmacological Synergy in Herbal Medicines with Applications to Cardiovascular Disease. *Evidence-Based Complement. Altern. Med.* 2012, 1–15. doi:10.1155/2012/519031

Wang, Y.-H., Suk, F.-M., Liu, C.-L., Chen, T.-L., Twu, Y.-C., Hsu, M.-H., et al. (2020b). Antifibrotic Effects of a Barbituric Acid Derivative on Liver Fibrosis by Blocking the NF-Kb Signaling Pathway in Hepatic Stellate Cells. *Front. Pharmacol.* 11, 388. doi:10.3389/fphar.2020.00388

Wang, Y.-X., Du, Y., Liu, X.-F., Yang, F.-X., Wu, X., Tan, L., et al. (2019b). A Hepatoprotection Study of Radix Bupleuri on Acetaminophen-Induced Liver Injury Based on CYP450 Inhibition. *Chin. J. Nat. Medicines* 17 (7), 517–524. doi:10.1016/S1875-5364(19)30073-1

Watanabe, A., Hashmi, A., Gomes, D. A., Town, T., Badou, A., Flavell, R. A., et al. (2007). Apoptotic Hepatocyte DNA Inhibits Hepatic Stellate Cell Chemotaxis via Toll-like Receptor 9. *Hepatology* 46 (5), 1509–1518. doi:10.1002/hep.21867

Wei, L., Chen, Q., Guo, A., Fan, J., Wang, R., and Zhang, H. (2018). Asiatic Acid Attenuates CCl 4 -induced Liver Fibrosis in Rats by Regulating the PI3K/AKT/mTOR and Bcl-2/Bax Signaling Pathways. *Int. Immunopharmacology* 60, 1–8. doi:10.1016/j.intimp.2018.04.016

Weiskirchen, R., and Tacke, F. (2016). Liver Fibrosis: From Pathogenesis to Novel Therapies. *Dig. Dis.* 34 (4), 410–422. doi:10.1159/000444556

Wilson, J. R., and Justin, N. (2015). Histone Recognition by WD40 Proteins. *Iran J. Pathol.* 10 (2), 83–100. doi:10.1007/978-3-319-18102-8_4

Wishart, D. S., Knox, C., Guo, A. C., Cheng, D., Shrivastava, S., Tzur, D., et al. (2008). DrugBank: a Knowledgebase for Drugs, Drug Actions and Drug Targets. *Nucleic Acids Res.* 36 (Database issue), D901–D906. doi:10.1093/nar/gkm958

Wu, Y., Zhang, F., Yang, K., Fang, S., Bu, D., Li, H., et al. (2019). SymMap: An Integrative Database of Traditional Chinese Medicine Enhanced By Symptom Mapping. *Nucleic. Acids Res.* 47 (D1), D1110–D1117. doi:10.1093/nar/gky1021

Xu, T., Huang, S., Huang, Q., Ming, Z., Wang, M., Li, R., et al. (2019). Kaempferol Attenuates Liver Fibrosis by Inhibiting Activin Receptor-like Kinase 5. *J. Cel Mol Med* 23 (9), 6403–6410. doi:10.1111/jcmm.14528

Xu, X., Zhang, W., Huang, C., Li, Y., Yu, H., Wang, Y., et al. (2012). A Novel Chemometric Method for the Prediction of Human Oral Bioavailability. *Ijms* 13 (6), 6964–6982. doi:10.3390/ijms13066964

Yan, Z., Qu, K., Zhang, J., Huang, Q., Qu, P., Xu, X., et al. (2015). CD147 Promotes Liver Fibrosis Progression via VEGF-A/VEGFR2 Signalling-Mediated Cross-Talk between Hepatocytes and Sinusoidal Endothelial Cells. *Clin. Sci. (Lond)* 129 (8), 699–710. doi:10.1042/CS20140823

Zadorozhna, M., Di Gioia, S., Conese, M., and Mangieri, D. (2020). Neovascularization Is a Key Feature of Liver Fibrosis Progression: Anti-angiogenesis as an Innovative Way of Liver Fibrosis Treatment. *Mol. Biol. Rep.* 47 (3), 2279–2288. doi:10.1007/s11033-020-05290-0

Zhang, Q., Xu, D., Guo, Q., Shan, W., Yang, J., Lin, T., et al. (2019a). Theranostic Quercetin Nanoparticle for Treatment of Hepatic Fibrosis. *Bioconjug. Chem.* 30 (11), 2939–2946. doi:10.1021/acs.bioconjchem.9b00631

Zhang, R., Zhu, X., Bai, H., and Ning, K. (2019b). Network Pharmacology Databases for Traditional Chinese Medicine: Review and Assessment. *Front. Pharmacol.* 10, 123. doi:10.3389/fphar.2019.00123

Zhao, X.-A., Chen, G., Liu, Y., Chen, Y., Wu, H., Xiong, Y., et al. (2018). Curcumin Reduces Ly6Chi Monocyte Infiltration to Protect against Liver Fibrosis by Inhibiting Kupffer Cells Activation to Reduce Chemokines Secretion. *Biomed. Pharmacother.* 106, 868–878. doi:10.1016/j.biopha.2018.07.028

Zhao, X. A., Chen, G. M., Liu, Y., Chen, Y. X., Wu, H. Y., Chen, J., et al. (2017). Inhibitory Effect of Silymarin on CCl4-Induced Liver Fibrosis by Reducing Ly6Chi Monocytes Infiltration. *Int. J. Clin. Exp. Pathol.* 10 (12), 11941–11951.

Zhao, Y., Ma, X., Wang, J., Zhu, Y., Li, R., Wang, J., et al. (2014). Paeoniflorin Alleviates Liver Fibrosis by Inhibiting HIF-1α through mTOR-dependent Pathway. *Fitoterapia* 99, 318–327. doi:10.1016/j.fitote.2014.10.009

Zhou, J., Huang, N., Guo, Y., Cui, S., Ge, C., He, Q., et al. (2019). Combined Obeticholic Acid and Apoptosis Inhibitor Treatment Alleviates Liver Fibrosis. *Acta Pharmaceutica Sinica B* 9 (3), 526–536. doi:10.1016/j.apsb.2018.11.004

Zhou, Y., Tong, X., Ren, S., Wang, X., Chen, J., Mu, Y., et al. (2016). Synergistic Anti-liver Fibrosis Actions of Total astragalus Saponins and Glycyrrhizic Acid via TGF-β1/Smads Signaling Pathway Modulation. *J. Ethnopharmacology* 190, 83–90. doi:10.1016/j.jep.2016.06.011

Zhu, F., Han, B., Kumar, P., Liu, X., Ma, X., Wei, X., et al. (2010). Update of TTD: Therapeutic Target Database. *Nucleic Acids Res.* 38 (Database issue), D787–D791. doi:10.1093/nar/gkp1014

Zhu, F., Li, Y.-M., Feng, T.-T., Wu, Y., Zhang, H.-X., Jin, G.-Y., et al. (2019). Freeze-dried Si-Ni-San Powder Can Ameliorate High Fat Diet-Induced Non-alcoholic Fatty Liver Disease. *Wjg* 25 (24), 3056–3068. doi:10.3748/wjg.v25.i24.3056

10

A Novel Systems Pharmacology Method to Investigate Molecular Mechanisms of *Scutellaria barbata* D. Don for Non-Small Cell Lung Cancer

*Jianling Liu[1], Meng Jiang[1], Zhihua Li[1], Xia Zhang[1], XiaoGang Li[1], Yuanyuan Hao[1], Xing Su[2], Jinglin Zhu[1], Chunli Zheng[1], Wei Xiao[3] and Yonghua Wang[1]**

[1] Key Laboratory of Resource Biology and Biotechnology in Western China, Ministry of Education, School of Life Sciences, Northwest University, Xi'an, China, [2] Pharmacology Department, School of Pharmacy, Shihezi University, Shihezi, China, [3] State Key Laboratory of New-tech for Chinese Medicine Pharmaceutical Process, Jiangsu Kanion Parmaceutical, Co., Ltd., Lianyungang, China

Correspondence:
Yonghua Wang
yh_wang@nwsuaf.edu.cn

Non-small cell lung cancer (NSCLC) is the most ordinary type of lung cancer which leads to 1/3 of all cancer deaths. At present, cytotoxic chemotherapy, surgical resection, radiation, and photodynamic therapy are the main strategies for NSCLC treatment. However, NSCLC is relatively resistant to the above therapeutic strategies, resulting in a rather low (20%) 5-year survival rate. Therefore, there is imperative to identify or develop efficient lead compounds for the treatment of NSCLC. Here, we report that the herb *Scutellaria barbata* D. Don (SBD) can effectively treat NSCLC by anti-inflammatory, promoting apoptosis, cell cycle arrest, and angiogenesis. In this work, we analyze the molecular mechanism of SBD for NSCLC treatment by applying the systems pharmacology strategy. This method combines pharmacokinetics analysis with pharmacodynamics evaluation to screen out the active compounds, predict the targets and assess the networks and pathways. Results show that 33 compounds were identified with potential anti-cancer effects. Utilizing these active compounds as probes, we predicted that 145 NSCLC related targets mainly involved four aspects: apoptosis, inflammation, cell cycle, and angiogenesis. And *in vitro* experiments were managed to evaluate the reliability of some vital active compounds and targets. Overall, a complete overview of the integrated systems pharmacology method provides a precise probe to elucidate the molecular mechanisms of SBD for NSCLC. Moreover, baicalein from SBD effectively inhibited tumor growth in an LLC tumor-bearing mice models, demonstrating the anti-tumor effects of SBD. Our findings further provided experimental evidence for the application in the treatment of NSCLC.

Keywords: non-small cell lung cancer, *Scutellaria barbata* D. Don, systems pharmacology, the molecular mechanism, baicalein

---

Abbreviations: ADME, absorption, distribution, metabolism, and excretion; LPSs, lipopolysaccharides; NSCLC, non-small cell lung cancer; SBD, *Scutellaria barbata* D. Don; TCMs, traditional Chinese medicines.

INTRODUCTION

Non-small cell lung cancer (NSCLC) is one of the leading causes of cancer death worldwide (Jemal et al., 2003). Faced with palliative care, chemotherapy is one of the main methods, but may cause severe side-effects and often leads to multidrug resistance (Ho et al., 2007). Therefore, the future of NSCLC treatment depends on the exploration and development of more effective drugs. In recent years, a large number of therapies, such as platinum therapies still represent the most common first-line treatment for NSCLC, however, it's still difficult to achieve the most ideal treatment effect.

Traditional Chinese medicines (TCMs) are effective to relieve complicated diseases in a multi-target/multi-component manner, which makes them unique among all traditional medicines (Qiu, 2015), and have been used to treat various human diseases for over 4,000 years (Tang et al., 2009). For instance, *Scutellaria barbata* D. Don (SBD), is a perennial herb which is natively distributed in northeast Asia. This herb is known as Ban-Zhi Lian in TCMs which has been used to inhibit inflammatory (Dai et al., 2013) and block tumor (Wang, 2012) growth. Although SBD has been proven to be dramatically efficient in curing NSCLC (Wang Q. et al., 2018), the fundamental molecular action mechanisms are still not systematically explored. The bioactive compounds, the potential targets and the related pathways of SBD remain unknown. With the advancement of analytical tools such as systems biology (Kitano, 2002), network biology (Barabási and Oltvai, 2004) and network pharmacology (Hopkins, 2008), the intricate and holistic mechanisms of TCMs may be elucidated in a fast and highly effective way.

Recently, as a novelty discipline, systems pharmacology provides a new manner that integrates pharmacology and systems biology pharmacology, provides a new approach to explore TCMs across multiple scales of complexity ranging from molecular and cellular levels to tissue and organism levels (Berger and Iyengar, 2009). Systems pharmacology contains pharmacokinetics (ADME properties of drugs) evaluation, target prediction as well as network analysis (Huang et al., 2014), which offers a platform for identifying multiple mechanisms of action of medicine. In our previous work, the systems pharmacology method has been successfully applied to uncover the underlying function mechanisms of TCM formulas for cancer, depression, and cardiovascular diseases treatment (Li et al., 2014; Zhang et al., 2014; Zheng et al., 2014).

Here, we introduce the method of systems pharmacology to resolve the underlying action mechanisms of herbal medicines in the treatment of NSCLC. Firstly, we filtered active compounds from the constructed SBD compound database by calculating pharmacokinetic properties and evaluating their oral bioavailability (OB) and drug-likeness (DL). Then, based on the integrated target prediction methods which united the biological and mathematical models, homologous targets of these active compound were predicted. Subsequently, obtained targets were validated by function enrichment analysis and target-disease interactions analysis. Ultimately, the network pharmacology and NSCLC-related signaling pathways evaluation were carried out to systematically disclose the underlying reciprocity between active compounds, active targets and pathways. The results not only significantly improved our understanding of NSCLC treatment mechanism, but also dissected the molecular mechanism of action of SBD, which promoted the exploitation of TCM in the treatment of sophisticated diseases. And *in vitro* experiments were conducted to evaluate the reliability of some vital active compounds and targets. Additionally, our *in vivo* results, which we subsequently confirmed using *in vitro* mechanism based assays, demonstrate that the significant anti-tumor activity of baicalein from SBD is associated with a direct impact of baicalein on improving tumor-inflammatory microenvironment. Our characterization of baicalein mediated changes in enzymes, cytokines, chemokines, and other growth factors associated with a tumor-inflammatory microenvironment offer multiple candidates to serve as potential biomarkers for ongoing clinical trials. In this paper, the detailed flow chart is shown in **Figure 1**.

MATERIALS AND METHODS

Candidate Compound Database

All candidate compounds of SBD were manually collected from a wide scale text mining and our in-house developed database: the Traditional Chinese Medicine Systems Pharmacology Database (TCMSP[1]) (Ru et al., 2014). We got a total of 80 candidate compounds including flavonoids, terpenoids, and others. Glycosides were easy to hydrolyze into free glycosides absorbed by intestinal mucosa (Németh et al., 2003). Therefore, two aglycone compounds of glycosides in herbs were also added into the compound database for SBD. Eventually, we obtained 82 related compounds of SBD.

ADME Screening

To investigate the active compounds of SBD that play a role in anti-NSCLC, we predicted the OB (predicted OB) and DL (predicted drug-likeness) values of them.

Oral Bioavailability

Oral bioavailability is considered to be an important indicator of the efficiency of active drug delivery to the systemic circulation, and OB is therefore one of the most important ADME of oral drugs. In this article, OB screening is calculated by a powerful internal system, OBioavail1.1 (Xu et al., 2012), we set the OB value mainly considering the following two factors as the basic principle. First, the information extracted from the studied medicines should be as much as probable with a minimum of molecules. Second, reasonably explaining the obtaining model by the reported pharmacological data (Wang et al., 2013). In this work, we have obtained an OB value of 30%, and the selected active compounds will be analyzed in the next step.

Drug-Likeness

Drug-likeness (DL) is used to estimate the similarity of physical properties of compounds with known drugs. In order to pick out the drug-like active molecules from SBD, based on molecular

[1] http://lsp.nwu.edu.cn/index.php

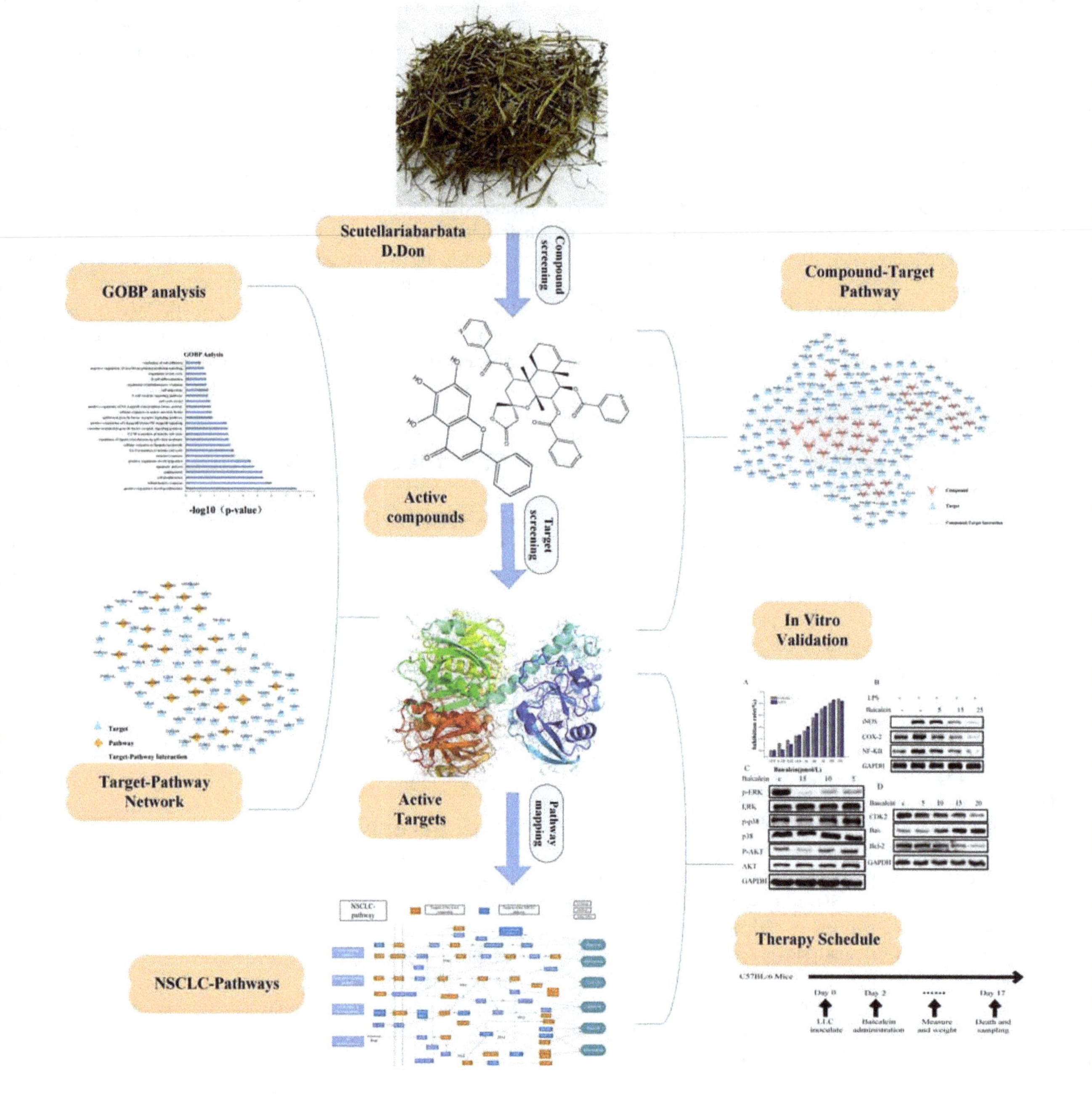

FIGURE 1 | Systems pharmacology approach workflow.

descriptors and Tanimoto similarity (Yamanishi et al., 2010; Liu et al., 2013), we used a self-constructed model DL to calculate the drug-likeness index of these compounds. The Drug-likeness evaluation method is as follows:

$$T(A, B) = (A * B) / (|A|^2 + |B|^2 - A * B)$$

Here, A is defined as a molecular descriptor for herbal compounds and B is defined as the average molecular properties of all compounds in Drug Bank database[2] (Wishart et al., 2008). In this work, a compound with DL $\geq$ 0.18 was selected as the active compound for further study.

In order to acquire the potential active compounds, the screening principle was defined as follows: OB $\geq$ 30%; DL $\geq$ 0.18.

Target Prediction

To establish a direct link between the potential active compounds of SBD and the target, target selection for active compounds remains an urgent step. Therefore, compounds were further

[2]http://www.drugbank.ca/

analyzed at the gene level. Firstly, targets exploration was fulfilled based on the weighted ensemble similarity (WES) and systematic drug targeting tool (SysDT). SysDT is a powerful computational model combining mathematics and bioinformatics. However, WES is a *in silico* model to pinpoint the drug direct targets of the actual bioactive ingredients (Liu et al., 2017). Secondly, we have mapped targets for UniProt[3], unifying their names and organisms. Normalized compound targets are mapped to the CTD database[4] (Davis et al., 2013), Therapeutic Target Database (TTD[5]) (Zhu et al., 2012), and Pharmacogenomics Knowledgebase (PharmGKB[6]) (Thorn et al., 2013) to obtain their associated diseases, providing a clearly defined target-disease relationship.

GOBP

To probe the involved biological processes of the obtained targets, in this work, gene ontology (GO) enrichment analysis was performed by linking targets to DAVID (The Database for Annotation, Visualization and Integrated Discovery[7]) (Wang J. et al., 2018). Terms from "Biological Process" (GOBP) were utilized to symbol gene function (Yang et al., 2018). Only GO terms with p-value ≤ 0.05 were chosen. The false discovery rate (FDR) was introduced to reveal a multiple-hypothesis testing faulty measure of p-values by utilizing the web tool DAVID. We employed a 0.05 FDR criteria as an important cut off in our analysis.

Network Construction

Currently, we have completed the screening and mapping of the active compounds and active targets. In order to investigate the multiple action mechanism of active compounds against NSCLC, and further clarify the relationship between active targets and active compounds. The Cytoscape 3.6.0 (Liu et al., 2016), a popular bioinformatics software package for biological network visualization and data integration was used. Two types of global networks were constructed: compound-target (C-T) network and target-pathway network (T-P) (Yu et al., 2012). In the magic network, compounds, targets, and pathways were represented by nodes, and the relationship between them was represented by the edges. In addition, degree (a vital topological parameter) was analyzed by the plug in Network Analyzer of Cytoscape (Shannon et al., 2003). The degree of a node is defined as the number of edges connected to that node.

In order to explore the integrative mechanisms of the formula for NSCLC, firstly, the activity target was mapped to the KEGG database[8] (Kanehisa et al., 2017) and we got the basic information of the pathway. Secondly, according to the latest NSCLC pathological information, an integrated "NSCLC-Pathway" was assembled by integrating the key pathways that obtained through the T-P network and C-P network analysis.

Experimental Validation

Cell and Mice

Human NSCLC H1975, RAW264.7 and Lewis lung carcinoma (LLC) cells were obtained from Chinese Academy of Sciences Shanghai cell bank. H1975 cells were cultured in RPMI1640 (Gibco) media complemented with 10% heat inactivated fetal bovine serum (FBS). RAW264.7 and LLC cells were cultured in DMEM (Gibco, United States) with 10% FBS. Cells were cultured at 37°C with 5% CO_2 for all experiments. Mice were maintained under specific pathogen-free conditions at the Institute of Laboratory Animals, Jiangsu Kanion Parmaceutical, Co., Ltd. and used under protocols approved by the respective Institute of pharmacology and toxicology institutional review board (IRB), all animal experiments were performed in accordance with national and European guidelines. C57BL/6 mice (6–8 week-old) were purchased from the Comparative Medicine Centre of Yangzhou University. Female C57BL/6 wild type mice (6–8 week-old) were inoculated subcutaneously in the right flank with 5×10^5 LLC cells per mouse (day 0). Before treatment, mice were then randomized into two groups: control ($n = 6$), Baicalein ($n = 6$). Baicalein (1.5 mg/kg, Yuan ye, Shanghai) was treated every day administration after the tumor inoculation (day 2). For untreated mice, an isotype control for physiological saline was intraperitoneally (i.p.) injected. Tumors were measured on every alternate day, and tumor volumes were calculated using the formula for a typical ellipsoid length $\times$ (width^2) $\times$ 0.5(mm^3). For survival decomposition, mice with tumors greater than the length limit of 20 mm were sacrificed and counted as dead. To examine the requirement of the priming and effector phases of tumor mass, the mice were sacrificed and tumors harvested for analysis, following 17 day observations and measurements.

Cell Viability Assay

Baicalein was purchased from Shanghai Yuanye Bio-Technology, Co., Ltd. (HPLC $\geq$ 98%, shanghai, China). Test samples were dissolved in dimethylsulfoxide (DMSO) (Sigma, United States) to get 100 mM, as a stock solution, and then stored at 4°C, it was not degrade due to high concentration of DMSO. The final dilutions of DMSO added to the culture medium never exceeded 0.1% what insured there was no effect on cell viability.

H1975 cells in the logarithmic phase were seeded at a density of 1×10^5 cells/ml in 96-well culture plates. After incubated 48 h, cells were exposed to different concentrations of baicalein (1.675, 3.125, 6.25, 12.5, 25, 50, 100, and 150 μmol/L), RAW264.7 and H1975 cells have the same experimental protocol. After treatment for 48 h, then, 10 μl of CCK-8 assay (Best Bio, Shanghai, China) was added to each well and the cells were incubated for 1–4 h at 37°C and 5% CO_2. A plate reader was used to detect the optical density (OD) absorbance at 450 nm. The cell viability was calculated as: OD of treatment/OD of control $\times$ 100%.

[3] http://www.uniprot.org
[4] http://ctdbase.org/
[5] http://database.idrb.cqu.edu.cn/TTD
[6] https://www.pharmgkb.org
[7] http://david.abcc.ncifcrf.gov
[8] http://www.genome.jp/kegg/

Western Blotting

Cells were scraped, collected by centrifugation and lysis in Qproteome^{TM} Mammalian Protein Prep Kit (Qiagen, Germany). The protein concentration of lysate was measured by a Quick Stari Bradford Protein Assay Kit (Bio-Rad, United States). Equal amount of protein taken from each sample was electrophoresis by 10% SDS-page gel electrophoresis and electroblotted onto nitrocellulose membranes, which were then incubated in a blocking buffer of 5% bovine serum albumin (BSA) in Tris-buffered saline. Primary antibody incubations were done overnight at 4°C in blocking buffer. After washing, secondary antibody incubations was done at room temperature for 1–1.5 h in blocking buffer. Primary antibodies recognizing the following proteins were obtained from ABcam: COX-2, iNOS, NF-κB, p38, ERK, p-p38, P-ERK, AKT, p-AKT, Bcl-2, CDK2, Bax, GAPDH. The membranes were detected by using the Clarity^{TM} Western ECL substrate (Bio-Rad) and labeling were visualized by Imagelab software (Bio-Rad).

Flow Cytometry Staining and Analysis

Tumors were digested with collagenase and hyaluronidase for 1 h at 37°C. After lysising of red blood cell, the dissociated cells were incubated on ice for 10 min, and then spun down at 300 g, 4°C for 7 min, cells from these tumors were either used for flow cytometry analysis or further processed and used for functional analyses. Tumor cell suspensions, were washed, blocked with Fc Block (anti-mouse CD16/32 mAb; BD Biosciences) at 4°C on ice for 15 min, and stained with fluorescence conjugated antibodies against surface markers CD49b, CD3E, CD8a, and CD25. These antibodies were purchased from BioLegend, eBioscience, or BD Biosciences. Cells were then fixed in Fixation/Permeabilization buffer (eBioscience) and stained with antibodies against intracellular proteins, including FoxP3 (BioLegend), granzyme B and interferon-γ (IFN-γ) (BD Pharmingen). Stained cells and isotype-control-stained cells, were assayed using a BD FACSVerse (BD Biosciences, United States). Data analysis was performed using the FlowJo (Tree Star) software.

Statistical Analysis

All Data are rendered as means ± standard error and the statistical results are analyzed by a one-way ANOVA and Student's t-test. p-Values below 0.05 were considered as statistically significant.

RESULTS

Active Compounds Screening

In this work, a total of 82 SBD related candidate compounds were collected from the SBD. To screen out the active compounds, it is significant to evaluate the compounds' ADME properties including oral bioavailability (OB $\geq$ 30%) and drug-likeness (DL $\geq$ 0.18). As a result, based on the satisfactory screening conditions: 33 active components have been identified by us. In order to acquire more comprehensive results and make up for the theoretical screening deficiencies, some certain unqualified compounds, which have relatively poor pharmacokinetic properties, but are the most abundant and active compounds of certain herbs, were also selected as the active components for further study. For example, quercetin has poor OB (25%) property, it has been retained for further analysis as it is the main component of SBD and has anticancer and anti-inflammatory effects (Mukherjee and Khuda-Bukhsh, 2015). Also, luteolin with relatively poor OB (26.5%) was retained for further analysis since it exerts remarkable tumor suppressive activity on various types of cancers, including NSCLC (Jiang J et al., 2018). In the end, we obtained all 33 candidate components (**Supplementary Table 1**) (The structures of the compounds were derived from NCBI[9]) of SBD. Thereinto, flavonoids compounds have been reported to demonstrate significant biologic activity including anti-inflammatory, inhibit tumor angiogenesis, and cell cycle arrest (Zhang L. et al., 2017; Anwar et al., 2018). Such as, apigenin (MOL001 OB = 33.6% DL = 0.25), baicalein (MOL070 0B = 44.6% DL = 0.21). According to reports, diterpene compounds have activity test results, indicating that diterpene alkaloids have good cytotoxicity and can effectively inhibit the growth of a variety of human tumor cells (Lee and Ychoi, 2010), for example, Scutebarbatine F. In addition to the above components, SBD also contains ursolic acid, β-sitosterol, which has significant antitumor activity (Song et al., 2017; Rajavel et al., 2018). These active compounds could be the main elements for curing NSCLC.

Target and Function Analysis

To get the targets related to NSCLC we firstly identified 225 targets of these active compounds by means of the WES and SysDT algorithms. The results shown that the candidate compounds act on multiple targets, and one target can also be linked to multiple candidate molecules. For example, target Nitric oxide synthase 2 (NOS2) corresponds to 15 compounds accounting for 45% of the total active compounds. Subsequently, as we know, increasing evidence has identified that improving the inflammatory microenvironment plays a crucial role in the research progress of NSCLC (Lee et al., 2017). Hence, the targets involved in the biological progress of NSCLC will be further preserved. Then, 225 candidate targets were mapping to the CTD, TTD, PharmGKB database to obtain the corresponding target related diseases. After screening, we finally retrieved 145 potential targets (**Supplementary Table 2**).

GOBP Analysis

To identify and analyze whether the biological process corresponding to the active target corresponds to NSCLC. GO (p-value $\leq$ 0.05) enrichment analysis was used to obtain 24 vital biological processes (**Figure 2**) by mapping targets to DAVID and screening. The results shown that the majority of these targets were strongly associated with various biological processes, including negative regulation of apoptosis process, positive regulation of cell proliferation, positive regulation of cell migration, inflammatory response, and angiogenesis. These

[9]https://pubchem.ncbi.nlm.nih.gov

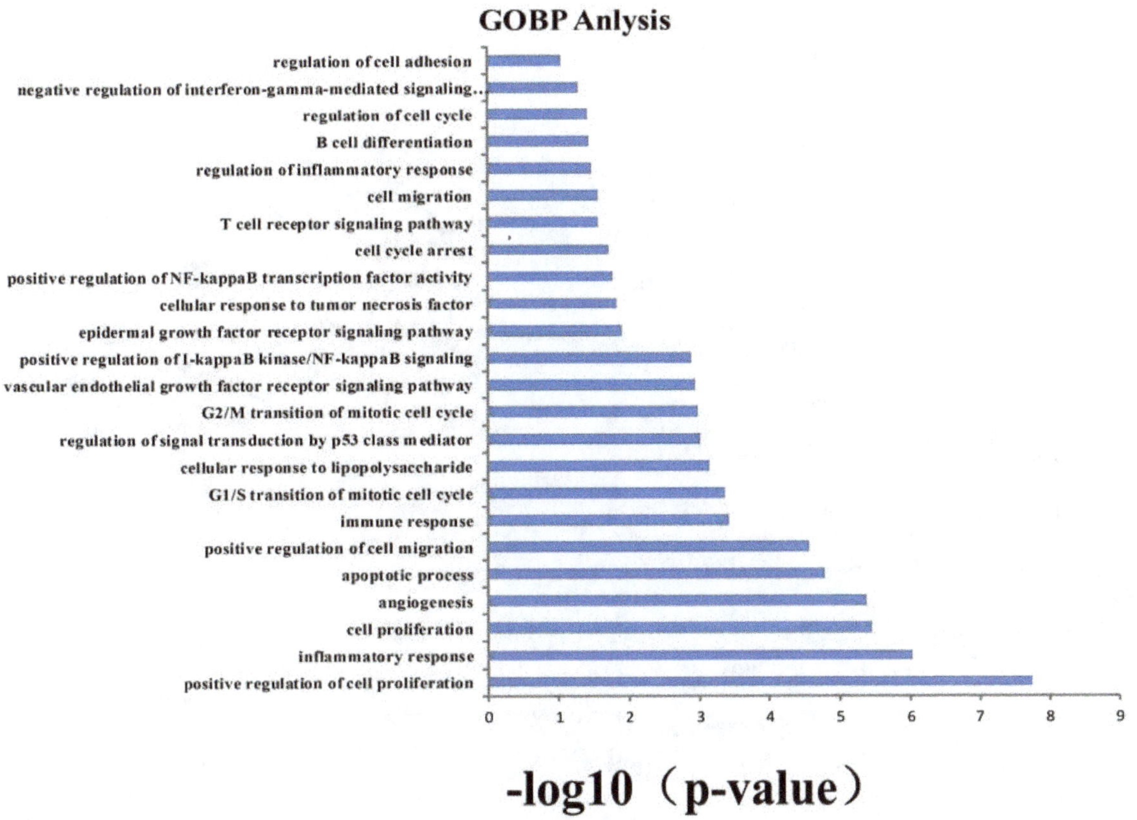

FIGURE 2 | Gene ontology (GO) analysis of potential target genes. *y*-axis shows significantly enriched "biological process" (BP) categories in GO relative to the target genes, and *x*-axis shows the counts of targets.

biological processes are related to the research mechanism of NSCLC.

Compound-Target Network Evaluation

In order to more directly reflect the relationship between targets and compounds, we have used Cytoscape 3.6.0 to map out the C-T relation network diagram. As shown in **Figure 3**, C-T diagram consist of 187 nodes (33 active compound nodes and 145 active target nodes) and 684 edges. Subsequently, C-T network topology analysis showed that the average degree of targets for each target was 4.7, illustrating the multi-target nature of SBD. Among the 33 active compounds, 25 of them show a high degree (degree > 10), which may play a key role in the network. Meanwhile, each active compound is associated with multiple targets, manifesting the potential synergistic effects among them.

Here, baicalein (MOL070) is the core component of SBD and display the highest number of target interactions (degree = 46). Previously, baicalein has been shown to have anti-cancer activities in several human cancer cell types including breast cancer, ovarian cancer, and colonic cancer (Yu et al., 2014; Wang et al., 2017; Dou et al., 2018). But beyond that, scutellarin (MOL036, degree = 39), a flavonoid used in Chinese herbal medicine, inhibited the proliferation and migration of human NSCLC cells (Sun et al., 2018). Also, wogonin (MOL007, degree = 27) is one of the active components of favonoids that are present in extracts from SBD. Recently, regulating immune function, anticancer and anti-inflammatory effects of wogonin have been discovered (Wang et al., 2010; Shi et al., 2017; Zhao et al., 2018). So, we speculate that the top three compounds might be the crucial elements in the treatment of NSCLC, which might exhibit anti-tumor and anti- inflammatory effects of SBD in the treatment of NSCLC. For instance, phosphatidylinositol-4,5-bisphosphate 3-kinase catalytic subunit gamma (PIK3CG, degree = 7) is targeted by seven active compounds from SBD. PIK3CG induces a transcription process that promotes immune suppression tumor growth and inflammation (Kaneda et al., 2017). Then, prostaglandin G/H synthase 2 (PTGS2, degree = 10) is simultaneously targeted by 10 active compounds, and has high expression in various tumors, which can promote tumor growth and regulates inflammatory response (Liu et al., 2018; Zhu et al., 2018). All of these suggest that SBD probably treat NSCLC by anti-inflammatory, inhibiting tumor angiogenesis, cell cycle arrest, and promoting apoptosis.

Target-Pathway Network Evaluation

The result displays that 145 targets are further mapped to 108 pathways, which show an average degree of 6.85 per pathway and 2.8 per target pathway. Then, we discover that several target proteins (71/145) are mapped to multiple pathways (≥ 5),

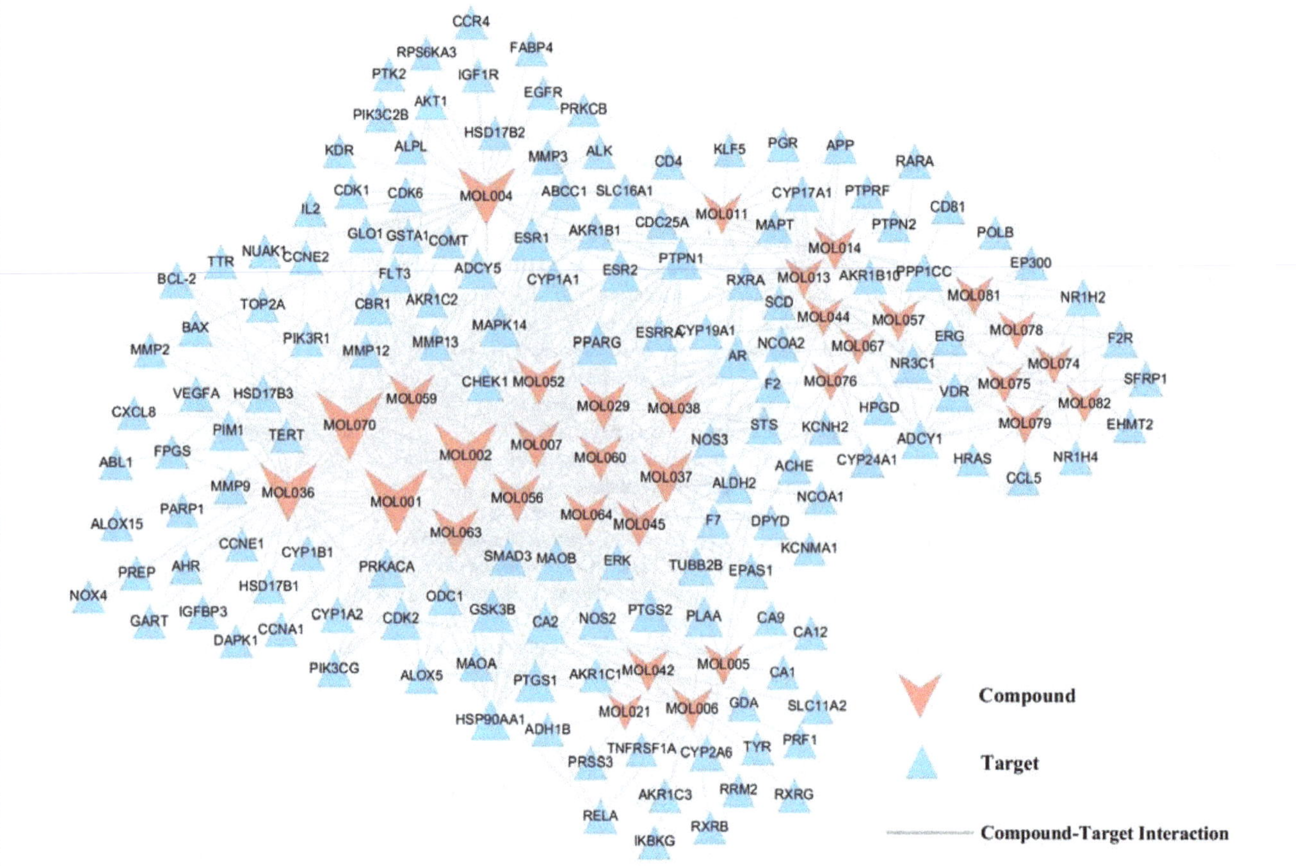

FIGURE 3 | C-T network. A compound node and a target node are connected, if the gene is targeted by the consistent compound. Node size is relative to its degree.

exhibiting that these targets might intercede the interactions and cross-talk between different pathways. Meanwhile, numerous pathways (70/108), also regulated by multiple target proteins ($\geq$8), might be the main factors for NSCLC. As shown in **Figure 4**, those pathways were tightly interacted with targets. Such as, PI3K-Akt signaling pathway (degree = 21), VEGF signaling pathway (degree = 11). For instance, The PI3K-Akt pathway is an important signaling pathway that may activate downstream of a series of extracellular signals and impact on cellular processes including cell proliferation, apoptosis, and survival (Jiang Z. Q. et al., 2018; Tan et al., 2018), which can be targeted by numerous active compound like wogonin (MOL007), baicalein (MOL070) quercetin (MOL002), apigenin (MOL001), and so forth. Hence, PI3K-Akt signaling pathway with the highest degree may be a significant pathway involved in the proliferation, apoptosis against NSCLC. Also, tumor angiogenesis, apoptosis, and migration related pathways were also enriched, like VEGF signaling pathway mediates the absolute dependence of tumor cells on the continuous supply of blood vessels to nourish their growth and to facilitate metastasis (Li et al., 2012). Hence, tumor vascularization is a vital process for tumor growth, invasion, and metastasis. SBD may be served as an attractive herb in anti-NSCLC therapy. In addition, P53 signaling pathway also stands out in the enriched pathway list, which can mediate cell cycle arrest and cell proliferation (Hsua et al., 2001). Therefore, it is concluded that SBD opportunity regulates the treatment of NSCLC through anti-inflammation, cell cycle arrest, tumor angiogenesis, cell apoptosis, and other pathways.

NSCLC-Pathway Construction

Considering the complex mechanism of SBD in the treatment of NSCLC, an integrated "NSCLC-pathway" was constructed by integrating the key pathways that obtained through the T-P network analysis. NSCLC-pathway (**Figure 5**) that comprises of four signaling pathways such as hsa04370: VEGF signaling pathway, hsa04151:PI3K-Akt signaling pathway, hsa04115: p53 signaling pathway and hsa04064: NF-kappa B signaling pathway. The target proteins of the integrated "NSCLC-pathway" exhibit markedly close functional relationship with the NSCLC related proteins. As shown in **Figure 5**, the NSCLC-pathway can be separated into two represent therapeutic modules (Inflammation related module and tumor related module). Inflammation related module consists of hsa04064: NF-kappa B signaling pathway. Then, tumor related module including hsa04370: VEGF signaling pathway, hsa04151:

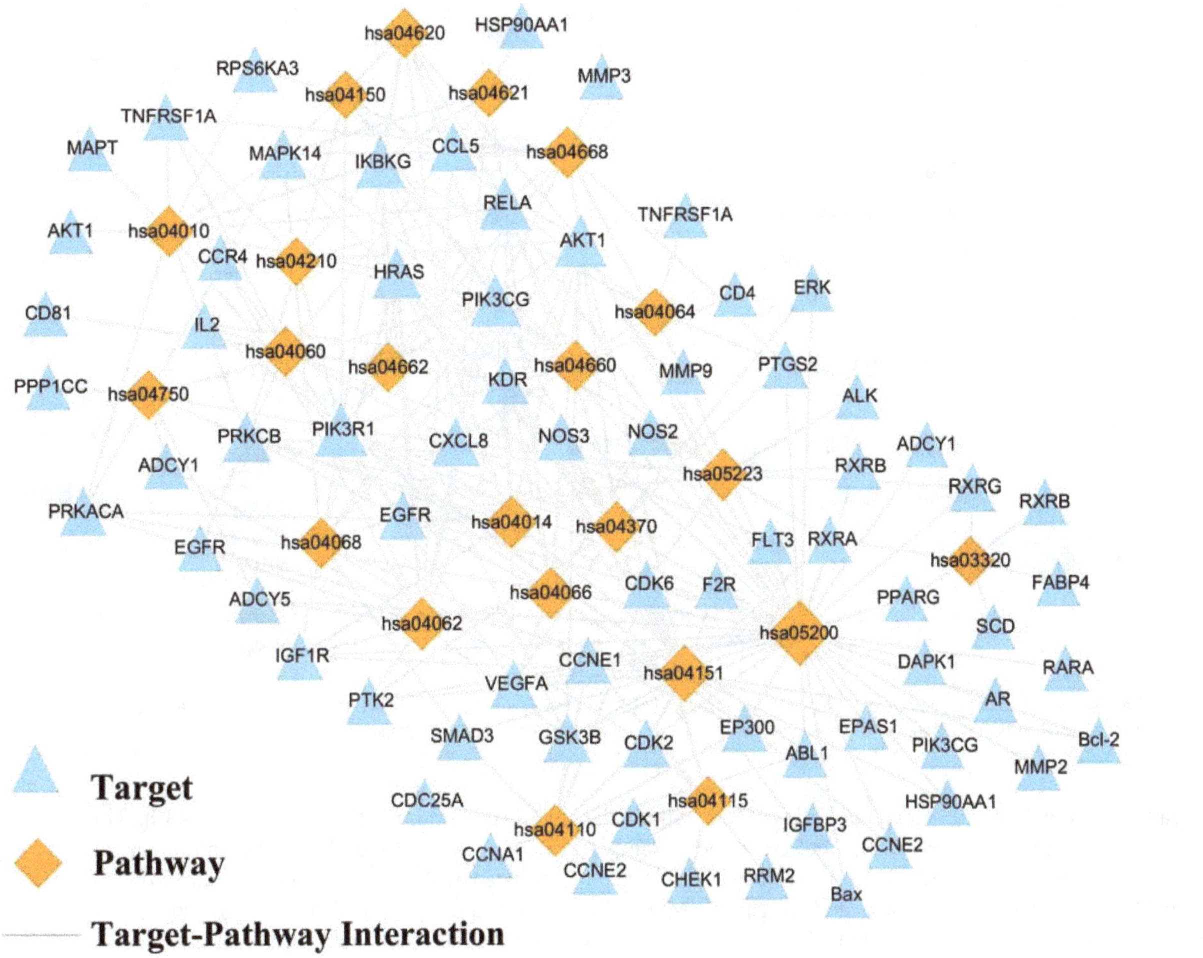

FIGURE 4 | T-P network. The T-P network was consisted of targets and pathways, if the pathway is linked to the target. Node size is related to the degree.

PI3K-Akt signaling pathway and hsa04115; p53 signaling pathway.

Inflammation Related Module

Inflammatory microenvironment plays a very important role in all stages of tumor development. Many important cytokines and chemical factors participate in this process. At the same time, the tumor microenvironment promotes the continuous response of the inflammation. Thus, it is necessary to control the development of the tumor by targeting the key signaling pathway in the tumor-inflammatory microenvironment. In **Figure 5**, baicalein (MOL070) activates transcription factor p65 (NF-κB), which reduces the expression of the downstream proteins prostaglandin G/H synthase 2 (COX-2) and Nitric oxide synthase (iNOS). For example, The NF-κB family of transcription factors is involved in the activation of a wide range of genes associated with inflammation, differentiation, tumorigenesis, embryonic development, and apoptosis (Ozawa et al., 2018; Zakaria et al., 2018). Then, COX-2 is not expressed in most normal tissues at high levels but is strongly induced by LPS and many cytokines, playing a crucial role in the development of various inflammatory responses (Zhang Q. et al., 2017). The results showed that baicalein form SBD could be utilized to treat NSCLC by regulating the anti-inflammatory activities of NF-κB, COX-2, and iNOS.

Tumor Related Module

As shown in the **Figure 5**, tumor related targets in the active targets are mapped to three pathways, including P53 signaling pathway, PI3K-AKT signaling pathway and VEGF signaling pathway. These pathways control tumor development by inhibiting cell proliferation and cell cycle. For example, in the P53 signaling pathway, baicalein (MOL070) can extensively act on cdk-Cyclin complexes and inhibit their activity, especially G1 phase cdk2-CyclinE (CDK2). It has been reported that the cell cycle is blocked by baicalein therapy, thus inhibiting cell proliferation (Hsua et al., 2001). These results suggested that baicalein from SBD inhibits NSCLC proliferation by incomplete DNA synthesis and cell division. Additionally, some targets in the PI3K-AKT signaling pathway engage in equaling the levels between the cell cycle and apoptosis. The apoptosis signaling can be initiated either at face through

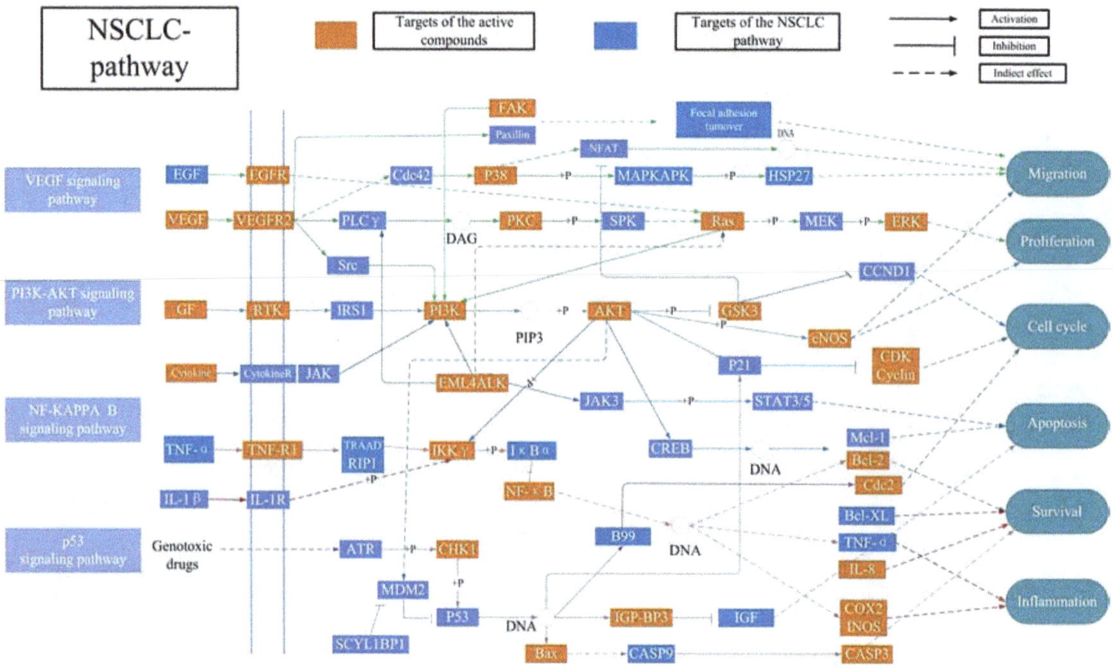

FIGURE 5 | Distribution of target proteins of SBD on the compressed 'NSCLC-pathway.' Four pathways form the tubular NSCLC pathway. Arrows show activation active, T-arrows show inhibition active and segments represent indirectly activation effect or inhibition effect.

a death receptor-induced signaling pathway or within the cell via the release of proapoptotic molecules. For example, Apoptosis regulator Bcl-2 (Bcl-2) can be regulated by baicalein (MOL070), scutellarin (MOL036), and wogonin (MOL007). Previous data *in vivo* indicated that Caspases are linked to Bcl-2 family which is the key regulator of apoptosis in cancer (Timucin et al., 2018). Furthermore, tumor vascularization is an important process of tumor growth, invasion, and metastasis. Anti-angiogenesis has been considered to be an attractive target anti-tumor treatment (Ferrara and Kerbel, 2005; Cooney et al., 2006; Tran et al., 2007). Such as, In the VEGF signaling pathway was modulated by wogonin (MOL007) and baicalein (MOL070). It has been reported in the literature that inhibition of the activation of VEGF downstream protein kinases Mitogen-activated protein kinase 14 (p38) and Mitogen-activated protein kinase 3 (ERK) can inhibit cell proliferation, survival, and migration (Galaria et al., 2004). Thus, all above suggest that SBD may treat NSCLC by regulating the cell cycle, apoptosis, and anti-angiogenesis.

In vitro Experimental Validation

CCK-8 Assay

In our pre-experiment, the RAW 264.7 cell viability as affected by the baicalein from SBD at various doses was determined by CCK-8 assay (**Figure 6A**), and the outcome showed that high cell viability (>70%) was attained for baicalein at <25 μmol/L, respectively. Thus, three doses of baicalein were taken (5, 15, and 25 μmol/L) for subsequent experiments.

H1975 cells (1×10^5 cells/ml) are cultured with the concentrations of 1.675 to 150 μmol per liter culture media with no serum of the baicalein for 48 h. Then, We performed CCK-8 assay to evaluate the inhibitory effects of baicalein induced proliferation of H1975 cells. Growth of H1975 cells was significantly inhibited by different concentrations of baicalein, and the 30% concentration of inhibition (IC30) of baicalein was 15 μmol/L respectively at 48 h (**Figure 6A**). Since lower doses baicalein had no inhibitory effect on the viability of H1975 cells, concentrations of baicalein (5, 10, 15, and 20 μmol/L) were chosen for subsequent experiments.

Targets Validation

To further assess the obtained results in systems pharmacology analysis, we have chosen baicalein from SBD to examine the compound potential anti-inflammatory effect using RAW264.7 cells treated with LPSs (1 ug/ml). In particular, we conduct western blot analysis for iNOS, NF-κB, and COX-2 protein expression to confirm anti-inflammatory effects of the predicted compounds.

As shown in **Figure 6B**, the levels of iNOS, NF-κB, and COX-2 proteins in the panel of RAW264.7 cell lines tested are reported. We observe that after baicalein treatment, the protein expressions of iNOS, NF-κB, and COX-2 in RAW264.7 cells are significantly declined. **Figure 6B** illustrates that baicalein treatment, as a single agent, causing a decrease of the iNOS, NF-κB, and COX-2 expression. To sum up, *in vitro* study provides additional information for screening compound with potentially anti-inflammatory effect and demonstrates the reliability of in systems pharmacology screen strategy.

To verify the reliability of anti-tumor related targets screened from systems pharmacology, we observe that baicalein treatment,

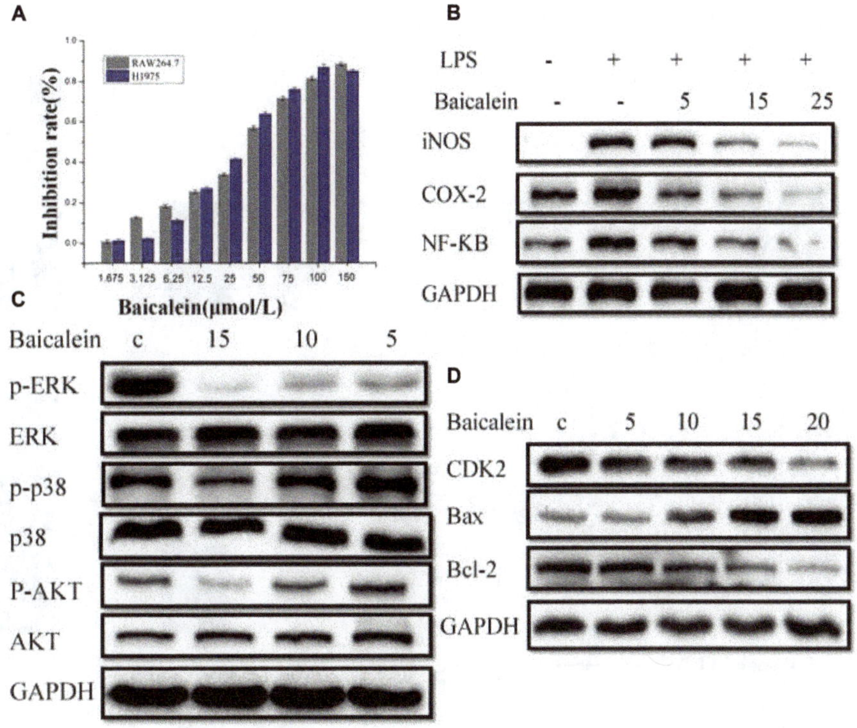

FIGURE 6 | *In vitro* Experimental validation. **(A)** Cell viability of RAW264.7 and H1975 cells. The determination of cell viability of RAW264.7 and H1975 cells was carried out by CCK-8 assay after treated with control or baicalein for 48 h. **(B)** RAW264.7 cells were pretreated with (5, 15, or 25 μM), or the combinations for 2 h, vehicle as the control. The exposure to LPS (1 μg/ml) for 20 h, then iNOS, NF-κB and COX-2 accumulation of cytoplasm were measured by western blot. GAPDH was used as loading control. **(C)** H1975 cells were treated with baicalein (5, 10, or 15 μM) for 2 h, next, cell lysates were used to assess the phosphorylation of ERK, p38, and AKT. The total ERK, p38, and AKT are shown as a loading control. **(D)** Western blot analysis of CDK2, Bax, and Bcl-2 expression in H1975 cells. Cells were treatment with or without baicalein (5, 10, 15, or 20 μM) for 24 h. All results are repeated at least three independent experiments with the same tendency.

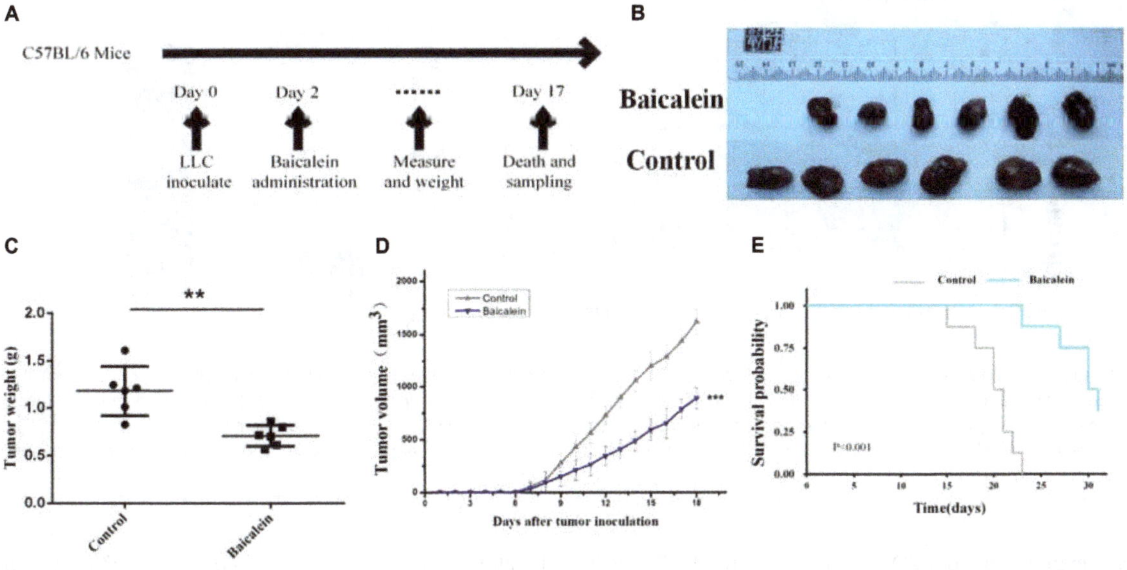

FIGURE 7 | *In vivo* Experimental validation. **(A)** Schematic diagram of *in vivo* experimental schedule. **(B,C)** LLC-tumors derived from control and baicalein (5×10^5 cells per C57B/L6 mice, six mice for each group) were photographed and weighed immediately after tumor extraction (mean ± SD; $^{**}p < 0.01$). **(D,E)** LLC-bearing mice were treated with control and baicalein. Tumor volume and survival rates are shown in **(D,E)**. Data represent the means ± SEM of six mice. $^{*}p < 0.05$, two-tailed Student's *t*-test.

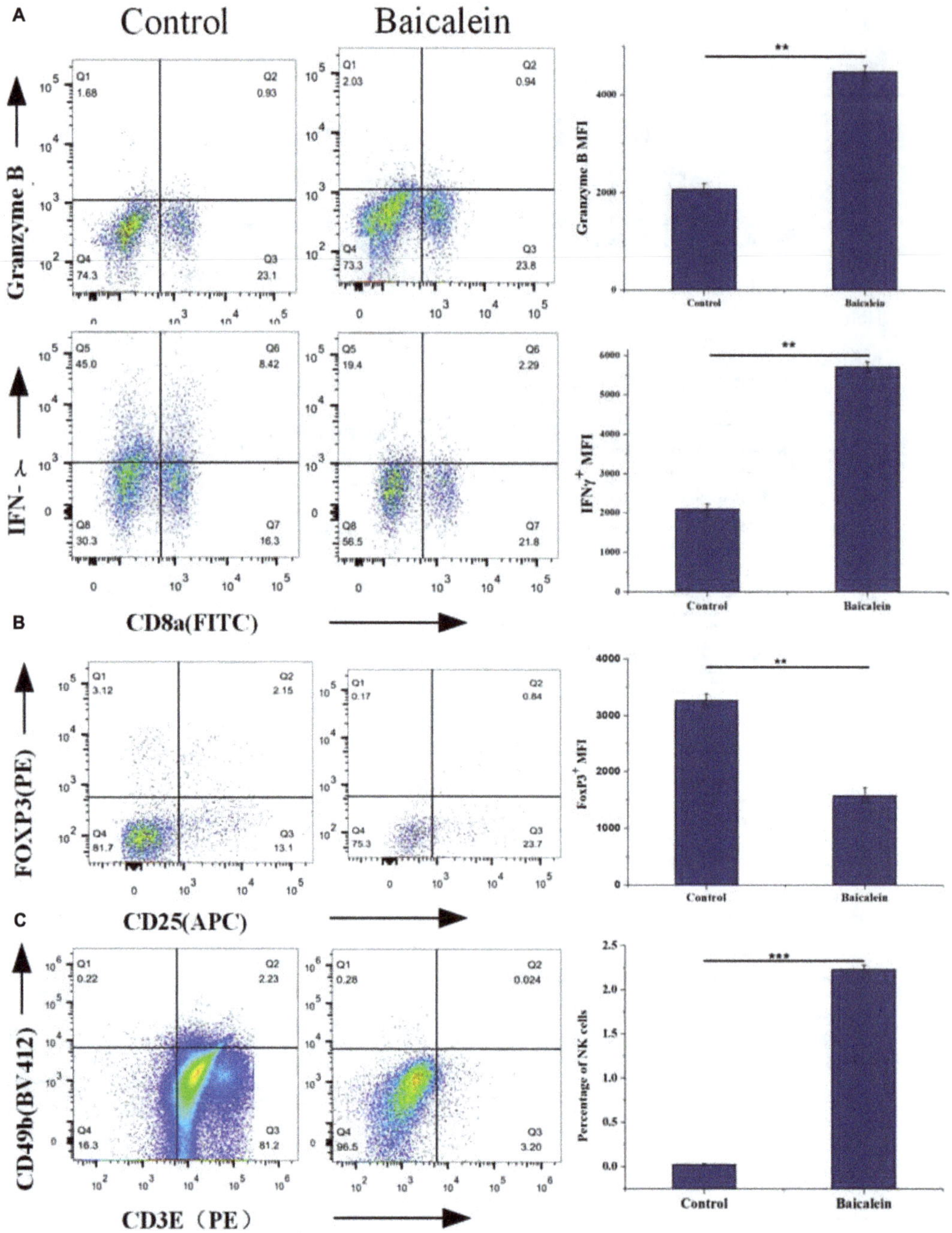

FIGURE 8 | *In vivo* Experimental validation, tumor samples were isolated from LLC-bearing mice at the end of the study and processed for flow cytometry analysis. **(A)** Percentage of CD8+ Granzyme B+ and CD8+ IFNγ+ T cells of CD45+ cells were measured by Flow cytometry, and protein expression shown as mean fluorescence intensity (MFI). **(B)** Flow cytometry analysis of tumor samples shows the effect of control and baicalein treatment on Foxp3 levels. **(C)** FACS analysis of tumor-cell suspensions from LLC-bear mice after control or baicalein treatment. Quantification of NK cell present in the tumor samples. Results are shown as mean ± SEM (***p* < 0.01; ****p* < 0.001).

the protein expressions of CDK2 and Bax in H1975 cells were both declined significantly at different dose levels. Our results show that after 24 h, an increase in Bax levels and a decrease in the level of CDK2 were detected in the P53 signaling pathway (**Figure 6D**), indicating that activating Bax and inhibiting CDK2 were vital for anti-NSCLC. Then, in the VEGF signaling pathway the phosphorylation of p38 was significantly down-regulated in baicalein-induced H1975 cells compared to those of the control group. Also, we examined the activation of ERK, baicalein inhibited phosphorylation of ERK in H1975 cells. However, total protein levels were not affected (**Figure 6C**), suggesting baicalein inhibited angiogenesis and cell proliferation by regulating VEGF signaling pathways. Next, we found that the p-AKT expression was down-regulated in H1975 cells treated with baicalein. In addition, the expression of Bcl-2 was decreased by baicalein treatment. The above results indicates that baicalein may suppress the PI3K/Akt pathway by down-regulating p-AKT (**Figure 6C**). Taken together, these data suggest that baicalein from SBD may treat the NSCLC by cell cycle arrest, promote apoptosis, and anti-angiogenesis.

In vivo Experiments

To elucidate the molecular mechanism of SBD in treating LLC tumor-bearing mice, we sought evidential insight for the driver of anti-tumor by improving the tumor-inflammatory microenvironment after baicalein from SBD administration (**Figure 7A**). LLC tumor-bearing mice were significantly more resistant to the development of baicalein mediate sarcoma than control mice and observed decreased tumor out growth (**Figures 7B–D**) and a significant survival benefit (**Figure 7E**) in baicalein-treated mice. Here, to evaluate the *in vivo* therapeutic effect of baicalein on NSCLC, tumor samples were collected from LLC tumor-bearing mice and subjected to fluorescence-activated cell sorting analysis. In the tumor-inflammatory microenvironment, we observed a significant increase in the proportion of cytotoxic CD8 + T cells in baicalein-treated mice, a sixfold of the proportion of CD8+/FoxP3+ cells compared to the control group. Also, reduction in the MFI of FoxP3+ Treg cells was observed in baicalein treatment group (**Figure 8B**), suggesting that an inhibition of Treg function associated with the reduction of FoxP3 protein expression (Ho et al., 2018) may be the direct result of the baicalein. Meanwhile, the baicalein therapy induced expansion of an IFNG and GZB-producing activated CD8+ T cell population in the tumor of mice (**Figure 8A**). Then, we examined the density of natural killer (NK) cells in the tumor sample. Significant positive correlations were observed between control and baicalein natural killer cells (**Figure 8C**). These results firmly establish that the baicalein from SBD therapy improves tumor inflammatory microenvironment mediated tumor control, resulting in a striking benefit in these advanced mouse models relevant to clinical.

DISCUSSION

Non-small cell lung cancer has a high degree of malignancy and it has the characteristics of an early metastasis, and the prognosis of NSCLC patients remains low despite the many advances that have occurred in early diagnosis and comprehensive therapies (Testa et al., 2018; Wang Z. et al., 2018). Therefore, search for antitumor drugs has become an important problem to be solved urgently.

Recently, SBD has been reported to possess vital biological activities, for instance anticancer activities (Zheng et al., 2018). In our work, the complex mechanism of SBD in the treatment of NSCLC was explored based on the system pharmacological work principle. Firstly, with the aid of the evaluation method, 33 active compounds were obtained from SBD and 145 active targets were predicted. These results reveal that the characteristics of SBD are multi-compounds and multi-targets anti-tumor effects. Then, target and C-T network analysis together display that some vital compounds of SBD such as wogonin, baicalein, and scutellarin may play an important role in the treatment of NSCLC, and SBD positively aiming for some targets like Bax, iNOS, and P38 exhibits the therapeutic effects against NSCLC by anti-inflammatory, promote apoptosis and anti-angiogenesis. In addition, The T-P network and the integrated NSCLC-relates pathway indicate that the major compounds of SBD might exert anti-NSCLC effect by modulating plenty different pathways including hsa04370:VEGF signaling pathway, hsa04151:PI3K-Akt signaling pathway, hsa04115:p53 signaling pathway and hsa04064:NF-kappa B signaling pathway. Based on our present study, the *in vitro* experiments further confirm that the baicalein from SBD combat NSCLC via regulating the critical proteins of our integrated NSCLC-pathway including COX-2, NF-κB, Bax, ERK, CDK1 and so on, attesting that NSCLC can be treated through a complex system with multi- compound-target-disease interactions. So, SBD exhibits anti-NSCLC effects in various aspects, including cell cycle arrest, anti-inflammatory, promoting apoptosis, and anti-angiogenesis in response to active compound. *In vivo*, additive therapeutic effects of baicalein were investigated for a tumor-bearing mouse model, where baicalein from SBD was demonstrated to possess high efficiency compared with control in the inhibition of tumor growth.

In summary, our study systematically indicated the inhibitory effect of SBD on anti-tumor *in vitro* and *in vivo*. These molecular mechanisms, including improve tumor inflammatory microenvironment, cell cycle arrest, promote apoptosis, and anti-angiogenesis are potentially those by which SBD exhibits its effectiveness in cancer treatment.

AUTHOR CONTRIBUTIONS

JL, MJ, and ZL contributed conception and design of the study. XZ and XL organized the database. JZ, YH, and XS performed the statistical analysis. MJ wrote the first draft of the manuscript. CZ, MJ, and WX wrote sections of the manuscript. All authors contributed to manuscript revision, read and approved the submitted version.

FUNDING

This work was supported by grants from Northwest University, National Natural Science Foundation of China (Grant Nos. 81803960 and U1603285). It also was supported by the Key Project of Natural Science Fund of Science and Technology Department of Shaanxi Province (Grant No. 2018JZ3007).

REFERENCES

Anwar, A., Uddin, N., Siddiqui, B. S., Siddiqui, R. A., Begum, S., and Choudhary, M. I. (2018). A natural flavonoid lawsonaringenin induces cell cycle arrest and apoptosis in HT-29 colorectal cancer cells by targeting multiple signalling pathways. *Mol. Biol. Rep.* 45, 1339–1348. doi: 10.1007/s11033-018-4294-5

Barabási, A., and Oltvai, Z. (2004). Network biology: understanding the cell's functional organization. *Nat. Rev. Genet.* 5, 101–113. doi: 10.1038/nrg1272

Berger, S. I., and Iyengar, R. (2009). Network analyses in systems pharmacology. *Bioinformatics* 25, 2466–2472. doi: 10.1093/bioinformatics/btp465

Cooney, M. M., Van, H. W., Bhakta, S., Ortiz, J., and Remick, S. C. (2006). Drug insight: vascular disrupting agents and angiogenesis–novel approaches for drug delivery. *Nat. Clin. Pract. Oncol.* 3, 682–692. doi: 10.1038/ncponc0663

Dai, Z. J., Lu, W. F., Jie, G., Kang, H. F., Ma, Y. G., Zhang, S. Q., et al. (2013). Anti-angiogenic effect of the total flavonoids in *Scutellaria barbata D. Don. BMC Complement. Altern. Med.* 13:150. doi: 10.1186/1472-6882-13-150

Davis, A. P., King, B. L., Mockus, S., Murphy, C. G., Saraceni-Richards, C., Rosenstein, M., et al. (2013). The comparative toxicogenomics database: update 2011. *Nucleic Acids Res* .41, D1104–D1114. doi: 10.1093/nar/gkq813

Dou, J., Wang, Z., Ma, L., Peng, B., Mao, K., Li, C., et al. (2018). Baicalein and baicalin inhibit colon cancer using two distinct fashions of apoptosis and senescence. *Oncotarget* 9, 20089–20102. doi: 10.18632/oncotarget.24015

Ferrara, N., and Kerbel, R. S. (2005). Angiogenesis as a therapeutic target. *Nature* 438, 967–974. doi: 10.1038/nature04483

Galaria, I. I., Fegley, A. J., Nicholl, S. M., Roztocil, E., and Davies, M. G. (2004). Differential regulation of ERK1/2 and p38(MAPK) by components of the Rho signaling pathway during sphingosine-1-phosphate-induced smooth muscle cell migration. *J. Surg. Res.* 114, 173–179. doi: 10.1016/j.jss.2004.05.012

Ho, M. M., Ng, A. V., Lam, S., and Hung, J. Y. (2007). Side population in human lung cancer cell lines and tumors is enriched with stem-like cancer cells. *Cancer Res.* 67, 4827–4833. doi: 10.1158/0008-5472.CAN-06-3557

Ho, W. S., Wang, H., Maggio, D., Kovach, J. S., Zhang, Q., Song, Q., et al. (2018). Pharmacologic inhibition of protein phosphatase-2A achieves durable immune-mediated antitumor activity when combined with PD-1 blockade. *Nat. Commun.* 9:2126. doi: 10.1038/s41467-018-04425-z

Hopkins, A. L. (2008). Network pharmacology: the next paradigm in drug discovery. *Nat. Chem. Biol.* 4, 682–690. doi: 10.1038/nchembio.118

Hsua, S. L., Hsieh, W. C., and Chou, C. J. (2001). Baicalein induces a dual growth arrest by modulating multiple cell cycle regulatory molecules. *Eur. J. Pharmacol.* 425, 165–171. doi: 10.1016/S0014-2999(01)01144-X

Huang, C., Zheng, C., Li, Y., Wang, Y., Lu, A., and Yang, L. (2014). Systems pharmacology in drug discovery and therapeutic insight for herbal medicines. *Brief. Bioinform.* 15, 710–733. doi: 10.1093/bib/bbt035

Jemal, A., Murray, T., Ward, E., Samuels, A., Tiwari, R. C., Ghafoor, A., et al. (2003). Cancer Statistics, 2005. *Ca A Cancer J. Clin.* 53, 5–26. doi: 10.3322/canjclin.53.1.5

Jiang, J., Xu, Y., Ren, H., Wudu, M., Wang, Q., Song, X., et al. (2018). MKRN2 inhibits migration and invasion of non-small-cell lung cancer by negatively regulating the PI3K/Akt pathway. *J. Exp. Clin. Cancer Res.* 37:189. doi: 10.1186/s13046-018-0855-7

Jiang, Z. Q., Li, M. H., Qin, Y. M., Jiang, H. Y., Zhang, X., and Wu, M. H. (2018). Luteolin inhibits tumorigenesis and induces apoptosis of non-small cell lung cancer cells via regulation of MicroRNA-34a-5p. *Int. J. Mol. Sci.* 19:E447. doi: 10.3390/ijms19020447

Kaneda, M., Messer, K., Ralainirina, N., Li, H., Leem, C., Gorjestani, S., et al. (2017). PI3K gamma is a molecular switch that controls immune suppression. *Nature* 539, 437–442. doi: 10.1038/nature19834

Kanehisa, M., Furumichi, M., Tanabe, M., and Sato, Y. (2017). Morishima, K., KEGG: new perspectives on genomes, pathways, diseases and drugs. *Nucleic Acids Res.* 45, D353–D361. doi: 10.1093/nar/gkw1092

Kitano, H. (2002). Systems biology: a brief overview. *Science* 295, 1662–1664. doi: 10.1126/science.1069492

Lee, H., and Ychoi, K. (2010). Two novel neo-clerodane diterpenoids from *Scutellaria barbata. Cheminform* 20, 288–290. doi: 10.1016/j.bmcl.2009.10.116

Lee, H. A., Koh, E. K., Sung, J. E., Kim, J. E., Song, S. H., Kim, D. S., et al. (2017). Ethyl acetate extract from *Asparagus cochinchinensis* exerts anti-inflammatory effects in LPS-stimulated RAW264. 7 macrophage cells by regulating COX-2/iNOS, inflammatory cytokine expression, MAP kinase pathways, the cell cycle and anti-oxidant activity. *Mol. Med. Rep.* 15, 1613–1623. doi: 10.3892/mmr.2017.6166

Li, B., Tao, W., Zheng, C., Shar, P. A., Huang, C., Fu, Y., et al. (2014). Systems pharmacology-based approach for dissecting the addition and subtraction theory of traditional Chinese medicine: an example using Xiao-Chaihu-Decoction and Da-Chaihu-decoction. *Comput. Biol. Med.* 53, 19–29. doi: 10.1016/j.compbiomed.2014.05.007

Li, X., Wang, X., Ye, H., Peng, A., and Chen, L. (2012). Barbigerone, an isoflavone, inhibits tumor angiogenesis and human non-small-cell lung cancer xenografts growth through VEGFR2 signaling pathways. *Cancer Chemother. Pharmacol.* 70, 425–437. doi: 10.1007/s00280-012-1923-x

Liu, H., Wang, J., Zhou, W., Wang, Y., and Yang, L. (2013). Systems approaches and polypharmacology for drug discovery from herbal medicines: an example using licorice. *J. Ethnopharmacol.* 146, 773–793. doi: 10.1016/j.jep.2013.02.004

Liu, J., Pei, T., Mu, J., Zheng, C., Chen, X., Huang, C., et al. (2016). Systems pharmacology uncovers the multiple mechanisms of xijiao dihuang decoction for the treatment of viral hemorrhagic fever. *Evid. Based Complement. Altern. Med.* 2016, 1–17. doi: 10.1155/2016/9025036

Liu, J., Zhu, J., Xue, J., Qin, Z., Shen, F., Liu, J., et al. (2017). In silico -based screen synergistic drug combinations from herb medicines: a case using *Cistanche tubulosa. Sci. Rep.* 7:16364. doi: 10.1038/s41598-017-16571-3

Liu, Q., Tong, D., Liu, G., Gao, J., Wang, L., Xu, J., et al. (2018). Metformin inhibits prostate cancer progression by targeting tumor-associated inflammatory infiltration. *Clin. Cancer Res.* 16, 1078–1432. doi: 10.1158/1078-0432.CCR-18-0420

Mukherjee, A., and Khuda-Bukhsh, A. R. (2015). Quercetin down-regulates IL-6/STAT-3 signals to induce mitochondrial-mediated apoptosis in a nonsmall-cell lung-cancer cell line, A549. *J. Pharmacopuncture* 18, 19–26. doi: 10.3831/KPI.2015.18.002

Németh, K., Plumb, G. W., Berrin, J. G., Juge, N., Jacob, R., Naim, H. Y., et al. (2003). Deglycosylation by small intestinal epithelial cell β-glucosidases is a critical step in the absorption and metabolism of dietary flavonoid glycosides in humans. *Eur. J. Nutr.* 42, 29–42. doi: 10.1007/s00394-003-0397-3

Ozawa, T., Arora, S., Szulzewsky, F., Juric-Sekhar, G., Miyajima, Y., Bolouri, H., et al. (2018). A de novo mouse model of C11orf95-RELA fusion-driven ependymoma identifies driver functions in addition to NF-κB. *Cell Rep.* 23, 3787–3797. doi: 10.1016/j.celrep.2018.04.099

Qiu, J. (2015). When the East meets the West: the future of traditional Chinese medicine in the 21st century. *Nat. Sci. Rev.* 2:377. doi: 10.1093/nsr/nwv049

Rajavel, T., Packiyaraj, P., Suryanarayanan, V., Singh, S. K., Ruckmani, K., and Pandima, D. K. (2018). β-Sitosterol targets Trx/Trx1 reductase to induce apoptosis in A549 cells via ROS mediated mitochondrial dysregulation and p53 activation. *Sci. Rep.* 8:2071. doi: 10.1038/s41598-018-20311-6

Ru, J., Li, P., Wang, J., Zhou, W., Li, B., Huang, C., et al. (2014). TCMSP: a database of systems pharmacology for drug discovery from herbal medicines. *J. Cheminform.* 6:13. doi: 10.1186/1758-2946-6-13

Shannon, P., Markiel, A., Ozier, O., Baliga, N. S., Wang, J. T., Ramage, D., et al. (2003). Cytoscape: a software environment for integrated models of biomolecular interaction networks. *Genome Res.* 13:2498. doi: 10.1101/gr.1239303

Shi, G., Wang, Q., Zhou, X., Li, J., Liu, H., Gu, J., et al. (2017). Response of human non-small-cell lung cancer cells to the influence of Wogonin with SGK1 dynamics. *Acta Biochim. Biophys. Sin.* 49, 302–310. doi: 10.1093/abbs/gmx006

Song, B., Zhang, Q., Yu, M., Qi, X., Wang, G., Xiao, L., et al. (2017). Ursolic acid sensitizes radioresistant NSCLC cells expressing HIF-1α through reducing endogenous GSH and inhibiting HIF-1α. *Oncol. Lett.* 13, 754–762. doi: 10.3892/ol.2016.5468

Sun, C., Zhu, Y., Li, X., Wang, X., Tang, L., Su, Z., et al. (2018). Scutellarin increases cisplatin-induced apoptosis and autophagy to overcome cisplatin resistance in non-small cell lung cancer via ERK/p53 and c-met/AKT signaling pathways. *Front. Pharmacol.* 9:92. doi: 10.3389/fphar.2018.00092

Tan, X., Zhang, Z., Yao, H., and Shen, L. (2018). Tim-4 promotes the growth of colorectal cancer by activating angiogenesis and recruiting tumor-associated macrophages via the PI3K/AKT/mTOR signaling pathway. *Cancer Lett.* 436, 119–128. doi: 10.1016/j.canlet.2018.08.012

Tang, F., Zhang, Q., Nie, Z., Yao, S., and Bo, C. (2009). Sample preparation for analyzing traditional Chinese medicines. *TrAC Trends Anal. Chem.* 28, 1253–1262. doi: 10.1002/rcm.6235

Testa, U., Castelli, G., and Pelosi, E. (2018). Lung cancers: molecular characterization, clonal heterogeneity and evolution, and cancer stem cells. *Cancers* 10:248. doi: 10.3390/cancers10080248

Thorn, C. F., Klein, T. E., and Altman, R. B. (2013). PharmGKB: the pharmacogenomics knowledge base. *Methods Mol. Biol.* 1015:311. doi: 10.1007/978-1-62703-435-7_20

Timucin, A. C., Basaga, H., and Kutuk, O. (2018). Selective targeting of antiapoptotic BCL-2 proteins in cancer. *Med. Res. Rev.* doi: 10.1002/med.21516 [Epub ahead of print].

Tran, T. C., Sneed, B., Haider, J., Blavo, D., White, A., Aiyejorun, T., et al. (2007). Automated, quantitative screening assay for antiangiogenic compounds using transgenic zebrafish. *Cancer Res.* 67:11386. doi: 10.1158/0008-5472.CAN-07-3126

Wang, H., Lin, C., Jh, J. H., Chow, K., Kuo, K., Lin, C., et al. (2010). Reversal of inflammation-associated dihydrodiol dehydrogenases (AKR1C1 and AKR1C2) overexpression and drug resistance in nonsmall cell lung cancer cells by wogonin and chrysin. *Int. J. Cancer* 120, 2019–2027. doi: 10.1002/ijc.22402

Wang, J., Chen, Y., Liu, B., Wang, Q., Zhang, L., Wang, Z., et al. (2018). Systematic investigation of the erigeron breviscapus mechanism for treating cerebrovascular disease. *J. Ethnopharmacol.* 224, 429–440. doi: 10.1016/j.jep.2018.05.022

Wang, Q., Acharya, N., Liu, Z., Zhou, X., Cromie, M., Zhu, J., et al. (2018). Enhanced anticancer effects of *Scutellaria barbata D. Don* in combination with traditional Chinese medicine components on non-small cell lung cancer cells. *J. Ethnopharmacol.* 217, 140–151. doi: 10.1016/j.jep.2018.02.020

Wang, T. S. (2012). A review of phytochemistry and antitumor activity of a valuable medicinal species: *Scutellaria barbata*. *J. Med. Plants Res.* 6, 4259–4275.

Wang, X., Xu, X., Li, Y., Li, X., Tao, W., Li, B., et al. (2013). Systems pharmacology uncovers Janus functions of botanical drugs: activation of host defense system and inhibition of influenza virus replication. *Integr. Biol.* 5, 351–371. doi: 10.1039/c2ib20204b

Wang, Y. F., Xu, Y. L., Tang, Z. H., Li, T., Zhang, L. L., Chen, X., et al. (2017). Baicalein induces beclin 1- and extracellular signal-regulated kinase-dependent autophagy in ovarian cancer cells. *Am. J. Chin. Med.* 45, 123–136. doi: 10.1142/S0192415X17500094

Wang, Z., Fang, M., Li, J., Yang, R., Du, J., and Luo, Y. (2018). High platelet levels attenuate the efficacy of platinum-based treatment in non-small cell lung cancer. *Cell. Physiol. Biochem.* 48, 2456–2469. doi: 10.1159/000492683

Wishart, D. S., Knox, C., Guo, A. C., Cheng, D., Shrivastava, S., Dan, T., et al. (2008). DrugBank: a knowledgebase for drugs, drug actions and drug targets. *Nucleic Acids Res.* 36, 901–906. doi: 10.1093/nar/gkm958

Xu, X., Zhang, W., Huang, C., Li, Y., Yu, H., Wang, Y., et al. (2012). A novel chemometric method for the prediction of human oral bioavailability. *Int. J. Mol. Sci.* 13, 6964–6982. doi: 10.3390/ijms13066964

Yamanishi, Y., Kotera, M., Kanehisa, M., and Goto, S. (2010). Drug-target interaction prediction from chemical, genomic and pharmacological data in an integrated framework. *Bioinformatics* 26, i246–i254. doi: 10.1093/bioinformatics/btq176

Yang, Y., Huang, C., Su, X., Zhu, J., Chen, X., Fu, Y., et al. (2018). Deciphering the multicomponent synergy mechanism from a systems pharmacology perspective: application to Gualou Xiebai Decoction for coronary heart disease. *J. Funct. Foods* 47, 143–155. doi: 10.1016/j.jff.2018.02.030

Yu, H., Chen, J., Xu, X., Li, Y., Zhao, H., Fang, Y., et al. (2012). A systematic prediction of multiple drug-target interactions from chemical, genomic, and pharmacological data. *PLoS One* 7:e37608. doi: 10.1371/journal.pone.0037608

Yu, X., Lu, K., Xia, J., and Mao, X. (2014). Baicalein induces HeLa cell growth inhibition by down-regulation of matrix metalloproteinases and activating extracellular signal-regulated kinase. *Chin. J. Cell. Mol. Immunol.* 30, 798–801.

Zakaria, N., Yusoff, N. M., Zakaria, Z., Widera, D., and Yahaya, B. H. (2018). Inhibition of NF-κB signaling reduces the stemness characteristics of lung cancer stem cells. *Front. Oncol.* 8:166. doi: 10.3389/fonc.2018.00166

Zhang, J., Li, Y., Chen, X., Pan, Y., Zhang, S., and Wang, Y. (2014). Systems pharmacology dissection of multi-scale mechanisms of action for herbal medicines in stroke treatment and prevention. *PLoS One* 9:e102506. doi: 10.1371/journal.pone.0102506

Zhang, L., Ren, B., Zhang, J., Liu, L., Liu, J., Jiang, G., et al. (2017). Anti-tumor effect of *Scutellaria barbata D. Don* extracts on Ovarian Cancer and its phytochemicals characterisation. *J. Ethnopharmacol.* 206, 184–192. doi: 10.1016/j.jep.2017.05.032

Zhang, Q., Jiang, X., He, W., Wei, K., Sun, J., Qin, X., et al. (2017). MCL plays an anti-inflammatory role in mycobacterium tuberculosis-induced immune response by inhibiting NF-κB and NLRP3 inflammasome activation. *Med. Inflamm.* 2017:2432904. doi: 10.1155/2017/2432904

Zhao, Y., Zhang, L., Wu, Y., Dai, Q., Zhou, Y., Li, Z., et al. (2018). Selective anti-tumor activity of wogonin targeting the warburg effect through stabilizing p53. *Pharmacol. Res.* 135, 49–59. doi: 10.1016/j.phrs.2018.07.011

Zheng, C., Wang, J., Liu, J., Pei, M., Huang, C., and Wang, Y. (2014). System-level multi-target drug discovery from natural products with applications to cardiovascular diseases. *Mol. Divers.* 18:621. doi: 10.1007/s11030-014-9521-y

Zheng, X., Kang, W., Liu, H., and Guo, S. (2018). Inhibition effects of total flavonoids from *Sculellaria barbata D. Don* on human breast carcinoma bone metastasis via downregulating PTHrP pathway. *Int. J. Mol. Med.* 41, 3137–3146. doi: 10.3892/ijmm.2018.3515

Zhu, F., Shi, Z., Qin, C., Tao, L., Liu, X., Xu, F., et al. (2012). Therapeutic target database update 2012: a resource for facilitating target-oriented drug discovery. *Nucleic Acids Res.* 40, 1128–1136. doi: 10.1093/nar/gkr797

Zhu, J., Zhu, J., Zhao, J., Zhao, J., Yu, Z., Yu, Z., et al. (2018). Epoxymicheliolide, a novelguaiane-type sesquiterpene lactone, inhibits NF-κB/COX-2 signaling pathways by targeting leucine 281 and leucine 25 in IKKβ in renal cell carcinoma. *Int. J. Oncol.* 53, 987–1000. doi: 10.3892/ijo.2018.4460

11

Xuebijing Injection Maintains GRP78 Expression to Prevent *Candida albicans*–Induced Epithelial Death in the Kidney

Ting Shang[1,2], Qilin Yu[3], Tongtong Ren[3], Xin-Tong Wang[1,2], Hongyan Zhu[1,2], Jia-Ming Gao[1,2], Guixiang Pan[1,2], Xiumei Gao[1], Yan Zhu[1,2], Yuxin Feng[1,2] and Ming-Chun Li[3]**

[1] *Tianjin State Key Laboratory of Modern Chinese Medicine, Tianjin University of Traditional Chinese Medicine, Tianjin, China,*
[2] *Research and Development Center of TCM, Tianjin International Joint Academy of Biomedicine, TEDA, Tianjin, China,*
[3] *Key Laboratory of Molecular Microbiology and Technology for Ministry of Education, College of Life Sciences, Nankai University, Tianjin, China*

***Correspondence:**
Yuxin Feng
fengyn@live.com
Ming-Chun Li
nklimingchun@163.com

Sepsis and septic shock threaten the survival of millions of patients in the intensive care unit. Secondary fungal infections significantly increased the risk of mortality in sepsis patients. Chinese medicine Xuebijing injection (XBJ) has been routinely used as an add-on treatment to sepsis and septic shock in China. Our network pharmacology analysis predicted that XBJ also influences fungal infection, consisting with results of pioneer clinical studies. We conducted *in vivo* and *in vitro* experiments to verify this prediction. To our surprise, XBJ rescued mice from lethal *Candida* sepsis in a disseminated *Candida albicans* infection model and abolished the colonization of *C. albicans* in kidneys. Although XBJ did not inhibit the growth and the virulence of *C. albicans in vitro*, it enhanced the viability of 293T cells upon *C. albicans* insults. Further RNA-seq analysis revealed that XBJ activated the endoplasmic reticulum (ER) stress pathway upon *C. albicans* infection. Western blot confirmed that XBJ maintained the expression of GRP78 in the presence of *C. albicans*. Interestingly, key active ingredients in XBJ (C0127) mirrored the effects of XBJ. C0127 not only rescued mice from lethal *Candida* sepsis and prevented the colonization of *C. albicans* in kidneys, but also sustained the survival of kidney epithelial cells partially by maintaining the expression of GRP78. These results suggested that XBJ may prevent fungal infection in sepsis patients. Pre-activation of ER stress pathway is a novel strategy to control *C. albicans* infection. Network pharmacology may accelerate drug development in the field of infectious diseases.

Keywords: fungal infection, *C. albicans*, Xuebijing injection, endoplasmic reticulum stress, GRP78, Chinese medicine

HIGHLIGHTS

1. Xuebijing (XBJ) prevented *Candida* sepsis in a murine model.
2. XBJ maintained GRP78 expression to prevent *C. albicans*–induced kidney epithelial death.
3. The key compounds in XBJ suppressed *Candida* sepsis and kidney failure partially by regulating GRP78.

INTRODUCTION

Fungal infection causes an annual mortality of 1.5 million people worldwide (Wirnsberger et al., 2016). The cost of treating invasive fungal infection is over 2 billion dollars in the US (Pfaller and Diekema, 2010). As the leading pathogen in patients suffering invasive fungal infections, *Candida albicans* fostered 50% of candida sepsis cases (Pfaller and Diekema, 2010; Brown et al., 2012). Associated with a mortality rate exceeding 40%, past decades witnessed a dramatic rise in the incidence of invasive candidiasis (Kullberg and Arendrup, 2015).

Limited choices of antifungal drugs are available to treat fungal infections with only two non-toxic antifungal classes for candidiasis (Diekema et al., 2012). Azoles are applied in clinical practice to treat *C. albicans*–related infections (Sakagami et al., 2018). Nevertheless, invasive *C. albicans* infection still claims mortality of 45% to 75% (Brown et al., 2012). Emerging drug-resistant fungal infections are also calling for novel management strategies to restrain fungal sepsis (Healey et al., 2016).

C. albicans–induced kidney failure is a major cause of mortality in *C. albicans* sepsis (Spellberg et al., 2005). Enhancing the function of the innate immune system rescued lethal *C. albicans* infections in murine models (Xiao et al., 2016; Dominguez-Andres et al., 2017). Other potential mechanisms remain elusive. Administrating mirR-124 and mirR-204 mimics prevented *C. albicans*–induced acute kidney injury (Li et al., 2014b; Li et al., 2018).

Secretory and membrane proteins are synthesized and modified in the endoplasmic reticulum (ER) of mammalian cells (Yu et al., 2015; Zhu and Lee, 2015). Activating ER stress signaling renders survival advantage for tissues and cells upon *C. albicans* infection. Glucose-regulated proteins (GRPs) are constitutively expressed in cells to maintain cellular homeostasis, belonging to the heat shock protein family as stress-inducible chaperones. Infections activate GRPs to translocate in the cells to assume functions such as regulating signaling transduction, proliferation and immunity (Zhu and Lee, 2015; Lewy et al., 2017). Conserved from yeast to human, GRP78 (BiP) is one of such proteins that regulate homeostasis of organs from endoderm, mesoderm, and ectoderm. Interestingly, GRP78 cross-talks with PI3K/AKT pathway, which sustains cell survival (Shani et al., 2008; Gray et al., 2013; Liu et al., 2013).

Xuebijing (XBJ) injection was prepared with extracts from five different Chinese herbs [*Carthamus tinctorius* flowers (Honghua), *Paeonia lactiflora* roots (Chishao), *Ligusticum chuanxiong* rhizomes (Chuanxiong), *Angelica sinensis* roots (Danggui), and Salvia miltiorrhiza roots (Danshen)] (Cheng et al., 2016; Li et al., 2016; Li et al., 2019; Zhang et al., 2018). Approved by the Food and Drug Administration of China in 2004, XBJ has been frequently used as an add-on therapy for multiple organ dysfunction syndromes, sepsis, and septic shock in China for over a decade (Chen et al., 2018a; Gao et al., 2015; Shi et al., 2017). It rendered a series of benefits for sepsis patients, including reducing 28-day mortality and incidence of complications, shortening dwelling time in the intensive care unit (Gao et al., 2015; Shi et al., 2017; Song et al., 2019). Pre-clinical studies indicated XBJ might be a treatment option for sepsis and septic shock individually (Jiang et al., 2013; Chen et al., 2018). Four classes of compounds from five different herbs in XBJ may be important for its antiseptic effect (Li et al., 2016). Intensive research is going on to identify major active compounds in XBJ that can effectively treat sepsis (Cheng et al., 2016; Li et al., 2016). Combining Xuebijing with anti-fungal agents or antibiotics had positive impacts on the quality of life of patients suffering invasive fungal infections in several clinical studies and may improve the survival of patients (Gao, 2010; Wang, 2010; Cao, 2017). However, it was not clear whether XBJ can influence fungal infection individually.

Our network pharmacology analysis predicted that XBJ not only affects therapeutic targets of sepsis but also influences fungal infection, suggesting XBJ may prevent fungal infection in sepsis patients. Here we reported that XBJ prevented systemic *C. albicans* infections. Notably, XBJ pretreatment protected 70% of mice from mortality after systemic *C. albicans* infection. It prevented the colonization of *C. albicans* in kidneys and enhanced the viability of kidney epithelial cells by sustaining ER stress signaling.

METHODS

Chemicals and Reagents

Xuebijing injection (catalog number: z20039833, batch number: 1606121) was manufactured by Tianjin Chase Sun Pharmaceutical Co., Ltd (Tianjin, China). This Chinese medicine is approved by the China Food and Drug Administration (CFDA) for treating sepsis and septic shock with the CFDA ratification number of GuoYaoZhunZi-Z20039833 for market approval as a drug product. It is routinely used as an add-on to conventional therapy for treating sepsis and septic shock in China (Jiang et al., 2013; Chen et al., 2018; Li et al., 2019). This injection contains extracts of five herbs, including *Carthamus tinctorius* flowers (Honghua in Chinese), *Paeonia lactiflora* roots (Chishao in Chinese), *Ligusticum chuanxiong* rhizomes (Chuanxiong in Chinese), *Angelica sinensis* roots (Danggui in Chinese), and Salvia miltiorrhiza roots (Danshen in Chinese).

Methods of extraction, preparation, and quality control of XBJ were the same as previously reported (Huang et al., 2011; Chen et al., 2016; Li et al., 2016; Zhang et al., 2018). Briefly, ingredients from *Carthamus tinctorius flowers* ("Honghua" in Chinese) were first extracted with ethanol then with water. Ingredients from the other four herbs were extracted with water. Finally, XBJ was standardized to contain 1.0 to 1.7 mg/ml of paeoniflorin and 0.2 to 0.5 mg/ml of hydroxysafflor yellow A as described (Huang et al., 2011; Chen et al., 2016; Li et al., 2016).

GRP78 inhibitor HA15 and other chemicals used in the experiments were ordered from Sigma-Aldrich (Shanghai, China) unless indicated. Paeoniflorin (Cas #: 23180-57-6), hydroxysafflor yellow A (Cas#: 78281-02-4), ferulic acid (Cas #:537-98-4), and protocatechualdehyde (Cas#:139-85-5) were purchased from Shanghai Yuanye Biotechnology Co., Ltd. (Shanghai, China). C0127 was prepared with paeoniflorin, hydroxysafflor yellow A, ferulic acid, and protocatechualdehyde according to reported concentrations in XBJ and manufacturer's quality control information (Liu et al., 2015; Zuo et al., 2017; Zuo et al., 2018). The structures of the four compounds in C0127 were presented in **Supplementary Figure 1**. Western blotting was performed using the GRP78 monoclonal antibody and tubulin monoclonal antibodies (Abcam, USA).

C. albicans Strain and Growth Conditions

C. albicans strain SC5314 (ATCC, USA), which was routinely cultivated in YPD (1% yeast extract, 2% peptone, 2% glucose), was used for all experiments in this study. The *C. albicans* cells were cultured overnight at 30°C and washed twice with PBS for further use.

Animal Experiments and Ethics Statement

This study was carried out in accordance with the recommendations of the Guide for the Care and Use of Laboratory Animals (NIH Publication No. 85-23, revised 1996, USA) and the recommendations in the Guidance for the Care and Use of Laboratory Animals issued by the Ministry of Science and Technology of China. All experiments were approved by the Institutional Animal Care and Use Committee of Nankai University and the Laboratory Animal Ethics Committee of the Tianjin University of Traditional Chinese Medicine (Tianjin, China) and were performed in accordance with its guidelines (Permit Number: TCM-LAE-20170017). Five to six week-old ICR female mice were used for *in vivo* experiments (Dong et al., 2017). The mice were provided with free access to food and sterile water and were caged under controlled temperature (23°C ± 2°C) and humidity (60% ± 5%) with an artificial 12 h light/dark cycle. The mice were randomly divided into six groups (n = 15 in each group) as follows: Control group injected with normal saline; CA group was infected with 5×10^6 colony-forming units of *C. albicans via* tail-vein injection. XBJ group treated with XBJ (6 ml/kg; Chase Sun Pharmaceutical, Ltd., Tianjin, China) by subcutaneous injection; CA+XBJ group infected with *C. albicans* and co-treated with XBJ (6 ml/kg); C0127 group infected with C. *albicans* after 3 injections of C0127 (6 ml/kg). XBJ and C0127 were administered once/day from Day -3 to Day -1 before the C. albicans infection. The *C. albicans* strain SC5314 was cultivated in YPD (1% yeast extract, 2% peptone, and 2% dextrose) broth with overnight shaking at 30°C. The systemic fungal infection and virulence assays were performed as described (Dong et al., 2017; Liang et al., 2018).

Database Construction and Network Analysis

Fungal infection-related targets were mainly integrated from literature mining, GeneCards (Stelzer et al., 2011) and Ingenuity Pathway Analysis (IPA, http://www.ingenuity.com) database (Kramer et al., 2014). Repetitive genes were automatically identified and removed by IPA software. In addition, ingredients derived from XBJ were collected from literature mining (Huang et al., 2011; Jiang et al., 2013; Guo et al., 2014; Han et al., 2017; Zuo et al., 2017; Zuo et al., 2018) and several TCM databases, such as TCMID (Xue et al., 2013) and TCMSP (Ru et al., 2014). Compounds that had more than 10 targets in mammalians were selected for further analysis. The chemical name of each compound was transferred into PubChem CID or CAS number which could be recognized by the IPA software. Furthermore, corresponding targets of XBJ ingredients that were not recorded by the IPA database were supplemented by literature from PubChem and databases of TCMID and TCMSP. In total, three datasets including XBJ ingredients, fungal infection associated targets, and corresponding targets of XBJ's major ingredients were constructed and then uploaded into the IPA system to visualize the discovery. The relationships between fungal infection-related targets and XBJ ingredients were discovered by "Build-Path Explorer" module. "Build-Connection" module was implemented to interpret the relationship between targets. "Overlay-Canonical Pathway" module was used to generate the resulting canonical pathways. "Build-Diseases & Functions" module was exploited to build the targets-related diseases and functions. We utilized the "Core analysis" module to analyze the correlation of the established network to acquire top diseases, top functions, top pathways, and top upstream regulators. Certain top upstream regulators were defined by the "Upstream Regulator" module. The "Path designer" module was performed to clarify the network. Upstream regulators analyses were performed to elucidate the causal inference of upstream biological causes and probable downstream effects on cellular and organismal biology (Kramer et al., 2014). "Path designer" module was used to demonstrate the network. The algorithm of the network analysis was based on Fisher's exact test with the enrichment score of P-values in this study.

RNA Isolation, RNA-seq, and Quantitative Real-Time Polymerase Chain Reaction

Total RNA was extracted by the phenol-chloroform method as previously described (Dong et al., 2017). The overall quality of RNA was determined by A260/A280 and analyzed by agarose gel electrophoresis. Roche GS-FLX 454 pyrosequencing was carried out using Illumina HiSeq™ 2000 (Oebiotech Company, China). Reverse transcriptions were conducted with an Oligo (dT)-primed RT reagent Kit (Promega, USA). Quantitative real-time polymerase chain reaction (PCR) was performed in triplicate and repeated in three independent experiments with the Mastercycler ep realplex system. Independent reaction mixtures were carried out with the same DNA template for both the genes of interest and the GAPDH reference gene using the RealMasterMix (SYBR Green) Kit (Trans-Gen Biotech, China) according to the instructions. The relative fold changes in gene expression were determined by the 2-delta delta Ct method. Data were presented as means ± SD of three independent experiments.

Hematoxylin and Eosin Staining

Hematoxylin and eosin (H&E) staining was conducted as described (Dong et al., 2017). Briefly, kidney tissues were collected 4 days after *C. albicans* infection and were fixed with 4% formalin at room temperature for 24 h, dehydrated with alcohol, and paraffin–embedded. The tissues were then cut into 5-μm-thick sections, which were stained with H&E at room temperature for 1 to 2 min and visualized under a microscope (BX53, Olympus, Japan).

Western Blotting

Protein was extracted from 293T cells using the RIPA solution. The protein concentration of the lysates was measured with the Bradford assay. Western blotting was conducted as described (Fu et al., 2007).

Statistical Analysis

Data were presented as the mean ± standard deviation for each group. All statistical analyses were performed using PRISM version 5.0 (GraphPad Software, Inc., La Jolla, CA, USA). Inter-group differences were analyzed using one-way analysis of variance, followed by Tukey's post-hoc test for multiple comparisons. The log-rank test was used to compare group survival trends. $P < 0.05$ was considered to indicate a statistically significant difference.

RESULTS

Network Pharmacology Analysis Predicted That XBJ May Regulate Fungal Infection

Effective in controlling systemic bacterial infection, XBJ has potentials in treating a series of diseases related to infections and tissue injuries (Wang et al., 2015; Xu et al., 2015; Chen et al., 2018; Hu et al., 2018; Tian et al., 2018). We conducted network pharmacology analysis to explore novel applications of XBJ. A library of 170 proteins/molecules related to fungal infection was built and top upstream regulators of these proteins were identified by IPA software (**Figure 1A** and **Supplementary Table 1**). Toll-like receptors (TLR2, TLR4), pro-inflammatory cytokines [tumor necrosis factor, interleukin 6 (IL-6), IL-1, and interferons], nuclear factor κB signaling, and HMGB1 were among top upstream regulators of the targets in fungal infection (**Figures 1B, C**). Interestingly, many of these molecules are known as Xuebijing targets (Jiang et al., 2013; Chen et al., 2018). These results indicated that XBJ may impact fungal infection. Pathway analysis revealed that HMGB1 signaling is among the top 4 pathways in fungal infection (**Figure 2A**). This echoes the reports that XBJ may target HMGB1 to attenuate organ injuries (Wang et al., 2007; Wang et al., 2015; Chen et al., 2016). In addition, multiple potential targets are related to inflammation and cell survival in the functional analysis (**Figure 2B**).

A further analysis predicted that 36 compounds derived from five herbs in XBJ regulate over 70 molecules related to fungal infection (**Figure 3A**). Indeed, many key upstream regulators among these molecules were XBJ targets (**Figures 3B, C**). IPA

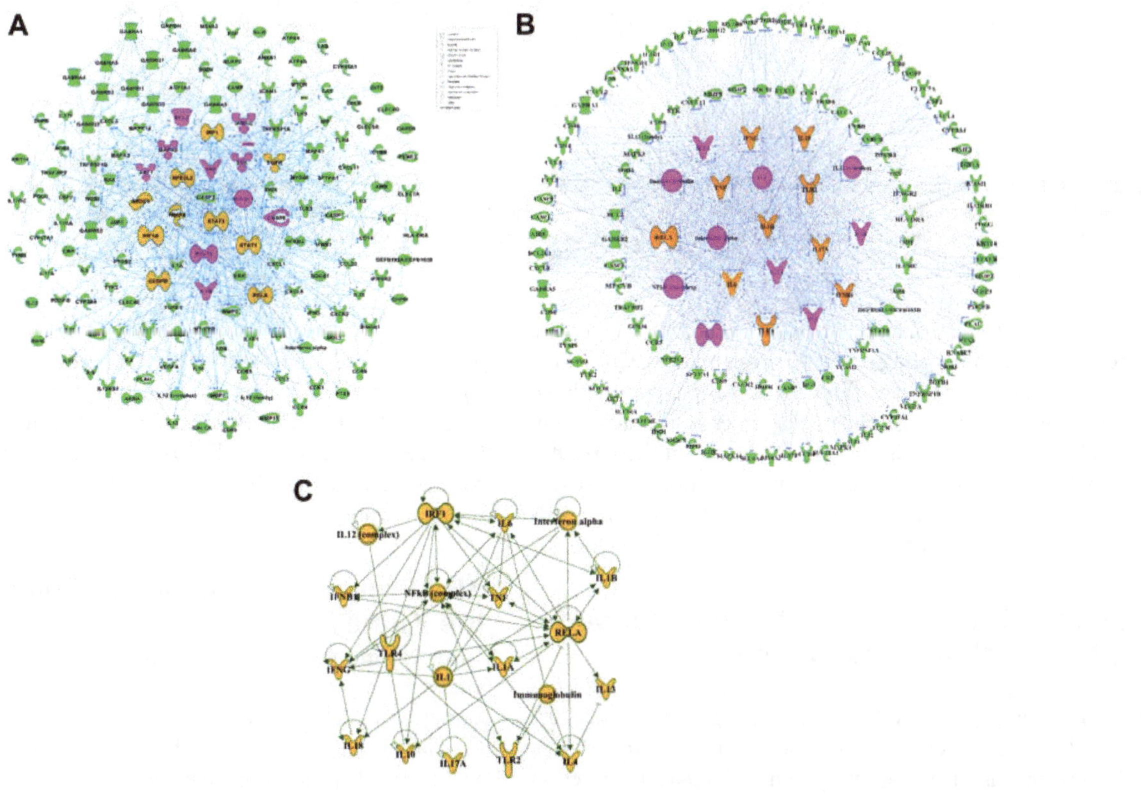

FIGURE 1 | Target proteins related to fungal infection were identified in network pharmacology analysis. **(A)** Protein-protein interactions of the potential and proved therapeutic targets in fungal infection. The top ten targets predicted by IPA were marked in saffron yellow and the top 20 molecules were labeled with purple-red. **(B)** Top 20 upstream regulators of the potential and proved therapeutic targets in fungal infection and their relationships with the related targets. The top ten upstream regulators predicted by IPA were marked in saffron yellow and the top 20 targets were marked in purple-red. **(C)** The network among top 20 upstream regulators of the potential and proved therapeutic targets in fungal infection predicted by IPA.

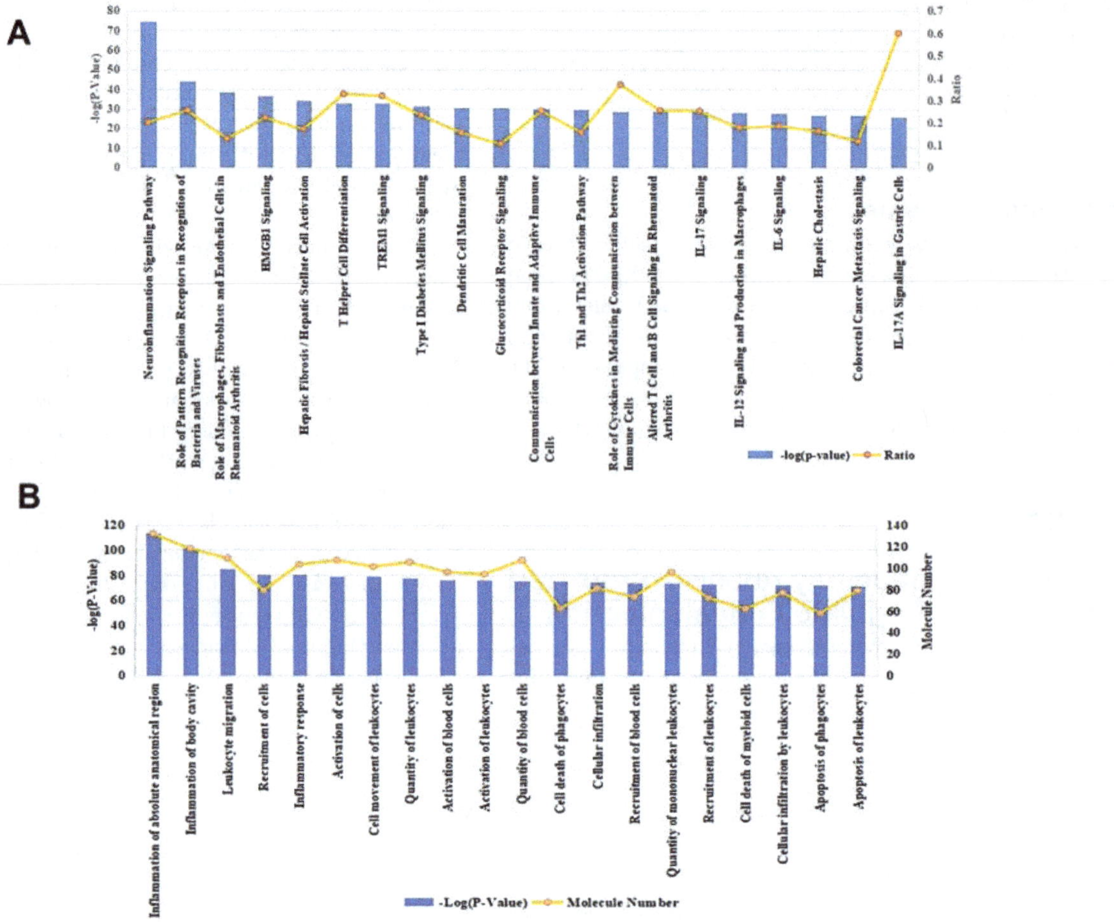

FIGURE 2 | Functional analysis and pathway analysis of 170 potential therapeutic targets in fungal infection. **(A)** The top 20 related pathways among molecules relevant to fungal infection. **(B)** Functional analysis of the 170 fungal infection target proteins. The top 20 pathways/functions were ranked from left to right by –log (*P* value) and the ratio (yellow line) referred to the proportion of 170 molecules in the respective pathway.

pathway analysis foretold that these 36 compounds targeted HMGB1, IL-6, and signaling related to organ injuries which were among the top 20 pathways (**Figures 4A, B**). Our functional analysis predicted that XBJ targets play roles in cell activation, survival, and apoptosis (**Figures 4C, D**). Based on these results, we hypothesized that XBJ prevents fungal infection and decided to test this hypothesis in a well-established *C. albicans* sepsis model (Dominguez-Andres et al., 2017; Zhao et al., 2017).

Xuebijing Prevented *C. albicans*–Induced Septic Shock in a Murine Model

All infected mice died 8 days after systemic *C. albicans* infection. 6 ml/kg XBJ pre-treatment for 3 days rescued ~70% of *C. albicans* infected mice from acute death (**Figure 5A**), indicating that it may prevent systemic *C. albicans* infection to arrest the consequent acute death. To address the question of whether XBJ directly affects the growth of *C. albicans*, we treated *C. albicans* in culture with different dilutions of XBJ (from 1:100 to 1:1000). However, XBJ did not affect the growth of *C. albicans* and hyphal development (data not shown), indicating the mechanism is related to the defense system in hosts. The functional analysis by IPA predicted that XBJ targets signaling pathways involved in organ damage and cell death (**Figures 4C, D**). This is consistent with clinical observations (Shi et al., 2017; Song et al., 2018). Thus, we hypothesized that XBJ improves the survival of *C. albicans*–infected mice partially through protecting kidneys.

XBJ Prevented *C. albicans* Colonization in the Kidney

To determine whether *C. albicans* colonizes kidney after XBJ intervention, we conducted a histopathological analysis of mouse kidneys, and determined the fungal load in kidneys 4 days after *C. albicans* infection. While hyphae, neutrophil penetration, and tissue damages were detected in kidneys of the control group, few hyphae were detected in the XBJ treated group. Neutrophil penetration and tissue damage were also reduced in the XBJ treated group (**Figure 7C**), suggesting XBJ inhibited *C. albicans* colonization in kidneys. Consistently, the kidney fungal burden decreased threefold in XBJ treated mice in the

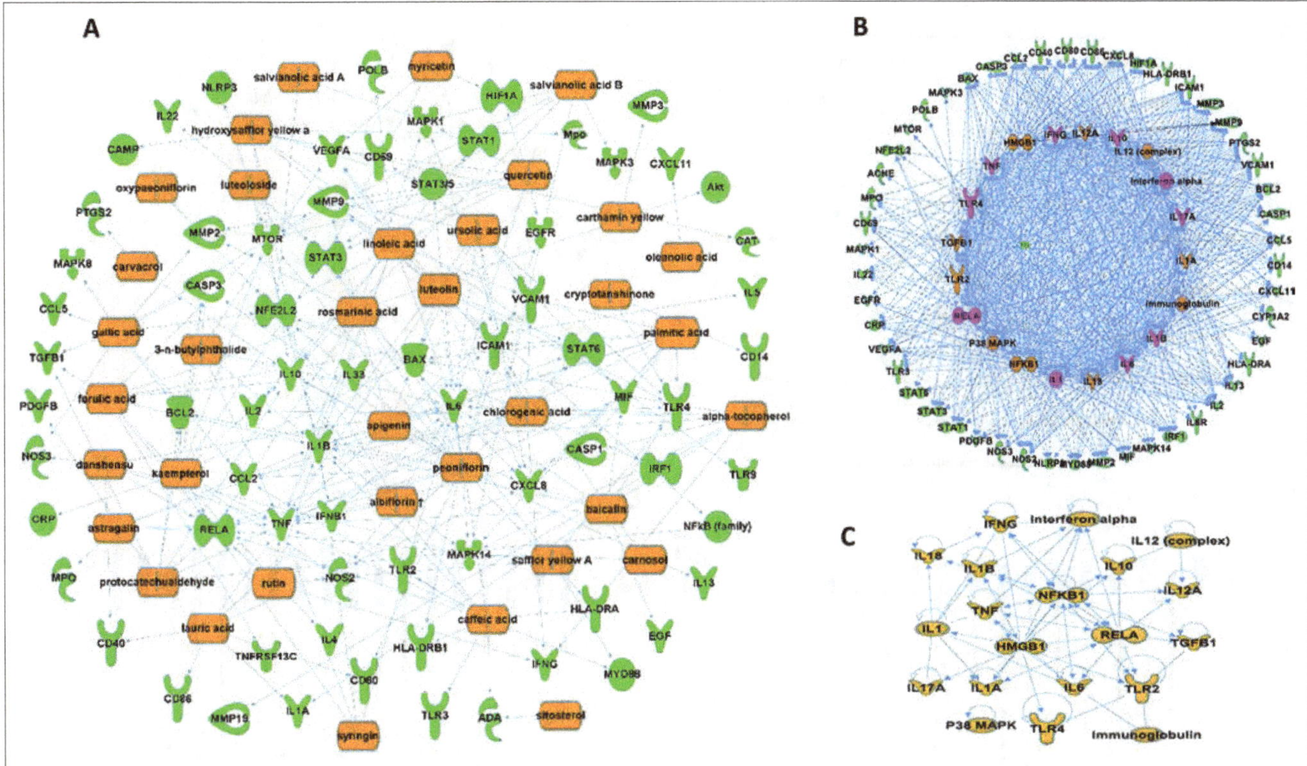

FIGURE 3 | XBJ ingredients regulate potential therapeutic targets of fungal infection. **(A)** XBJ ingredient-target network predicted by IPA. Thirty-six compounds from XBJ were predicted to cooperatively modulate 72 fungal infection-related targets. **(B)** Top 20 upstream regulators of potential XBJ targets in fungal infection (top 20 regulators were marked with saffron yellow and top 10 key molecules were labeled with purple-red). **(C)** The IPA-predicted network of top 20 upstream regulators of potential XBJ targets shown in **Figure 3B**.

colony-forming assay (**Figure 5B**). No *C. albicans* was detected in blood and kidney tissues 3 weeks after the infection in XBJ treated mice (data not shown). Next, we determined the effect of XBJ on kidney epithelial cell survival in different conditions. XBJ treatment at 1:100 dilution did not affect the survival of 293T cells. However, it significantly reduced cell death from ~35% to 15% upon *C. albicans* infection (**Figure 5C**).

XBJ Up-Regulated the ER Stress Signaling Pathway During *C. albicans* Infection

To determine how XBJ protects kidney cells, 293T cells under different treatments were subjected to RNA-seq analysis, including cells treated with saline, cells treated with XBJ only, cells infected with *C. albicans* only, and cells infected with *C. albicans* in the presence of XBJ (1:100 dilution). While *C. albicans* infection inhibited the ER stress signaling, XBJ treatment restored the expression of ER stress signaling. XBJ up-regulated the ATF6B and GRP170 on the mRNA level (**Figures 6A, B**). This was further confirmed by Western blot of GRP78. XBJ restored GRP78 expression to a similar level as control groups (non-infected 293T cells and non-infected 293T cells treated with XBJ) (**Figure 6C**). Therefore, XBJ may maintain the expression of the key factors in the ER stress signaling pathway to improve kidney epithelial cell survival.

Key Ingredients in XBJ Rescued Mice From Septic Shock and Prevented the Colonization of *C. albicans* in the Kidney

Network pharmacology analysis suggested that four major compounds in XBJ may regulate most XBJ targets related to fungal infection (**Supplementary Figure 2**). To understand the mechanism of XBJ on improving the survival in *C. Albicans* sepsis, C0127, a formula comprised of the four major active compounds from XBJ, was used to treat mice before the systemic *C. albicans* infection. Similar to XBJ, pre-treatment with C0127 not only significantly improved the survival of *C. albicans* infected mice but also decreased fungal loads in kidneys (**Figures 7A, B**). Similarly, hyphae and neutrophils infiltration can hardly be detected 4 days after *C. albicans* infection following the C0127 pre-treatment (**Figure 7C**).

Key Ingredients in XBJ Up-Regulated GRP78 to Improve 293T Cell Survival Upon *C. albicans* Infection

Like XBJ, C0127 maintained GRP78 expression on the protein level in 293T cells upon the *C. albicans* insult (**Figures 8A, B**). In our preliminary study, HA15, a GRP78 specific inhibitor (Cerezo et al., 2016; Ruggiero et al., 2018), induced apoptosis in 293T cells

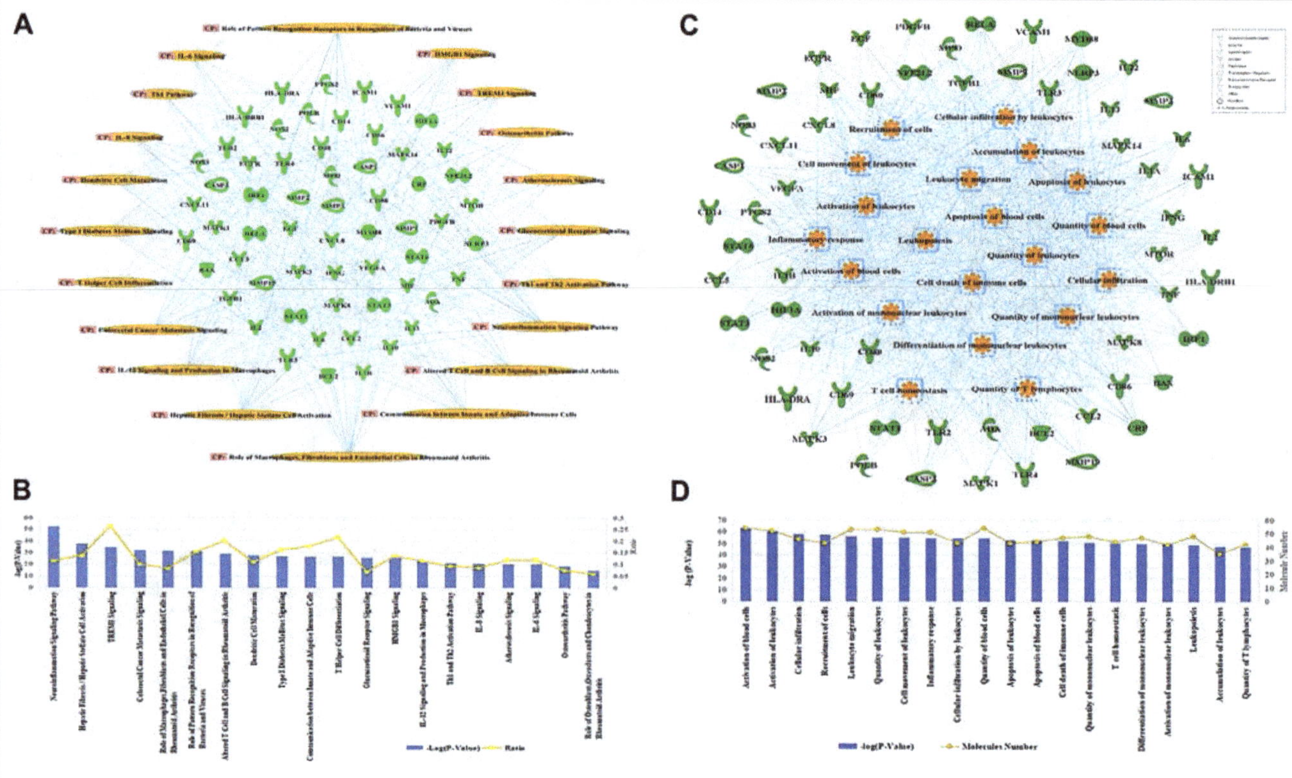

FIGURE 4 | Functional and pathway analysis of potential XBJ targets in fungal infection. **(A, B)** Pathway analysis of XBJ targets in fungal infection. **(A)** The relationships of potential XBJ targets and top 20 related pathways. **(B)** The ranking of the top 20 signaling pathways of potential XBJ targets was presented. The top 20 signaling pathways of potential XBJ targets in fungal infection were ranked from left to right by –log (*P* value). **(C, D)** Functional analysis of XBJ targets in fungal infection. **(C)** The target-function network was presented with the top 20 functions marked in saffron yellow. **(D)** The ranking of the top 20 functions of potential XBJ targets was presented. The top 20 related functions were ranked from left to right by –log (*P* value).

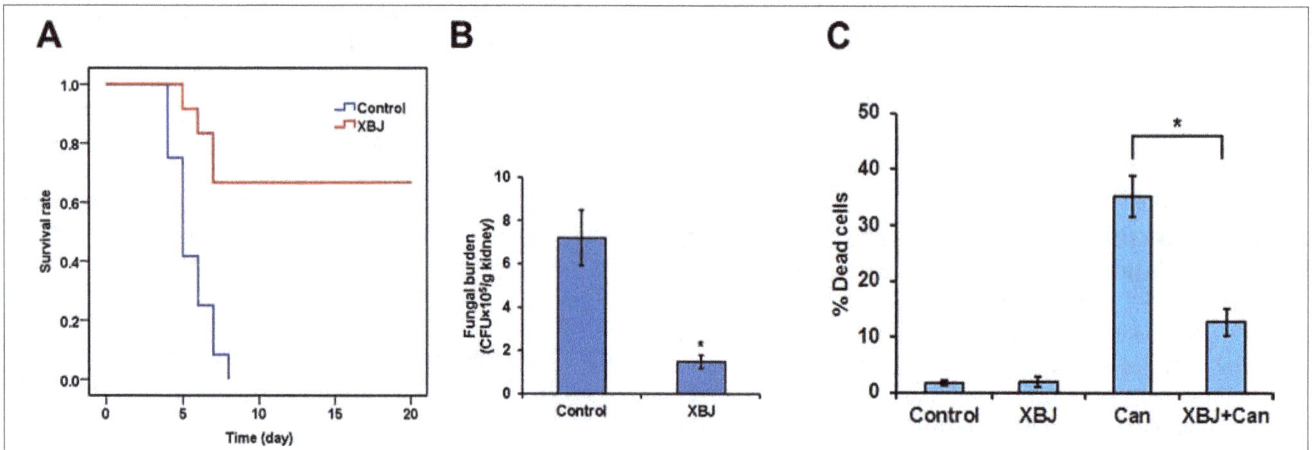

FIGURE 5 | XBJ pre-treatment inhibits the colonization of *C. albicans* in the kidney. **(A)** The survival curves of XBJ pre-treated and control mice after systemic *C. albicans* infection. XBJ (6 ml/kg) or 0.9% NaCl was administered by abdominal injections once/day for 3 days before systemic *C. albicans* infection to the treatment group or the control group. **(B)** The colony-forming assay to determine the fungal loads in the kidneys of control and XBJ treated mice. Kidney tissues from control and XBJ treated kidneys were harvested and subjected to *C. albicans* culture 4 days after the infection. Colonies were counted after 48 h of culture. **(C)** PI staining was used to determine the effect of XBJ on the survival of 293T cells 8 h after the *C. albicans* infection. $^{*}P < 0.05$.

in low-serum culture (data not shown). To determine whether GRP78 is required for the protective effect of XBJ and C0127, 293T cells were treated with HA15 upon *C. albicans* infection. It induced cell death in the presence of XBJ and C0127, indicating GRP78 is an important downstream effector of XBJ and C0127 for the survival of kidney cells (**Figure 8D**).

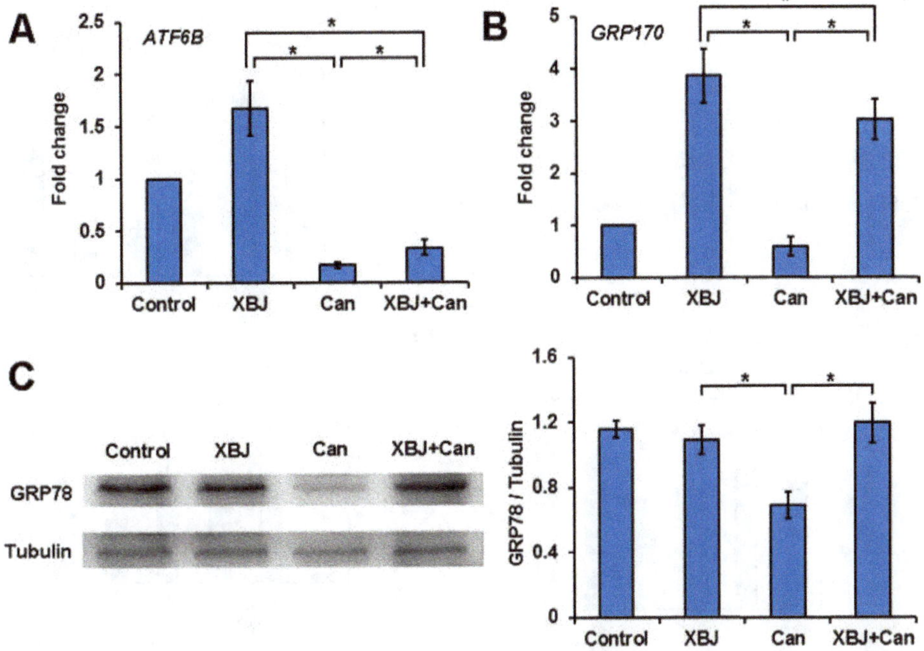

FIGURE 6 | XBJ up-regulates the ER stress signaling pathway during *C. albicans* infection. Six groups of 293T cells in different conditions were subjected to RNA-seq analysis, including cells treated with XBJ only, infected with *C. albicans*, 293T cells infected with *C. albicans* in the presence of XBJ (1:100 dilution). **(A, B)** RNA-seq results of ATF6B and GRP170, two genes in the ER stress pathway. **(C)** Western blot to determine the expression of GRP78 expression in different conditions in 293T cells. Data were representative of at least three independent experiments. *P < 0.05.

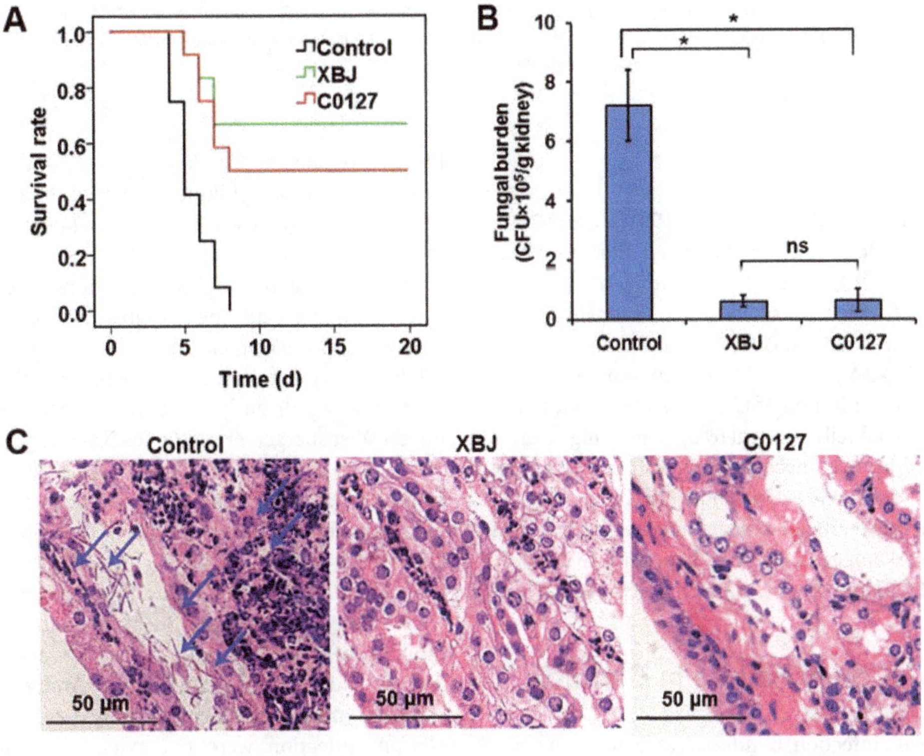

FIGURE 7 | Key compounds (C0127) in XBJ rescued mice from lethal infection of *C. albicans*. **(A)** Survival curves of different groups of mice in *Candida* infected (Control) and treatment groups. Control vs. XBJ and Control vs. C0127: $P < 0.05$. Control group: N = 11; XBJ and C0127 group: N = 12. **(B)** Colony-forming assay to evaluate fungal load in kidneys 4 days after *Candida* infection. $^{*}P < 0.05$. **(C)** Hematoxylin and eosin staining to determine the histology in kidneys. Arrows indicated fungal hyphae in an infected kidney.

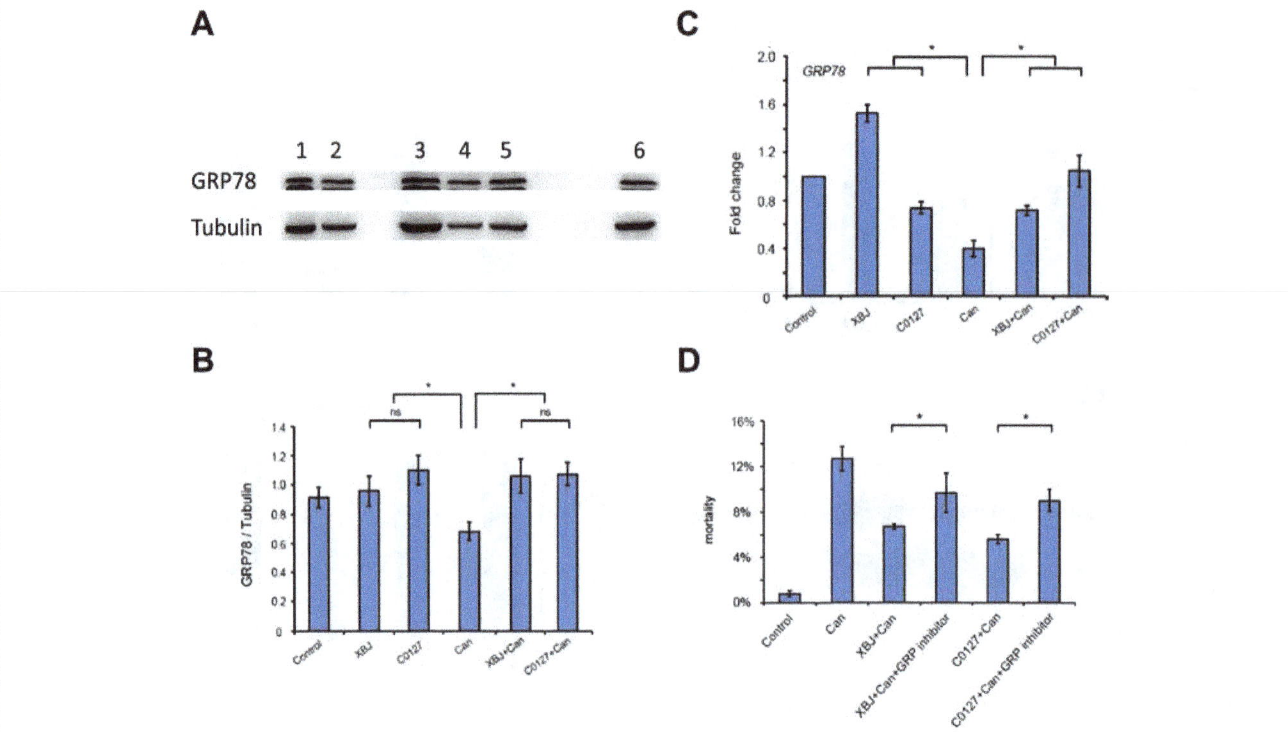

FIGURE 8 | XBJ and C0127 sustained GRP78 expression to improve the survival of 293T cells. **(A)** C0127 maintained GRP78 expression on protein level in 293T cells upon *C. albicans* infection. Western blot experiments were conducted to determine the expression of GRP78. Tubulin was used as an internal control. Lane 1. Control 293T cells; lane 2. *C. Albicans* infected 293T cells; lane 3. XBJ treated 293T cells; lane 4. *C. albicans* infected 293T cells treated with C0127; lane 5. *C. albicans* infected 293T cells treated with XBJ; lane 6. C0127 treated 293T cells. **(B)** Quantification of the GRP78 protein in 293T cells upon different treatments. Data were representative of at least three independent experiments with similar results. **(C)** Real-time PCR to determine the mRNA expression of GRP78 in 293T cells upon different treatments. **(D)** The influence of HA15, a GRP78 inhibitor, on the survival of 293T cells in low serum culture under different conditions by PI staining. Data were representative of at least three independent experiments with similar results. $^{*}P < 0.05$.

DISCUSSION

Summary of the Results and Significance

Our network pharmacology analysis predicted that XBJ may impact fungal infection. XBJ rescued lethal *Candida* sepsis and improved kidney epithelial cell survival by maintaining the expression of GRP78. In addition, C0127, a combination of four key compounds in XBJ also prevented *C. albicans*-induced acute death in mice and the colonization of *C. albicans* in the kidney. It improved kidney epithelial cells' survival by up-regulating GRP78. These results revealed a novel mechanism of XBJ in preventing organ failure and cell death. GRP78 was identified as a potential novel target of XBJ in preventing *C. albicans* infection. Our results suggested that network pharmacology is beneficial to identify novel applications of XBJ and other Chinese medicine formulas.

Mechanism of Kidney Failure in *Candida* Sepsis

During the bloodstream infection, *C. albicans* attaches to the host and then penetrates the host defense system to attack the target organs such as the kidney. It is characterized by the presence of hyphae and the damages to host cells (Brunke and Hube, 2013). The innate immune system plays an important role in controlling the progression of *Candida* sepsis. The damaged cells secrete pro-inflammation cytokines to recruit innate immune cells such as neutrophils to clear *C. albicans* (Wirnsberger et al., 2016; Dominguez-Andres et al., 2017).

Enhancing/activating the function of the innate immune system counteracts the progression of *Candida* sepsis by improving *C. albicans* clearance. Switching off a series of immune inhibitory regulators such as the E3 ubiquitin ligase CBLB, Sts, and Jnk1 significantly improved resistance to *C. albicans* in mice (Wirnsberger et al., 2016; Xiao et al., 2016; Zhao et al., 2017). The E3 ubiquitin ligase CBLB in the innate immune system negatively impacts the phagocytosis of neutrophils and macrophages (Wirnsberger et al., 2016; Xiao et al., 2016). The type I interferon-induced IL-15 production in the Ly6C^{high} monocytes is also required for *C. albicans* clearance by innate immune cells (Dominguez-Andres et al., 2017). In contrast, compromising the function of the innate immune system accelerates *C. albicans*-induced kidney failure (Dominguez-Andres et al., 2017).

Other mechanisms that enhance host defense against *C. albicans* infection were not extensively studied. Both global and local inflammation contribute to *C. albicans*-induced kidney failure. Li et al. showed the systematic expression of microRNAs prevented *C. albicans* infection (Li et al., 2014b; Li et al., 2018). They found *C. albicans* induced acute kidney injury by attenuating miR-124 expression and up-regulating MIP-1 in the kidney (Li et al., 2018), indicating local inflammation in the kidney contributed to kidney failure. Administrating miR-124 mimic inhibited MIP-1 expression in the kidney and restored kidney functions (Li et al., 2018). It is still not clear how miR-124 and miR-204 regulate innate immune system. However, global inflammation in the absence of *C. albicans* may not be sufficient to induce kidney failure. *C. albicans* kills kidney epithelial cells directly, while XBJ partially rescued 293T cell survival upon *C. albicans* exposures (**Figure 6**). This is consistent with our previous result that XBJ improved RAW264.7 cells survival upon the insult of LPS (Lyu et al., 2018).

XBJ and Organ Failure

XBJ has been approved to treat multiple organ dysfunction syndrome and sepsis in China for over a decade (Gao et al., 2015; Shi et al., 2017). A Meta-analysis by Song et al. demonstrated that combining XBJ with conventional intervention is superior to conventional intervention alone in treating MODS (Song et al., 2018). The benefits of XBJ to different organs (including lung, kidney, heart, and liver) were reported in a series of clinical studies (Fang and Wang, 2013; Wang et al., 2015; Zhang et al., 2016; Gao et al., 2018; Song et al., 2018) (Song et al., 2019). In a small-scale prospective, single-center, randomized double-blinded trial, Gao et al. found XBJ significantly lowered IL-1β, IL-8, and C-reactive protein in blood and up-regulated IL-10 in blood and decreased adverse events in patients with lung injury (Gao et al., 2018). Zhang et al. found XBJ improved myocardial function in patients with septic myocardial injury, indicated by improving cardiac troponin I, N-terminal proB-type natriuretic peptide, and procalcitonin in blood samples of patients (Zhang et al., 2016).

The major causes of organ failure in sepsis are disseminated intravascular coagulation (DIC), dysfunction of circulation, and cytokine storm. Results from basic research confirmed clinical observations and provided clues to the working mechanism of XBJ in preventing and treating different types of organ injuries systemically. It improves microcirculation partially by inhibiting blood-clotting to prevents/treats organ injuries (Wang et al., 2015; Xu et al., 2015; Jin et al., 2018). This is reflected in reversing abnormalities of metabolic biomarkers in sepsis (Shi et al., 2017).

XBJ is also likely to prevent/reverse organ injuries by improving cell survival and regulating cell functions (Chen et al., 2013; Li et al., 2014a). Li et al. reported XBJ enhanced survival of hematopoietic stem cells and mono-nuclear cells upon radiation insults *in vitro* and *in vivo*. XBJ also regulated the secretory function of Kupffer cells in heat stroke rats (Chen et al., 2013).

At the molecular level, XBJ regulates multiple signaling pathways to combat organ injuries. It down-regulated TLR4 signaling and stimulated the expression of Toll-interacting protein to improve organ functions (Liu et al., 2014b; Liu et al., 2014c; He et al., 2018). XBJ reduced ROS production in rats to attenuate pulmonary injury (Chen et al., 2017). P38 MAPK might be a XBJ target in a lung injury model (Liu et al., 2014a). HMGB1, a nuclear protein related to organ injury, is a biomarker of organ injury and a potential therapeutic target of organ injury (Wang et al., 1999; Musumeci et al., 2014). A series of publications indicated XBJ attenuates HMGB1 expression in sepsis organ injuries (Li et al., 2007; Wang et al., 2007; Wang et al., 2015; Chen et al., 2016). However, no gain-of-function and loss-of-function study has been conducted *in vivo* to determine the influences of XBJ on these pathways.

XBJ was used to treat and prevent different types of kidney injuries in the clinic and pre-clinical studies. In a clinical study, XBJ improved clinical symptoms of sepsis-induced acute kidney injury (Yuxi et al., 2017). In addition, XBJ attenuated herbicide paraquat-induced acute kidney injury in rats (Xu et al., 2017). It also prevented paraquat-induced apoptosis in human kidney cell line HK-2 (Tian et al., 2018). However, mechanisms of these effects remain to be illustrated. In this study, we revealed that XBJ may regulate GRP78 to improve the survival of kidney epithelial cells upon *C. albicans* insult and the combination of four compounds in XBJ can maintain GRP78 expression. This mechanism may also apply to other organs and cell types.

The Advantages of Utilizing Different Methods to Understand the Working Mechanism of XBJ in Preventing Invasive *C. albicans* Infection

Network pharmacology predictions are based on our current knowledge. The experimental pharmacology has value to supplement network pharmacology to expand our knowledge. Our results showed that combining both methods provides advantages to advance medicine. RNA-seq, real-time PCR, and Western blot were used to identify novel signaling that impacts kidney failure during invasive *C. albicans* infection. Glucose-Regulated Protein 78 (GRP78, BiP) was identified by Western Blot in 293T cells. Results of real-time PCR confirmed the influence of XBJ on GRP78 at the transcription level. However, this result remains to be confirmed *in vivo*. ATF6B and GRP170, two ER stress-related proteins were influenced by XBJ in RNA-seq. But we did not find their changes on protein level (data not shown). Whether XBJ influences the expression of GRP94, another important ER stress protein that shares a similar function with GRP78 (Zhu and Lee, 2015), is under investigation. Overall, combining multiple methods is superior to a single method approach in understanding the working mechanism of XBJ in preventing invasive *C. albicans* infection.

ER Stress Pathway in Cell Death and Organ Failure

GRP78 is a negative regulator of the unfolded protein response (UPR). Knocking down GRP78 triggered the UPR in un-stressed cells (Pyrko et al., 2007; Li et al., 2008). GRP78 represses apoptosis by inhibiting BIK and caspase-7 activation (Reddy et al., 2003; Fu et al., 2007). The function of GRP78 was not determined in a kidney-specific knockout animal model yet. However, its liver-specific knockdown induced liver injury, suggesting GRP78 plays a role in organ protection and may render protection for the kidney upon *C. albicans* insults (Ji et al., 2011; Chen et al., 2014; Zhu and Lee, 2015). Consistent with the literature, inhibiting the function of GRP78 increased the death of 293T cells (**Figure 8**). HA15, a specific GRP78 inhibitor, did not induce a dramatic increase of 293T cell death. This may due to the redundant function of GRP78 and GRP94 (Zhu and Lee, 2015). This hypothesis remains to be tested.

Network Pharmacology in Developing Novel Regimens to Prevent Fungal Infection

Network pharmacology may shed light on developing novel Chinese medicine (Lyu et al., 2017; Suo et al., 2017). In this study, it also provided hints for a potential application of XBJ. Our aim was to take the advantages of network pharmacology to reveal a novel mechanism of XBJ in preventing invasive fungal infection. ER stress signaling was not predicted as top signaling related to invasive fungal infection by our network pharmacology analysis. In addition, our literature mining did not retrieve strong evidence indicating an important role of ER stress signaling in invasive fungal infection. It emerged from our RNA-seq analysis using RNA extracted from 293T cells in the presence of *C. albicans* and XBJ treatments. The alteration of GRP78 was more pronounced on the protein level rather than the transcription level in *C. albicans*–infected 293T cells treated by XBJ. However, Western Blot confirmed XBJ and C0127 did sustain the expression of GRP78 (**Figures 6** and **8**). Hence, our new finding indicated network pharmacology analysis and experiments complemented each other in illustrating the mechanism of compound Chinese medicine in treating human diseases.

C0127 Prevents *C. albicans*–Induced Kidney Failure

Our network pharmacology analysis predicted that four compounds in XBJ regulated 2/3 of predicted XBJ targets in fungal infection (**Figure 3A** and **Supplementary Figure 2**). This prediction was confirmed in our *in vivo* study (**Figure 7**). C0127 not only prevented *Candida* sepsis but also prevented *C. albicans* colonization in the kidney. Paeoniflorin and hydroxysafflor yellow A, the top two high-concentration compounds in XBJ, may play major roles in preventing kidney failure upon systemic *C. albicans* infection. Paeoniflorin which claims the highest concentration in XBJ was isolated from Chishao (Liu et al., 2015; Han et al., 2017). Several groups reported that paeoniflorin attenuates ER stress in different tissues and organs (Chen et al., 2018a; Gu et al., 2016; Jiang et al., 2014; Zhu et al., 2018). Gu et al. indicated paeoniflorin exerted protection for MCAO rats by regulating ER stress. Zhu et al. reported that paeoniflorin attenuates ER stress in retinal pigment epithelial cells *via* triggering Ca(2+)/CaMKII-dependent activation of AMPK (Zhu et al., 2018). It is likely that paeoniflorin plays a major role in regulating the expression of GRP78 in kidney epithelial cells. However, this was not verified by our *in vitro* experiments. Paeoniflorin did not significantly enhance the expression of GRP78 individually (data not shown). Consistent with our results, Gu et al. found that a combination of *L. chuanxiong* and *Radix paeoniae*, two herbs in XBJ, attenuated ER stress–dependent apoptotic signaling pathway in MCAO rats (Gu et al., 2016). Hydroxysafflor yellow A (HSYA) plays a role in preventing tissue injuries (Han et al., 2017). Bai et al. reported the protective effect of HSYA on acute kidney injury in an ischemia/reperfusion (I/R) model. They found HSYA prevented I/R induced apoptosis in kidney epithelial cells *in vivo* and *in vitro*. HSYA may attenuate TLR4 signaling to prevent apoptosis in kidney epithelial cells (Bai et al., 2018). Increasing the stability of HSYA in XBJ may further enhance the protection to the kidney (Pu et al., 2017). In our experiment, XBJ or C0127 does not inhibit *C. albicans* growth *in vitro*. This is consistent with the observation of Canturk which showed 1mg/ml ferulic acid-induced necrosis in *C. albicans* and it synergistically enhanced the anti-fungal effect of caspofungin (Canturk, 2018). Thus, low conc. of ferulic acid is unlikely to influence the survival of *C. albicans* in systematic infection. The combination of four compounds does not have a synergistic inhibition on the growth of *C. albicans in vitro* either (data not shown).

Future Directions

Our network pharmacology analysis predicted that XBJ regulates type I interferon and its upstream regulators such as interferon α, TLR2, and TLR4 in invasive fungal infection (**Figures 3B, C**). Thus, we hypothesized that XBJ may regulate type I interferon signaling in the innate immune system to enhance the clearance of *C. albicans* in invasive *C. albicans* infection. XBJ and C0127 may regulate innate immune system to enhance the survival of *Candida* infected mice while enhancing the survival of kidney epithelial cells. We also aim to determine how XBJ and C0127 regulate the innate immune cells and whether type I interferon signaling mediates their effects.

CONCLUSIONS

In conclusion, XBJ may prevent systemic *C. albicans* infection in sepsis patients. Compounds with higher concentrations in XBJ played major roles in preventing *Candida* induced kidney failure. GRP78 is a novel target of XBJ and C0127 in kidney epithelial cells. Members of ER stress signaling might be novel therapeutic targets in organ protection and sepsis.

ETHICS STATEMENT

This study was carried out in accordance with the recommendations of the Guide for the Care and Use of Laboratory Animals (NIH Publication No. 85-23, revised 1996, USA) and the recommendations in the Guidance for the Care and Use of Laboratory Animals issued by the Ministry of Science and Technology of China. All experiments were approved by the Institutional Animal Care and Use Committee of Nankai University and the Laboratory Animal Ethics Committee of the Tianjin University of Traditional Chinese Medicine (Tianjin, china) and were performed in accordance with its guidelines (Permit Number: TCM-LAE-20170017).

AUTHOR CONTRIBUTIONS

QY, YF, and M-CL designed the study and developed the methodologies. TS, QY, YF, TR, X-TW, HZ and J-MG conducted research. QY, YF, TS, TR, HZ, X-TW, J-MG, GP, XG, YZ and M-C.L. analyzed the data and contributed critical reagents. QY, YF, YZ, TS, and M-CL wrote and revised the manuscript.

FUNDING

This project was supported by the National Science Foundation of China (Grant number: 81774018, 81973581, 81873037, 31670146, 81873961); Tianjin University of Traditional Chinese Medicine (Startup Grant for Y.F.); Nankai University (The Open Fund of Ministry of Education Key Laboratory of Molecular Microbiology and Technology); Tianjin Municipal Education Commission (Grant number: TD13-5046).

ACKNOWLEDGMENTS

We thank our colleagues for their supports. We thank Zhengcan Zhou, Dr. Shuang He, Ming Lyu, Yu-Le Wang, Guang-Xu Xiao, and Xin-Yan Liu for their technical supports and constructive discussions. We thank Dr. John Orgh for editing our manuscript.

REFERENCES

Bai, J., Zhao, J., Cui, D., Wang, F., Song, Y., Cheng, L., et al. (2018). Protective effect of hydroxysafflor yellow A against acute kidney injury via the TLR4/NF-kappaB signaling pathway. *Sci. Rep.* 8, 9173. doi: 10.1038/s41598-018-27217-3

Brown, G. D., Denning, D. W., Gow, N. A., Levitz, S. M., Netea, M. G., and White, T. C. (2012). Hidden killers: human fungal infections. *Sci. Transl. Med.* 4, 165rv113. doi: 10.1126/scitranslmed.3004404

Brunke, S., and Hube, B. (2013). Two unlike cousins: candida albicans and C. glabrata infection strategies. *Cell Microbiol.* 15, 701–708. doi: 10.1111/cmi.12091

Canturk, Z. (2018). Evaluation of synergistic anticandidal and apoptotic effects of ferulic acid and caspofungin against Candida albicans. *J. Food Drug Anal.* 26, 439–443. doi: 10.1016/j.jfda.2016.12.014

Cao, Y. (2017). 27 Cases of fungal pneumonia treated with xuebijing and fluconazole modern journal of integrative traditional chinese and western medicine. 17 (64), 125. doi: 10.19613/j.cnki.1671-3141.2017.64.107

Cerezo, M., Lehraiki, A., Millet, A., Rouaud, F., Plaisant, M., Jaune, E., et al. (2016). Compounds triggering ER stress exert anti-melanoma effects and overcome BRAF inhibitor resistance. *Cancer Cell* 29, 805–819. doi: 10.1016/j.ccell.2016.04.013

Chen, G., Gao, Y., Jiang, Y., Yang, F., Li, S., Tan, D., et al. (2018a). Efficacy and safety of xuebijing injection combined with ulinastatin as adjunctive therapy on sepsis: a systematic review and meta-analysis. *Front. Pharmacol.* 9, 743.

Chen, Y., Tong, H., Zhang, X., Tang, L., Pan, Z., Liu, Z., et al. (2013). Xuebijing injection alleviates liver injury by inhibiting secretory function of Kupffer cells in heat stroke rats. *J. Tradit. Chin. Med.* 33, 243–249. doi: 10.1016/S0254-6272(13)60133-8

Chen, W. T., Zhu, G., Pfaffenbach, K., Kanel, G., Stiles, B., and Lee, A. S. (2014). GRP78 as a regulator of liver steatosis and cancer progression mediated by loss of the tumor suppressor PTEN. *Oncogene* 33, 4997–5005. doi: 10.1038/onc.2013.437

Chen, S., Dai, G., Hu, J., Rong, A., Lv, J., Su, L., et al. (2016). Discovery of xuebijing injection exhibiting protective efficacy on sepsis by inhibiting the expression of HMGB1 in septic rat model designed by cecal ligation and puncture. *Am. J. Ther.* 23, e1819–e1825. doi: 10.1097/MJT.0000000000000296

Chen, Y., Tong, H., Pan, Z., Jiang, D., Zhang, X., Qiu, J., et al. (2017). Xuebijing injection attenuates pulmonary injury by reducing oxidative stress and proinflammatory damage in rats with heat stroke. *Exp. Ther. Med.* 13, 3408–3416. doi: 10.3892/etm.2017.4444

Chen, X., Feng, Y., Shen, X., Pan, G., Fan, G., Gao, X., et al. (2018). Anti-sepsis protection of Xuebijing injection is mediated by differential regulation of pro- and anti-inflammatory Th17 and T regulatory cells in a murine model of polymicrobial sepsis. *J. Ethnopharmacol.* 211, 358–365. doi: 10.1016/j.jep.2017.10.001

Cheng, C., Lin, J. Z., Li, L., Yang, J. L., Jia, W. W., Huang, Y. H., et al. (2016). Pharmacokinetics and disposition of monoterpene glycosides derived from Paeonia lactiflora roots (Chishao) after intravenous dosing of antiseptic XueBiJing injection in human subjects and rats. *Acta Pharmacol. Sin.* 37, 530–544. doi: 10.1038/aps.2015.103

Diekema, D., Arbefeville, S., Boyken, L., Kroeger, J., and Pfaller, M. (2012). The changing epidemiology of healthcare-associated candidemia over three decades. *Diagn. Microbiol. Infect. Dis.* 73, 45–48. doi: 10.1016/j.diagmicrobio.2012.02.001

Dominguez-Andres, J., Feo-Lucas, L., Minguito de la Escalera, M., Gonzalez, L., Lopez-Bravo, M., and Ardavin, C. (2017). Inflammatory Ly6C(high) monocytes protect against candidiasis through IL-15-driven NK cell/neutrophil Activation. *Immunity* 46, 1059–1072 e1054. doi: 10.1016/j.immuni.2017.05.009

Dong, Y., Zhang, D., Yu, Q., Zhao, Q., Xiao, C., Zhang, K., et al. (2017). Loss of Ssq1 leads to mitochondrial dysfunction, activation of autophagy and cell cycle arrest due to iron overload triggered by mitochondrial iron-sulfur cluster assembly defects in Candida albicans. *Int. J. Biochem. Cell Biol.* 85, 44–55. doi: 10.1016/j.biocel.2017.01.021

Fang, K., and Wang, X. L. (2013). Treatment of multiple organ dysfunction syndrome by Xuebijing Injection: a clinical research. *Zhongguo Zhong Xi Yi Jie He Za Zhi* 33, 205–207.

Fu, Y., Li, J., and Lee, A. S. (2007). GRP78/BiP inhibits endoplasmic reticulum BIK and protects human breast cancer cells against estrogen starvation-induced apoptosis. *Cancer Res.* 67, 3734–3740. doi: 10.1158/0008-5472.CAN-06-4594

Gao, J., Kong, L., Liu, S., Feng, Z., Shen, H., Liu, Q., et al. (2015). A prospective multicenter clinical study of Xuebijing injection in the treatment of sepsis and multiple organ dysfunction syndrome. *Zhonghua Wei Zhong Bing Ji Jiu Yi Xue* 27, 465–470. doi: 10.3760/cma.j.issn.2095-4352.2015.06.010

Gao, W., Li, N., and Cui, X. G. (2018). Efficacy of xuebijing injection on cardiopulmonary bypass-associated pulmonary injury: a prospective, single-center, randomized, double blinded trial. *Chin. J. Integr. Med.* 24, 815–821. doi: 10.1007/s11655-018-2933-7

Gao, S. (2010). The therapeutic effect of Xuebijing on fungal pneumonia. *Nei Mongol J. Tradit. Chin. Med.* 2, 62–63. doi: 10.16040/j.cnki.cn15-1101.2010.09.132

Gray, M. J., Mhawech-Fauceglia, P., Yoo, E., Yang, W., Wu, E., Lee, A. S., et al. (2013). AKT inhibition mitigates GRP78 (glucose-regulated protein) expression and contribution to chemoresistance in endometrial cancers. *Int. J. Cancer* 133, 21–30. doi: 10.1002/ijc.27994

Gu, J., Chen, J., Yang, N., Hou, X., Wang, J., Tan, X., et al. (2016). Combination of ligusticum chuanxiong and radix paeoniae ameliorate focal cerebral ischemic in MCAO rats via endoplasmic reticulum stress-dependent apoptotic signaling pathway. *J. Ethnopharmacol.* 187, 313–324. doi: 10.1016/j.jep.2016.04.024

Guo, Y., Wang, Y., Huang, X., Lv, H., Fan, R., Huang, W., et al. (2014). Determination of hydroxysafflor yellow a in biological fluids of patients with traumatic brain injury by UPLC-ESI-MS/MS after injection of Xuebijing. *BioMed. Chromatogr.* 28, 1090–1095. doi: 10.1002/bmc.3124

Han, J. Y., Li, Q., Ma, Z. Z., and Fan, J. Y. (2017). Effects and mechanisms of compound Chinese medicine and major ingredients on microcirculatory dysfunction and organ injury induced by ischemia/reperfusion. *Pharmacol. Ther.* 177, 146–173. doi: 10.1016/j.pharmthera.2017.03.005

He, F., Wang, J., Liu, Y., Wang, X., Cai, N., Wu, C., et al. (2018). Xuebijing injection induces anti-inflammatory-like effects and downregulates the expression of TLR4 and NF-kappaB in lung injury caused by dichlorvos poisoning. *BioMed. Pharmacother.* 106, 1404–1411. doi: 10.1016/j.biopha.2018.07.111

Healey, K. R., Zhao, Y., Perez, W. B., Lockhart, S. R., Sobel, J. D., Farmakiotis, D., et al. (2016). Prevalent mutator genotype identified in fungal pathogen Candida glabrata promotes multi-drug resistance. *Nat. Commun.* 7, 11128. doi: 10.1038/ncomms11128

Hu, H. X., Zhu, M. Q., Sun, Y. C., Ma, C., Wang, X., and Liu, X. L. (2018). Xuebijing enhances neuroprotective effects of ulinastatin on transient cerebral ischemia via Nrf2-are signal pathways in the hippocampus. *J. Biol. Regul. Homeost. Agents* 32, 1143–1149.

Huang, H., Ji, L., Song, S., Wang, J., Wei, N., Jiang, M., et al. (2011). Identification of the major constituents in Xuebijing injection by HPLC-ESI-MS. *Phytochem. Anal.* 22, 330–338. doi: 10.1002/pca.1284

Ji, C., Kaplowitz, N., Lau, M. Y., Kao, E., Petrovic, L. M., and Lee, A. S. (2011). Liver-specific loss of glucose-regulated protein 78 perturbs the unfolded protein response and exacerbates a spectrum of liver diseases in mice. *Hepatology* 54, 229–239. doi: 10.1002/hep.24368

Jiang, M., Zhou, M., Han, Y., Xing, L., Zhao, H., Dong, L., et al. (2013). Identification of NF-kappaB Inhibitors in Xuebijing injection for sepsis treatment based on bioactivity-integrated UPLC-Q/TOF. *J. Ethnopharmacol.* 147, 426–433. doi: 10.1016/j.jep.2013.03.032

Jiang, Z., Chen, W., Yan, X., Bi, L., Guo, S., and Zhan, Z. (2014). Paeoniflorin protects cells from GalN/TNF-alpha-induced apoptosis *via* ER stress and mitochondria-dependent pathways in human L02 hepatocytes. *Acta. Biochim. Biophys.* Sin (Shanghai) 46 (5), 357–367 doi: 10.1093/abbs/gmu010

Jin, H., Chen, Y., Ding, C., Lin, Y., Chen, Y., Jiang, D., et al. (2018). Microcirculatory disorders and protective role of Xuebijing in severe heat stroke. *Sci. Rep.* 8, 4553. doi: 10.1038/s41598-018-22812-w

Kramer, A., Green, J., Pollard, J.Jr., and Tugendreich, S. (2014). Causal analysis approaches in ingenuity pathway analysis. *Bioinformatics* 30, 523–530. doi: 10.1093/bioinformatics/btt703

Kullberg, B. J., and Arendrup, M. C. (2015). Invasive candidiasis. *N. Engl. J. Med.* 373, 1445–1456. doi: 10.1056/NEJMra1315399

Lewy, T. G., Grabowski, J. M., and Bloom, M. E. (2017). BiP: master regulator of the unfolded protein response and crucial factor in flavivirus biology. *Yale J. Biol. Med.* 90, 291–300.

Li, Y. P., Qiao, Y. J., Wu, Z. X., Yao, Y. M., Yu, Y., and Wu, Y. (2007). Effects of Xuebijing injection on high-mobility group box chromosomal protein 1 in septic rats. *Zhongguo Wei Zhong Bing Ji Jiu Yi Xue* 19, 239–241. doi: 10.3760/j.issn:1003-0603.2007.04.013

Li, J., Ni, M., Lee, B., Barron, E., Hinton, D. R., and Lee, A. S. (2008). The unfolded protein response regulator GRP78/BiP is required for endoplasmic reticulum integrity and stress-induced autophagy in mammalian cells. *Cell Death Differ.* 15, 1460–1471. doi: 10.1038/cdd.2008.81

Li, D., Lu, L., Zhang, J., Wang, X., Xing, Y., Wu, H., et al. (2014a). Mitigating the effects of Xuebijing injection on hematopoietic cell injury induced by total body irradiation with gamma rays by decreasing reactive oxygen species levels. *Int. J. Mol. Sci.* 15, 10541–10553. doi: 10.3390/ijms150610541

Li, X. Y., Zhang, K., Jiang, Z. Y., and Cai, L. H. (2014b). MiR-204/miR-211 downregulation contributes to candidemia-induced kidney injuries *via* derepression of Hmx1 expression. *Life Sci.* 102, 139–144. doi: 10.1016/j.lfs.2014.03.010

Li, X., Cheng, C., Wang, F., Huang, Y., Jia, W., Olaleye, O. E., et al. (2016). Pharmacokinetics of catechols in human subjects intravenously receiving XueBiJing injection, an emerging antiseptic herbal medicine. *Drug Metab. Pharmacokinet.* 31, 95–98. doi: 10.1016/j.dmpk.2015.10.005

Li, X. Y., Zhang, Y. Q., Xu, G., Li, S. H., and Li, H. (2018). miR-124/MCP-1 signaling pathway modulates the protective effect of itraconazole on acute kidney injury in a mouse model of disseminated candidiasis. *Int. J. Mol. Med.* 41, 3468–3476. doi: 10.3892/ijmm.2018.3564

Li, J., Olaleye, O. E., Yu, X., Jia, W., Yang, J., Lu, C., et al. (2019). High degree of pharmacokinetic compatibility exists between the five-herb medicine XueBiJing and antibiotics comedicated in sepsis care. *Acta Pharm. Sin. B.* 9, 1035–1049. doi: 10.1016/j.apsb.2019.06.003

Liang, C., Zhang, B., Cui, L., Li, J., Yu, Q., and Li, M. (2018). Mgm1 is required for maintenance of mitochondrial function and virulence in Candida albicans. *Fungal Genet. Biol.* 120, 42–52. doi: 10.1016/j.fgb.2018.09.006

Liu, R., Li, X., Gao, W., Zhou, Y., Wey, S., Mitra, S. K., et al. (2013). Monoclonal antibody against cell surface GRP78 as a novel agent in suppressing PI3K/AKT signaling, tumor growth, and metastasis. *Clin. Cancer Res.* 19, 6802–6811. doi: 10.1158/1078-0432.CCR-13-1106

Liu, M. W., Su, M. X., Zhang, W., Wang, Y. Q., Chen, M., Wang, L., et al. (2014a). Protective effect of Xuebijing injection on paraquat-induced pulmonary injury via down-regulating the expression of p38 MAPK in rats. *BMC Complement Altern. Med.* 14, 498. doi: 10.1186/1472-6882-14-498

Liu, Y. K., He, J. B., Chen, H. E., Chen, D., Miao, Y. F., Ying, L., et al. (2014b). Effect of Xuebijing Injection on TLR4-NF-kappaB-TNF-alpha pathway of rats' myocardial anoxia/reoxygenation. *Zhongguo Zhong Xi Yi Jie He Za Zhi* 34, 1463–1468. doi: 10.7661/CJIM.2014.12.1463

Liu, Y. K., Huang, L. J., Zhao, S., Lin, W., He, J. B., Ying, L., et al. (2014c). Effect of Xuebijing injection on TLR4-NF-kappaB-IL-1beta pathway of myocardial hypoxia/reoxygenation in rats. *Zhongguo Ying Yong Sheng Li Xue Za Zhi* 30, 55–59. doi: 10.13459/j.cnki.cjap.2014.01.007

Liu, Y. C., Yao, F. H., Chai, Y. F., Dong, N., Sheng, Z. Y., and Yao, Y. M. (2015). Xuebijing injection promotes M2 polarization of macrophages and improves survival rate in septic mice. *Evid. Based Complement Alternat. Med.* 2015, 352642. doi: 10.1155/2015/352642

Lyu, M., Yan, C. L., Liu, H. X., Wang, T. Y., Shi, X. H., Liu, J. P., et al. (2017). Network pharmacology exploration reveals endothelial inflammation as a common mechanism for stroke and coronary artery disease treatment of Danhong injection. *Sci. Rep.* 7, 15427. doi: 10.1038/s41598-017-14692-3

Lyu, M., Zhou, Z., Wang, X., Lv, H., Wang, M., Pan, G., et al. (2018). Network pharmacology-guided development of a novel integrative regimen to prevent acute graft-vs.-host disease. *Front. Pharmacol.* 9, 1440. doi: 10.3389/fphar.2018.01440

Musumeci, D., Roviello, G. N., and Montesarchio, D. (2014). An overview on HMGB1 inhibitors as potential therapeutic agents in HMGB1-related pathologies. *Pharmacol. Ther.* 141, 347–357. doi: 10.1016/j.pharmthera.2013.11.001

Pfaller, M. A., and Diekema, D. J. (2010). Epidemiology of invasive mycoses in North America. *Crit. Rev. Microbiol.* 36, 1–53. doi: 10.3109/10408410903241444

Pu, W., Zhang, H., Wang, M., Liu, Y., Sun, L., and Ren, X. (2017). Superior stability of hydroxysafflor yellow a in xuebijing injection and the associated mechanism. *Molecules* 22 (12), 2129. doi: 10.3390/molecules22122129

Pyrko, P., Schonthal, A. H., Hofman, F. M., Chen, T. C., and Lee, A. S. (2007). The unfolded protein response regulator GRP78/BiP as a novel target for increasing chemosensitivity in malignant gliomas. *Cancer Res.* 67, 9809–9816. doi: 10.1158/0008-5472.CAN-07-0625

Reddy, R. K., Mao, C., Baumeister, P., Austin, R. C., Kaufman, R. J., and Lee, A. S. (2003). Endoplasmic reticulum chaperone protein GRP78 protects cells from apoptosis induced by topoisomerase inhibitors: role of ATP binding site in suppression of caspase-7 activation. *J. Biol. Chem.* 278, 20915–20924. doi: 10.1074/jbc.M212328200

Ru, J., Li, P., Wang, J., Zhou, W., Li, B., Huang, C., et al. (2014). TCMSP: a database of systems pharmacology for drug discovery from herbal medicines. *J. Cheminform.* 6, 13. doi: 10.1186/1758-2946-6-13

Ruggiero, C., Doghman-Bouguerra, M., Ronco, C., Benhida, R., Rocchi, S., and Lalli, E. (2018). The GRP78/BiP inhibitor HA15 synergizes with mitotane action against adrenocortical carcinoma cells through convergent activation of ER stress pathways. *Mol. Cell Endocrinol.* 474, 57–64. doi: 10.1016/j.mce.2018.02.010

Sakagami, T., Kawano, T., Yamashita, K., Yamada, E., Fujino, N., Kaeriyama, M., et al. (2018). Antifungal susceptibility trend and analysis of resistance mechanism for Candida species isolated from bloodstream at a Japanese university hospital. *J. Infect. Chemother* 25 (1), 34–40. doi: 10.1016/j.jiac.2018.10.007

Shani, G., Fischer, W. H., Justice, N. J., Kelber, J. A., Vale, W., and Gray, P. C. (2008). GRP78 and Cripto form a complex at the cell surface and collaborate to inhibit transforming growth factor beta signaling and enhance cell growth. *Mol. Cell Biol.* 28, 666–677. doi: 10.1128/MCB.01716-07

Shi, H., Hong, Y., Qian, J., Cai, X., and Chen, S. (2017). Xuebijing in the treatment of patients with sepsis. *Am. J. Emerg. Med.* 35, 285–291. doi: 10.1016/j.ajem.2016.11.007

Song, R., Dong, C., Wang, C., Zhang, H., and Yang, Z. (2018). Effectiveness of Xuebijing in treatment of multiple organ dysfunction syndrome: a Meta analysis. *Zhonghua Wei Zhong Bing Ji Jiu Yi Xue* 30, 848–854. doi: 10.3760/cma.j.issn.2095-4352.2018.09.006

Song, Y., Yao, C., Yao, Y., Han, H., Zhao, X., Yu, K., et al. (2019). XueBiJing Injection Versus Placebo for Critically Ill Patients With Severe Community-Acquired Pneumonia: A Randomized Controlled Trial. *Crit. Care Med.* 47, e735–e743. doi: 10.1097/CCM.0000000000003842

Spellberg, B., Ibrahim, A. S., Edwards, J. E.Jr., and Filler, S. G. (2005). Mice with disseminated candidiasis die of progressive sepsis. *J. Infect. Dis.* 192, 336–343. doi: 10.1086/430952

Stelzer, G., Dalah, I., Stein, T. I., Satanower, Y., Rosen, N., Nativ, N., et al. (2011). *In-silico* human genomics with GeneCards. *Hum. Genomics* 5, 709–717. doi: 10.1186/1479-7364-5-6-709

Suo, T., Liu, J., Chen, X., Yu, H., Wang, T., Li, C., et al. (2017). Combining chemical profiling and network analysis to investigate the pharmacology of complex prescriptions in traditional chinese medicine. *Sci. Rep.* 7, 40529. doi: 10.1038/srep40529

Tian, X., Zhang, W. L., Hu, L. L., She, X. R., Hong, G. L., Chen, L. M., et al. (2018). The protective effect of Xuebijing on paraquat-induced HK-2 cells apoptosis and the underlying mechanisms. *Zhonghua Lao Dong Wei Sheng Zhi Ye Bing Za Zhi* 36, 1–6. doi: 10.3760/cma.j.issn.1001-9391.2018.01.001

Wang, H., Bloom, O., Zhang, M., Vishnubhakat, J. M., Ombrellino, M., Che, J., et al. (1999). HMG-1 as a late mediator of endotoxin lethality in mice. *Science* 285, 248–251. doi: 10.1126/science.285.5425.248

Wang, Q., Yao, Y. M., Wang, W. J., Xian, L. M., Dong, N., Xu, S., et al. (2007). Effect of Xuebijing injection on renal high mobility group box-1 protein expression and acute kidney injury in rats after scald injury. *Zhongguo Yi Xue Ke Xue Yuan Xue Bao* 29, 478–483. doi: 10.3760/j.issn:0529-5815.2007.17.018

Wang, Q., Wu, X., Tong, X., Zhang, Z., Xu, B., and Zhou, W. (2015). Xuebijing Ameliorates Sepsis-Induced Lung Injury by Downregulating HMGB1 and RAGE Expressions in Mice. *Evid. Based Complement Alternat. Med.* 2015, 860259. doi: 10.1155/2015/860259

Wang, J. W. (2010). Efficiency and security of amphotericin b plus xuebijing injection in early empirical treatment of invasive fungal infection in ICU. *Chin. J. Med. Guide* 12, 2. doi: 10.3969/j.issn.1009-0959.2010.11.055

Wirnsberger, G., Zwolanek, F., Asaoka, T., Kozieradzki, I., Tortola, L., Wimmer, R. A., et al. (2016). Inhibition of CBLB protects from lethal Candida albicans sepsis. *Nat. Med.* 22, 915–923. doi: 10.1038/nm.4134

Xiao, Y., Tang, J., Guo, H., Zhao, Y., Tang, R., Ouyang, S., et al. (2016). Targeting CBLB as a potential therapeutic approach for disseminated candidiasis. *Nat. Med.* 22, 906–914. doi: 10.1038/nm.4141

Xu, Q., Liu, J., Guo, X., Tang, Y., Zhou, G., Liu, Y., et al. (2015). Xuebijing injection reduces organ injuries and improves survival by attenuating inflammatory responses and endothelial injury in heatstroke mice. *BMC Complement Altern. Med.* 15, 4. doi: 10.1186/s12906-015-0519-5

Xu, J. J., Zhen, J. T., Tang, L., and Lin, Q. M. (2017). Intravenous injection of Xuebijing attenuates acute kidney injury in rats with paraquat intoxication. *World J. Emerg. Med.* 8, 61–64. doi: 10.5847/wjem.j.1920-8642.2017.01.011

Xue, R., Fang, Z., Zhang, M., Yi, Z., Wen, C., and Shi, T. (2013). TCMID: Traditional Chinese Medicine integrative database for herb molecular mechanism analysis. *Nucleic Acids Res.* 41, D1089–D1095. doi: 10.1093/nar/gks1100

Yu, Q., Jia, C., Dong, Y., Zhang, B., Xiao, C., Chen, Y., et al. (2015). Candida albicans autophagy, no longer a bystander: Its role in tolerance to ER stress-related antifungal drugs. *Fungal Genet. Biol.* 81, 238–249. doi: 10.1016/j.fgb.2015.02.008

Yuxi, Q., Zhang, H., Baili, Y., and Shi, S. (2017). Effects of Xuebijing Injection for Patients With Sepsis-induced Acute Kidney Injury After Wenchuan Earthquake. *Altern. Ther. Health Med.* 23, 36–42.

Zhang, H., Wei, L., Zhao, G., Liu, S., Zhang, Z., Zhang, J., et al. (2016). Protective effect of Xuebijing injection on myocardial injury in patients with sepsis: a randomized clinical trial. *J. Tradit. Chin. Med.* 36, 706–710. doi: 10.1016/S0254-6272(17)30003-1

Zhang, N., Cheng, C., Olaleye, O.E., Sun, Y., Li, L., Huang, Y., et al. (2018). Pharmacokinetics-Based Identification of Potential Therapeutic Phthalides from XueBiJing, a Chinese Herbal Injection Used in Sepsis Management. *Drug Metab. Dispos.* 46, 823–834.

Zhao, X., Guo, Y., Jiang, C., Chang, Q., Zhang, S., Luo, T., et al. (2017). JNK1 negatively controls antifungal innate immunity by suppressing CD23 expression. *Nat. Med.* 23, 337–346. doi: 10.1038/nm.4260

Zhu, G., and Lee, A. S. (2015). Role of the unfolded protein response, GRP78 and GRP94 in organ homeostasis. *J. Cell Physiol.* 230, 1413–1420. doi: 10.1002/jcp.24923

Zhu, X., Wang, K., Zhou, F., and Zhu, L. (2018). Paeoniflorin attenuates atRAL-induced oxidative stress, mitochondrial dysfunction and endoplasmic reticulum stress in retinal pigment epithelial cells via triggering Ca(2+)/CaMKII-dependent activation of AMPK. *Arch. Pharm. Res.* 41, 1009–1018. doi: 10.1007/s12272-018-1059-6

Zuo, L., Zhong, Q., Wang, Z., Sun, Z., Zhou, L., Li, Z., et al. (2017). Simultaneous determination and pharmacokinetic study of twelve bioactive compounds in rat plasma after intravenous administration of Xuebijing injection by UHPLC-Q-Orbitrap HRMS. *J. Pharm. BioMed. Anal.* 146, 347–353. doi: 10.1016/j.jpba.2017.09.010

Zuo, L., Zhou, L., Xu, T., Li, Z., Liu, L., Shi, Y., et al. (2018). Antiseptic activity of ethnomedicinal Xuebijing revealed by the metabolomics analysis using UHPLC-Q-Orbitrap HRMS. *Front. Pharmacol.* 9, 300. doi: 10.3389/fphar.2018.00300

12

Network Pharmacology-Based Validation of Caveolin-1 as a Key Mediator of Ai Du Qing Inhibition of Drug Resistance in Breast Cancer

Neng Wang[1], Bowen Yang[1,2], Xiaotong Zhang[1], Shengqi Wang[1,2], Yifeng Zheng[1,2], Xiong Li[1,2], Shan Liu[1], Hao Pan[1], Yingwei Li[1,3], Zhujuan Huang[1], Fengxue Zhang[1] and Zhiyu Wang[1,2]**

[1] The Research Center of Basic Integrative Medicine, Guangdong Provincial Academy of Chinese Medical Sciences, Guangzhou University of Chinese Medicine, Guangzhou, China, [2] Integrative Research Laboratory of Breast Cancer, Discipline of Integrated Chinese and Western Medicine, The Second Affiliated Hospital of Guangzhou University of Chinese Medicine, Guangzhou, China, [3] Tropical Medicine Institute, Guangzhou University of Chinese Medicine, Guangzhou, China

***Correspondence:**
Fengxue Zhang
zhangfengxue@gzucm.edu.cn
Zhiyu Wang
wangzhiyu976@126.com

Chinese formulas have been paid increasing attention in cancer multidisciplinary therapy due to their multi-targets and multi-substances property. Here, we aim to investigate the anti-breast cancer and chemosensitizing function of Ai Du Qing (ADQ) formula made up of *Hedyotis diffusa*, *Curcuma zedoaria (Christm.) Rosc.*, *Astragalus membranaceus (Fisch.) Bunge,* and *Glycyrrhiza uralensis Fisch*. Our findings revealed that ADQ significantly inhibited cell proliferation in both parental and chemo-resistant breast cancer cells, but with little cytotoxcity effects on the normal cells. Besides, ADQ was found to facilitate the G2/M arresting and apoptosis induction effects of paclitaxel. Network pharmacology and bioinformatics analysis further demonstrated that ADQ yielded 132 candidate compounds and 297 potential targets, and shared 22 putative targets associating with breast cancer chemoresponse. Enrichment analysis and experimental validation demonstrated that ADQ might improve breast cancer chemosensitivity *via* inhibiting caveolin-1, which further triggered expression changes of cell cycle-related proteins p21/cyclinB1 and apoptosis-associated proteins PARP1, BAX and Bcl-2. Besides, ADQ enhanced *in vivo* paclitaxel chemosensitivity on breast cancer. Our study not only uncovers the novel function and mechanisms of ADQ in chemosensitizing breast cancer at least partly *via* targeting caveolin-1, but also sheds novel light in utilizing network pharmacology in Chinese Medicine research.

Keywords: breast cancer chemosensitivity, network pharmacology, bioinformatics analysis, Ai Du Qing, caveolin-1

Abbreviations: ADQ, Ai Du Qing; CAV1, caveolin-1; DAD, diode array detection; DAPI, 4′,6-diamidino-2-phenylindole; DAVID, Database for Annotation, Visualization and Integrated Discovery; DEGs, differentially expressed genes; DL, drug-likeness; GEO, Gene Expression Omnibus; GO, Gene Ontology; H&E staining, hematoxylin-eosin staining; HPLC, high-performance liquid chromatography; HUMECs, the primary human mammary epithelial cells; HUVECs, the human umbilical vein endothelial cells; IC50, the half maximal inhibitory concentration; IHC, immunohistochemistry; KEGG, Kyoto Encyclopedia of Genes and Genomes; NCBI, National Center for Biotechnology Information; OB, oral bioavailability; PARP1, Poly (ADP-ribose) polymerase 1; PI, propidium iodide; PPI, protein–protein interaction; TCM, traditional Chinese medicine; TCMID, Traditional Chinese Medicine Integrated Database; TCMSP, Traditional Chinese Medicine Systems Pharmacology; TUNEL, terminal dexynucleotidyl transferase(TdT)-mediated dUTP nick end labeling.

INTRODUCTION

Breast cancer is the most common female malignancy and one of the leading causes of cancer-related deaths, with 252,710 new cases of invasive breast cancer and 40,610 breast cancer-related deaths diagnosed in women in the United States in 2017 (DeSantis et al., 2017). Chemotherapy is one of the main therapeutic approaches for treating this disease, but it remains non-selectively toxic to normal tissues (Li et al., 2005). Paclitaxel (taxol) is the first-line treatment for metastatic breast cancer. The activity of paclitaxel is primarily due to its inhibitory effects on microtubule assembly, which leads to arrest of the mitotic phase of the cell cycle and subsequent apoptosis. Nevertheless, paclitaxel application is still limited due to its systemic toxicity and acquired resistance (Janczar et al., 2017; Stage et al., 2018). Thus, there is an urgent need for novel and safe chemosensitizing strategies. Currently, increasing attention has been paid to the synergistic effects of natural phytochemicals in enhancing the chemoresponse and relieving cytotoxic effects (Wang et al., 2014).

Traditional Chinese Medicine (TCM) has attracted worldwide attention from clinicians and researchers due to its multi-target and multi-substance characteristics and good safety profile (Gupta et al., 2013). In contrast to Western medicine, TCM prescriptions are composed of several herbs and are called formulas. Originating from Yellow Emperor's Classic theory (Chinese name Huang Di Nei Jing), the golden principle of formula composition should be based on Jun-Chen-Zuo-Shi (Lu, 1985; Fan et al., 2006). The ADQ formula was created by Prof. Zhiyu Wang based on the Jun-Chen-Zuo-Shi principle and long-term clinical experience. The ADQ formula is mainly composed of four herbs: Jun (Emperor) herb *Hedyotis diffusa* (Chinese name Bai Hua She Cao, BHSSC), Chen (Minister) herb *Curcuma zedoaria (Christm.) Rosc.* (Chinese name E Zhu, EZ), Zuo (adjuvant) herb *Astragalus membranaceus (Fisch.) Bunge* (Chinese name Huang Qi, HQ), and Shi (courier) herb *Glycyrrhiza uralensis Fisch* (Chinese name Gan Cao, GC). Each herb in the formula can inhibit cancer growth *via* cell cycle arrest, apoptosis induction, and immune regulation (Fu et al., 2014a; Gao et al., 2014; Wang et al., 2014, 2015b; Feng et al., 2017). In addition, each herb is a drug that is frequently prescribed to cancer patients according to statistical analyses of the medication rules of national TCM masters (Song et al., 2015). However, the multi-target and multi-substance properties of this formula have made it very challenging to explore its underlying mechanisms.

In the past decade, multi-omic technologies including genomics, transcriptomic, proteomics, metabolomics, and serum pharmacokinetics have been developed for the high-throughput screening and identification of targets involved in TCM formulas (Li et al., 2014). However, these traditional approaches are expensive and require multidisciplinary collaboration and complex analytical procedures (Xu et al., 2017). With the development of bioinformatics, systems biology is emerging as a more holistic approach for integrating compound–target interactions from a molecular to system level. One of the most significant applications of systems biology is to use network pharmacology to understand the complex mechanism of actions of TCM formulas. Following ingredient collection and screening, pharmacokinetic evaluation (absorption, distribution, and metabolism), target prediction, and network analysis (Liu et al., 2013), it is becoming faster and easier to present an entire drug-target interaction network and determine the involved core molecule and pathways. In addition, by intersecting with a disease target database, it is more efficient to elucidate how formulas intervene with critical targets that facilitate disease occurrence and progression (Ru et al., 2014).

The current study was designed to determine the preclinical efficacy of ADQ against breast cancer *in vitro* and *in vivo*. To this end, we investigated the anti-cancer and chemosensitizing functions of ADQ extracts in this disease. The results showed that ADQ effectively and safely enhanced breast cancer chemosensitivity *in vitro* and *in vivo*. To determine the mechanism of action, we constructed a "drug–target–disease" network among ADQ components (drug), ADQ targets (target), and genes in breast cancer chemoresistance (disease). The results of the network analysis and biological experimental findings suggested that ADQ mainly targets CAV1 to induce chemosensitizing effects. The results of this study not only provide scientific evidence to support the application of ADQ formula in the treatment of breast cancer but also highlight the novel role of network pharmacology in the modernization of TCM.

MATERIALS AND METHODS

Preparation and Quality Control of ADQ

For ADQ preparation, BHSSC, EZ, HQ, and GC were mixed at a 1:1:1:1 ratio and then subjected to a grinding machine. The mixture was extracted with 95% alcohol by reflux extraction for 1 h and repeated three times. Then the supernatants were concentrated by rotary evaporation and evaporated to dryness in a water bath to obtain raw ethanol extract powder. The production ratio was calculated as 7.2–9.6%. For quality control analysis, the Agilent 1260 System (Agilent, Palo Alto, CA, United States) with DAD was applied for HPLC analysis. The Agilent C_{18} Column (5 μm, 250 mm × 4.6 mm) with the SecurityGuard Cartridge System (Phenomenex, Sacramento, CA, United States) was applied for HPLC analysis. The mobile phases consisted of acetonitrile (A) and 0.05% (v/v) phosphoric acid (B) using a gradient program of 15% A in 0–23 min, 15–38% A in 23–40 min, 38% A in 40–50 min, 38–61% A in 50–60 min, and 61% in 60–75 min. The flow rate was 1.0 mL/min and the column temperature was set to 30°C The DAD detector was set at 216, 236, 260, 276, and 308 nm. P-coumaric acid, calycosin-7-glucoside, liquiritin, glycyrrhizic acid, and curcumol were prepared and diluted with methanol for the preparation of standard solutions. A volume of 10 μL of these solutions was analyzed with HPLC, and the calibration curves were finally established. For the preparation of sample solutions, 0.1 g ADQ was dissolved in 20 mL methanol. After sonicating for 60 min, the sample solution was filtrated through a 0.2 μm membrane filter for HPLC analysis.

Cell Culture

The human breast cancer cell lines MDA-MB-231 and MCF-7 were purchased from the American Type Culture Collection (Manassas, VA, United States). MDA-MB-231/T and MCF-7/T cells were derived from parental cells by gradually increasing paclitaxel (taxol) treatments for 6 months in the laboratory. MDA-MB-231, MCF-7, MDA-MB-231/T, and MCF-7/T cells were maintained in Dulbecco's Modified Eagle Medium (DMEM) containing 10% fetal bovine serum (FBS) and 1% penicillin and streptomycin (Gibco Life Technologies, Lofer, Austria). Primary human mammary epithelial cells (HUMECs) and its Ready Medium (Catalog No. 12752010) were purchased from Gibco, and human umbilical vein endothelial cells (HUVECs) were purchased from the National Infrastructure of Cell Line Resource[1]. The cells were maintained in DMEM supplemented with 10% FBS, 1% penicillin, 1% streptomycin (Gibco), 40 U/L insulin (Sigma, St. Louis, MO, United States), 40 U/mL heparin (Sigma), and 1% non-essential amino acids (Cyagen Biosciences, Santa Clara, CA, United States).

Cell Number and Colony Formation Assay

After the indicated drug treatment, cell numbers were counted using trypan blue exclusion on a Cellometer Mini device (Nexcelom, Boston, MA, United States). Experiments were performed in triplicate. For the colony formation assay, cells at a density of 1×10^3 cells/well were seeded into 6-well plates. After cell attachment, paclitaxel or ADQ was added to the wells alone or in combination for 4 h. Then the cells were cultured with fresh medium for 2 weeks. The colonies were fixed in 4% paraformaldehyde, stained with Coomassie Blue, photographed, and counted under a microscope.

Flow Cytometry Analysis

For the drug efflux assay, MDA-MB-231 or MCF-7 cells were pretreated with ADQ for 24 h, followed by incubation with epirubicin for 60 min at 37°C. After dug exposure and washing, the cells were released in drug-free medium for 90 min and harvested for flow cytometry analysis. For cell cycle analysis, cells were fixed in ice-cold 70% ethanol at −20°C overnight. Then cells were washed with phosphate-buffered saline, stained with 50 mg/mL propidium iodide (Sigma), and dissolved in 100 mg/L RNase A (Sigma). For apoptosis analysis, the cells were stained with the Annexin V-FITC Apoptosis Staining/Detection Kit (BD Biosciences, San Jose, CA, United States). All flow cytometry analyses were conducted with FACSAria SORP (BD Biosciences) and analyzed by Modifit LT or FlowJo software.

Immunofluorescence Analysis and Hoechst 33258 Staining

For measurements of phosphorylated histone *p*-H2AX expression, cells were incubated with 4% paraformaldehyde and 0.2% triton X-100 for 10 min. Following blocking in goat serum for 60 min, the samples were co-incubated with primary antibodies against *p*-H2AX (ABclonal Technology, Boston, MA, United States) at 4°C overnight and subsequently labeled with fluorescence-conjugated secondary antibodies for 2 h at room temperature. Then DAPI was applied for nuclear staining, and the signals were detected by fluorescence microscopy (TS2R; Nikon, Tokyo, Japan). With regard to Hoechst 33528 detection, cells were seeded at 60–70% confluency in 6-well plates, and then treated with the indicated drug for 48 h. Then Hoechst 33258 staining was conducted according to the manufacturer's instructions.

Establishment of the Herb–Ingredient–Target Interaction

The chemical ingredients were collected from TCM databases including the TCMSP Database[2] the TCMID[3], and the BATMAN-TCM[4]. The ingredients were screened according to drug likeness (DL) and OB values, and the ingredients were retained if DL $\geq$ 0.18 and OB $\geq$ 30, a criterion suggested by the TCMSP database. The ingredient–target networks were constructed for these herbs using Cytoscape software (version 3.2.1).

Gene Ontology and Pathway Enrichment Analysis

Gene expression data were retrieved from the NCBI GEO database[5], and then analyzed with the GEO2R online analysis tool[6]. The dataset GSE41112 includes 24 tumors of breast cancer patients with chemotherapy and 37 without chemotherapy, and the GSE87455 dataset includes human breast cancer samples with "no treatment" (n = 122) and "chemo only" (n = 83) groups. The DEGs were screened with $P \leq 0.05$ and fold control (FC) $\geq$ 1.5 criteria, delivered to the Search Tool for the Retrieval of Interacting Genes/Protines (STRING) database to evaluate the PPI information, and also submitted to the DAVID[7] for enrichment analysis. The significant enrichment analysis of DEGs was assessed based on the GO and KEGG[8].

Plasmids and Small Interfering RNA Construction and Transfection

The pcDNA 3.1(+)-CAV1 was provided by Vigene Company (Jinan, China) and transfected into cells using Lipofectamine 2000 (Invitrogen, Carlsbad, CA, United States). After 24 h, the transfected cells were passaged and selected for 2 weeks with 10 μg/mL puromycin (Invitrogen). Pooled populations of positive cells were used for subsequent experiments. Negative control cell lines were generated by transfecting cells with scrambled plasmids. The small interfering RNAs (siRNAs) targeting CAV1 or scrambled siRNAs were purchased from

[1] http://www.cellresource.cn

[2] http://lsp.nwu.edu.cn/tcmsp.php

[3] https://academic.oup.com/nar/article/41/D1/D1089/1057998

[4] http://bionet.ncpsb.org/batman-tcm/

[5] http://www.ncbi.nlm.nih.gov/geo

[6] http://www.ncbi.nlm.nih.gov/geo/geo2r/

[7] http://david.abcc.ncifcrf.gov/

[8] http://www.genome.jp/kegg/kegg2.html

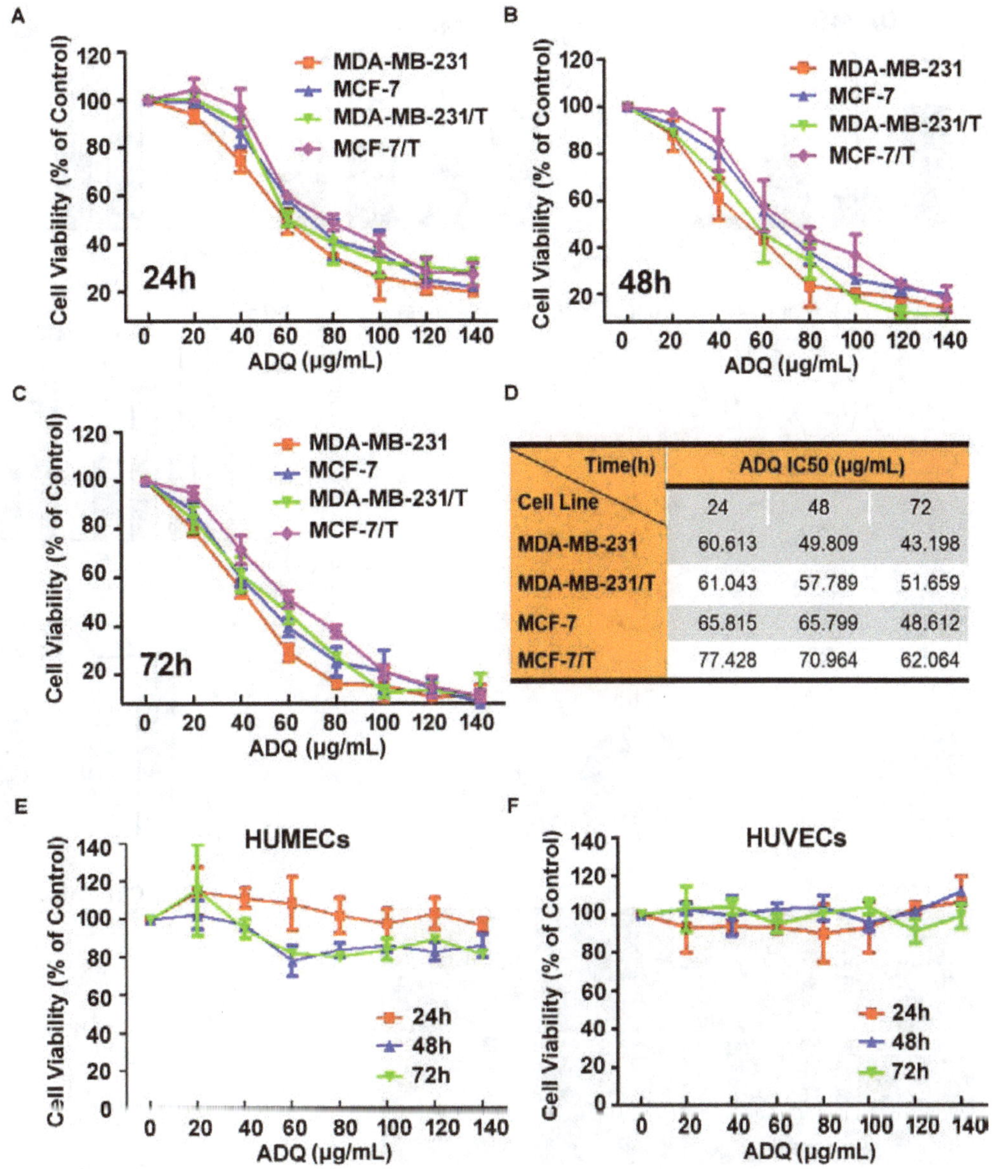

Cell Line \ Time(h)	ADQ IC50 (µg/mL)		
	24	48	72
MDA-MB-231	60.613	49.809	43.198
MDA-MB-231/T	61.043	57.789	51.659
MCF-7	65.815	65.799	48.612
MCF-7/T	77.428	70.964	62.064

FIGURE 1 | Effects of ADQ on cell proliferation in the paclitaxel-sensitive breast cancer cells and paclitaxel-resistant human breast cancer cells. **(A–C)** Exponentially growing cells of MDA-MB-231, MCF-7, MDA-MB-231/T, and MCF-7/T were treated with ADQ at the indicated concentrations (0–140 µg/mL) for 24, 48, and 72 h; **(D)** The IC50s of ADQ for MDA-MB-231, MDA-MB-231/T, MCF-7, and MCF-7/T cells; **(E,F)** Exponentially growing cells of HUMECs and HUVECs were treated with ADQ at the indicated concentrations (0–140 µg/mL) for 24, 48, and 72 h.

Invitrogen (Carlsbad) and transfected using the X-tremeGENE siRNA transfection reagent (Roche Diagnostics, Indianapolis, IN, United States) according to the manufacturer's instructions.

Western Blotting

To determine the protein concentration, cells were lysed in RIPA buffer (Sigma) containing a protease inhibitor mixture (Roche Diagnostics). The protein concentration was measured with the bicinchoninic acid assay (Thermo Fisher Scientific, Bonn, Germany). Quantified protein lysates (15 µg) were subjected to sodium dodecyl sulfate polyacrylamide gel electrophoresis and resolved on 12% polyacrylamide gels. Then the proteins were transferred onto a PVDF membrane (GE Healthcare, Freiburg, Germany). The membrane was probed with primary antibodies including CAV1, p21, cyclin B1, cleaved poly (ADP-ribose) polymerase (PARP), Bcl2-associated X protein (BAX), B-cell lymphoma 2 (Bcl-2), p53, and phosphorylated p53 (p-p52, ser 15), and β-actin (Cell Signaling Technology, Beverly, MA, United States) at 4°C overnight. After washing three times with Tris-buffered saline and 0.05% Tween-20, the membrane was incubated with secondary anti-rabbit or anti-mouse antibodies for 2 h at room temperature. The signals were visualized using the ECL Advance Western Blotting Detection Reagent (GE Healthcare) and quantified with FlowJo software.

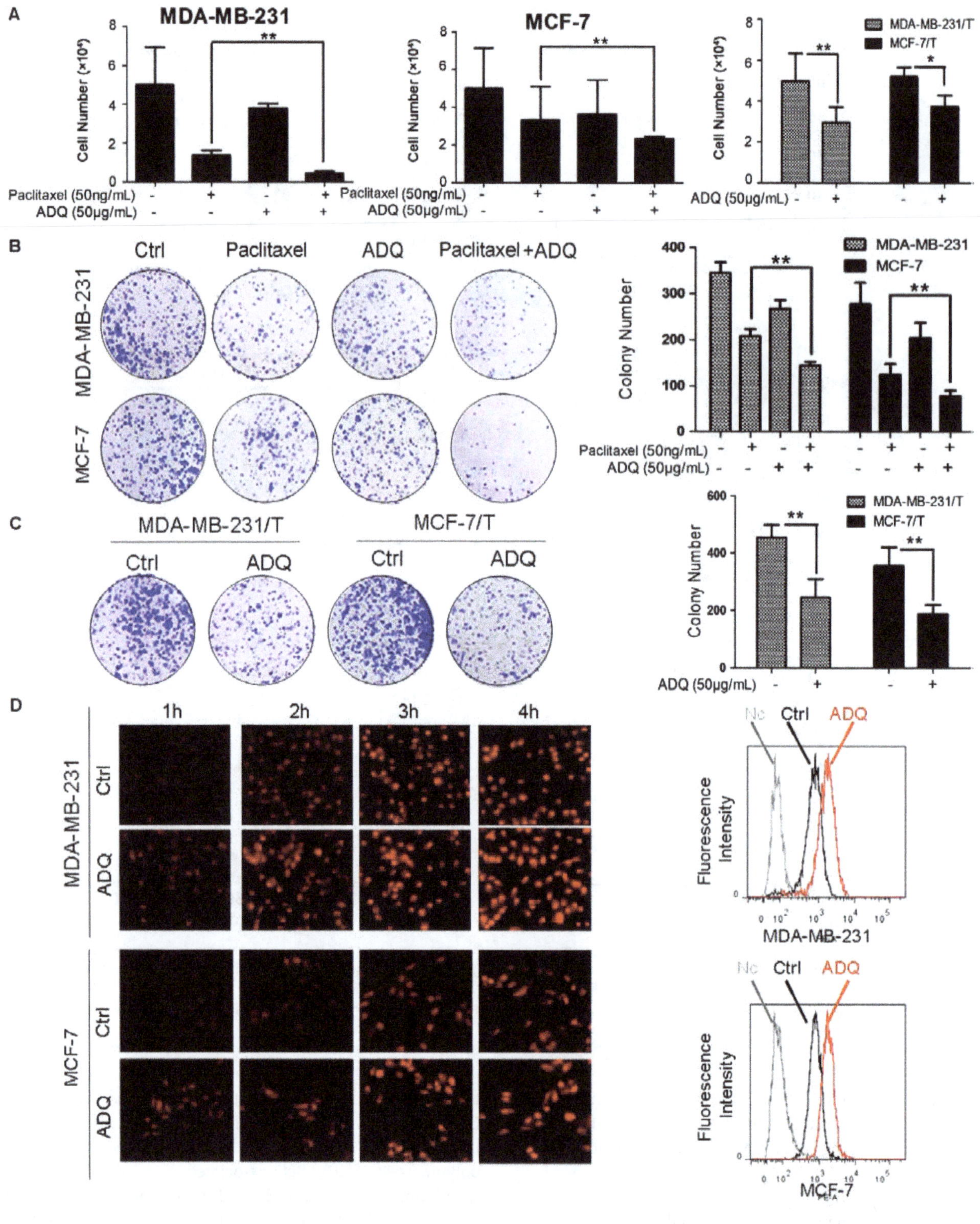

FIGURE 2 | ADQ significantly enhances the chemosensitivity of breast cancer cells. **(A)** The synergistic effects of ADQ (50 μg/mL) with paclitaxel (50 ng/mL) on MDA-MB-231 and MCF-7 cells, and the inhibitory effects of ADQ (50 μg/mL) on MDA-MB-231/T and MCF-7/T cells were studied by the cell counting assay after 48h treatment (*$P < 0.05$ *v.s.* control, **$P < 0.01$ *v.s.* control, values represented as the mean ± SD, $n = 3$); **(B)** Colony formation assay for evaluating the long-term inhibitory effects of ADQ (50 μg/mL) with or without paclitaxel (50 ng/mL) on MDA-MB-231 and MCF-7 cells; **(C)** Colony formation assay for evaluating the long-term inhibitory effects of ADQ (50 μg/mL) on MDA-MB-231/T and MCF-7/T cells (*$P < 0.05$ *v.s.* control, **$P < 0.01$ *v.s.* control, values represented as the mean ± SD, $n = 3$); **(D)** the drug efflux assay revealed that ADQ (50 μg/mL) could enhance the epirubicin intake into breast cancer cells, as shown by increased fluorescence intensity of epirubicin in ADQ-treated cells by flow cytometry analysis.

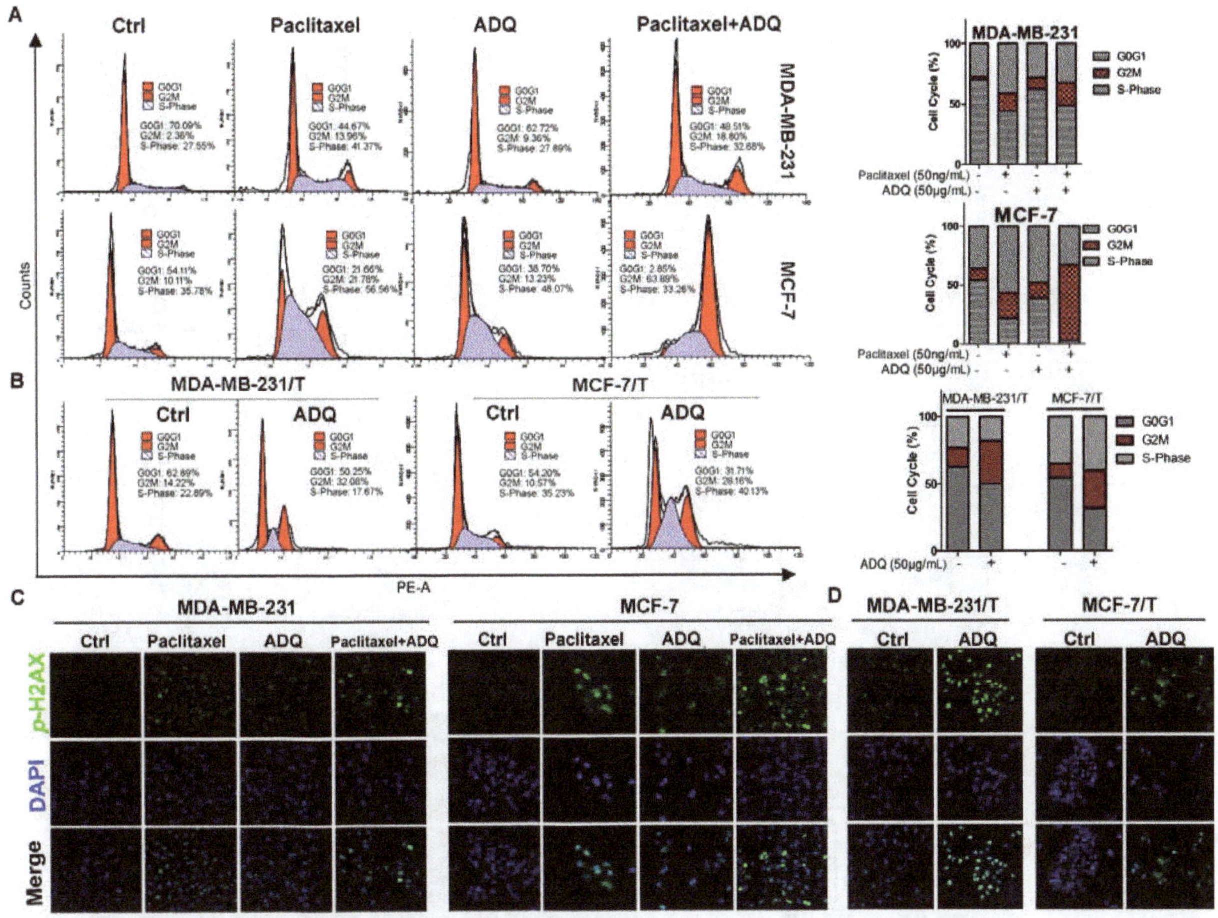

FIGURE 3 | ADQ and paclitaxel induce breast cancer cell cycle arrest at the G2/M phase. Representative cell cycle analysis of **(A)** the MDA-MB-231 and MCF-7 cells treated with ADQ (50 μg/ml) and/or paclitaxel (50 ng/mL), as well as **(B)** the MDA-MB-231/T and MCF-7/T cells treated with ADQ (50 μg/mL) for 48 h using flow cytometry. The length of each cell cycle phase was calculated; The immunofluorescence assay was performed to examine *p*-H2A.X **(C)** in the MDA-MB-231 and MCF-7 cells treated with ADQ (50 μg/mL) and/or paclitaxel (50 ng/mL), as well as **(D)** in the MDA-MB-231/T and MCF-7/T cells treated with ADQ (50 μg/mL) for 48 h.

Breast Cancer Mice Models and Drug Treatment

All animal procedures were performed in accordance with institutional guidelines for the care and use of laboratory animals approved by the Animal Care and Use Committee of Guangzhou University of Chinese Medicine and the National Institutes of Health guide for the care and use of laboratory animals. The mouse mammary tumor virus (MMTV)-PyMT mouse model of breast cancer spontaneously develops 100% multiple and luminal-like breast tumors from normal mammary epitheliums by 8–12 weeks, similar to the pathological processes and characteristics in human breast cancer (Lin et al., 2003; Wang et al., 2013). In this study, 9-week-old MMTV-PyMT mice were randomly divided into four groups, and treated with saline (Ctrl group), 10 mg/kg paclitaxel (paclitaxel group), 100 mg/kg ADQ (ADQ group), or 10 mg/kg paclitaxel plus 100 mg/kg ADQ (paclitaxel + ADQ group) for 26 days ($n = 6$ mice, total of 60 glands), respectively. Paclitaxel was given by intraperitoneal injection at 10 mg/kg every 3 days, and ADQ was given by oral gavage at 100 mg/kg once a day. The body weight and tumor volumes were recorded throughout the whole experimental period.

Hematoxylin and Eosin Staining, Immunohistochemistry, and Terminal Deoxynucleotidyl Transferase dUTP Nick End Labeling

Hematoxylin and eosin staining and IHC were conducted according to the protocol provided by Wang et al. (2017a). The terminal dexynucleotidyl transferase dUTP nick end labeling (TUNEL) assay was conducted according to the manufacturer's instructions (Catalog No. KGA7051; KeyGen Biotech, Nanjing, China).

Statistical Analysis

The data are shown as the mean ± standard deviation. The two-tailed Student's *t*-test or one-way analysis of variance

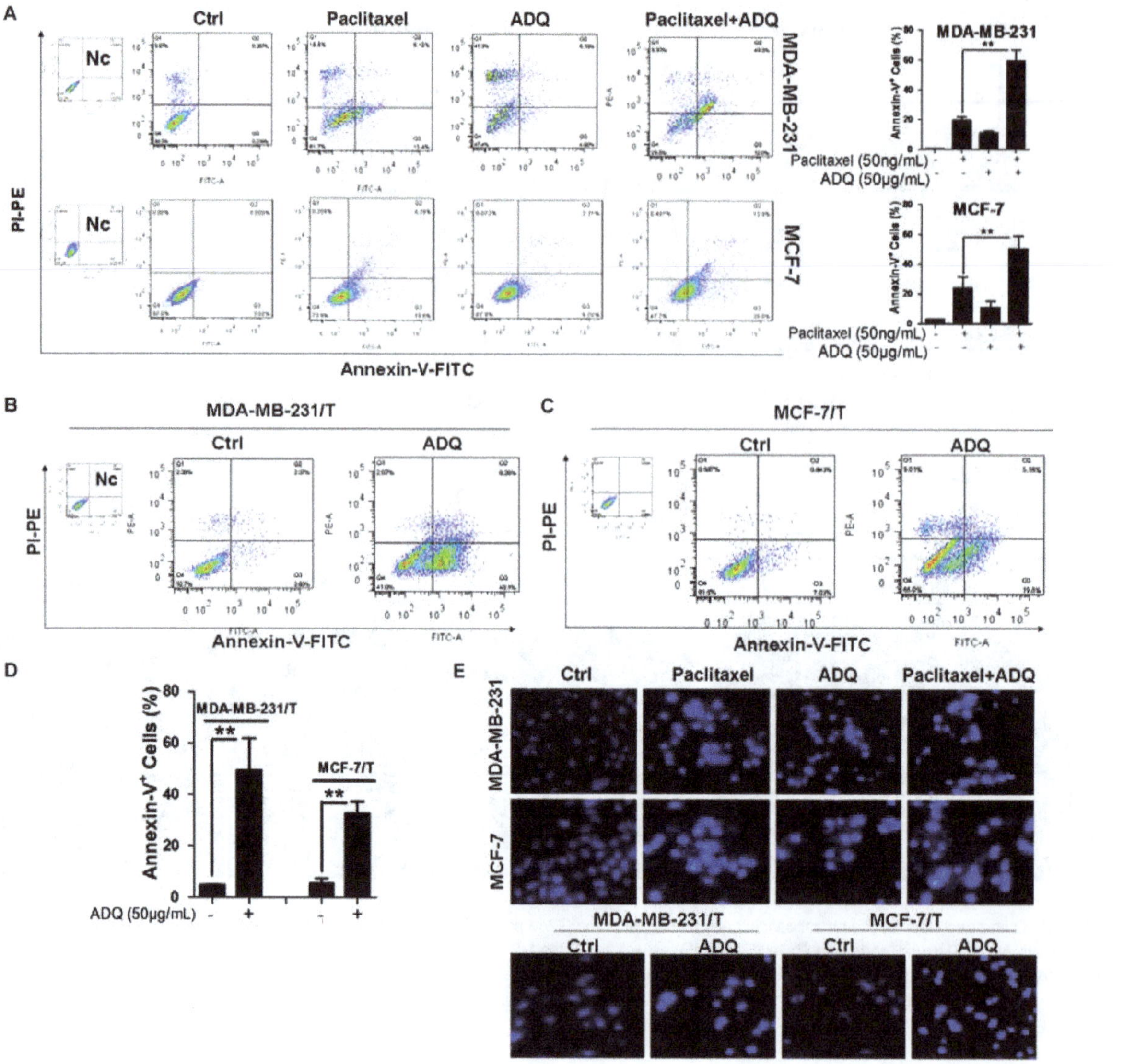

FIGURE 4 | ADQ augments paclitaxel-induced apoptosis in breast cancer cells. Representative apoptosis analysis of **(A)** the MDA-MB-231 and MCF-7 cells treated with ADQ (50 μg/mL) and/or paclitaxel (50 ng/mL), as well as **(B–D)** the MDA-MB-231/T and MCF-7/T cells treated with ADQ (50 μg/mL) for 48h using flow cytometry (*P < 0.05 *v.s.* control, **P < 0.01 *v.s.* control, values represented as the mean ± SD, n = 3); **(E)** Hoechst 33258 staining showed typical apoptotic morphology changes of cells after indicated treatment.

was used to determine the significance of the data between groups. P-values less than 0.05 were considered statistical significant.

RESULTS

ADQ Markedly Inhibits Growth in Paclitaxel-Sensitive and Paclitaxel-Resistant Human Breast Cancer Cells

For quality control of ADQ, the chromatographic fingerprinting of ADQ was conducted and quantitative analysis of *p*-coumaric acid (peak 1), calycosin-7-glucoside (peak 2), liquiritin (peak 3), glycyrrhizic acid (peak 4), and curcumol (peak 5) in ADQ was compared among different batches (**Supplementary Figure S1**). Based on an established HPLC method, good linearity of five compounds was achieved with a correlation coefficient of $R^2 \geq 0.9995$ (**Supplementary Table S1**). The retention times of these compounds were determined to be 19.8, 23.9, 25.8, 50.7, and 69.5 min, respectively. The contents of the five compounds in the ADQ samples were also determined (**Supplementary Table S2**). We evaluated the influence of ADQ on the proliferation of breast cancer cell lines including MDA-MB-231 and MCF-7, as well as their derived paclitaxel-resistant cell lines MDA-MB-231/T and MCF-7/T. Significant inhibition of growth was observed in both parental and resistant cells at 24 h (**Figure 1A**),

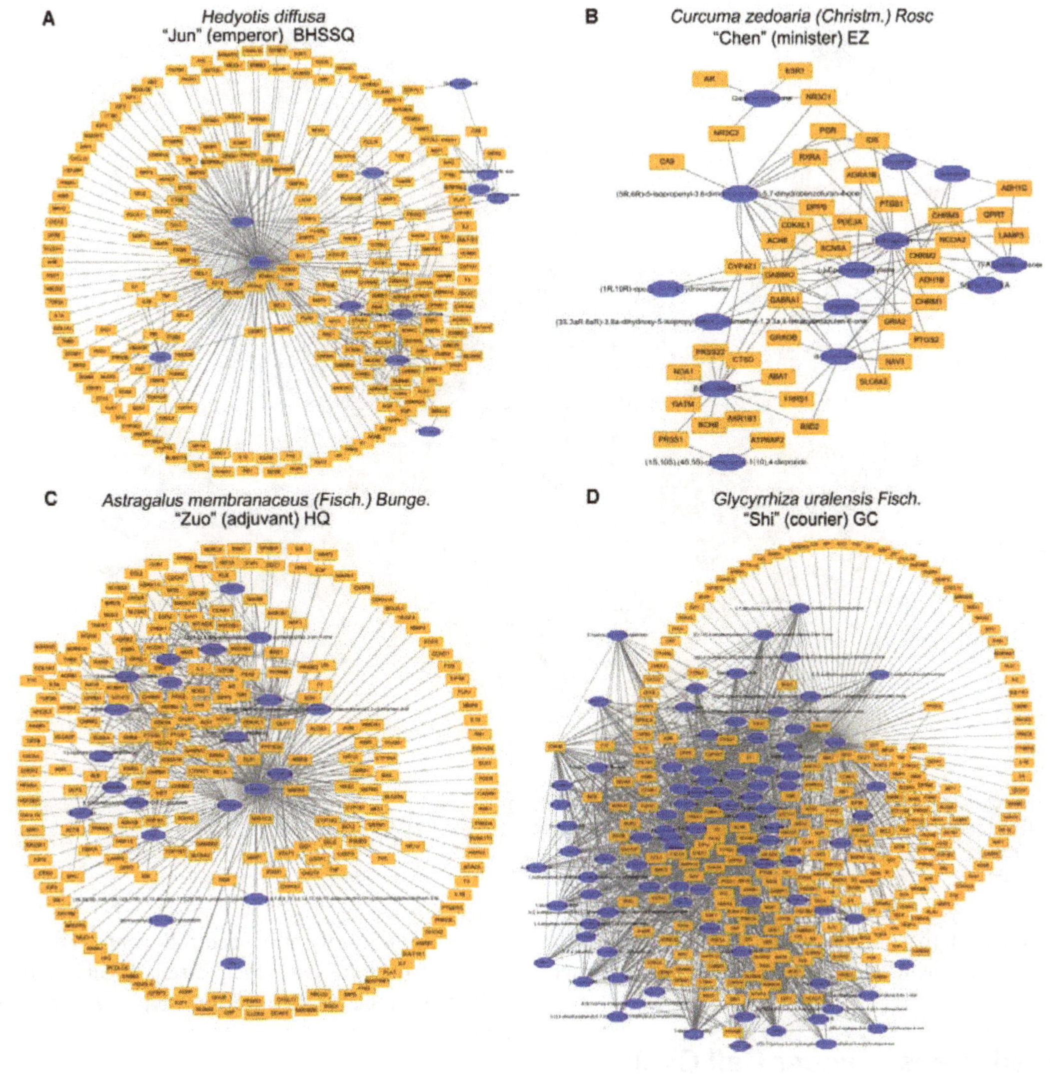

FIGURE 5 | The ingredient-target network of single herb in ADQ. **(A)** BHSSQ; **(B)** EZ; **(C)** HQ; and **(D)** GC. The blue diamond nodes represent ingredients, and the orange rectangle nodes represent targets.

48 h (**Figure 1B**), and 72 h (**Figure 1C**). IC_{50} of ADQ was shown in **Figure 1D** for the indicated cell lines. Specifically, the IC_{50} values of ADQ at 48 h for MDA-MB-231, MDA-MB-231/T, MCF-7, and MCF-7/T were 49.809, 57.789, 65.799, and 70.964 μg/mL, respectively, suggesting that ADQ had similar suppressive effects on both sensitive and resistant breast cancer cells. To determine the cytotoxic effects of ADQ on normal cells, we also investigated its effects on HUMECs and HUVECs, and found that ADQ did not have cytotoxic inhibitory effects on both types of normal cells (**Figures 1E,F**). These findings indicated that ADQ exerted selective toxic effects on breast cancer cells.

ADQ Significantly Enhances the Chemosensitivity of Breast Cancer Cells

To determine the synergistic activities of ADQ with paclitaxel in breast cancer, MDA-MB-231 and MCF-7 cells were treated with ADQ and paclitaxel for 48 h. As presented in **Figure 1** and **Supplementary Figure S2**, the tested concentrations of taxol and ADQ were set according to their IC_{50} at 48 h. ADQ significantly enhanced paclitaxel-induced death in MDA-MB-231 and MCF-7 cells. Interestingly, ADQ administration at 50 μg/mL also caused a clear reduction in the number of resistant breast cancer cells (**Figure 2A**). We also evaluated the long-term inhibitory effects of ADQ on the colony formation capabilities of breast cancer cells with or without paclitaxel. The results showed that the combination group exhibited a substantial reduction in the colony numbers of parental MDA-MB-231 and MCF-7 cells (**Figure 2B**). In addition, the growth of paclitaxel-resistant MDA-MB-231/T and MCF-7/T cells was greatly suppressed in the presence of ADQ (**Figure 2C**). The drug efflux assay revealed that ADQ could enhance epirubicin influx into breast cancer cells, as shown by the increased fluorescence intensity of epirubicin in ADQ-treated cells (**Figure 2D**).

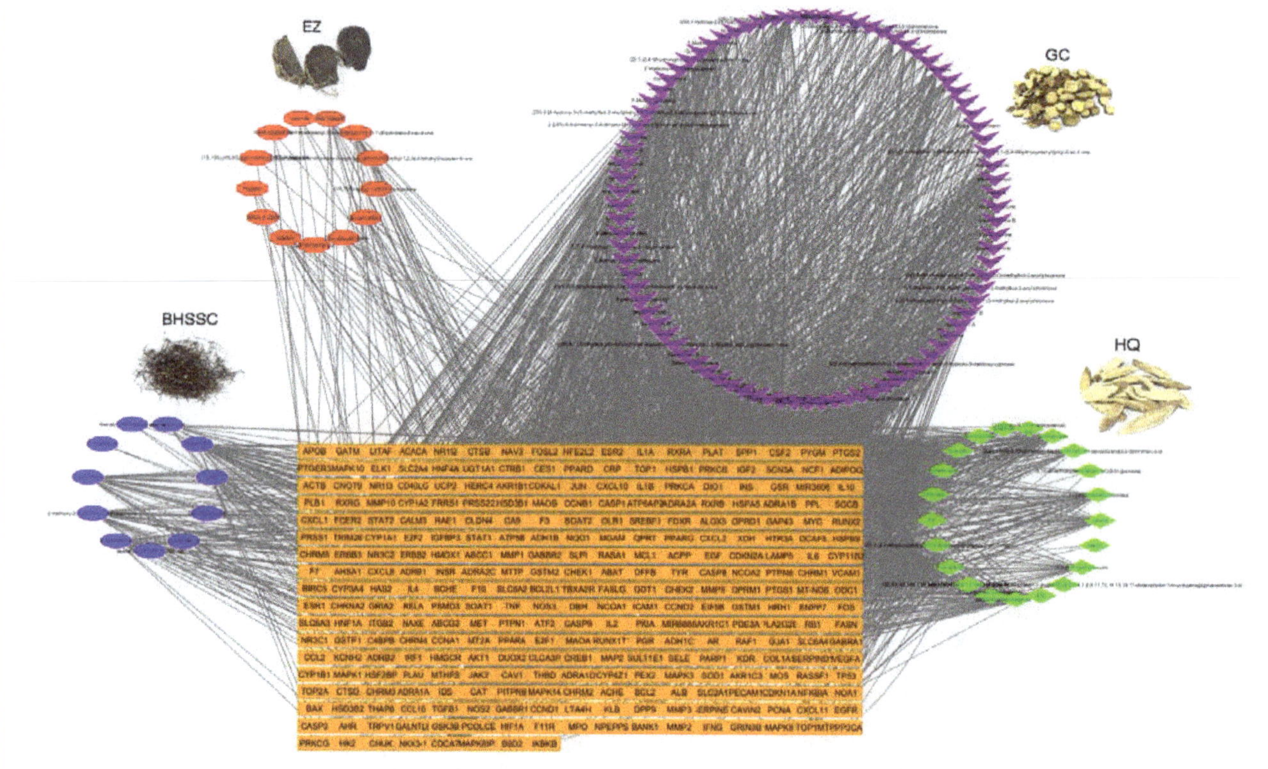

FIGURE 6 | The ingredient-target network of ADQ. The compound-target network was constructed by linking the herbs, candidate compounds and all their potential targets. The nodes represent ingredients of herbs (blue for BHSSC, red for EZ, purple for GC, and green for HQ), and the orange rectangle nodes represent the shared targets of these four herbs.

These results indicated that ADQ could chemosensitize both paclitaxel-sensitive and paclitaxel-resistant human breast cancer cells.

ADQ Induced Breast Cancer Cell Cycle Arrest at the G2/M Checkpoint

Uncontrolled cell mitosis represents one of the hallmarks of cancer. Thus, we used PI staining to examine the effects of ADQ on the cell cycle distribution of both paclitaxel-sensitive and paclitaxel-resistant cells. As labeled in **Figure 3A**, the flow cytometry results revealed that paclitaxel or ADQ alone could induce G2/M checkpoint arrest in both breast cancer cell lines. In addition, ADQ and paclitaxel combination increased G2/M arrest by 26% in MDA-MB-231 cells and by 66% in MCF-7 cells (**Figure 3A**). Furthermore, the G2/M population of MDA-MB-231/T and MCF-7/T cells was also arrested by ADQ with a 56 and 63% increase, respectively (**Figure 3B**). Previous studies have shown that perturbation of the G2/M transition was largely due to DNA damage, and *p*-H2AX could be a marker for monitoring DNA damage (Sancar et al., 2004). The immunofluorescence results showed that *p*-H2AX intensity was significantly elevated following paclitaxel or ADQ treatment in both breast cancer cell lines. Consistent with the cell cycle findings, ADQ synergistically interacted with paclitaxel to enhance *p*-H2AX expression in both breast cancer cell lines (**Figure 3C**). Furthermore, the expression of *p*-H2AX in MDA-MB-231/T and MCF-7/T cells was also significantly enhanced following ADQ administration, indicating that the chemosensitizing effects of ADQ might be attributed to DNA damage-induced G2/M checkpoint arrest (**Figure 3D**).

ADQ Augmented Paclitaxel-Induced Apoptosis in Breast Cancer Cells

Apoptosis is another important mechanism that causes cell death induced by chemotherapy drugs (Johnstone et al., 2002; Li et al., 2010). To determine if ADQ could synergistically aggravate paclitaxel-induced apoptosis, Annexin V/PI staining was applied to detect the apoptotic events. As shown in **Figure 4A**, the percentage of early and late apoptotic events in MDA-MB-231 and MCF-7 cells reached about 20 and 25%, respectively, after exposure to 50 ng/mL paclitaxel. Interestingly, when ADQ was administrated with paclitaxel concurrently, the percentage of MDA-MB-231 and MCF-7 apoptotic cells was increased to approximately 60% and 51%, respectively. Notably, ADQ was also capable of inducing apoptosis in paclitaxel-resistant breast cancer cells. The percentage of apoptotic cells in MDA-MB-231/T reached 45% following ADQ treatment after 48 h, and MCF-7/T cells reached 30% (**Figures 4B–D**). Based on flow cytometry results, Hoechst 33258 staining was utilized to observe the morphological changes of apoptotic cells by fluorescence imaging (Zhang et al., 2010). In paclitaxel-sensitive breast cancer cells, ADQ

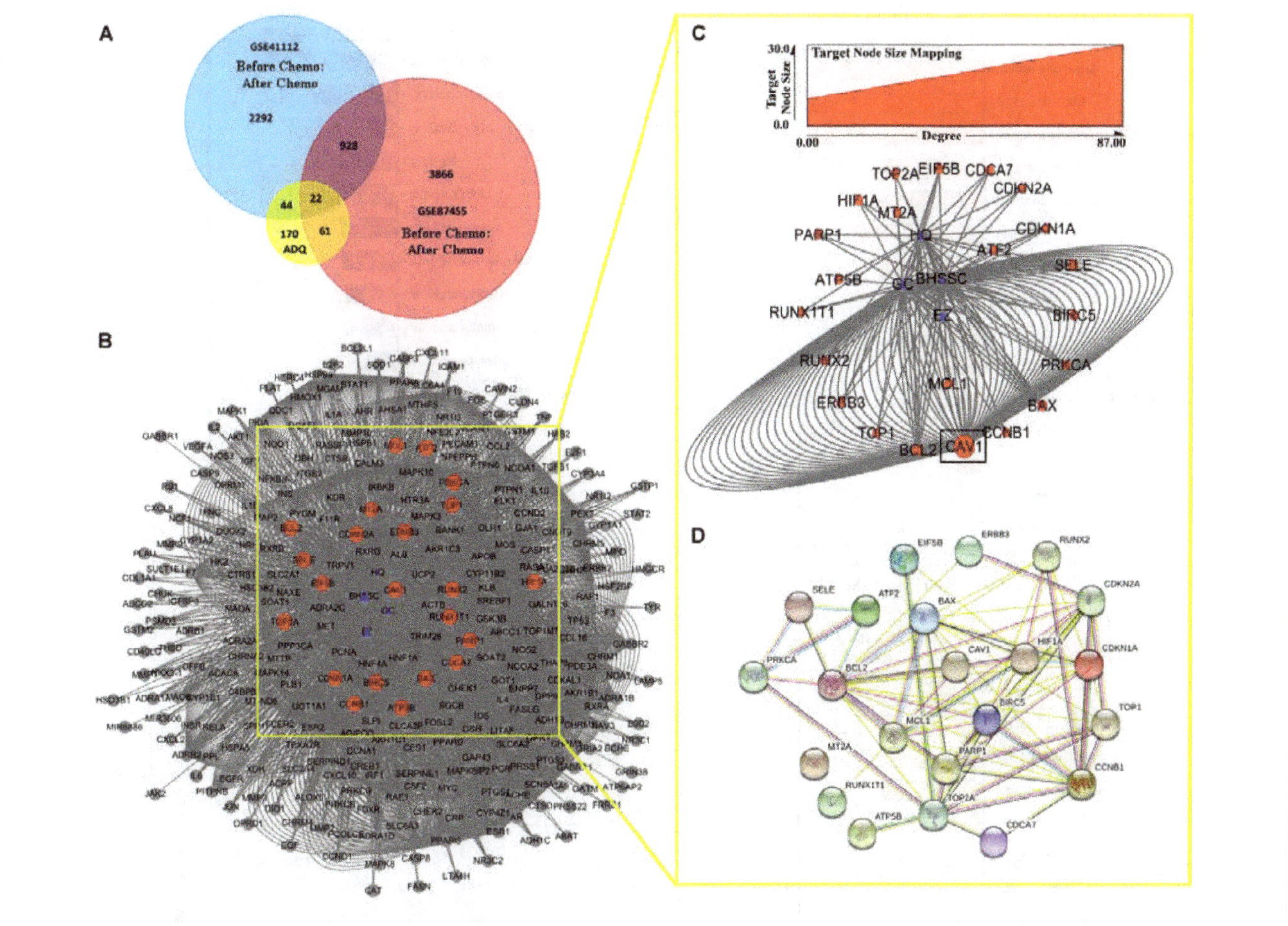

FIGURE 7 | Potential genes involved in the chemosensitizing effects of ADQ against breast cancer. **(A,B)** The venn analysis showed the crosstalk of DEGs in ADQ and datasets GSE5764/GSE87455 of breast cancer patients before and after chemotherapy; **(C)** CAV1 was the key target with the largest node size according to "Degree" in the node size mapping; **(D)** The PPI of hub targets involved in the chemosensitizing effects of ADQ. The blue triangle nodes represent ADQ herbs, and the red rectangle nodes represent the 22 hub targets.

synergistically enhanced Hoechst 33258 staining intensity induced by paclitaxel in both MDA-MB-231 and MCF-7 cells. In paclitaxel-resistant cell models, typical morphological characteristics of apoptosis, such as chromatin condensation and cell pyknosis, were more easily observed following ADQ treatment (**Figure 4E**). Together, these findings confirmed that ADQ promoted paclitaxel-induced apoptosis in breast cancer cells.

Network Pharmacology Analysis of ADQ

ADQ consists of four herbs including BHSSC, EZ, HQ, and GC. To establish the ingredient-target network of ADQ, we screened candidate compounds for (OB $\geq$ 30%) and DL (DL $\geq$ 0.1) in each herb. There were 12 compounds in BHSSC targeting 225 genes (**Figure 5A**), 14 compounds in EZ targeting 41 genes (**Figure 5B**), 21 compounds in HQ targeting 222 genes (**Figure 5C**), and 94 compounds in GC targeting 241 genes (**Figure 5D**). The "candidate active compounds" are listed in **Supplementary Table S3**. Overall, our results showed that ADQ yielded 132 candidate compounds and 297 potential targets after eliminating all duplicates (**Figure 6**). Specifically, the network included 429 nodes and 2874 ingredient–target interactions, of which 132 candidate compounds had a median of 10 target correlations, suggesting the existence of complex correlations among different compounds and targets.

Establishment of the Compound–Target–Disease Network of ADQ

To determine the pharmacological mechanisms of ADQ against chemoresistance, the DEGs of breast cancer patients before and after chemotherapy were extracted from GSE41112 and GSE87455 microarray sets. A total of 3286 genes in GSE5764 and 4877 genes in GSE87455 were identified using the GEO2R analysis tool ($P \leq 0.05$, FC $\geq$ 1.5). The Venn diagram analysis showed that ADQ shared 22 putative targets with the two datasets (**Figure 7A**). These hub genes included CAV1, HIF1A, CCNB1, BAX, BCL2, PARP1, ERBB3, MCL1, PRKCA, CDCA7, CDKN1A,

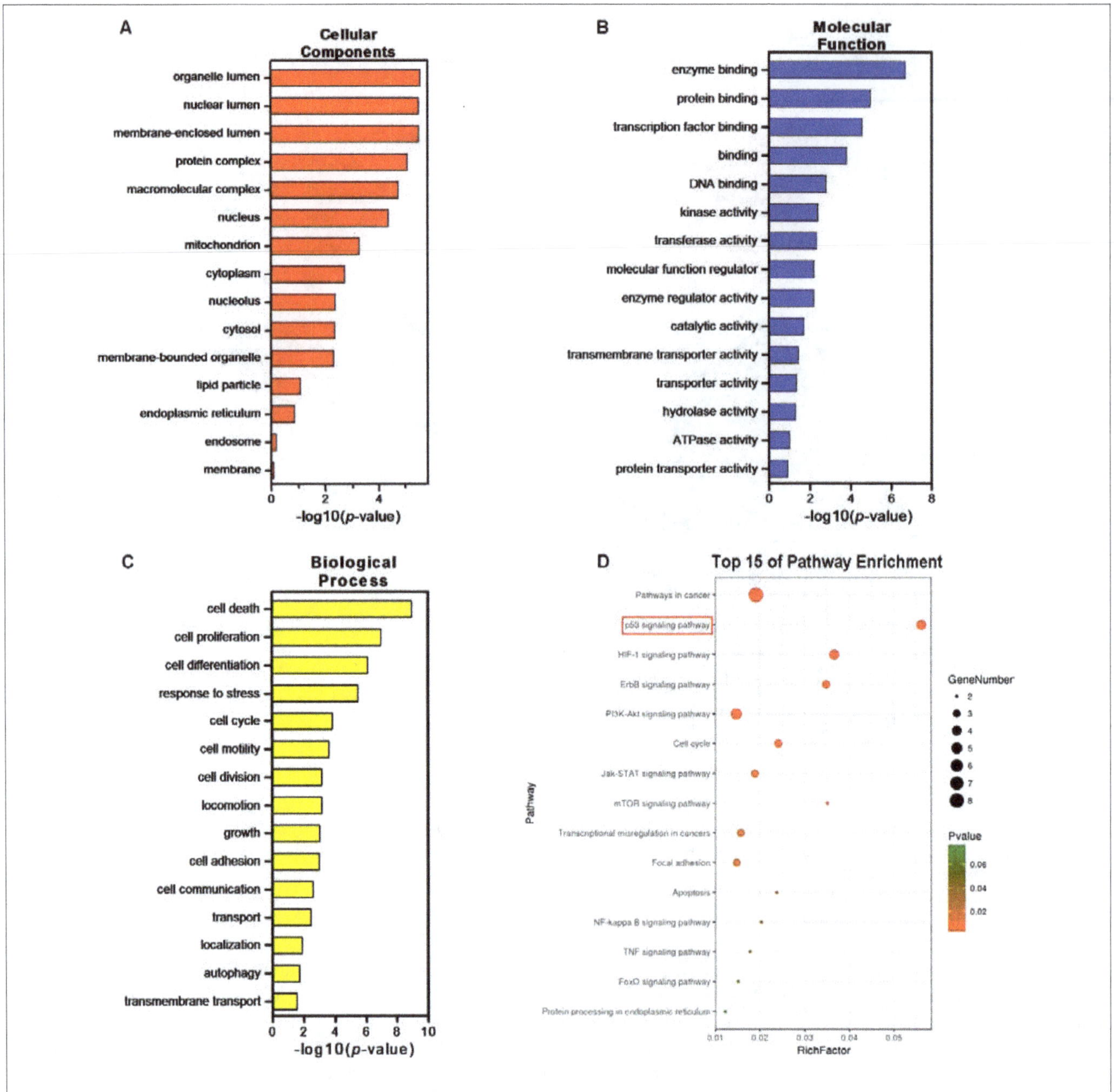

FIGURE 8 | Gene Ontology (GO) and Pathway enrichment analysis of the crosstalk targets. GO terms analysis of the 22 hub genes containing 3 aspects including **(A)** cellular components, **(B)** molecular function, and **(C)** biological process. **(D)** Pathway enrichment analysis of the 22 hub genes.

CDKN2A, TOP1, TOP2A, SELE, ATP5B, RUNX2, BIRC5, ATF2, RUNX1T1, MT2A, and EIF5B (**Figure 7B**), among which CAV1 was the key target with the largest node size according to "Degree" in the node size mapping (**Figure 7C**). We further extracted the 22 significant targets to construct the PPI containing 22 nodes and 71 edges based on the STRING database, and the PPI enrichment *P*-value of these hub genes was 2.22×10^{-16}, indicating that they were at least partially biologically connected (**Figure 7D**). All of these findings suggested that CAV1 might be one of the the most likely mechanisms affecting ADQ regulation network.

Thus, we continued to identify candidate targets by setting all human genes as background, and using GO and pathway enrichment analysis. GO classified function into categories of cellular components, molecular function, and biological process. The top three enrichments in the cellular components category were organelle lumen, nuclear lumen, and membrane-enclosed lumen (**Figure 8A**); in the molecular function category were enzyme binding, protein binding, and transcription factor binding (**Figure 8B**); and in the biological process category were cell death, cell proliferation, and cell differentiation (**Figure 8C**). In **Figure 8D**, KEGG analysis ($P < 0.05$) indicated that

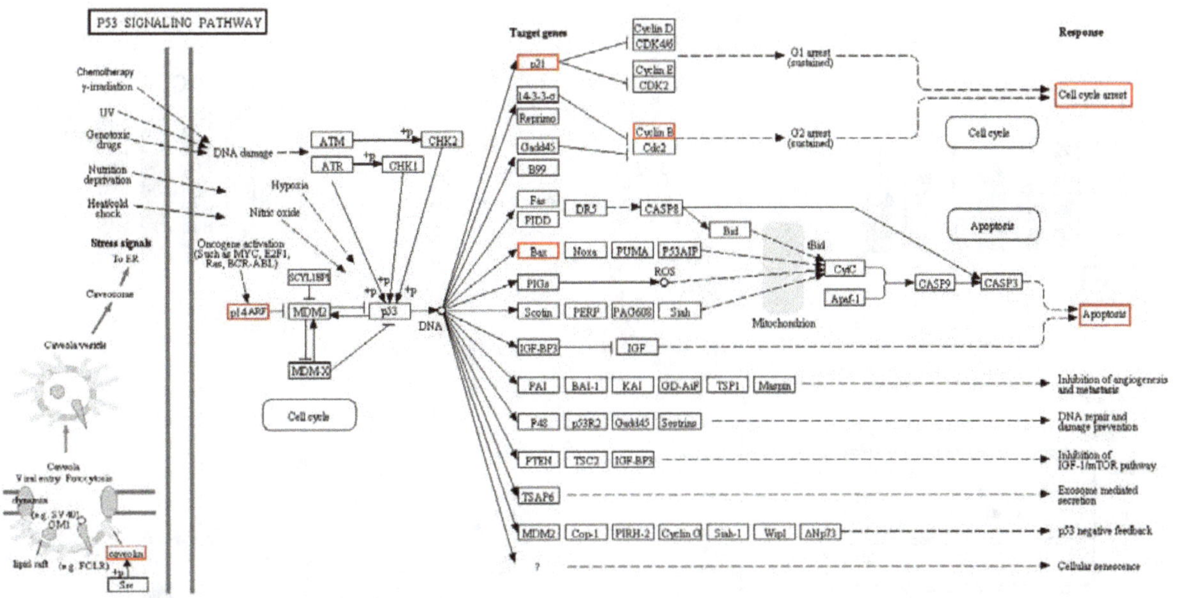

FIGURE 9 | KEGG pathway suggested that various targets in p53 signaling were tightly associated with ADQ pharmacological action. The red rectangle nodes represent the most significant genes or biological pathways associated with ADQ pharmaoclogical action (*P* = 0.00003896097).

multiple cancer-related pathways were significantly involved in the mechanisms of ADQ including focal adhesion, apoptosis, cell cycle, p53, HIF-1, ErbB, phosphoinositide 3-kinase (PI3K)/Akt, Janus kinase/signal transducer and activator of transcription, mammalian target of rapamycin, NF-kappa B, and tumor necrosis factor signaling pathways. Notably, It was various targets in p53 signaling were tightly associated with ADQ pharmacological action (*P* = 0.00003896097, red rectangle, **Figure 8D**). P53 signaling can be stimulated by a number of stress signals including DNA damage, oxidative stress, and activated oncogenes, consequently leading to cell cycle arrest and apoptosis (Mello and Attardi, 2017). Meanwhile, accumulating evidence has demonstrated that CAV1, the leading hub target of ADQ, is correlated with various stressors including chemotherapy, radiotherapy, fluid shear, oxidative stress, and ultraviolet exposure (Wang et al., 2015c). This novel stress response protein plays significant roles in modulating cell survival, proliferation, and apoptosis (Wang et al., 2017d). In **Figure 9**, we postulated that CAV1 might be activated in response to ADQ treatment, subsequently influencing the cell cycle regulatory proteins p21 and cyclin B1, and apoptotic markers such as BAX.

Validation of CAV1 as a Major Chemosensitizing Target of ADQ in Breast Cancer

We continued to validate whether the chemosensitizing activity of ADQ was *CAV1*-dependent. Among the multiple breast cancer cell lines tested, ZR75-1, SKBR3, and MCF7 had no or low CAV1 expression, whereas MDA-MB-231 and MDA-MB-436 had strong CAV1 expression (Shi et al., 2015). In this study, we detected the expression of CAV1 among a series of breast cancer and normal mammary cell lines. The results showed that CAV1 expression was significantly downregulated in the MDA-MB-231 and MCF-7 breast cancer cells, and was enhanced in their taxol-resistant counterparts (**Supplementary Figure S3**). This phenomenon was consistent with the oncogenic and tumor suppressor roles of CAV1 in breast cancer development (Wang et al., 2015c). To directly examine whether CAV1 was critical for ADQ action, we elevated CAV1 levels by transfecting recombinant CAV1 plasmid in *CAV1*-deficient MCF-7 cells, and decreased its expression with si*CAV1* in *CAV1*-expressing MDA-MB-231 cells. CAV1 expression in the gene-modified cells was confirmed by western blot analysis (**Supplementary Figure S4A**). Then we determined if CAV1 overexpression abrogated the anti-cancer and chemosensitizing effects induced by ADQ in breast cancer cells. As shown in **Figure 10A**, ADQ synergistically interacted with paclitaxel to suppress MCF-7 cell proliferation, whereas CAV1 overexpression obviously abrogated the synergistic effects of ADQ with paclitaxel in suppressing breast cancer growth ($p \leq 0.01$). To determine if CAV1 signaling was involved in ADQ chemosensitizing activity, the indicated proteins were analyzed (**Figure 10B**). Western blot analysis revealed that ADQ alone could inhibit CAV1 expression, accompanied by the increased expression of p21 and decreased expression of cyclin B1. In addition, the expression of cleaved PARP1 and BAX were enhanced by ADQ, whereas Bcl-2 expression was decreased following ADQ treatment. Notably, CAV1 overexpression resulted in decreased p21 and increased cyclin B1 expression. Furthermore, CAV1 overexpression inhibited apoptosis, as shown by the decreased expression of cleaved PARP1 and BAX and increased Bcl-2 expression. Cell cycle analysis further revealed that CAV1

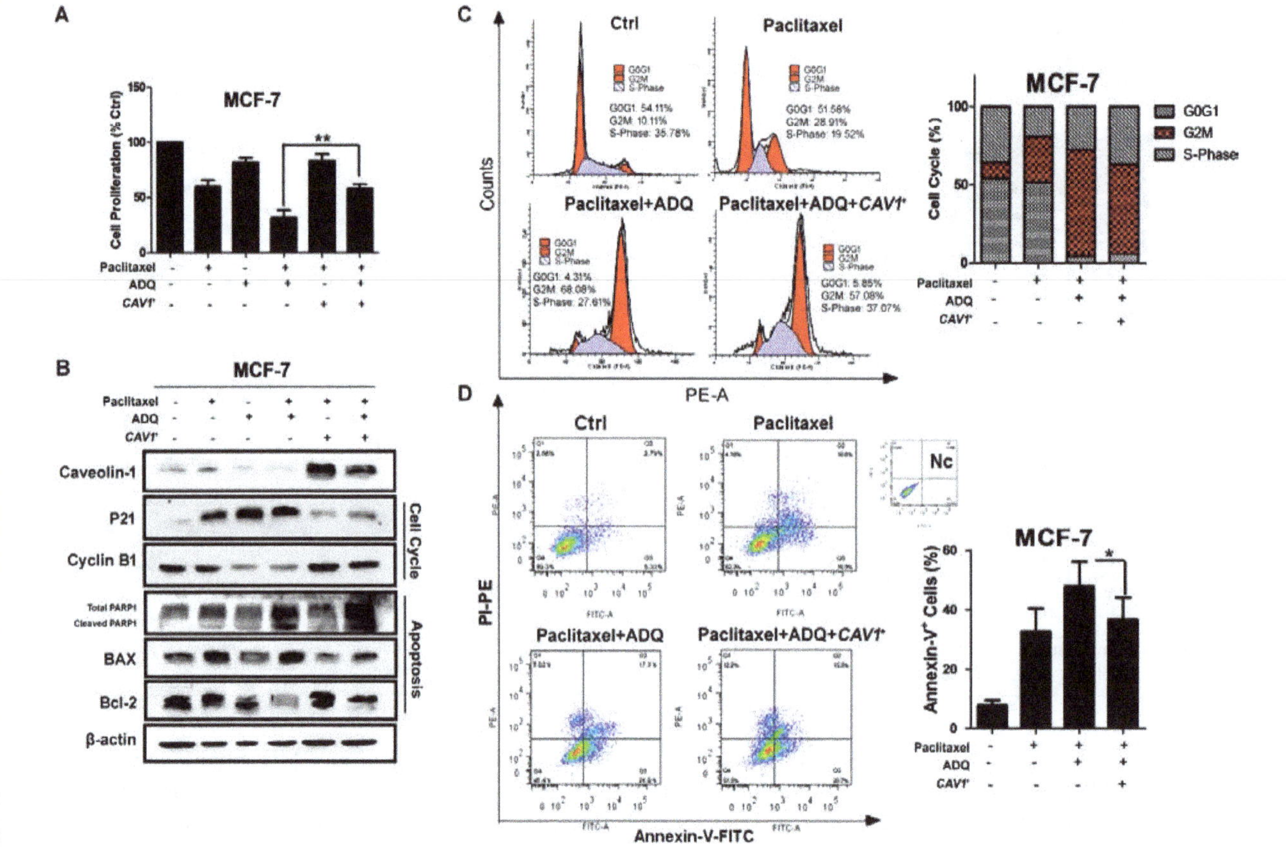

FIGURE 10 | *CAV1* overexpression abrogated the anti-cancer and chemosensitizing effects induced by ADQ on breast cancer cells. *CAV1*-deficient MCF-7 cells were transfected with caveolin-1 recombinant plasmids and treated with ADQ (50 μg/ml) and/or paclitaxel (50 ng/ml) for 48 h. **(A)** The cell counting assay revealed that *CAV1* overexpression obviously abrogated the synergistic effects of ADQ with paclitaxel in suppressing breast cancer growth ($^{**}P < 0.01$ *v.s.* control, values represented as the mean ± SD, $n = 3$); **(B)** The expressions of CAV1, p21, cyclinB1, PARP1, BAX and Bcl-2 using western blotting analysis after indicated treatment; **(C)** Representative cell cycle demonstrated CAV1 overexpression relieved the G2/M arresting effects of ADQ from 68.08 to 57.08% in MCF-7 cells using flow cytometry. The length of each cell cycle phase was calculated; **(D)** Representative apoptosis analysis indicated *CAV1* overexpression reduced the apoptotic events induced by paclitaxel plus with ADQ treatment from 47.890 to 36.780% using flow cytometry ($^{*}P < 0.05$ *v.s.* control, values represented as the mean ± SD, $n = 3$).

overexpression relieved the G2/M arresting effects of ADQ from 68.08 to 57.08% in MCF-7 cells (**Figure 10C**). CAV1 overexpression also significantly reduced the apoptotic events induced by paclitaxel with ADQ treatment from 47.89 to 36.78% (**Figure 10D**). These data showed that ADQ inhibited CAV1 to improve breast cancer chemosensitivity.

In *CAV1*^{high} MDA-MB-231 cells, CAV1 knockdown did not significantly aggravate the inhibitory ability of ADQ in the presence of paclitaxel, suggesting that ADQ might target CAV1 to chemosensitize breast cancer (**Figure 11A**). Similarly, si*CAV1* did not significantly change the expression levels of p21, cyclin B1, PARP1, BAX, and Bcl-2 when administrated together with paclitaxel and ADQ (**Figure 11B**), nor were significant changes observed in cell cycle distribution and apoptotic cells (**Figures 11C,D**). Furthermore, MDA-MB-231/T and MCF-7/T showed strong CAV1 expression compared with their parental cell lines (**Supplementary Figure S4B**). In paclitaxel-resistant breast cancer cell models, both CAV1 silencing and ADQ treatment resulted in the significant suppression of cell proliferation, but CAV1 silencing did not increase the effects of ADQ, namely inhibition of proliferation, cell cycle arrest, or apoptosis induction in MDA-MB-231/T and MCF-7/T cells (**Figures 12A–D**). These findings demonstrated that ADQ could target CAV1 to induce cell cycle arrest and apoptosis, thereby chemosensitizing paclitaxel-resistant breast cancer cells.

ADQ Enhanced *in vivo* Paclitaxel Chemosensitivity on Breast Cancer

We finally evaluated the *in vivo* efficacy of ADQ on breast cancer with the MMTV-PyMT transgenic mouse model, which spontaneously develops 100% multiple and luminal-like breast tumors from normal mammary epitheliums by 8–12 weeks, similar to the pathological processes and characteristics in human breast cancer (Lin et al., 2003; Wang et al., 2013). Therefore, it is an appropriate preclinical model for investigating the chemosensitivity effects of ADQ with paclitaxel (**Figure 13A**). The results of the *in vivo* experiments revealed that ADQ alone could significantly inhibit breast tumor growth ($^{*}P = 0.0444$, **Figure 13C**) and reduce tumor volume ($^{*}P = 0.0104$, **Figure 13D**), while with little influence

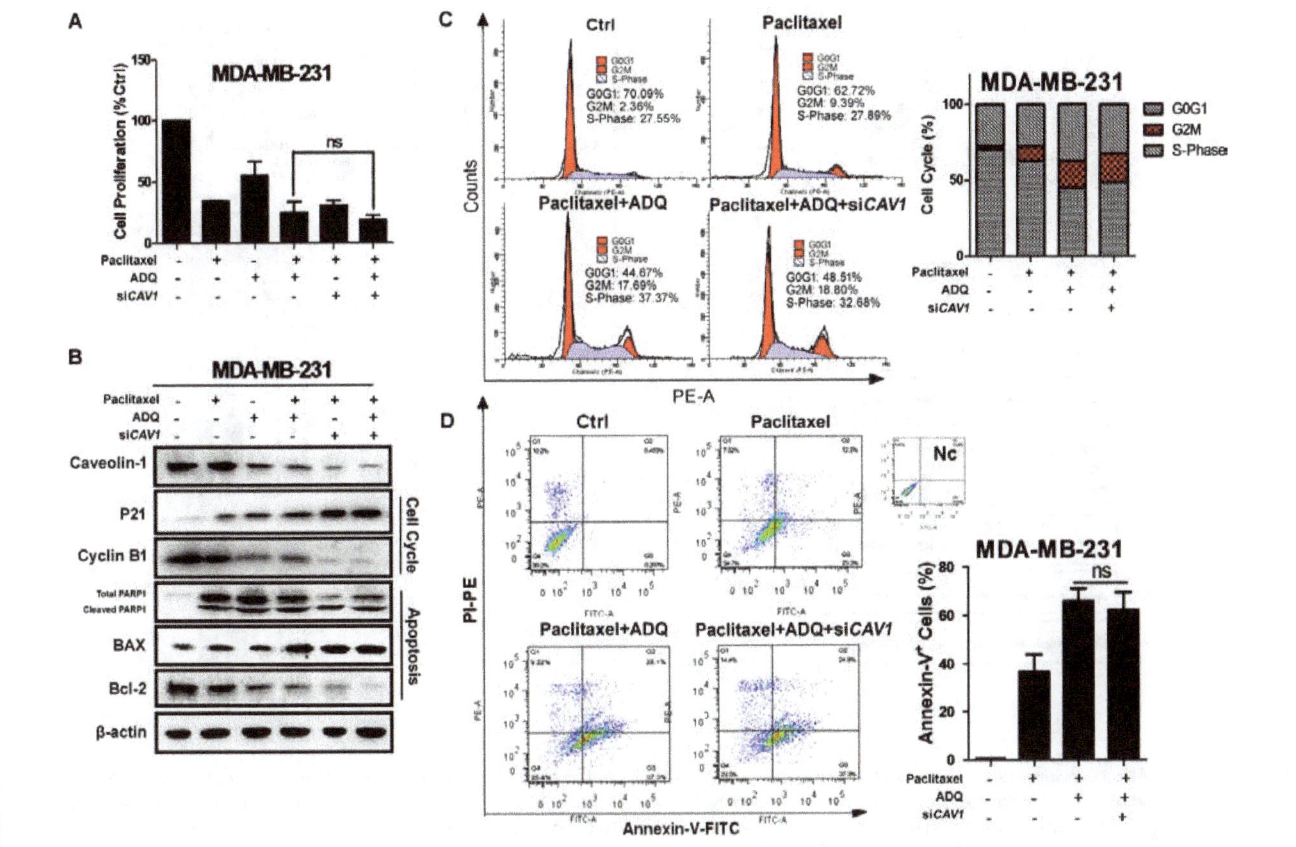

FIGURE 11 | *CAV1* knockdown exerted no additive anti-cancer and chemosensitivity effects induced by ADQ on breast cancer cells. *CAV1*-expressing MDA-MB-231 cell were exposed to si*CAV1* for 24 h and treated with or without ADQ (50 μg/ml) and/or paclitaxel (50 ng/ml) for additional 24 h. **(A)** the cell counting assay demonstrated that si*CAV1* administration did not further increase the chemosensitivity of ADQ; **(B)** The expressions of CAV1, p21, cyclinB1, PARP1, BAX and Bcl-2 using western blotting analysis after indicated treatment; si*CAV1* did not significantly enhance the chemosensitivity of ADQ by altering **(C)** cell cycle distribution and **(D)** apoptotic population with flow cytometry assay.

on mouse body weight (**Figure 13B**). Meanwhile, ADQ alone caused an increase in the apoptotic ratio and a decrease in ki67 expression, further demonstrating its tumor suppressive functions (**Figure 13E**). The results also revealed that the combination of paclitaxel and ADQ exerted stronger inhibitory effects on overall tumor growth than paclitaxel alone (**Figure 13C**). Notably, ADQ did not lead to significant weight loss throughout the experiment, whereas a slight reduction of body weight was found in the paclitaxel-treated mice (**Figure 13B**). Furthermore, both H&E staining and the TUNEL assay revealed that the synergistic use of paclitaxel and ADQ resulted in significant increases of apoptosis in tumor tissues, accompanied by the decreased expression of Ki67 and CAV1 (**Figure 13E**). These results indicate that ADQ is a potential adjuvant drug for breast cancer treatment with good safety.

DISCUSSION

With increasing attention being paid to multi-target strategies for cancer treatment, TCM has become a valuable resource. In this study, we investigated the anti-cancer and chemosensitizing functions of ADQ extracts in breast cancer. Our findings revealed that ADQ significantly inhibited the growth of breast cancer cells by cell cycle arrest and apoptosis induction. In particular, ADQ did not cause cytotoxic effects in normal cells. Similar findings have also been shown for other herbs including Huangqi, Ginseng, Banzhilian, Huachansu injection, TJ-48, Shenqi fuzheng injection, and Kanglaite injection (Qi et al., 2015). Notably, the four-herb formula PHY906 was developed as an adjuvant therapy with chemosensitizing effects. Currently, three phase I and one phase II clinical trial on PHY906 have been completed in the United States. In these clinical studies, PHY906 administration led to the reduction of chemotherapy-associated side effects in patients with metastatic colorectal cancer (PHY906+CPT-11/5FU/LV) and advanced pancreatic cancer (PHY906+capecitabine) (Lam et al., 2015). Omics studies have demonstrated that PHY906 can inhibit colon cancer growth by modulating cell apoptosis by intervening interferon-gamma production and responses to steroid hormone stimulus. Our study also demonstrated that ADQ could increase breast cancer chemosensitivity to paclitaxel by increasing breast cancer cell apoptosis and cell cycle arrest at the G2/M checkpoint. In addition, *in vivo* findings further confirmed the anti-breast

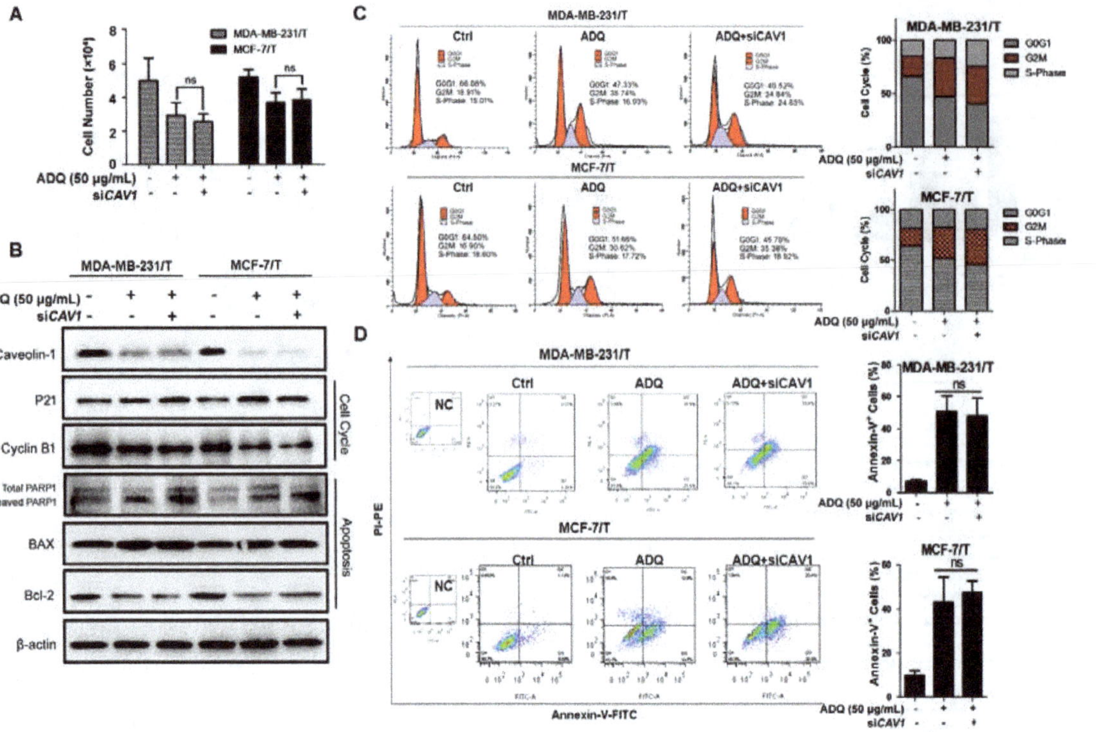

FIGURE 12 | *CAV1* knockdown exerted no additive effects induced by ADQ on Reversal of multidrug-resistance in paclitaxel-resistant breast cancer cells. MDA-MB-231/T and MCF-7/T cell were exposed to si*CAV1* for 24 h and treated with or without ADQ (50 μg/ml) for additional 24 h, respectively. **(A)** the cell counting assay demonstrated that si*CAV1* administration did not further increase the inhibition ratio when ADQ was added; **(B)** The expressions of CAV1, p21, cyclinB1, PARP1, BAX and Bcl-2 using western blotting analysis after indicated treatment; si*CAV1* did not significantly enhance the suppressive activities of ADQ by altering **(C)** cell cycle distribution and **(D)** apoptotic population with flow cytometry assay.

cancer and chemosensitizing effects of ADQ with good safety. Therefore, it is of great value to explore the effects and mechanisms of ADQ in breast cancer.

The development of network pharmacology has shifted our traditional view from the "one drug, one target" model to the "drug–target network" (Hopkins, 2008). Bioinformatics analysis has further optimized the high-throughput screening strategy to validate candidate targets associated with diseases (Eichler, 2012). A target fishing approach has been applied by a number of TCM studies. For example, Wang et al. (2017b) identified tumor-associated macrophages/C-X-C motif chemokine ligand 1 as key modulators of XIAOPI formula in the prevention of breast cancer metastasis based on network pharmacology analysis and cytokine array screening. Chemoinformatics, bioinformatics, and network biology were applied together to predict the active compounds of Tianfoshen oral liquid and to validate its therapeutic targets against colorectal cancer (Wang et al., 2017c). In this study, network analysis revealed a total of 132 active compounds and 297 genes in the ADQ formula, and bioinformatics analysis further identified 22 genes closely correlated with the chemosensitizing activities of ADQ through Venn diagram analysis with breast cancer chemoresponsive genes extracted from GSE41112 and GSE87455. These results suggested that ADQ efficacy was through the synergistic effect of multi-compounds, multi-targets, and multi-pathways. Among these hub molecules, CAV1 was the key target node with the largest "Degree," indicating that it may be one of the most likely mechanisms affecting the ADQ regulation network. Meanwhile, pathway enrichment analysis demonstrated that CAV1 acted as a key upstream node influencing cell cycle, apoptosis, and p53 signaling. Interestingly, CAV1 has also been considered an important stress-responsive molecule by recent studies and our previous report (Lavie et al., 1998; Yang et al., 1998; Glait et al., 2006; Wang et al., 2015c). Therefore, it was selected for subsequent validation. Interestingly, a lot of work has demonstrated that CAV1 is necessary for p53 activation. For example, Volonte et al. (2009) validated that CAV1 expression is required for the activation of ATM-p53-p21 pathway, and Bartholomew et al. (2009) indicated that CAV1 is a novel binding protein for mouse double minute 2 homolog, thereby preventing p53 proteasome degradation and stabilizing its cellular expression. Our study demonstrated that p53 expression in both MDA-MB-231 and MCF-7 cells was downregulated compared with primary mammary epithelial cells, accompanied by CAV1 reduction (**Supplementary Figure S5**). However, although ADQ administration led to CAV1 inhibition, the expression of p53 and p-p53 (ser15) did not significantly change, indicating that ADQ-induced p21 and apoptosis activation might not be related to p53 (**Supplementary Figure S6**). With regard to the genetic status of p53, MDA-MB-231 was mutated and MCF-7

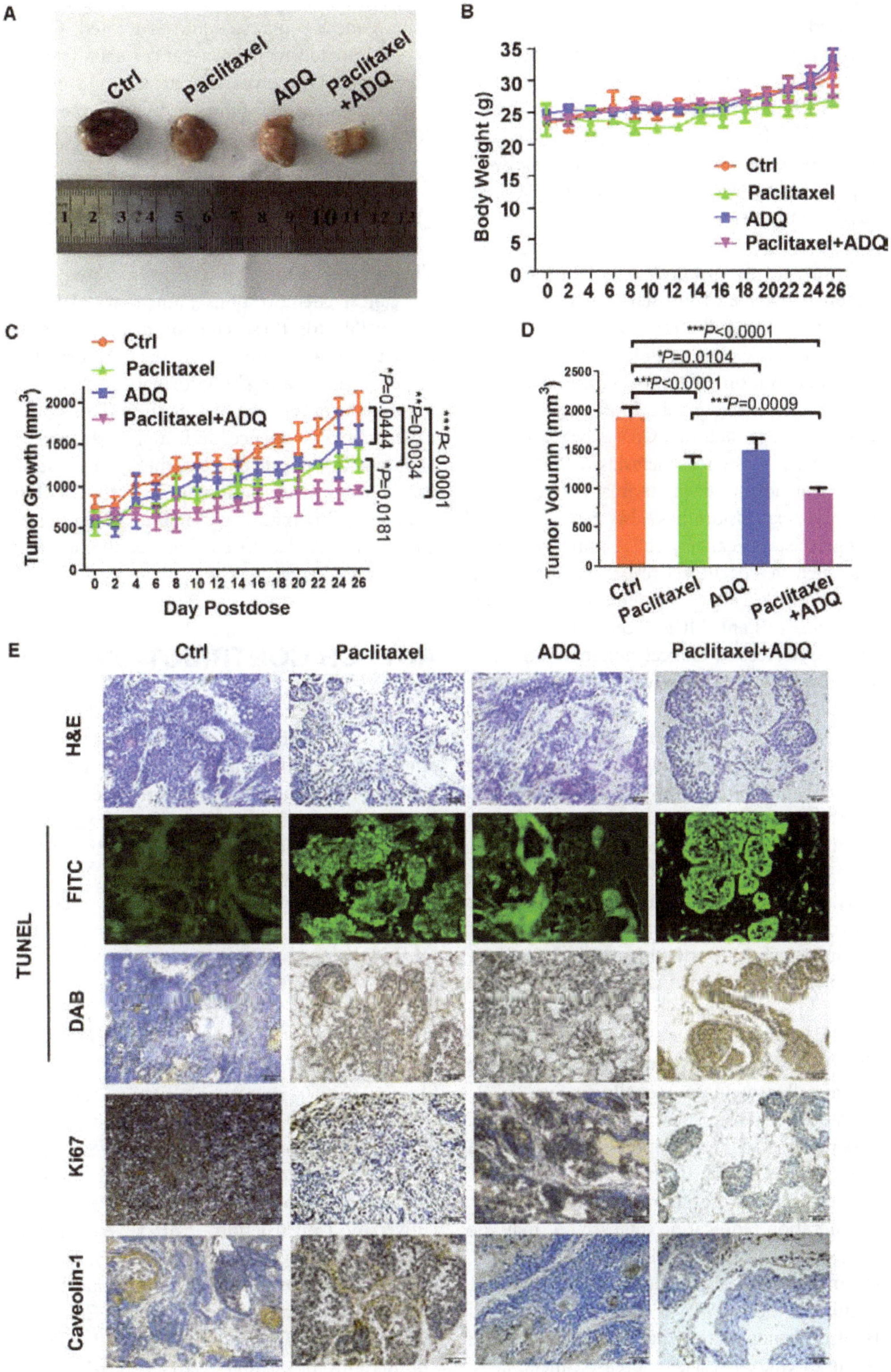

FIGURE 13 | ADQ enhanced *in vivo* paclitaxel chemosensitivity on breast cancer. 9-week-old MMTV-PyMT mice were randomly divided into four groups, and were treated with vehicle (Ctrl group), 10 mg/kg paclitaxel (Paclitaxel group), 100 mg/kg ADQ (ADQ group), or 10mg/kg paclitaxel plus 100 mg/kg ADQ (Paclitaxel + ADQ group) according to designated treatment schedule. **(A)** Representative images of tumors dissected, **(B)** Body weight, and **(C,D)** Tumor volumes, and **(E)** H&E staining, TUNEL detection, and IHC detection of Ki67 and CAV1 expressions from the indicated groups (n = 6 mice, total of 60 glands, $^{*}P < 0.05$, $^{**}P < 0.01$, $^{***}P < 0.0001$ *v.s.* control).

was wild type. Because the degradation speed of mutated p53 was significantly reduced, p53 expression was highly elevated in MDA-MB-231 cells compared with MCF-7 cells (**Supplementary Figure S5**); however, ADQ had little effect on p53 expression in both breast cancer cells (**Supplementary Figure S6**), indicating that the susceptibility of MDA-MB-231 or MCF-7 cells to ADQ was not related to p53 genetic status. Overall, network pharmacology has provided us with a highly efficient strategy to identify key targets and their complex correlation in the development of TCM formulas.

CAV1 plays dual roles in the progression of breast, lung, cervical, gastric, glioma liver, and prostate cancers (Wang et al., 2017d). During tumor initiation, its loss not only triggers tumor-survival signals including PI3K/Akt and MAPK, but also leads to the inactivation of tumor suppressor genes such as BRCA1 and PTEN (Glait et al., 2006). By contrast, accumulating evidence has suggested that CAV1 overexpression correlates with cancer drug resistance, metastasis, the survival of cancer stem cells, and advanced carcinoma (Wang et al., 2015c). Increased CAV1 expression has also been observed in a series of drug-resistant cancer cells compared with their parental cells such as paclitaxel-resistant A549 cells, vinblastine-resistant SKVLB1 cells, colchicine-resistant HT-29 cells, and adraimycin-resistant MCF-7 cells (Lavie et al., 1998; Yang et al., 1998). Moreover, clinical investigations have revealed that CAV1 expression is positively correlated with chemotherapy response in gastric cancer (Yuan et al., 2013) and non-small lung cancer (Brodie et al., 2014). Therefore targeting CAV1 is a promising strategy for overcoming cancer drug resistance. Interestingly, our study demonstrated that ADQ could inhibit CAV1 to improve breast cancer chemosensitivity. In addition, CAV1-overexpressing MDA-MB-231 cells were more susceptible to ADQ than low CAV1-expressing MCF-7 cells. Consistent with our findings, previous studies have revealed that multiple active compounds in ADQ exerted anti-cancer effects partly by mediating CAV1 expression. For example, it was shown that quercetin reversed tamoxifen resistance in breast cancer cells, and its metabolites likely suppressed CAV1 expression (Wang et al., 2015a; Kamada et al., 2016). Calycosin glycoside regulates nitric oxide/CAV1/matrix metalloproteinase signaling (Fu et al., 2014b). The CAV1-mediated anti-cancer effects of ADQ in this study were possibly due to the complex interaction and synergistic/neutralizing effects among the involved compounds. However, ADQ also exhibited a significant inhibitory effects on MCF-7 cell proliferation, indicating that there may be other molecular targets responsible for the effects of ADQ. Because the phytochemicals in Chinese formula are too complex to analyze, it is unlikely that CAV1 is the only target of ADQ. Our results also demonstrated that CAV1 expression was highly elevated in paclitaxel-resistant breast cancer cells, and ADQ chemosensitized breast cancer cells by inhibiting CAV1, consistent with the oncogenic role of CAV1. This phenomenon might be explained by the property of the stress-related function of CAV1, which plays a key role in protecting cells from hazardous stimuli. During cancer initiation, malignant transformation may be accelerated due to CAV1 loss, which would sensitize normal cells to oncogenic events. In contrast, when cancer progresses and is treated, CAV1 expression may be upregulated to protect cancer cells from escaping death by speeding aerobic glycolysis, increasing stem cell populations, or overexpressing ATP-binding cassette transporters (Wang et al., 2015c).

CONCLUSION

The results of our study demonstrated that ADQ improved the cancer chemoresponse, and that CAV1 was at least in part responsible for these chemosensitizing effects. Our work has great implications for the discovery of breast cancer therapeutic targets by integrating bioinformatics and network pharmacology followed by experimental validation. This study not only provides experimental evidence and molecular mechanisms that may facilitate the safe and effective therapeutic use of herbal medicines for breast cancer, and may lead to CAV1-based therapeutic strategies for mammary malignancies. However, preclinical studies are needed to confirm its chemosensitizing effects and active ingredients.

AUTHOR CONTRIBUTIONS

NW and ZW conducted the design of the experiments and wrote the manuscript. FZ contributed to the revised manuscript. NW conducted network pharmacology analysis and bioinformatics analysis. BY, XL, and XZ contributed to the drug preparation and quality control of ADQ. SW, YZ, and SL carried out cell culture and molecular biology experiments. ZH, HP, and YL conducted flow cytometry analysis.

FUNDING

This work was supported by the National Natural Science Foundation of China (81703764, 81573651, 81873306, and 81703749), Guangdong Science and Technology Department (2016A030306025), Pearl River S&T Nova Program of Guangzhou (201506010098), Combined Scientific Project Funded by Guangdong Provincial Science and Technology Agency and Guangdong Provincial Academy of Traditional Chinese Medicine (2014A020221047), Guangdong High-level University Construction Project (A1-AFD018161Z1510, A1-AFD018171Z11102, and A1-AFD018171Z11101), Guangdong High-level Personnel of Special Support Program (A1-3002-16-111-003), Guangdong traditional Chinese medicine bureau project (20181132 and 20182044), the Post-doctoral Science Foundation of China (2017M612644, 2017M622669, and 2018T110861), the Ph.D. Start-up Fund of Natural Science Foundation of Guangdong Province (2017A030310213) and Guangdong provincial key project (2016kzdxm032), and the Specific Research Fund for TCM Science and Technology of Guangdong Provincial Hospital of Chinese Medicine (YN2018MJ07 and YN2018QJ08).

ACKNOWLEDGMENTS

We thank LetPub (www.letpub.com) for the linguistic assistance.

SUPPLEMENTARY MATERIAL

FIGURE S1 | The chromatographic fingerprints of ADQ. HPLC chromatograms on 216 nm detection for **(A)** standard compounds, **(B)** ADQ (1: p-Coumaric acid; 2: Calycosin-7-glucoside; 3: Liquiritin; 4: Glycyrrhizic acid; 5: Curcumol).

FIGURE S2 | The IC50s of paclitaxel for MDA-MB-231, MDA-MB-231/T, MCF-7, and MCF-7/T cells. The parental/resistant cells of **(A)** MDA-MB-231 and **(B)** MCF-7 were treated with paclitaxel at the indicated concentrations (0–200 ng/mL) for 48 h.

FIGURE S3 | The expressions of CAV1 were determined by western blot among MDA-MB-231, MDA-MB-231/T, MCF-7, MCF-7/T, HUMECs, and HUVECs.

FIGURE S4 | The expressions of CAV1 using western blotting analysis. **(A)** MCF-7 cells were transfected with the recombinant plasmid of CAV1, and MDA-MB-231 cells were transfected with si*CAV1* for 48 h. The CAV1 levels were then confirmed by western blot analysis; **(B)** The expressions of CAV1 on the indicated parental breast cancer cells and the paired paclitaxel-resistant cells ($^{**}P < 0.01$ *v.s.* control, values represented as the mean ± SD, $n = 3$).

FIGURE S5 | The expressions of CAV1, p53 and p-p53 (ser15) were determined by western blot among MDA-MB-231, MCF-7, and HUMECs ($^{**}P < 0.01$ *v.s.* control, values represented as the mean ± SD, $n = 3$).

FIGURE S6 | The expressions of CAV1, p53 and p-p53 (ser15) were determined by western blot with or without ADQ in MDA-MB-231 and MCF-7 ($^{**}P < 0.01$ *v.s.* control, values represented as the mean ± SD, $n = 3$).

TABLE S1 | The establishment of calibration curves for HPLC analysis.

TABLE S2 | The contents of five components in ADQ.

TABLE S3 | Information on candidate active compounds from BHSSC, EZ, HQ and GC herbs of ADQ decoration.

REFERENCES

Bartholomew, J. N., Volonte, D., and Galbiati, F. (2009). Caveolin-1 regulates the antagonistic pleiotropic properties of cellular senescence through a novel Mdm2/p53-mediated pathway. *Cancer Res.* 69, 2878–2886. doi: 10.1158/0008-5472.CAN-08-2857

Brodie, S. A., Lombardo, C., Li, G., Kowalski, J., Gandhi, K., You, S., et al. (2014). Aberrant promoter methylation of caveolin-1 is associated with favorable response to taxane-platinum combination chemotherapy in advanced NSCLC. *PLoS One* 9:e107124. doi: 10.1371/journal.pone.0107124

DeSantis, C. E., Ma, J., Goding Sauer, A., Newman, L. A., and Jemal, A. (2017). Breast cancer statistics, 2017, racial disparity in mortality by state. *CA Cancer J. Clin.* 67, 439–448. doi: 10.3322/caac.21412

Eichler, G. S. (2012). Bioinformatics/biostatistics: microarray analysis. *Methods Mol. Biol.* 823, 347-358. doi: 10.1007/978-1-60327-216-2_22

Fan, T. P., Yeh, J. C., Leung, K. W., Yue, P. Y., and Wong, R. N. (2006). Angiogenesis: from plants to blood vessels. *Trends Pharmacol. Sci.* 27, 297–309. doi: 10.1016/j.tips.2006.04.006

Feng, J., Jin, Y., Peng, J., Wei, L., Cai, Q., Yan, Z., et al. (2017). *Hedyotis Diffusa* Willd extract suppresses colorectal cancer growth through multiple cellular pathways. *Oncol. Lett.* 14, 8197–8205. doi: 10.3892/ol.2017.7244

Fu, J., Wang, Z., Huang, L., Zheng, S., Wang, D., Chen, S., et al. (2014a). Review of the botanical characteristics, phytochemistry, and pharmacology of *Astragalus membranaceus* (Huangqi). *Phytother. Res.* 28, 1275–1283. doi: 10.1002/ptr.5188

Fu, S., Gu, Y., Jiang, J. Q., Chen, X., Xu, M., and Shen, J. (2014b). Calycosin-7-O-beta-D-glucoside regulates nitric oxide /caveolin-1/matrix metalloproteinases pathway and protects blood-brain barrier integrity in experimental cerebral ischemia-reperfusion injury. *J. Ethnopharmacol.* 155, 692–701. doi: 10.1016/j.jep.2014.06.015

Gao, X. F., Li, Q. L., Li, H. L., Zhang, H. Y., Su, J. Y., Wang, B., et al. (2014). Extracts from *Curcuma zedoaria* inhibit proliferation of human breast cancer cell MDA-MB-231 in vitro. *Evid. Based Complement. Alternat. Med.* 2014:730678. doi: 10.1155/2014/730678

Glait, C., Ravid, D., Lee, S. W., Liscovitch, M., and Werner, H. (2006). Caveolin-1 controls BRCA1 gene expression and cellular localization in human breast cancer cells. *FEBS Lett.* 580, 5268–5274. doi: 10.1016/j.febslet.2006.08.071

Gupta, S. C., Prasad, S., Sethumadhavan, D. R., Nair, M. S., Mo, Y. Y., and Aggarwal, B. B. (2013). Nimbolide, a limonoid triterpene, inhibits growth of human colorectal cancer xenografts by suppressing the proinflammatory microenvironment. *Clin. Cancer Res.* 19, 4465–4476. doi: 10.1158/1078-0432.CCR-13-0080

Hopkins, A. L. (2008). Network pharmacology: the next paradigm in drug discovery. *Nat. Chem. Biol.* 4, 682–690. doi: 10.1038/nchembio.118

Janczar, S., Nautiyal, J., Xiao, Y., Curry, E., Sun, M., Zanini, E., et al. (2017). WWOX sensitises ovarian cancer cells to paclitaxel via modulation of the ER stress response. *Cell Death Dis.* 8:e2955. doi: 10.1038/cddis.2017.346

Johnstone, R. W., Ruefli, A. A., and Lowe, S. W. (2002). Apoptosis: a link between cancer genetics and chemotherapy. *Cell* 108, 153–164.

Kamada, C., Mukai, R., Kondo, A., Sato, S., and Terao, J. (2016). Effect of quercetin and its metabolite on caveolin-1 expression induced by oxidized LDL and lysophosphatidylcholine in endothelial cells. *J. Clin. Biochem. Nutr.* 58, 193–201. doi: 10.3164/jcbn.16-2

Lam, W., Jiang, Z., Guan, F., Huang, X., Hu, R., Wang, J., et al. (2015). PHY906(KD018), an adjuvant based on a 1800-year-old Chinese medicine, enhanced the anti-tumor activity of sorafenib by changing the tumor microenvironment. *Sci. Rep.* 5:9384. doi: 10.1038/srep09384

Lavie, Y., Fiucci, G., and Liscovitch, M. (1998). Up-regulation of caveolae and caveolar constituents in multidrug-resistant cancer cells. *J. Biol. Chem.* 273, 32380–32383.

Lin, E. Y., Jones, J. G., Li, P., Zhu, L., Whitney, K. D., Muller, W. J., et al. (2003). Progression to malignancy in the polyoma middle T oncoprotein mouse breast cancer model provides a reliable model for human diseases. *Am. J. Pathol.* 163, 2113–2126. doi: 10.1016/s0002-9440(10)63568-7

Li, P., Fu, Y., Ru, J., Huang, C., Du, J., Zheng, C., et al. (2014). Insights from systems pharmacology into cardiovascular drug discovery and therapy. *BMC Syst. Biol.* 8:141. doi: 10.1186/s12918-014-0141-z

Li, Q. Q., Wang, G., Huang, F., Banda, M., and Reed, E. (2010). Antineoplastic effect of beta-elemene on prostate cancer cells and other types of solid tumour cells. *J. Pharm. Pharmacol.* 62, 1018–1027. doi: 10.1111/j.2042-7158.2010.01135.x

Liu, H., Wang, J., Zhou, W., Wang, Y., and Yang, L. (2013). Systems approaches and polypharmacology for drug discovery from herbal medicines: an example using licorice. *J. Ethnopharmacol.* 146, 773–793. doi: 10.1016/j.jep.2013.02.004

Li, X., Wang, G., Zhao, J., Ding, H., Cunningham, C., Chen, F., et al. (2005). Antiproliferative effect of beta-elemene in chemoresistant ovarian carcinoma cells is mediated through arrest of the cell cycle at the G2-M phase. *Cell. Mol. Life Sci.* 62, 894–904. doi: 10.1007/s00018-005-5027-1

Lu, Z. J. (1985). The yellow emperor's internal classic, an ancient medical canon of traditional Chinese medicine. *J. Tradit. Chin. Med.* 5, 153–154.

Mello, S. S., and Attardi, L. D. (2017). Deciphering p53 signaling in tumor suppression. *Curr. Opin. Cell Biol.* 51, 65–72. doi: 10.1016/j.ceb.2017.11.005

Qi, F., Zhao, L., Zhou, A., Zhang, B., Li, A., Wang, Z., et al. (2015). The advantages of using traditional Chinese medicine as an adjunctive therapy in the whole course of cancer treatment instead of only terminal stage of cancer. *Biosci. Trends* 9, 16–34. doi: 10.5582/bst.2015.01019

Ru, J., Li, P., Wang, J., Zhou, W., Li, B., Huang, C., et al. (2014). TCMSP: a database of systems pharmacology for drug discovery from herbal medicines. *J. Cheminform.* 6:13. doi: 10.1186/1758-2946-6-13

Sancar, A., Lindsey-Boltz, L. A., Unsal-Kacmaz, K., and Linn, S. (2004). Molecular mechanisms of mammalian DNA repair and the DNA damage checkpoints. *Annu. Rev. Biochem.* 73, 39–85. doi: 10.1146/annurev.biochem.73.011303.073723

Shi, Y., Tan, S. H., Ng, S., Zhou, J., Yang, N. D., Koo, G. B., et al. (2015). Critical role of CAV1/caveolin-1 in cell stress responses in human breast cancer cells via modulation of lysosomal function and autophagy. *Autophagy* 11, 769–784. doi: 10.1080/15548627.2015.1034411

Song, L. M., Wu, J. R., and Jiang, D. (2015). Analysis of the medication rules of national TCM masters for the treatment of phymatosis based on data mining. *Chin. J. Inf. TCM* 22, 50–53.

Stage, T. B., Bergmann, T. K., and Kroetz, D. L. (2018). Clinical pharmacokinetics of paclitaxel monotherapy: an updated literature review. *Clin. Pharmacokinet.* 57, 7–19. doi: 10.1007/s40262-017-0563-z

Volonte, D., Kahkonen, B., Shapiro, S., Di, Y., and Galbiati, F. (2009). Caveolin-1 expression is required for the development of pulmonary emphysema through activation of the ATM-p53-p21 pathway. *J. Biol. Chem.* 284, 5462–5466. doi: 10.1074/jbc.C800225200

Wang, C., Schwab, L. P., Fan, M., Seagroves, T. N., and Buolamwini, J. K. (2013). Chemoprevention activity of dipyridamole in the MMTV-PyMT transgenic mouse model of breast cancer. *Cancer Prev. Res.* 6, 437–447. doi: 10.1158/1940-6207.capr-12-0345

Wang, H., Tao, L., Qi, K., Zhang, H., Feng, D., Wei, W., et al. (2015a). Quercetin reverses tamoxifen resistance in breast cancer cells. *J. BUON* 20, 707–713.

Wang, N., Wang, Q., Tang, H., Zhang, F., Zheng, Y., Wang, S., et al. (2017a). Direct inhibition of ACTN4 by ellagic acid limits breast cancer metastasis via regulation of beta-catenin stabilization in cancer stem cells. *J. Exp. Clin. Cancer Res.* 36:172. doi: 10.1186/s13046-017-0635-9

Wang, N., Wang, Z., Peng, C., You, J., Shen, J., Han, S., et al. (2014). Dietary compound isoliquiritigenin targets GRP78 to chemosensitize breast cancer stem cells via beta-catenin/ABCG2 signaling. *Carcinogenesis* 35, 2544–2554. doi: 10.1093/carcin/bgu187

Wang, N., Wang, Z., Wang, Y., Xie, X., Shen, J., Peng, C., et al. (2015b). Dietary compound isoliquiritigenin prevents mammary carcinogenesis by inhibiting breast cancer stem cells through WIF1 demethylation. *Oncotarget* 6, 9854–9876. doi: 10.18632/oncotarget.3396

Wang, N., Zheng, Y., Gu, J., Cai, Y., Wang, S., Zhang, F., et al. (2017b). Network-pharmacology-based validation of TAMS/CXCL-1 as key mediator of XIAOPI formula preventing breast cancer development and metastasis. *Sci. Rep.* 7:14513. doi: 10.1038/s41598-017-15030-3

Wang, S., Wang, H., and Lu, Y. (2017c). Tianfoshen oral liquid: a CFDA approved clinical traditional Chinese medicine, normalizes major cellular pathways disordered during colorectal carcinogenesis. *Oncotarget* 8, 14549–14569. doi: 10.18632/oncotarget.14675

Wang, S., Wang, N., Zheng, Y., Zhang, J., Zhang, F., and Wang, Z. (2017d). Caveolin-1: an oxidative stress-related target for cancer prevention. *Oxid. Med. Cell. Longev.* 2017:7454031. doi: 10.1155/2017/7454031

Wang, Z., Wang, N., Liu, P., Peng, F., Tang, H., Chen, Q., et al. (2015c). Caveolin-1, a stress-related oncotarget, in drug resistance. *Oncotarget* 6, 37135–37150. doi: 10.18632/oncotarget.5789

Xu, T., Pi, Z., Liu, S., Song, F., and Liu, Z. (2017). Chemical profiling combined with "omics" technologies (CP-omics): a strategy to understand the compatibility mechanisms and simplify herb formulas in traditional chinese medicines. *Phytochem. Anal.* 28, 381–391. doi: 10.1002/pca.2685

Yang, C. P., Galbiati, F., Volonte, D., Horwitz, S. B., and Lisanti, M. P. (1998). Upregulation of caveolin-1 and caveolae organelles in taxol-resistant A549 cells. *FEBS Lett.* 439, 368–372.

Yuan, G., Regel, I., Lian, F., Friedrich, T., Hitkova, I., Hofheinz, R. D., et al. (2013). WNT6 is a novel target gene of caveolin-1 promoting chemoresistance to epirubicin in human gastric cancer cells. *Oncogene* 32, 375–387. doi: 10.1038/onc.2012.40

Zhang, J., Guo, H., Qian, G., Ge, S., Ji, H., Hu, X., et al. (2010). MiR-145, a new regulator of the DNA fragmentation factor-45 (DFF45)-mediated apoptotic network. *Mol. Cancer* 9:211. doi: 10.1186/1476-4598-9-211

13

Wenfei Buqi Tongluo Formula Against Bleomycin-Induced Pulmonary Fibrosis by Inhibiting TGF-β/Smad3 Pathway

Lu Ding[1†], Yaxin Li[2†], Yingying Yang[3], Siyu Song[2], Hongyu Qi[1], Jing Wang[4], Ziyuan Wang[5], Jiachao Zhao[2], Wei Zhang[6], Linhua Zhao[7], Daqing Zhao[1], Xiangyan Li[1] and Zeyu Wang[6]**

[1]Jilin Ginseng Academy, Key Laboratory of Active Substances and Biological Mechanisms of Ginseng Efficacy, Ministry of Education, Jilin Provincial Key Laboratory of Bio-Macromolecules of Chinese Medicine, Changchun University of Chinese Medicine, Changchun, China, [2]College of Integrated Traditional Chinese and Western Medicine, Changchun University of Chinese Medicine, Changchun, China, [3]Graduate College, Beijing University of Chinese Medicine, Beijing, China, [4]Department of Respiratory, Affiliated Hospital of Changchun University of Chinese Medicine, Changchun, China, [5]College of Traditional Chinese Medicine, Changchun University of Chinese Medicine, Changchun, China, [6]Department of Scientific Research, Changchun University of Chinese Medicine, Changchun, China, [7]Molecular Biology Laboratory, Guang'anmen Hospital, China Academy of Chinese Medical Sciences, Beijing, China

***Correspondence:**
Xiangyan Li
xiangyan_li1981@163.com
Zeyu Wang
zeyu781022@163.com

†These authors have contributed equally to this work*

Pulmonary fibrosis (PF) is the end stage of various chronic and progressive interstitial lung diseases. TGF-β, a profibrotic cytokine, can promote epithelial–mesenchymal transition (EMT), extracellular matrix (ECM) accumulation, and fibroblast proliferation, which contribute to progressive lung remodeling in PF. The Wenfei Buqi Tongluo (WBT) formula has been certified to be effective in the prevention and treatment of PF in clinical practice and has inhibitory effects on EMT, inflammation, and profibrotic factors. However, the pharmacological mechanisms of WBT against PF need to be further explored. In this study, we first analyzed the chemical components of the WBT formula using the UHPLC/Q-TOF-MS analysis. The potential targets of the identified compounds from WBT were predicted by the network pharmacology, which was confirmed by *in vivo* and *in vitro* study. After screening by the PubChem database, we first identified the 36 compounds of WBT and predicted the TGF-β signaling pathway, with ECM degradation as potential mechanism of WBT against PF by the network pharmacology. Furthermore, WBT treatment inhibited the levels of TGF-β and Smad3 phosphorylation and subsequently alleviated EMT and ECM accumulation in the bleomycin-induced mouse model and TGF-β1–induced cell model. These findings indicate that WBT can block the progressive process of PF by inhibiting EMT and promoting ECM degradation *via* the TGF-β/Smad3 pathway. This study may provide new insights into the molecular mechanism of WBT for the prevention and treatment of PF in the clinical application.

Keywords: WBT formula, network pharmacology, pulmonary fibrosis, extracellular matrix accumulation, epithelial–mesenchymal transition, TGF-β1/Smad3 pathway

INTRODUCTION

Pulmonary fibrosis (PF) is an end stage for various chronic and progressive interstitial lung diseases and is accompanied by gradually worsening symptoms such as fatigue, weight loss, and shortness of breath (King et al., 2011). PF is caused by occupational factors, autoimmune disorders, infections, and genetic factors, but the cause of this disease generally cannot be identified, which is called idiopathic PF (IPF) (Glass et al., 2020). IPF is a specific and common type of PF, in which lung function inexorably declines, leading to respiratory failure and eventually death. The incidence of IPF is increasing every year, with approximately three million people worldwide suffering from the disease (Nalysnyk et al., 2012; Hutchinson et al., 2015). Currently, only two drugs, pirfenidone and nintedanib, are used for the treatment of IPF, which can slow the decline of lung function in patients with IPF (King et al., 2014; Flaherty et al., 2019). However, the effects of the two drugs on patient survival are uncertain and can produce many adverse reactions, such as nausea, diarrhea, dyspepsia, and rash (Pang et al., 2019). Therefore, it is essential to develop drugs to delay the progression of IPF.

As reported, epithelial–mesenchymal transition (EMT), myofibroblast activation, and collagen accumulation are main pathological characteristics of PF (Ohyashiki et al., 1976; Todd et al., 2012; Salton et al., 2019). During the development of PF, EMT is a pathological process where epithelial cells lose their phenotypes and acquire mesenchymal features. EMT is often detected for several biomarkers, including E-cadherin, N-cadherin, and α-smooth muscle actin (α-SMA) (Salton et al., 2019). An aberrant EMT event can induce extracellular matrix (ECM) accumulation and deposition, which contributes to the progression of lung remodeling in patients with PF (Philp et al., 2018). Myofibroblasts, differentiated from fibroblasts, are the main producers of ECM and are characterized by the presence of α-SMA (Todd et al., 2012). Importantly, TGF-β, as a profibrotic cytokine, can promote EMT, ECM accumulation, and fibroblast proliferation and differentiation to myofibroblasts to participate in PF, which may be mediated by the Smad2/3 signaling pathway (Kolahian et al., 2016; Walton et al., 2017; Lederer and Martinez, 2018).

Traditional Chinese medicine (TCM) has a long history in treating PF and its practitioners have accumulated rich experience in doing so. TCM considers the fact that the pathogenesis of PF is the obstruction of *Qi* and the stagnation of blood circulation, and the treatment for PF needs to promote *Qi* and activate blood circulation (Zhang et al., 2018). Moreover, many TCM drugs, including formulas (Fufang Biejia Ruangan Pills, Jinkui Shenqi Wan, etc.), single herbs (*Rheum palmatum* L., *Astragalus mongholicus* Bunge, etc.), and active components (gallic acid, quercetin, curcumin, gambogic acid, etc.) have been identified to be efficient in anti-fibrosis, improving lung function and reducing dyspnea (Zhang et al., 2021). The Wenfei Buqi Tongluo (WBT) formula is a hospital preparation for PF made by the Affiliated Hospital of Changchun University of Chinese Medicine that has been certified to be effective in anti-fibrosis treatment in clinical practice. As shown in **Table 1**, WBT is composed of 13 Chinese medicines. Our previous study showed that WBT could inhibit EMT in TGF-β1–induced A549 cells (Ding et al., 2021). In addition, the Xian-ke granule, a basic TCM formula of WBT, proved to be effective in anti-PF for bleomycin (BLM)–induced mice through the inhibition of the inflammatory response (Li et al., 2012) and the decrease of the connective tissue growth factor and integrin-linked kinase in the lung tissues (Yang et al., 2014). These results indicate that WBT has potential anti-fibrosis effect, but its pharmacological mechanisms and possible components need to be further explored.

The network pharmacology is a meaningful way to reveal the pharmacological mechanism of TCM formula, and the holistic view is a common characteristic between the TCM and the network pharmacology (Li and Zhang, 2013). Therefore, in this study, we used UHPLC/Q-TOF-MS to identify the possible components in WBT. The pharmacology network was used to predict the potential targets and mechanisms of WBT against PF, according to the guidance of the network pharmacology evaluation method (Li, 2021). Then, the pharmacological function and possible mechanism of WBT against PF was confirmed in animal and cell experiments. This study may provide new insights into the therapeutic effect and molecular mechanisms of WBT in the clinical applications aiming to delay PF progression.

TABLE 1 | The compositions of WBT formula.

Chinese name	Abbr	Latin name	Family	Weight (g)	Part used	Voucher specimen
Huang qi	HQ	*Astragalus mongholicus* Bunge	Fabaceae	40	Root	201910-01
Huang qin	HQN	*Scutellaria baicalensis* Georgi	Lamiaceae	20	Root	201910-02
Dan shen	DS	*Salvia miltiorrhiza* Bunge	Lamiaceae	20	Root	201910-03
Hu zhang	HZ	*Reynoutria japonica* Houtt.	Polygonaceae	15	Rhizome	201910-04
Dang gui	DG	*Angelica sinensis* (Oliv.) Diels	Apiaceae	15	Root	201910-05
Chuan xiong	CX	*Conioselinum anthriscoides 'Chuanxiong'*	Apiaceae	15	Root	201910-06
Di long	DL	*Pheretima aspergillum* (E.Perrier)	Megascolecidae	10	Whole animal	201910-07
Tao ren	TR	*Prunus persica* (L.) Batsch	Rosaceae	10	Seed	201910-08
Zi wan	ZW	*Aster tataricus* L.f.	Asteraceae	15	Rhizome	201910-09
Kuan donghua	KDH	*Tussilago farfara* L.	Asteraceae	15	Flower	201910-10
Jiang banxia	JBX	*Pinellia ternata* (Thunb.) Makino	Araceae	9	Rhizome	201910-11
Wei lingxian	WLX	*Clematis chinensis* Osbeck	Ranunculaceae	15	Rhizome	201910-12
Xi xiancao	XXC	*Sigesbeckia orientalis* L.	Asteraceae	15	Herba	20191013

MATERIALS AND METHODS

Materials and Reagents

Collagen I (ab34710), α-SMA (ab5694), E-cadherin (ab40772), N-cadherin (ab76011), TGF-β1 (ab215715), p-Smad3 (S423/S425, ab52903), and goat anti-rabbit/mouse antibodies (ab6721, ab6789) were purchased from Abcam (Cambridge, MA, USA). BLM (HY17565) and pirfenidone (PFD, HYB0673) were obtained from MedChemExpress (Princeton, NJ, USA). Calycosin-7-glucoside (ST08820120-5240), scutellarin (RS03111020-5839), apigenin-7-O-β-D-glucuronic acid (ST08920120-3075), oroxin B (ST09240120-5589), scutellarin methylester (ST15580120-4087), baicalin (RS01861020-5587), salvianolic acid A (ST005570120MG-4881), emodin glucoside (ST10890120-7823), wogonoside (ST08350120-5014), apigenin (RS000411020-5729), scutellarein (ST06340120-3414), baicalein (RS01871020-5699), isoastragaloside IV (ST81100105-6855), wogonin (RS01711020-5325), oroxylin A (ST23660220-6180), emodin (RS01401020-5940), salvianolic acid F (ST22410105mg-5189), salvianolic acid B (ST000500120mg-4065), and luteolin (RS00071020-5864) were purchased from Shanghai Shidande Standard Technical Service Co., Ltd. (Shanghai, China). Astragaloside I (DST190216-016), astragaloside II (DST180315-023), and astragaloside III (DST181118-018) were purchased from Chengdu Durst Biotechnology Co., Ltd. (Chengdu, China).

Preparation of WBT Extract

The 13 Chinese medicines (**Table 1**) constituting WBT were purchased from Beijing General Pharmaceutical Corporation (Beijing, China) and provided by the Department of Pharmacy, the Affiliated Hospital of Changchun University of Chinese Medicine (Changchun, China). The voucher specimens were deposited at the Jilin Ginseng Academy, Changchun University of Chinese Medicine. According to the preparation processing as traditional use, the standard procedure from Chinese Pharmacopoeia (2020 edition), and previous studies (Huang Q. et al., 2018; Yang et al., 2021), all drugs were blended, mixed, and extracted by 2,000 ml of distilled water (the drug solvent ration of this formula is 9.0) at 100°C for 30 min, which was repeated three times to obtain the aqueous extract of WBT formula. After centrifugation, the supernatant was dried under a vacuum to produce a powdery extract with the drug-extract ratio of 22.47% (obtained 48 g of powdery extract from 214 g of raw materials). The powder was stored at −20°C for further experiments.

UHPLC/Q-TOF-MS Analysis of WBT Extract

As previous described (Zuo et al., 2019; Yang et al., 2021), UHPLC analyses were carried out with a Waters ACQUITY UPLC I-Class Plus/Xevo G2-XS QTOF system (Waters, Milford, USA). Chromatographic separation was performed on a Waters ACQUITY UPLC BEH C18 (4.6 × 150 mm, 3.5 μm) at 30°C. The mobile phase was composed of 0.1% formic acid in water (A) and 0.1% formic acid in acetonitrile (B) running at 0.3 ml/min, consistent with the following optimal gradient elution program: 0–4 min, 1% B; 4–5 min, 1%–5 B; 5–10 min, 5%–17 B; 10–18 min, 17%–17 B; 18–23 min, 17%–22 B; 23–28 min, 22%–25 B; 28–34 min, 25%–32 B; 34–37 min, 32%–50 B; 37–40 min, 50%–95 B. The injection volume of WBT samples was 5 μl. The high-resolution MS data were recorded on a Xevo G2-XS QTOF mass spectrometer by MS^E in both the positive and negative ESI modes. The parameters of the electrospray ion source were set as follows: capillary voltage, 2.5 kV; cone voltage, 60 V; collision energy, 40–80 eV; scan mass range, 100–1,500 m/z; ion source temperature, 120°C; desolvation gas temperature, 500°C; cone gas flow rate, 50 L/h; desolvation gas flow rate, 800 L/h. The obtained MS^E data were conducted using UNIFI™ 1.9.3.0 software (Waters, Milford, USA).

Components and Disease Targets Collection

The PubChem database (https://pubchem.ncbi.nlm.nih.gov/) was used to obtain the molecular structure (SDF format) of each component that identified from WBT powder extract. Then, the molecular structural files were uploaded to the PharmaMapper (http://lilab-ecust.cn/pharmmapper/submitfile.html), ChemMapper (http://lilab-ecust.cn/chemmapper/), and SwissTarget (http://www.swisstargetprediction.ch/index.php) databases to predict the potential targets of each component from WBT (Huang H. et al., 2018; Yang et al., 2020; Mu et al., 2021). The GeneCards database (https://www.genecards.org/) was used to collect PF-related targets (Mu et al., 2021). Finally, the corresponding Gene and UniProt ID of each target were obtained from the UniProt database (https://www.uniprot.org/) (Shawky, 2019). The targets were used for the establishment of a component-target network.

Network Construction and Analysis

The targets of WBT and PF were combined so that the overlapping targets between PF and WBT could be obtained. Then, the overlapping targets were uploaded to the STRING database, and the information about protein–protein interaction was obtained. Meanwhile, the network of Chinese medicines, chemical ingredients, and potential targets was established and visualized by Cytoscape 3.8.0. The components of WBT and targets of the components were represented by hexagon and (or) rectangle, and the interaction was shown by a connecting line. Finally, depending on the overlapping targets, the significant Gene Ontology (GO) and Reactome Pathway were screened by the Metascape and DAVID databases.

Mouse Model Establishment and Drug Administration

All animal care and procedures were approved by the Experimental Animal Ethics Committee of Changchun University of Chinese Medicine (batch number: 20190134). Seventy of 8-week-old male C57BL/6 mice purchased from Beijing Weitong Lihua Experimental Animal Technology Co., Ltd. [License No. SCXK (Beijing) 2016-0006] were kept at the Animal Experimental Center of Changchun University of Chinese Medicine (Changchun, China) at an ambient temperature (20 ± 2°C) and 50%–60% humidity. In this study, mice were randomly divided into seven groups with 10 mice in each group, including the blank control, sham operation, BLM, BLM + WBT (3, 6, and 12 g/kg, among them, the dose of 6 g/kg/day is equal dosage of clinic, 12 g/kg/day is the higher dosage, and 3 g/kg/day is the lower dosage), and BLM + pirfenidone (PFD, 200 mg/kg) groups, according to the book named Experimental Methodolgy of Pharamacology (2002 version). Except for the control group, mice were intraperitoneally with pentobarbital sodium (10 ml/kg) and intratracheally injected with BLM (5 mg/kg) or 0.9% normal saline (sham operation group), according to the previous report (Shahbaz et al., 2021). WBT and PFD were administered by gavage on the second day after BLM or NS injection for 14 days (once a day). Mice in the blank control, sham, and model groups were given pure water in the same amount of WBT.

Micro-CT Imaging

Micro-CT imaging was performed with Quantum FX Micro CT (PerkinElmer, Inc., Waltham, MA, USA). After anesthetizing with isoflurane, the lungs were imaged with the help of cardiopulmonary gating techniques. The X-ray system of the scanner used a micro-focusing tube with a focal spot of 5 μm at 4 W and generated X-rays with cone beam geometry. The scanner's detection system was composed of an amorphous silicon digital X-ray plate, which could acquire projection radiographs at a rate of 30 frames per second. The X-ray tube was set at 90 kV and 80 μA and took the projection radiographs during a 360° gantry rotation, with a total scanning time of 4 min. The reconstructed visual field was 36 mm with a high-resolution scanning mode (Lv et al., 2013; Ruscitti et al., 2017).

Histopathological Examination and Assessment

H&E and Masson's trichrome stainings were performed to evaluate the pathological changes of mouse lung tissues from different groups, as previously described (Zhao et al., 2020). For H&E and Masson's trichrome staining, the exfoliated lung tissue of mice was fixed in 4% paraformaldehyde for 24 h, embedded in paraffin, cut into the 5-μm-thick sections, and stained with H&E and Masson's trichrome kits. The degrees of inflammatory and fibrotic injuries in the lung tissues were scored according to the Mikawar and Ashcroft methods, respectively (Katoh et al., 1998; Pedroza et al., 2016). Immunohistochemical (IHC) staining was used to analyze the levels of PF-related proteins, such as collagen I, α-SMA, E-cadherin, N-cadherin, and TGF-β1 in the lung tissues, according to the manufacturer's instructions (Kishi et al., 2018). After dewaxing and antigen repairing, the tissue was incubated with primary antibodies at 4°C overnight, followed by a conjugated secondary antibody and DAB staining. After counterstaining with hematoxylin, the images for antigenic sites were visualized and acquired by a Digital Microscope and Slide Scanner (M8, PreciPoint, Thuringia, Germany). The relative staining score of each protein was determined by calculating the areal density using Image-Pro Plus 6.0 software (Media Cybemetics, Inc., Rockville, MD, USA).

Hydroxyproline Analysis

The content of hydroxyproline (HYP) in mouse lung tissue was quantified by the HYP assay kit (Nanjing Jiancheng Institute of Bioengineering), according to a previous study (Lv et al., 2013).

Cell Culture and Model Establishment

The TC-1 cell line was bought from the iCell Bioscience, Inc. (Shanghai, China), and cultured in RPMI 1640 containing 10% fetal bovine serum (Clark Bioscience, Claymont, USA), penicillin (100 kU/L), and streptomycin (100 mg/L) (Biosharp, Hefei, China) at 37°C in a 5% CO_2 humidified incubator. When the cells were in good condition, in accordance with the previous study (Zeng et al., 2021), TGF-β1 (10 ng/ml) was added to induce TC-1 cells transformation into mesenchymal-like cells.

Cell Viability Assay

According to the previous study (Zeng et al., 2021), TC-1 cells were seeded into 96-well plates at a density of 6,000 cells/well, which were used to investigate the effect of WBT on cell viability after treatment for 48 h. To investigate the toxicity of WBT, TC-1 cells were treated with WBT at a concentration of 7.1–1,000 μg/ml for 48 h. In the TGF-β1–induced cell model, TC-1 cells were set as the control [dimethyl sulfoxide (DMSO) alone], model [TGF-β1 (10 ng/ml)], and treatment group [TGF-β1 (10 ng/ml) + WBT (7.1–1,000 μg/ml)] to examine the effect of WBT on the cell viability. After treatment for 48 h, MTT (0.5 mg/ml) was added (Solibol, Beijing, China), and DMSO (150 μl) was used to dissolve formazan crystals, which was measured as the absorbance at 490 nm using a microplate reader. The cell survival rate was calculated as the percentage of each group relative to the control group.

Quantitative Real-Time PCR Analysis

The total RNA of TC-1 cells in different groups was extracted by a total RNA kit. After that, 1 μg of total RNA was reverse-transcribed into cDNA with the iScript cDNA synthesis kit. The Bio-Rad CFX96 system was used to perform quantitative (qPCR) analysis, and the relative mRNA level was calculated using the $2^{-\Delta\Delta Ct}$ method and normalized by GAPDH (Zhang Z. et al., 2020). The primer sequences of N-Cadherin, E-cadherin, α-SMA, collagen I, and GAPDH are listed in **Supplementary Table S1**.

Western Blot Analysis

The total protein of TC-1 cells in different groups was obtained by an ice-cold RIPA buffer and separated by SDS-PAGE, transferred onto PVDF membranes. After blocking for 1 h at room temperature with a blocking buffer containing 5% BSA, the membranes were incubated with the primary antibody overnight at 4°C. After incubating with the HRP-conjugated secondary antibody for 2 h, the blots were visualized by a chemiluminescent imaging system (ChemiDoc XRS+, Bio-Rad, CA, USA) and quantified by ImageJ software (Jiang et al., 2021).

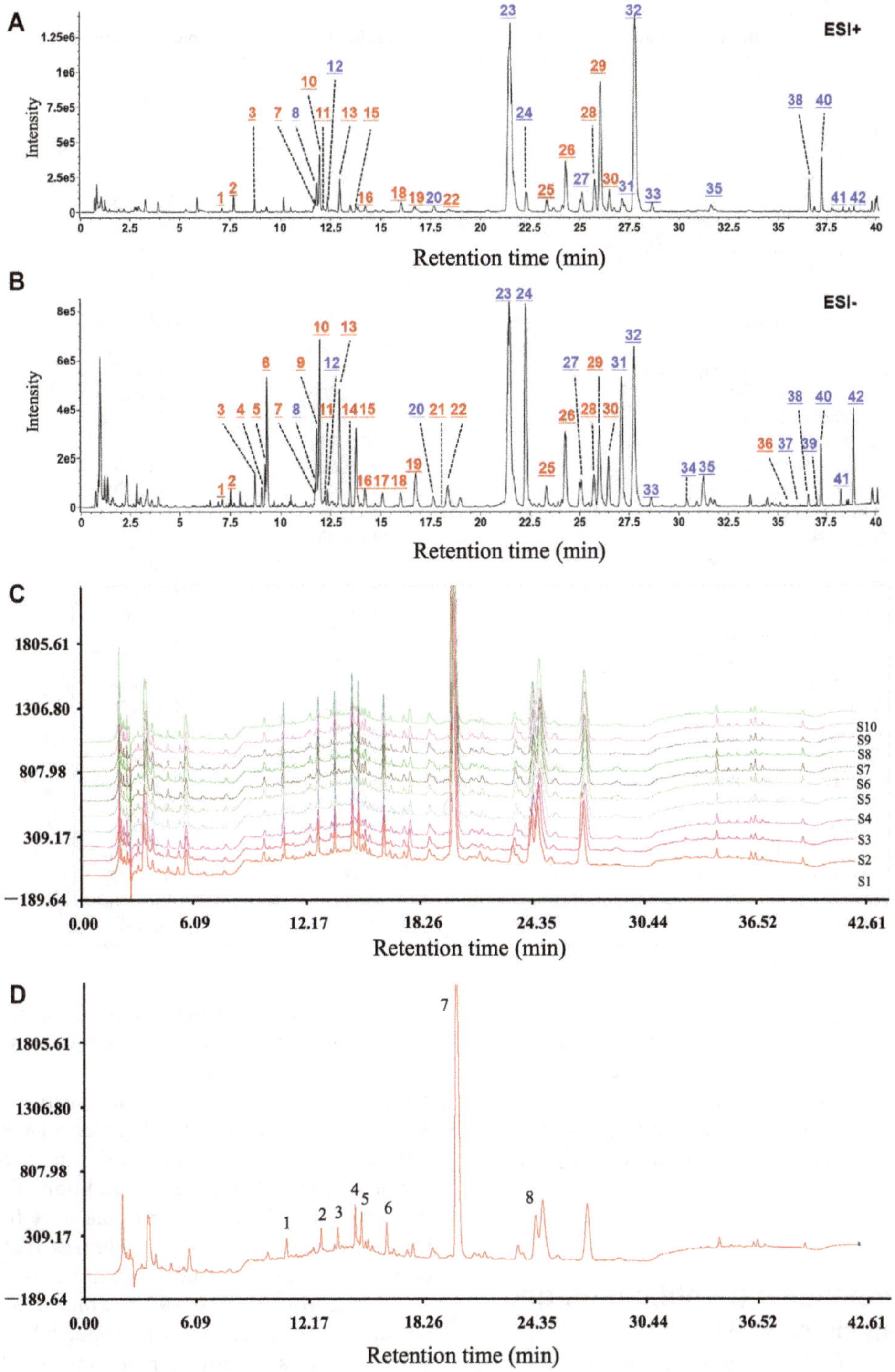

FIGURE 1 | The main active components and good reproducibility of the WBT formula were determined by UHPLC/Q-TOF-MS analysis. **(A,B)** The chromatograms of the WBT formula for 42 active components in positive and negative ion modes. Blue numbers represent the compounds confirmed with the reference standards. **(C and D)** The reproducible HPLC fingerprints of the 10 batches of WBT (S1–S10) were identified using the Similarity Evaluation System for Chromatographic Fingerprint of Traditional Chinese Medicine (2004 Edition).

TABLE 2 | The 36 components of WBT formula from UHPLC/Q-TOF-MS analysis screened according to PubChem database.

Component ID	Ingredient name	Molecular weight	Molecular formula	Herb source
1	Cryptochlorogenic acid	354.0951	$C_{16}H_{18}O_9$	Zi-wan/Kuan dong-hua
2	Chlorogenic acid	354.0951	$C_{16}H_{18}O_9$	Zi-wan/Kuan dong-hua
3	Amygdalin	457.1584	$C_{20}H_{27}NO_{11}$	Tao-ren
4	Caffeic acid	180.0423	$C_9H_8O_4$	Zi-wan
5	Viscidulin I	302.0427	$C_{15}H_{10}O_7$	Huang-qin
6	Calycosin-7-glucoside	446.1213	$C_{22}H_{22}O_{10}$	Huang-qin
7	Polydatin	390.1315	$C_{20}H_{22}O_8$	Hu-zhang
8	Chrysin 6-C-glucoside 8-C-arabinoside	548.153	$C_{26}H_{28}O_{13}$	Huang-qin
9	Baicalein 7-O-β-D-glucuronide	464.0955	$C_{21}H_{20}O_{12}$	Huang-qin
10	Scutellarin	462.0798	$C_{21}H_{18}O_{12}$	Huang-qin
11	Isochlorogenic acid A	516.1268	$C_{25}H_{24}O_{12}$	Kuan-dong-hua
12	Isochlorogenic acid B	516.1268	$C_{25}H_{24}O_{12}$	Kuan-dong-hua
13	5,4′-Dihydroxy-7-methoxyflavone	284.0685	$C_{16}H_{12}O_5$	Huang-qin
14	Isochlorogenic acid C	516.1268	$C_{25}H_{24}O_{12}$	Kuan-dong-hua
15	Scutellarin methylester	476.0955	$C_{22}H_{20}O_{12}$	Huang-qin
16	Viscidulin III	346.0689	$C_{17}H_{14}O_8$	Huang-qin
17	Emodin-8-β-D-glucoside	432.1056	$C_{21}H_{20}O_{10}$	Hu-zhang
18	Baicalin	446.0849	$C_{21}H_{18}O_{11}$	Huang-qin
19	Salvianolic acid B	718.1534	$C_{36}H_{30}O_{16}$	Dan-shen
20	Dihydrobaicalin	448.1006	$C_{21}H_{20}O_{11}$	Huang-qin
21	Norwogonin 7-O-glucuronide	446.0849	$C_{21}H_{18}O_{11}$	Huang-qin
22	Salvianolic acid A	494.1213	$C_{26}H_{22}O_{10}$	Dan-shen
23	Chrysin-7-O-β-D-glucuronide	430.09	$C_{21}H_{18}O_{10}$	Huang-qin
24	Oroxylin A 7-O-β-D-glucuronide	460.1006	$C_{22}H_{20}O_{11}$	Huang-qin
25	5,7-dihydroxy-6-methoxyflavone 7-O-β-D-glucuronide	460.0955	$C_{22}H_{20}O_{11}$	Huang-qin
26	Emodin glucoside	432.1056	$C_{21}H_{20}O_{10}$	Hu-zhang
27	Wogonoside	460.1006	$C_{22}H_{20}O_{11}$	Hu-zhang
28	Scutellarein	286.0477	$C_{15}H_{10}O_6$	Huang-qin
29	Baicalein	270.0528	$C_{15}H_{10}O_5$	Huang-qin
30	8-methyl-5,7,4′-trihydroxyisoflavone	284.0685	$C_{16}H_{12}O_5$	Huang-qin
31	Astragaloside III	784.4609	$C_{41}H_{68}O_{14}$	Huang-qi
32	Wogonin	284.0685	$C_{16}H_{12}O_5$	Huang-qin
33	Astragaloside II	826.4715	$C_{43}H_{70}O_{15}$	Huang-qi
34	Oroxylin A	284.0685	$C_{16}H_{12}O_5$	Huang-qin
35	Astragaloside I	868.482	$C_{45}H_{72}O_{16}$	Huang-qi
36	Emodin	270.0528	$C_{15}H_{10}O_5$	Hu-zhang

Statistical Analysis

The data are expressed as mean ± SD. All data were statistically analyzed by GraphPad prism 9.0 software (San Diego, CA, USA). Multiple groups were compared by one-way ANOVA (Tukey's post hoc) to determine the statistical significance. For all the statistical analyses, $p < 0.05$ was statistically significant.

RESULTS

Chemical Components Identification and Similarity Analysis of WBT

After optimization of the chromatographic and mass spectrometric conditions, a total of 42 compounds were identified or deduced from WBT formula, in which 16 components (expressed by * in **Supplementary Table S2**), including calycosin-7-glucoside, scutellarin/methylester, baicalin, and salvianolic acid A/B, were identified by the reference standards. The 42 compounds in WBT were characterized by comparing the retention time, accurate mass, and fragment ions with those of the standards or data reported by the literature. Furthermore, the attribution to the single herb was confirmed by the base peak intensity (BPI) chromatograms of the blank sample, WBT formula, and individual herbs. The BPI chromatograms of the WBT formula after collection in the positive and negative ion modes are shown in **Figures 1A,B**. The detailed information for 42 compounds in WBT is shown in **Supplementary Table S2**. In addition, the fingerprint and the similarity of the WBT formula were further analyzed by UHPLC method. As shown in **Figures 1C,D**, the percentages of the similarities from all 10 batches of WBT powdery extract were range from 91.0% to 99.3%, which indicates that the WBT powdery extract has good reproducibility. Importantly, we selected six standard compounds in WBT extract to perform quantitative analysis to avoid the risk of artifacts with higher dose in animal study. As shown in **Supplementary Figure S1** and **Supplementary Table S3**, the WBT extract included calycosin-7-glucoside (0.4499 mg/g), baicalin (17.2408 mg/g), salvianolic acid B (3.3389 mg/g), salvianolic acid A (0.96 mg/g), emodin-8-β-D-glucoside (1.0735 mg/g), and wogonoside (6.7344 mg/g), which were the dose range as indicated in the consensus document of clinical evidence-based ethnopharmacology.

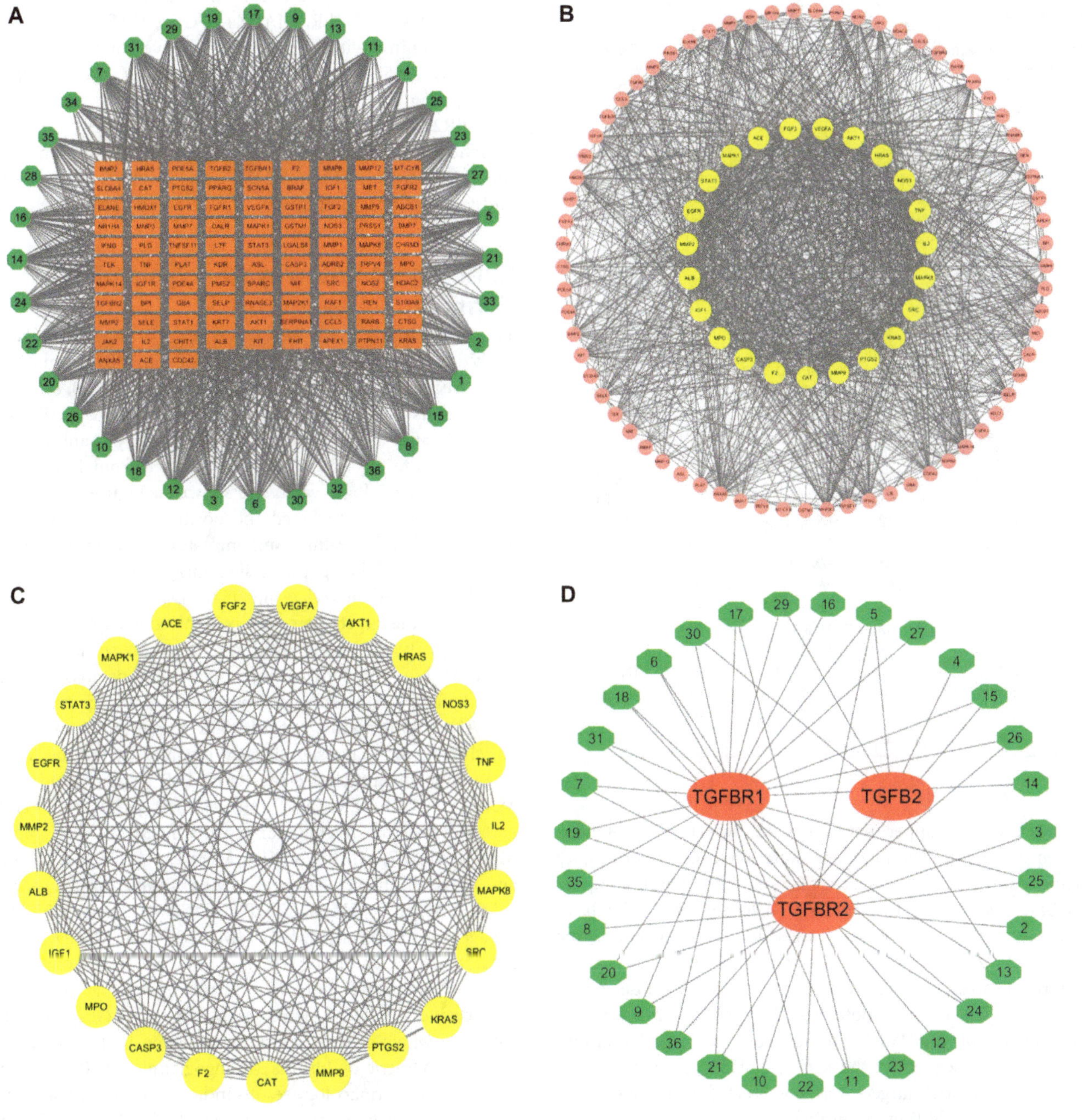

FIGURE 2 | Potential targets of WBT formula were predicted by network pharmacology. **(A)** The network of the 36 selected components of WBT formula and potential targets was constructed. The green octagons represent the components ID of 36 compounds, and the orange rectangles represent the potential targets participated in PF. **(B and C)** PPI networks of 93 potential targets and 23 core targets are shown after screening with the degree ≥27, betweenness ≥0.08, and closeness ≥0.58. The circle represents the all-potential targets, and the yellow circle represents the core targets **(D)**. The network of 31 active components and the targets in TGF-β pathway was analyzed. The red ovals represent the TGF-β–related targets, and the green hexagons represent the 31 screened components from WBT formula.

Potential Target Screening and Network Establishment for Components of WBT Formula and Pulmonary Fibrosis

According to the PubChem database, the 42 components in the WBT powdery extract were normalized, and those that had not been confirmed potential therapeutic targets were excluded, leaving 36 ingredients for further analysis of the network pharmacology (**Table 2**). The molecular structure files of the 36 components were obtained from the PubChem database, depending on which the potential targets of 36 components were obtained from several databases, such as PharmaMapper

TABLE 3 | The 93 hub targets between 36 active components of WBT formula and pulmonary fibrosis.

No	Gene name	No	Gene name	No	Gene name
1	ABCB1	32	HMOX1	63	PDE4A
2	ACE	33	HRAS	64	PDE5A
3	ADRB2	34	IFNG	65	PLAT
4	AKT1	35	IGF1	66	PLG
5	ALB	36	IGF1R	67	PMS2
6	ANXA5	37	IL2	68	PPARG
7	APEX1	38	JAK2	69	PRSS1
8	ASL	39	KDR	70	PTGS2
9	BMP2	40	KIT	71	PTPN11
10	BMP7	41	KRAS	72	RAF1
11	BPI	42	KRT7	73	RARB
12	BRAF	43	LGALS3	74	REN
13	CALR	44	LTF	75	Rnase3
14	CASP3	45	MAP2K1	76	S100A9
15	CAT	46	MAPK1	77	SCN5A
16	CCL5	47	MAPK14	78	SELE
17	CDC42	48	MAPK8	79	SELP
18	CHIT1	49	MET	80	SERPINA1
19	CHRM3	50	MIF	81	SLC6A4
20	CTSG	51	MMP1	82	SPARC
21	EGFR	52	MMP12	83	SRC
22	ELANE	53	MMP2	84	STAT1
23	F2	54	MMP3	85	STAT3
24	FGF2	55	MMP7	86	TEK
25	FGFR1	56	MMP8	87	TGFB2
26	FGFR2	57	MMP9	88	TGFBR1
27	FHIT	58	MPO	89	TGFBR2
28	GBA	59	MT-CYB	90	TNF
29	GSTM1	60	NOS2	91	TNFSF11
30	GSTP1	61	NOS3	92	TRPV4
31	HDAC2	62	NR1H4	93	VEGFA

database, ChemMapper database, and SwissTarget database. Moreover, the potential targets were screened according to many parameters (fit score ≥2.5 in the PharmaMapper database, score ≥0.01 in the ChemMapper database, probability ≥0.079 in the SwissTarget database). Afterward, the UniProt ID corresponding to each target was obtained from the UniProt database, and the reduplicative targets were deleted to obtain a total of 687 potential therapeutic targets of 36 components of the WBT powdery extract (**Supplementary Table S4**). Subsequently, the network of 36 components and their 687 potential targets was constructed (**Supplementary Figure S2**). In addition, according to the score >11.8, a total of 584 potential targets of PF were selected from the GeneCards database. On the basis of the 687 potential targets of WBT and the 584 potential targets of PF, 93 overlapping targets were obtained, and the network of 36 active components and 93 overlapping targets was established and is shown in **Figure 2A** and **Table 3**. Importantly, on the basis of the topological analysis for component-overlapping targets network, the top four components of WBT formula were screened out depending on the degree >48, including baicalein, oroxylin A 7-O-β-D-glucuronide, viscidulin I, and viscidulin III (**Supplementary Figure S3**). As shown in **Figure 2B**, the PPI network of potential targets from WBT formula has 93 nodes and 1,272 edges. The 23 main targets, represented by yellow circles, contained ALB, VEGFA, AKT1, TNF, MMP2, MMP9, STAT3, EGFR, MAPK1, FGF2, CASP3, and others after screening with degree ≥27, betweenness ≥0.08, and closeness ≥0.58 (**Figure 2C**). Importantly, among the 93 overlapping targets, TGF-β and its receptors (TGF-βR1 and TGF-βR2), as classical profibrotic indicators, were also enriched, which are potential targets of 31 components in the WBT formula (**Figure 2D**). Collectively, 36 components and their 93 potential targets for PF were predicted.

Enrichment Pathways Analysis of WBT Formula

The Metascape database was used to perform GO enrichment for analyzing the potential mechanisms of the WBT formula. For these mechanisms, the 390 biological processes (BPs), 80 cellular components (CCs), and 105 molecular functions (MFs) were obtained and are shown in **Supplementary Tables S5–S7**. Moreover, the top 20 entries were selected from BP, CC, and MF, in order of -log *p* value, are shown in **Figure 3A**. The BPs regulated by WBT included the positive regulation of kinase activity, wound healing, inflammatory response, cytokine production, and the apoptotic signaling pathway. For CCs, CC mainly contained the vesicle lumen, the ECM, and focal adhesion. In the MFs, the targets were mainly involved in peptidase activity, kinase activity, BMP receptor binding, cytokine receptor binding, and other bindings. Furthermore, the DAVID database was used to obtain 91 terms from the Reactome pathway enrichment analysis (**Supplementary Table S8**). Importantly, the top 20 enrichment pathways significantly involved in the mechanism of WBT formula included the RAF/MAP kinase cascade (KIT, MAPK1, KRAS, TEK, JAK2, HRAS, FGF2, EGFR, IL2, FGFR2, and FGFR1), the degradation of the ECM (MMP1, MMP2, MMP3, MMP7, MMP8, MMP9, MMP12, CASP3, CTSG, PLG, and ELANE), the activation of MMPs (PRSS1, MMP1, MMP2, MMP3, MMP7, MMP8, MMP9, CTSG, PLG, and ELANE), collagen degradation (MMP1, MMP2, MMP3, MMP7, MMP8, MMP9, MMP12, and ELANE), and other pathways (**Figure 3B**). Remarkably, these potential targets participating in the degradation of ECM were regulated by TGF-β signaling pathway, which is an important regulator in the occurrence and development of fibrosis (Frangogiannis, 2020). Together, the network pharmacology results indicate that WBT may inhibit the TGF-β signaling pathway to regulate ECM production and degradation or other downstream pathways for the blockade of PF progression. However, except for the TGF-β signaling pathway, the mechanisms and targets from the network pharmacology need to be further evaluated.

WBT Attenuates Pulmonary Fibrosis Progression in BLM-Induced Mice

To further assess the protective effect of WBT against PF, mice were treated with WBT or PFD for 14 days after intratracheal injection of BLM (**Figure 4A**). After the treatment, the lungs of mice in the different groups (Sham, BLM, BLM + WBT, and BLM + PFD) were observed in three different planes by micro-CT scanning.

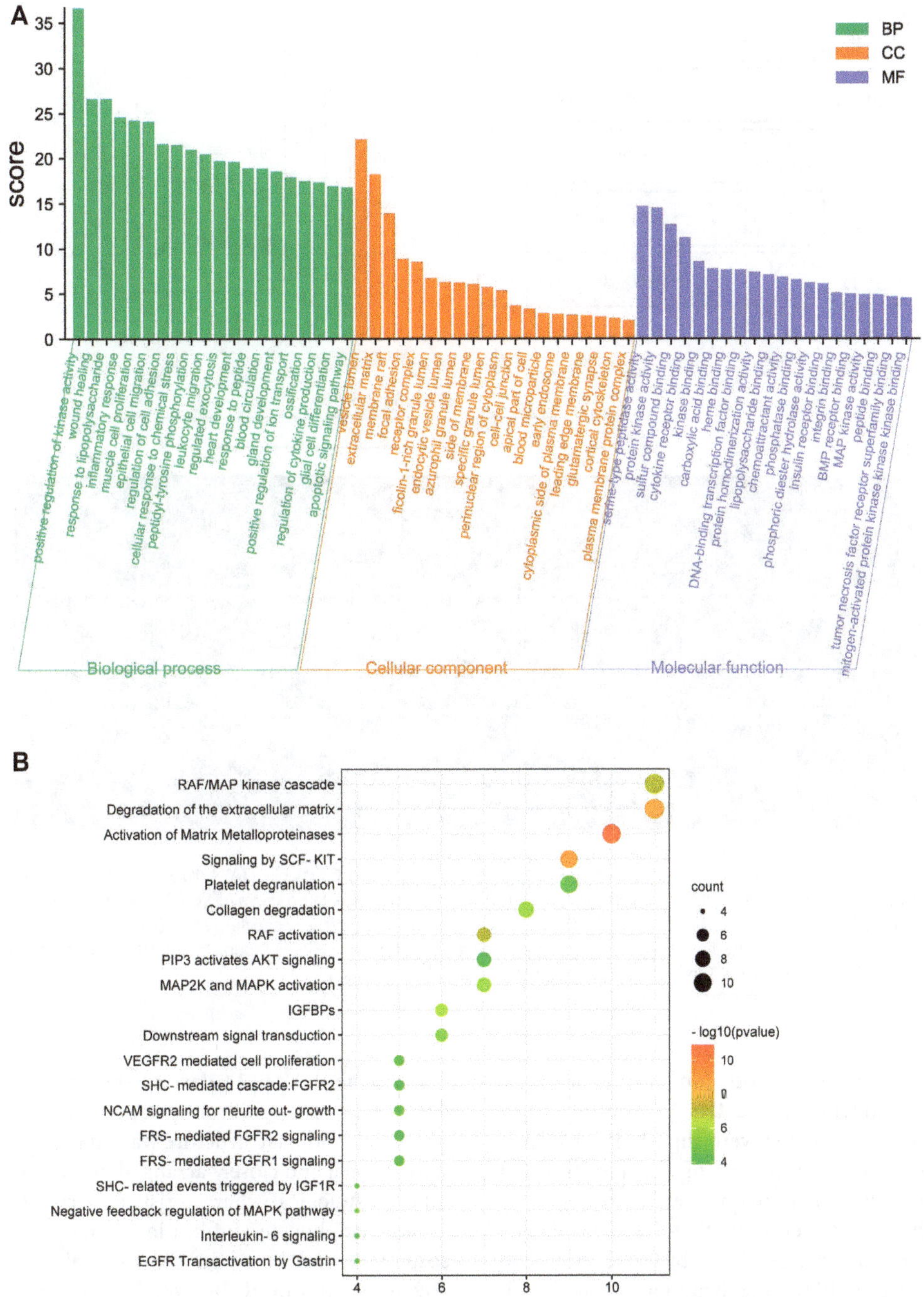

FIGURE 3 | Enrichment analysis of the potential targets of WBT formula against PF was performed by the Metascape and DAVID database. **(A)** The top 20 terms of biological process (BP), cellular component (CC), and molecular function (MF) of WBT formula are shown as a bar diagram. **(B)** The top 20 Reactome pathway terms participating in PF are shown as a bubble diagram by the DAVID database, according to the *p*-value of the calculation.

As shown in **Figure 4B**, the micro-CT imaging shows that lung tissues from blank and sham groups show clear texture, no abnormal density shadow, and a bronchial vascular bundle that runs normally. The interstitial thickening around bronchial vascular bundles in the axial fiber system and the diffuse interlobular septum thickening in the peripheral fiber system can be markedly observed in the both lungs from BLM-induced model group. Moreover, subpleural linear shadows are seen in many places, indicating that BLM-induced lungs have obvious characteristics of ground glass density and grid-like changes. Compared with model group, the lung texture is clearer, and the bronchial vascular bundles are not significantly thickened in the lungs from WBT-treated group. The original diffuse ground glass

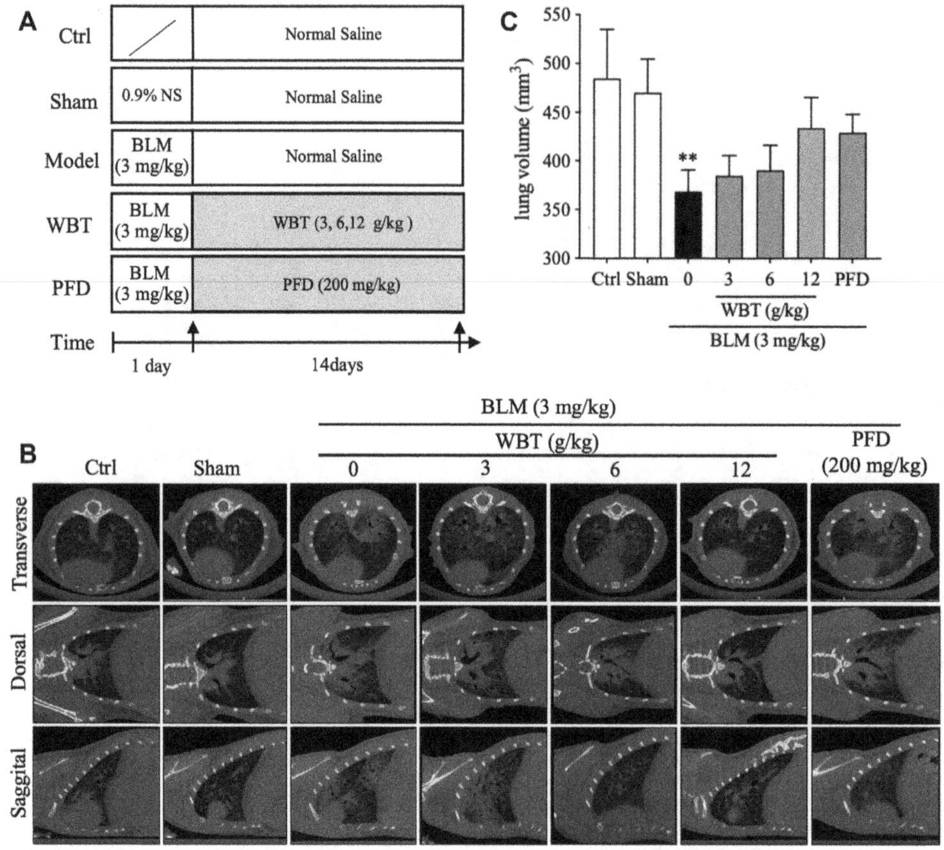

FIGURE 4 | The protective effect of WBT formula on BLM-induced lung injury was evaluated by micro-CT imaging. **(A)** A diagram for the mouse modeling process and WBT or PFD administration is shown. **(B)** After BLM induction and 14-day intervention, the representative *in vivo* micro-CT scans for the lungs from different groups of Ctrl, Sham, BLM, BLM + WBT (3, 6, and 12 g/kg), and BLM + PFD (200 mg/kg) in the transverse, dorsal, or sagittal planes. **(C)** The lung volume of different groups in the BLM-induced mouse model was quantified by the three-dimensional volume rendering technique (n = 4 per group). $^{**}p < 0.01$, compared to the Sham group. BLM, bleomycin; Ctrl, control; WBT, Wenfei Buqi Tongluo formula; PFD, pirfenidone.

density and grid-like change in both lungs were obviously inhibited by WBT treatment (**Figure 4B**). In addition, BLM-induced decreases of lung volume were slightly improved by WBT treatment, compared with that of the model group (**Figure 4C**). Moreover, the protective effect of WBT in 12 g/kg was significantly better than that in 6 and 3 g/kg. The improvement for the changes of PF by WBT at 12 g/kg was similar with that of PFD at 200 mg/kg. Therefore, in subsequent experiments, the WBT group of 12 g/kg was used for histopathological and IHC analysis.

H&E and Masson's trichrome stainings were performed and analyzed to investigate the effect of WBT on histological changes in the lung tissues from BLM-induced mice. The H&E staining results show that many alveolar walls were thickened and accompanied by infiltration of lymphocytes and macrophages in the BLM-induced group, compared with that in the sham group. BLM injection increased the number of inflammatory cells infiltrating around blood vessels and forming vascular sleeves, accompanied by acidic serous substance exudation in the local alveolar cavity (**Figure 5A**, upper panel). After 14 days of treatment, the extent of tissue destruction was significantly suppressed by WBT or PFD. The bronchial epithelial structure was intact, and the epithelial cells were normal and closely arranged in the WBT group. However, other histological characteristics, including thicker alveolar walls, lymphocyte infiltration, and a small amount of eosinophil and blood in the local alveolar cavity were not obviously improved by WBT (**Figure 5A**, upper panel). Masson's trichrome staining confirmed that the blue staining for fibrous collagen deposition as an index of PF in the lung tissues induced by BLM was significantly inhibited by WBT or PFD (**Figure 5A**, lower panel). The areas of collagen deposition in WBT or PFD-treated lung tissues were markedly lower than that in the BLM-induced group (**Figure 5B**). Notably, the scores from Mikawar and Ashcroft methods were reduced by WBT on the basis of H&E and Masson's trichrome stainings, which indicates that WBT can decrease the lung injury induced by BLM (**Figure 5C**). Together, WBT treatment can improve lung architecture and collagen deposition to block the progression of PF in the BLM-induced mouse model.

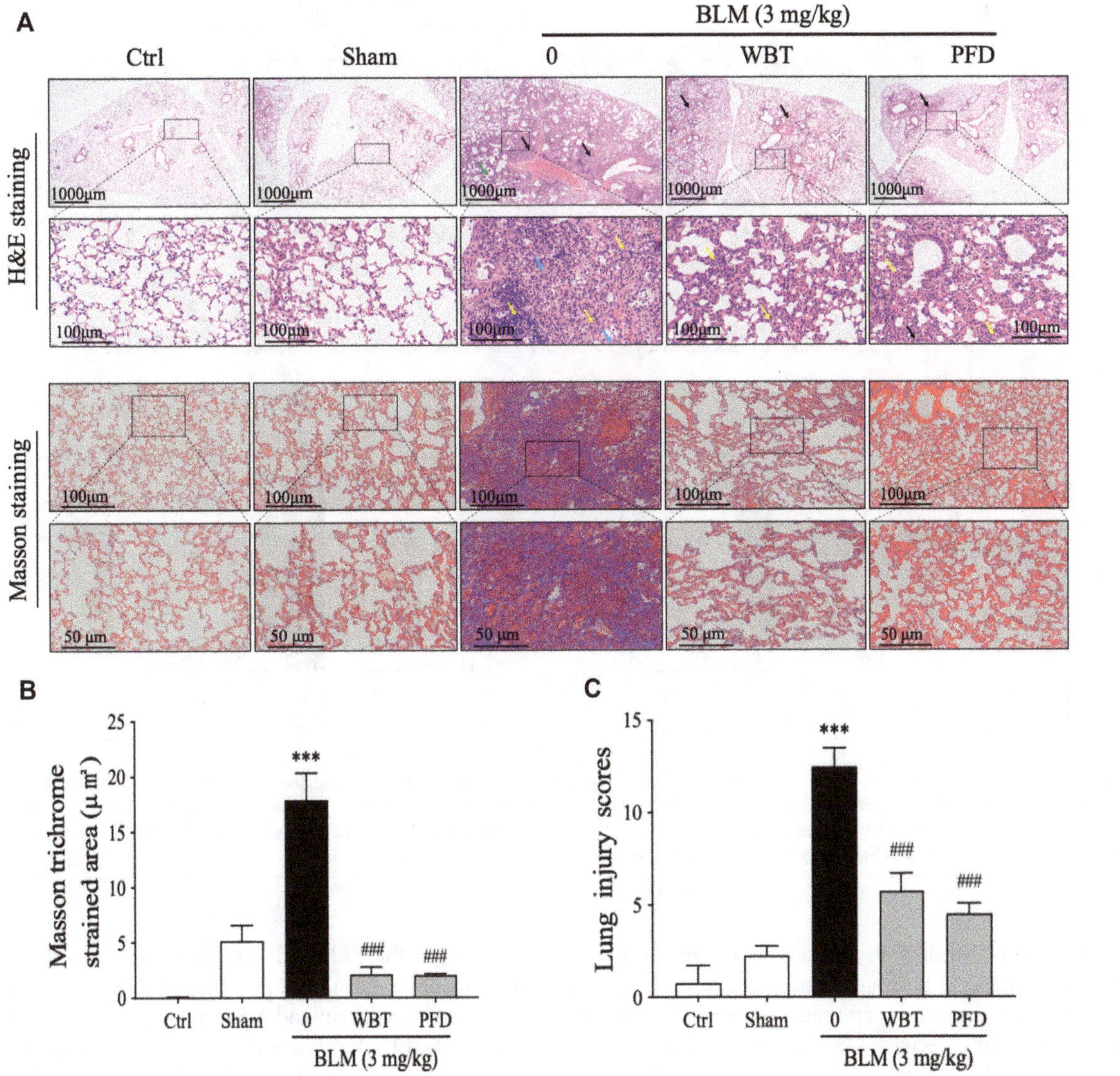

FIGURE 5 | WBT formula attenuated BLM-induced lung fibrosis after 14-day treatment. **(A)** H&E and Masson's trichrome stainings for the lung tissues from Ctrl, Sham, BLM, BLM + WBT (12 g/kg), and BLM + PFD (200 mg/kg) groups were presented (n = 5). The images in the lower panels (scale bar = 50 μm) of each staining were magnified from the inset of the photomicrographs in the upper panels (scale bar = 200 μm). **(B)** Quantitative analysis of Masson's trichrome staining in the sections of mouse lungs (n = 5). **(C)** The pathological score of lung injury was analyzed in different groups (n = 5). ***$p < 0.001$, compared to the sham group; ###$p < 0.001$, compared to the BLM group. BLM, bleomycin; Ctrl, control; WBT, Wenfei Buqi Tongluo formula; PFD, pirfenidone.

WBT Decreases the Level of TGF-β and Smad3 Phosphorylation in BLM-Induced Mice

As enriched by the network pharmacology, the TGF-β signaling pathway is critical for the protection of WBT against PF. Therefore, the expressions of TGF-β and p-Smad3 in different lung tissues from the sham, model, or WBT/PFD groups were determined by IHC staining. As shown in **Figures 6A,B**, the increase of TGF-β level induced by BLM is significantly down-regulated by WBT. Furthermore, the phosphorylation of Smad3 is significantly inhibited by the WBT treatment, compared with the BLM-induced model group (**Figure 6A**, lower panel, and **Figure 6C**). In addition, WBT and PFD have similar inhibitory effects in TGF-β and p-Smad3 expressions at the protein level. Collectively, WBT blocks the TGF-β/Smad3 pathway in the lung tissues of BLM-induced mice, which confirms the enrichment of TGF-β pathway for WBT by the network pharmacology.

WBT Reduces Collagen Accumulation in BLM-Induced Mice and TGF-β1–Induced TC-1 Cells

Collagen I is an important component of ECM accumulation, an important characteristic of PF (Long et al., 2018). As shown in **Figure 3**, the collagen degradation pathway is a potential

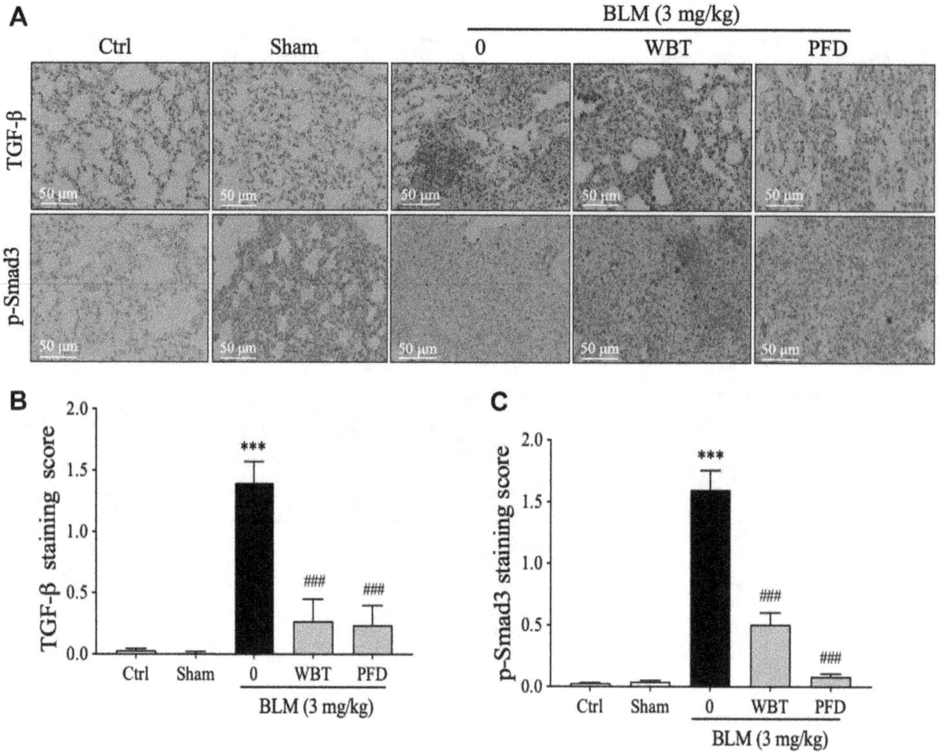

FIGURE 6 | The WBT formula inhibited the TGF-β/Smad3 pathway in the BLM-induced mouse model of lung fibrosis. **(A)** Immunohistochemical assay was used to detect the expression of TGF-β1 and p-Smad3 in the lungs from different groups of control, sham, model, and treatment. Scale bar = 50 μm. **(B,C)** Quantification of relative TGF-β1 and p-Smad3 levels from **(A)** was analyzed (n = 5); ***$p < 0.001$, compared to the sham group; ###$p < 0.001$, compared to the BLM group. BLM, bleomycin; Ctrl, control; WBT, Wenfei Buqi Tongluo formula; PFD, pirfenidone.

mechanism of WBT against PF, according to the results of network pharmacological analysis. In the BLM-induced mouse model, the level of collagen I was up-regulated by BLM induction, which was significantly decreased by the treatment of WBT or PFD (**Figures 7A,B**). Moreover, HYP, a special amino acid extracted from collagen, represents the content of total collagen, which is a theoretically guide for the diagnosis and prognosis of PF (Berisio et al., 2004). The measurement of HYP content in mouse lung tissues showed that the HYP level in BLM-induced model group was higher than that in the sham groups, whereas the content of HYP induced by BLM was significantly decreased by WBT treatment (**Figure 7C**). In addition, in TGF-β1–induced TC-1 cells (the cytotoxicity test of WBT to TC-1 cells is shown in **Supplementary Figure S4**), the expression of collagen I was also significantly down-regulated by WBT treatment (**Figure 7D**). Together, these results indicated that WBT can attenuate collagen accumulation *in vivo* and *in vitro.*

WBT Inhibited EMT in BLM-Induced Mice and TGF-β1–Induced TC-1 Cells

EMT is a common developmental process in the pathogenesis of PF, which can be induced by TGF-β (Nieto et al., 2016). Consistent with the previous study (Ding et al., 2021), the treatment of WBT significantly inhibited EMT *in vivo* and *in vitro*. In the BLM-induced mouse model, the IHC staining demonstrated that the EMT with the decreased E-cadherin and increased N-cadherin and α-SMA was promoted by BLM, which was blocked by WBT, compared with that of the model group (**Figure 8A**, middle and lower panels, and **Figures 8C,D**). In this BLM-induced mouse model, the regulation of WBT on EMT markers was similar to that of PFD (**Figure 8**). In addition, in TGF-β1–induced TC-1 cells, the changes of α-SMA, E-cadherin, and N-cadherin regulated by the WBT formula at the mRNA and protein levels were similar to those in the BLM-induced mouse model (**Figures 8E–G**). Together, these data indicate that WBT can inhibit EMT in the BLM-induced mouse model and the TGF-β1–induced cell model.

DISCUSSION

To explore the chemical components and mechanism of the WBT formula against PF, in this study, we performed UHPLC/Q-TOF-MS analysis, the network pharmacology prediction and experimental validation. According to PubChem database, a total of 36 chemical compounds in WBT powdery extract from UHPLC/Q-TOF-MS analysis were identified or tentatively characterized. Then, the potential targets and mechanisms of these compounds against PF were predicted by

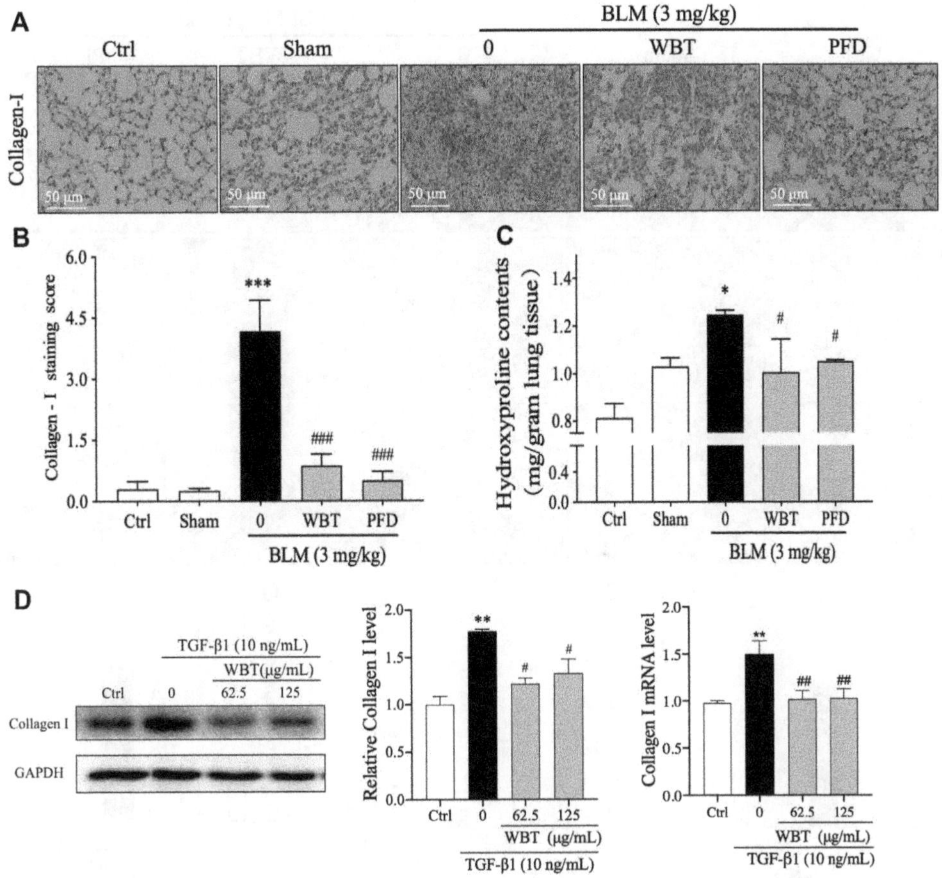

FIGURE 7 | WBT formula inhibited BLM-induced collagen deposition in the mouse and TC-1 cell model of lung fibrosis. **(A)** The level of collagen I was detected by immunohistochemical staining in the mouse lung from different groups. Scale bar = 50 μm. **(B)** The relative collagen I level from **(A)** was quantified (n = 5); ***$p < 0.001$, compared to the sham group; ###$p < 0.001$, compared to the BLM group. **(C)** The content of hydroxyproline in the lung tissues from different groups was determined by a commercial measurement kit. **(D)** After incubation with TGF-β1 and/or WBT for 48 h, qPCR and Western blot analysis were performed. The relative levels of collagen I in TC-1 cells were calculated and normalized to GAPDH. Data are from three independent experiments. *$p < 0.05$, **$p < 0.01$, and ***$p < 0.001$, compared to the sham group; #$p < 0.05$, ##$p < 0.05$, and ###$p < 0.001$, compared to the BLM or TGF-β1 group. BLM, bleomycin; WBT, Wenfei Buqi Tongluo formula; PFD, pirfenidone (TGF-β1, 10 ng/ml).

the network pharmacology. Furthermore, on the basis of the BLM-induced PF mouse model, the effect of WBT against PF was confirmed by micro-CT imaging and histopathological staining. Importantly, the effects of WBT on the TGF-β1 signaling pathway, EMT inhibition, and ECM degradation were investigated to verify the network pharmacology-based mechanism prediction. Overall, this study was the first to demonstrate that the WBT formula inhibited the TGF-β/ Smad3 pathway to reduce EMT and promote ECM degradation against PF.

On the basis of the theories of TCM with tonifying *Qi*, activating blood circulation, dredging collaterals, and clearing heat, the WBT formula was formed and used for the clinical applications of lung-related diseases. Among this formula, *Qi*-tonifying (Huang qi), blood-activating (Dan shen, Dang gui, Chuan xiong, and Di long), and heat-clearing (Huang qin) Chinese medicines are usually used in clinical practice for the treatment of PF, which is consistent with a previous report (Zhang et al., 2018). The anti-PF effect of Huang qi and Dang gui has been confirmed by a systematic review and meta-analysis for randomized controlled trials of IPF (Zhang Y. et al., 2020). In this study, we found that the main chemical components of WBT formula were present in four medicinal herbs: Huang qin, Huang qi, Hu zhang, and Kuan donghua. After UHPLC/Q-TOF-MS analysis and screening by the PubChem database, 36 potential compounds that have been reported as treating PF were obtained, including baicalein, baicalin, scutellarein, scutellarin, salvianolic acid B, polydatin, and chlorogenic acid. As reported previously, baicalein attenuates fibroblast differentiation and collagen production in fibroblasts and rat PF models, which may be mediated by regulating the connective tissue growth factor, miR-21, or the TGF-β/Smad signaling pathway (MacLusky et al., 1986; Gao et al., 2013; Sun et al., 2020). Baicalin ameliorates BLM-induced PF by regulating the PI3K/Akt and TGF-β signaling pathways (Huang et al., 2016; Zhao et al., 2020). The *in vitro* and *in vivo* evidence demonstrates that scutellarein and scutellarin can inhibit PF progression through regulation of the TGF-β/Smad, PI3K/Akt, Bax/Bcl2, or NF-κB/NLRP3

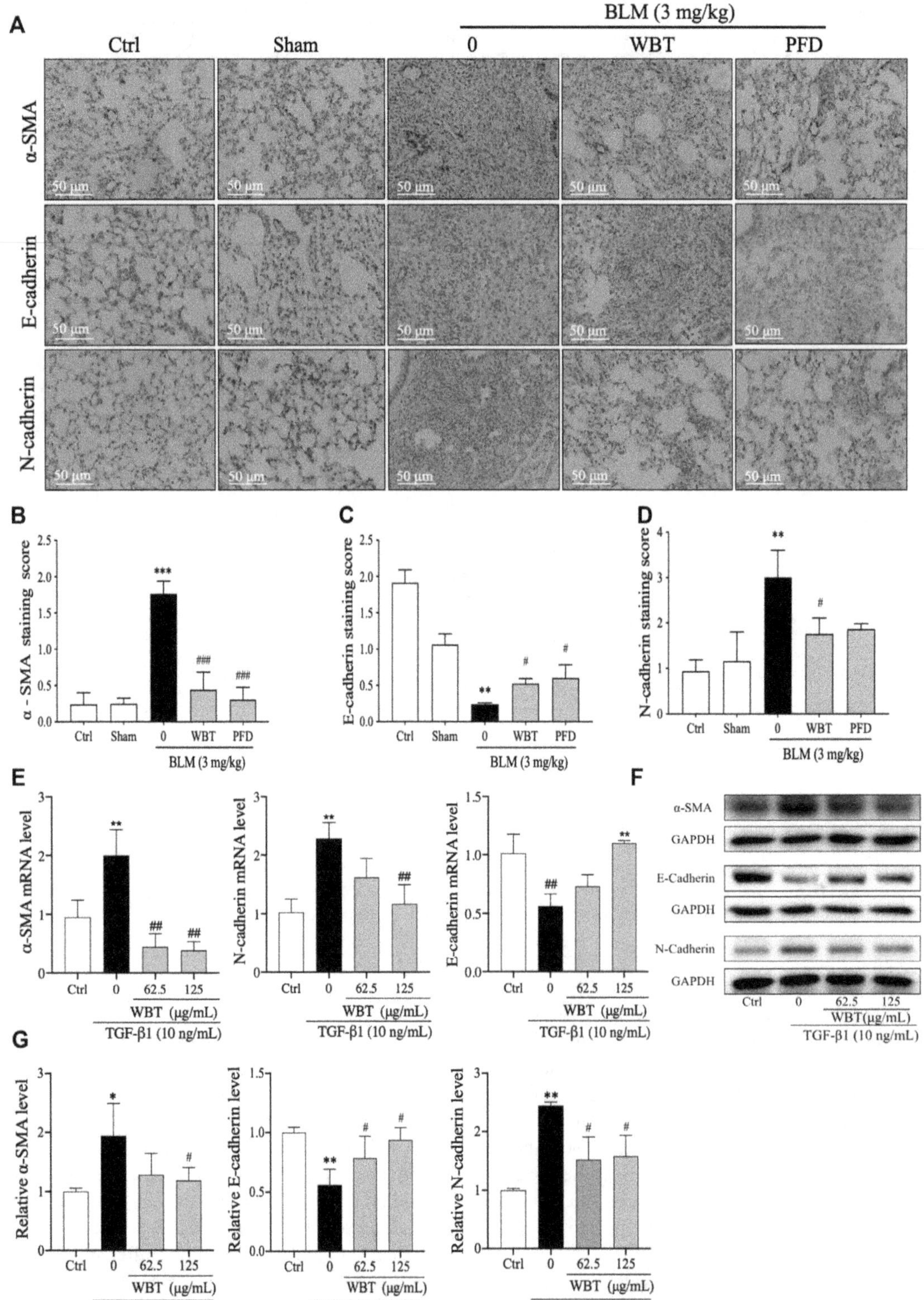

FIGURE 8 | WBT formula inhibited epithelial–mesenchymal transition induced by BLM in the mouse model and TGF-β1 in the TC-1 cell model. **(A)** The levels of α-SMA, E-cadherin, and N-cadherin in the lung tissues from control (Ctrl), sham, BLM, and BLM + WBT/PFD groups were determined by immunohistochemical assay. Scale bar = 50 μm. **(B,D)** The levels of α-SMA, E-cadherin, and N-cadherin from **(A)** were quantified (n = 5). **(E)** After incubation with TGF-β1 and/or WBT for 48 h, qPCR analysis was performed and the relative mRNA levels of α-SMA, E-cadherin, and N-cadherin in TC-1 cells were calculated and normalized to GAPDH. **(F,G)** The protein levels of α-SMA, E-cadherin, and N-cadherin in TC-1 cells treated with TGF-β1 and/or WBT for 48 h were determined by Western blot analysis. GAPDH was used as the loading control. Data are from three independent experiments. *$p < 0.05$, **$p < 0.01$, and ***$p < 0.001$, compared to the sham group; #$p < 0.05$, ##$p < 0.05$, and ###$p < 0.001$, compared to the BLM or TGF-β1 group. BLM, bleomycin; WBT, Wenfei Buqi Tongluo formula; PFD, pirfenidone (TGF-β1, 10 ng/ml).

pathways (Miao et al., 2020; Peng et al., 2020). Moreover, four compounds, namely, baicalein, 7-O-β-D-glucuronide, viscidulin I, and viscidulin III, were screened out as the top key compounds by topological property (**Supplementary Figure S3**) from the network pharmacology, which are from Huang qin (**Supplementary Table S1**). However, except for baicalein, the effect of other three compounds in anti-PF needs to be further verified by experimentation. Overall, the chemical components of Huang qin may have a potential function in treating PF. In addition, salvianolic acid B from Dan shen, polydatin from Hu zhang, and chlorogenic acid from Zi wan or Kuan donghua were reported to prevent and treat PF by multiple mechanisms, including anti-inflammation, endoplasmic reticulum stress inhibition, and TGF-β/Smad blockade (Hogan and Lee, 1987; Liu et al., 2016; Wang et al., 2017; Jiang et al., 2020). The above findings support the claims that these compounds, identified by UHPLC/Q-TOF-MS analysis, may be active components of WBT for treating PF.

The WBT formula had an obviously inhibitory effect on PF in the cell models (Ding et al., 2021), but the molecular mechanism of WBT remains unclear. According to the results of the PPI network, the potential targets of WBT against PF included ALB, VEGFA, STAT3, MAPK1, MMPs, TGFB2 and its receptors, and FGF2 and its receptors, which participate in many progressions of PF, such as ECM deposition, EMT, and myofibroblast differentiation. Critically, we also found that TGFB2 and its receptors (TGFBR1 and TGFBR2) were potential targets of 31 components identified from WBT. In our study, we evaluated the inhibitory effect of WBT against PF in the BLM-induced mouse model using micro-CT imaging and histopathological analysis and further assess the key roles of TGF-β signaling pathways to explain the molecular mechanism of WBT against PF. The images of micro-CT, H&E, and Masson's trichrome stainings have proved that WBT had significant inhibition for the lung fibrotic injury after BLM induction. Compared with the BLM-induced model group, the levels of TGF-β and p-Smad3 were significantly inhibited by WBT, which supported the predicted mechanism of WBT from the network pharmacology. For excessive ECM deposition, *in vivo* and *in vitro*, WBT could promote collagen degradation and decrease the content of lung HYP and the expression of collagen I, which could block the progress of PF. The role of WBT on ECM accumulation might be related to the activation of matrix metalloproteinases (MMPs), including collagenases (MMP1 and MMP8), gelatinases (MMP2 and MMP9), and stromelysins (MMP3 and MMP7) (Mahalanobish et al., 2020); however, the specific effect and mechanisms of MMPs need to be further investigated for supporting the prediction of the network pharmacology. Furthermore, some of the chemical components of WBT, such as amygdalin, scutellarin, and salvianolic acid B, have been reported to inhibit the EMT by regulating several markers, including α-SMA, E-cadherin, and N-cadherin (Liu et al., 2016; Wang et al., 2019; Peng et al., 2020). In addition, other signaling pathways, such as FGF, EGFR, VEGFA, and MAPK, play potential roles in the pathogenesis of PF (Iyer et al., 2015; Venkataraman and Frieman, 2017; Koo et al., 2018; Guo et al., 2021), which have been enriched as potential targets of WBT and are involved in cytokine production, cell proliferation, adhesion and migration, ECM degradation, and MMP activation. However, the regulatory effects of WBT on these pathways in anti-PF treatment should be further investigated. More importantly, the direct interaction of those potential compounds from WBT with TGF-β and other targets also needs to be detected in the future.

CONCLUSION

In summary, we first time identified 36 chemical compounds of WBT and predicted TGF-β signaling pathway and ECM degradation as potential mechanisms of WBT against PF by the network pharmacology. Furthermore, BLM-induced mouse model and TGF-β1–induced cell model were used to verify the prediction of the network pharmacology and found that WBT treatment can inhibit the levels of TGF-β and Smad3 phosphorylation and subsequently alleviate EMT and ECM accumulation *in vivo* and *in vitro*. These findings indicate that WBT could block the progressive process of PF by inhibiting EMT and prompting EMC degradation *via* TGF-β/Smad3 pathway. This study, for the first time, can provide new insights into the molecular mechanism of WBT for the prevention and treatment of PF in the clinical application.

AUTHOR CONTRIBUTIONS

LD, YL, SS, HQ, JW, ZW, and JZ performed the experiments. YY performed the network pharmacology analysis. WZ assisted with micro-CT imaging. LD, YL, and YY analyzed data and drafted the manuscript. LZ and DZ supervised the experiments and the manuscript. XL and ZW designed and revised the manuscript. All authors read and approved the final version of the manuscript.

FUNDING

This work was supported by the National Natural Science Foundation of China (81804013), the Key Research and Development Program of Jilin Province (20200404057YY), and the Special Project for Emergency of the Ministry of Science and Technology (2020YFC0845000).

ACKNOWLEDGMENTS

We thank the kind support from Dr. Wenzhi Yang (State Key Laboratory of Component-based Chinese Medicine, Tianjin Key Laboratory of TCM Chemistry and Analysis, Tianjin University of Traditional Chinese Medicine, Tianjin, China) for detecting active components. We thank the kind support from Xing Huang (PerkinElmer Inc., Waltham, MA) for micro-CT image interpretation. We thank LetPub (www.letpub.com) for its linguistic assistance during the preparation of this manuscript.

REFERENCES

Berisio, R., Granata, V., Vitagliano, L., and Zagari, A. (2004). Imino Acids and Collagen Triple helix Stability: Characterization of Collagen-like Polypeptides Containing Hyp-Hyp-Gly Sequence Repeats. *J. Am. Chem. Soc.* 126, 11402–11403. doi:10.1021/ja047069h

Ding, L., Song, S. Y., Li, Y. X., Li, X. Y., and Wang, Z. Y. (2021). Effect of Wenfei Buqi Tongluo Prescription on the Cell Proliferation, Morphology, and Epithelial-Mesenchymal Transition in the TGF-β1-Induced A549 Cells. *Chin. J. Gerontol.* 41, 1686–1690. doi:10.3969/j.issn.1005-9202.2021.08.037

Flaherty, K. R., Wells, A. U., Cottin, V., Devaraj, A., Walsh, S. L. F., Inoue, Y., et al. (2019). Nintedanib in Progressive Fibrosing Interstitial Lung Diseases. *N. Engl. J. Med.* 381, 1718–1727. doi:10.1056/NEJMoa1908681

Frangogiannis, N. (2020). Transforming Growth Factor-β in Tissue Fibrosis. *J. Exp. Med.* 217, e20190103. doi:10.1084/jem.20190103

Gao, Y., Lu, J., Zhang, Y., Chen, Y., Gu, Z., and Jiang, X. (2013). Baicalein Attenuates Bleomycin-Induced Pulmonary Fibrosis in Rats through Inhibition of miR-21. *Pulm. Pharmacol. Ther.* 26, 649–654. doi:10.1016/j.pupt.2013.03.006

Glass, D. S., Grossfeld, D., Renna, H. A., Agarwala, P., Spiegler, P., Kasselman, L. J., et al. (2020). Idiopathic Pulmonary Fibrosis: Molecular Mechanisms and Potential Treatment Approaches. *Respir. Investig.* 58, 320–335. doi:10.1016/j.resinv.2020.04.002

Guo, H., Jian, Z., Liu, H., Cui, H., Deng, H., Fang, J., et al. (2021). TGF-β1-induced EMT Activation via Both Smad-dependent and MAPK Signaling Pathways in Cu-Induced Pulmonary Fibrosis. *Toxicol. Appl. Pharmacol.* 418, 115500. doi:10.1016/j.taap.2021.115500

Hogan, Y., and Lee, C. M. (1987). Interaction of Trace Metal Contaminants on Hematological Responses: Influence of Infection with Trypanosoma Lewisi. *J. Natl. Med. Assoc.* 79, 521–531.

Huang, X., He, Y., Chen, Y., Wu, P., Gui, D., Cai, H., et al. (2016). Baicalin Attenuates Bleomycin-Induced Pulmonary Fibrosis via Adenosine A2a Receptor Related TGF-β1-Induced ERK1/2 Signaling Pathway. *BMC Pulm. Med.* 16, 132. doi:10.1186/s12890-016-0294-1

Huang, H., Zhang, G., Zhou, Y., Lin, C., Chen, S., Lin, Y., et al. (2018a). Reverse Screening Methods to Search for the Protein Targets of Chemopreventive Compounds. *Front. Chem.* 6, 138. doi:10.3389/fchem.2018.00138

Huang, Q., Lan, T., Lu, J., Zhang, H., Zhang, D., Lou, T., et al. (2018b). DiDang Tang Inhibits Endoplasmic Reticulum Stress-Mediated Apoptosis Induced by Oxygen Glucose Deprivation and Intracerebral Hemorrhage through Blockade of the GRP78-IRE1/PERK Pathways. *Front. Pharmacol.* 9, 1423. doi:10.3389/fphar.2018.01423

Hutchinson, J., Fogarty, A., Hubbard, R., and Mckeever, T. (2015). Global Incidence and Mortality of Idiopathic Pulmonary Fibrosis: a Systematic Review. *Eur. Respir. J.* 46, 795–806. doi:10.1183/09031936.00185114

Iyer, A. K., Ramesh, V., Castro, C. A., Kaushik, V., Kulkarni, Y. M., Wright, C. A., et al. (2015). Nitric Oxide Mediates Bleomycin-Induced Angiogenesis and Pulmonary Fibrosis via Regulation of VEGF. *J. Cel. Biochem.* 116, 2484–2493. doi:10.1002/jcb.25192

Jiang, L., Wang, J., Ju, J., and Dai, J. (2020). Salvianolic Acid B and Sodium Tanshinone II A Sulfonate Prevent Pulmonary Fibrosis through Anti-Inflammatory and Anti-fibrotic Process. *Eur. J. Pharmacol.* 883, 173352. doi:10.1016/j.ejphar.2020.173352

Jiang, L., Yin, X., Chen, Y. H., Chen, Y., Jiang, W., Zheng, H., et al. (2021). Proteomic Analysis Reveals Ginsenoside Rb1 Attenuates Myocardial Ischemia/Reperfusion Injury through Inhibiting ROS Production from Mitochondrial Complex I. *Theranostics* 11, 1703–1720. doi:10.7150/thno.43895

Katoh, T., Andoh, T., Mikawa, K., Tanizawa, M., Tanigawa, M., Suzuki, R., et al. (1998). Computed Tomographic Findings in Non-Specific Interstitial Pneumonia/Fibrosis. *Respirology* 3, 69–75. doi:10.1111/j.1440-1843.1998.tb00099.x

King, T. E., Jr., Pardo, A., and Selman, M. (2011). Idiopathic Pulmonary Fibrosis. *Lancet* 378, 1949–1961. doi:10.1016/S0140-6736(11)60052-4

King, T. E., Jr., Bradford, W. Z., Castro-Bernardini, S., Fagan, E. A., Glaspole, I., Glassberg, M. K., et al. (2014). A Phase 3 Trial of Pirfenidone in Patients with Idiopathic Pulmonary Fibrosis. *N. Engl. J. Med.* 370, 2083–2092. doi:10.1056/NEJMoa1402582

Kishi, M., Aono, Y., Sato, S., Koyama, K., Azuma, M., Abe, S., et al. (2018). Blockade of Platelet-Derived Growth Factor Receptor-β, Not Receptor-α Ameliorates Bleomycin-Induced Pulmonary Fibrosis in Mice. *PLoS One* 13, e0209786. doi:10.1371/journal.pone.0209786

Kolahian, S., Fernandez, I. E., Eickelberg, O., and Hartl, D. (2016). Immune Mechanisms in Pulmonary Fibrosis. *Am. J. Respir. Cel Mol Biol* 55, 309–322. doi:10.1165/rcmb.2016-0121TR

Koo, H. Y., El-Baz, L. M., House, S., Cilvik, S. N., Dorry, S. J., Shoukry, N. M., et al. (2018). Fibroblast Growth Factor 2 decreases Bleomycin-Induced Pulmonary Fibrosis and Inhibits Fibroblast Collagen Production and Myofibroblast differentiation. *J. Pathol.* 246, 54–66. doi:10.1002/path.5106

Lederer, D. J., and Martinez, F. J. (2018). Idiopathic Pulmonary Fibrosis. *N. Engl. J. Med.* 378, 1811–1823. doi:10.1056/NEJMra1705751

Li, S., and Zhang, B. (2013). Traditional Chinese Medicine Network Pharmacology: Theory, Methodology and Application. *Chin. J. Nat. Med.* 11, 110–120. doi:10.1016/S1875-5364(13)60037-0

Li, X., Gong, X. Y., Yang, G., Wang, S., Sui, X. D., and Yue, D. H. (2012). Research on the Effect of Xiankekeli on Pathomorphological Changes Influenced in Pulmonary Fibrosis Rats. *Lishizhen Med. Mater. Med. Res.* 23, 2449–2451. doi:10.3969/j.issn.1008-0805.2012.10.028

Li, S. (2021). Network Pharmacology Evaluation Method Guidance-Draft. *World J. Tradit. Chin. Med.* 7, 165–166+146154. doi:10.4103/wjtcm.wjtcm_11_21

Liu, Q., Chu, H., Ma, Y., Wu, T., Qian, F., Ren, X., et al. (2016). Salvianolic Acid B Attenuates Experimental Pulmonary Fibrosis through Inhibition of the TGF-β Signaling Pathway. *Sci. Rep.* 6, 27610. doi:10.1038/srep27610

Long, K. R., Newland, B., Florio, M., Kalebic, N., Langen, B., Kolterer, A., et al. (2018). Extracellular Matrix Components HAPLN1, Lumican, and Collagen I Cause Hyaluronic Acid-Dependent Folding of the Developing Human Neocortex. *Neuron* 99, 702–719.e6. doi:10.1016/j.neuron.2018.07.013

Lv, X. X., Wang, X. X., Li, K., Wang, Z. Y., Li, Z., Lv, Q., et al. (2013). Rupatadine Protects against Pulmonary Fibrosis by Attenuating PAF-Mediated Senescence in Rodents. *PLoS One* 8, e68631. doi:10.1371/journal.pone.0068631

MacLusky, N. J., Krey, L. C., Parsons, B., Merriam, G. R., Loriaux, D. L., Pfeiffer, D. G., et al. (1986). Are Catechol Oestrogens Obligatory Mediators of Oestrogen Action in the Central Nervous System? II. Potencies of Natural and Synthetic Oestrogens for Induction of Gonadotrophin Release and Female Sexual Behaviour in the Rat. *J. Endocrinol.* 110, 499–505. doi:10.1677/joe.0.1100499

Mahalanobish, S., Saha, S., Dutta, S., and Sil, P. C. (2020). Matrix Metalloproteinase: An Upcoming Therapeutic Approach for Idiopathic Pulmonary Fibrosis. *Pharmacol. Res.* 152, 104591. doi:10.1016/j.phrs.2019.104591

Miao, K., Pan, T., Mou, Y., Zhang, L., Xiong, W., Xu, Y., et al. (2020). Scutellarein Inhibits BLM-Mediated Pulmonary Fibrosis by Affecting Fibroblast differentiation, Proliferation, and Apoptosis. *Ther. Adv. Chronic Dis.* 11, 2040622320940185. doi:10.1177/2040622320940185

Mu, C., Sheng, Y., Wang, Q., Amin, A., Li, X., and Xie, Y. (2021). Potential Compound from Herbal Food of Rhizoma Polygonati for Treatment of COVID-19 Analyzed by Network Pharmacology: Viral and Cancer Signaling Mechanisms. *J. Funct. Foods* 77, 104149. doi:10.1016/j.jff.2020.104149

Nalysnyk, L., Cid-Ruzafa, J., Rotella, P., and Esser, D. (2012). Incidence and Prevalence of Idiopathic Pulmonary Fibrosis: Review of the Literature. *Eur. Respir. Rev.* 21, 355–361. doi:10.1183/09059180.00002512

Nieto, M. A., Huang, R. Y., Jackson, R. A., and Thiery, J. P. (2016). Emt: 2016. *Cell* 166, 21–45. doi:10.1016/j.cell.2016.06.028

Ohyashiki, T., Kanaoka, Y., and Sekine, T. (1976). Studies on Calcium Ion-Induced Conformation Changes in the Actin-Tropomyosin-Troponin System by Fluorimetry. III. Changes in the Conformation of Tropomyosin Associated with Functional States. *Biochim. Biophys. Acta* 420, 27–36. doi:10.1016/0005-2795(76) 90341-x

Pang, L. J., Liu, J. P., and Lv, X. D. (2019). Comparative Effectiveness of 3 Traditional Chinese Medicine Treatment Methods for Idiopathic Pulmonary Fibrosis: A Systematic Review and Network Meta-Analysis Protocol. *Medicine (Baltimore)* 98, e16325. doi:10.1097/MD.0000000000016325

Pedroza, M., Le, T. T., Lewis, K., Karmouty-Quintana, H., To, S., George, A. T., et al. (2016). STAT-3 Contributes to Pulmonary Fibrosis through Epithelial Injury and Fibroblast-Myofibroblast Differentiation. *FASEB J.* 30, 129–140. doi:10.1096/fj.15-273953

Peng, L., Wen, L., Shi, Q. F., Gao, F., Huang, B., Meng, J., et al. (2020). Scutellarin Ameliorates Pulmonary Fibrosis through Inhibiting NF-κB/NLRP3-Mediated Epithelial-Mesenchymal Transition and Inflammation. *Cel. Death Dis.* 11, 978. doi:10.1038/s41419-020-03178-2

Philp, C. J., Siebeke, I., Clements, D., Miller, S., Habgood, A., John, A. E., et al. (2018). Extracellular Matrix Cross-Linking Enhances Fibroblast Growth and Protects against Matrix Proteolysis in Lung Fibrosis. *Am. J. Respir. Cel. Mol. Biol.* 58, 594–603. doi:10.1165/rcmb.2016-0379OC

Ruscitti, F., Ravanetti, F., Essers, J., Ridwan, Y., Belenkov, S., Vos, W., et al. (2017). Longitudinal Assessment of Bleomycin-Induced Lung Fibrosis by Micro-CT Correlates with Histological Evaluation in Mice. *Multidiscip. Respir. Med.* 12, 8. doi:10.1186/s40248-017-0089-0

Salton, F., Volpe, M. C., and Confalonieri, M. (2019). Epithelial‑Mesenchymal Transition in the Pathogenesis of Idiopathic Pulmonary Fibrosis. *Medicina (Kaunas)* 55, 83. doi:10.3390/medicina55040083

Shahbaz, M., Kamran, S. H., and Anwar, R. (2021). Amelioration of Bleomycin and Methotrexate-Induced Pulmonary Toxicity by Serratiopeptidase and Fisetin. *Nutr. Cancer* 73 (11-12), 2774–2784. doi:10.1080/01635581.2020.1860242

Shawky, E. (2019). Prediction of Potential Cancer-Related Molecular Targets of North African Plants Constituents Using Network Pharmacology-Based Analysis. *J. Ethnopharmacol.* 238, 111826. doi:10.1016/j.jep.2019.111826

Sun, X., Cui, X., Chen, X., and Jiang, X. (2020). Baicalein Alleviated TGF β1-induced Type I Collagen Production in Lung Fibroblasts via downregulation of Connective Tissue Growth Factor. *Biomed. Pharmacother.* 131, 110744. doi:10.1016/ j.biopha.2020.110744

Todd, N. W., Luzina, I. G., and Atamas, S. P. (2012). Molecular and Cellular Mechanisms of Pulmonary Fibrosis. *Fibrogenesis Tissue Repair* 5, 11. doi:10.1186/1755-1536-5-11

Venkataraman, T., and Frieman, M. B. (2017). The Role of Epidermal Growth Factor Receptor (EGFR) Signaling in SARS Coronavirus-Induced Pulmonary Fibrosis. *Antivir. Res.* 143, 142–150. doi:10.1016/j.antiviral.2017.03.022

Walton, K. L., Johnson, K. E., and Harrison, C. A. (2017). Targeting TGF-β Mediated SMAD Signaling for the Prevention of Fibrosis. *Front. Pharmacol.* 8, 461. doi:10.3389/fphar.2017.00461

Wang, Y. C., Dong, J., Nie, J., Zhu, J. X., Wang, H., Chen, Q., et al. (2017). Amelioration of Bleomycin-Induced Pulmonary Fibrosis by Chlorogenic Acid through Endoplasmic Reticulum Stress Inhibition. *Apoptosis* 22, 1147–1156. doi:10.1007/ s10495-017-1393-z

Wang, Z., Fang, K., Wang, G., Guan, X., Pang, Z., Guo, Y., et al. (2019). Protective Effect of Amygdalin on Epithelial-Mesenchymal Transformation in Experimental Chronic Obstructive Pulmonary disease Mice. *Phytother Res.* 33, 808–817. doi:10.1002/ ptr.6274

Yang, G., Gong, X. Y., Li, X., Su, X., and Wang, S. (2014). Effect of Xianke Granules on Expression Levels of CTGF, ILK in Pulmonary Fibrosis Rats. *Chin. J. Exp. Tradit. Med. Formulae* 20, 141–145. doi:10.13422/j.cnki.syfjx.2014140141

Yang, K., Zeng, L., Ge, A., Shi, Y., Zhu, X., Liu, W., et al. (2020). The Effect of Hedysarum Multijugum Maxim.-Chuanxiong Rhizoma Compound on Ischemic Stroke: A Research Based on Network and Experimental Pharmacology. *Oxid. Med. Cel Longev.* 2020, 6072380. doi:10.1155/2020/6072380

Yang, Y., Ding, L., Bao, T., Li, Y., Ma, J., Li, Q., et al. (2021). Network Pharmacology and Experimental Assessment to Explore the Pharmacological Mechanism of Qimai Feiluoping Decoction against Pulmonary Fibrosis. *Front. Pharmacol.* 12. doi:10.3389/fphar.2021.770197

Zeng, H., Gao, H., Zhang, M., Wang, J., Gu, Y., Wang, Y., et al. (2021). Atractylon Treatment Attenuates Pulmonary Fibrosis via Regulation of the mmu_circ_0000981/miR-211-5p/TGFBR2 Axis in an Ovalbumin-Induced Asthma Mouse Model. *Inflammation* 44, 1856–1864. doi:10.1007/s10753-021-01463-6

Zhang, S., Wu, H., Liu, J., Gu, H., Li, X., and Zhang, T. (2018). Medication Regularity of Pulmonary Fibrosis Treatment by Contemporary Traditional Chinese Medicine Experts Based on data Mining. *J. Thorac. Dis.* 10, 1775–1787. doi:10.21037/jtd.2018.03.11

Zhang, Y., Gu, L., Xia, Q., Tian, L., Qi, J., and Cao, M. (2020a). Radix Astragali and Radix Angelicae Sinensis in the Treatment of Idiopathic Pulmonary Fibrosis: A Systematic Review and Meta-Analysis. *Front. Pharmacol.* 11, 415. doi:10.3389/fphar.2020.00415

Zhang, Z., Zhai, L., Lu, J., Sun, S., Wang, D., Zhao, D., et al. (2020b). Shen-Hong-Tong-Luo Formula Attenuates Macrophage Inflammation and Lipid Accumulation through the Activation of the PPAR-γ/LXR-α/ABCA1 Pathway. *Oxid. Med. Cel. Longev.* 2020, 3426925. doi:10.1155/2020/3426925

Zhang, Y., Lu, P., Qin, H., Zhang, Y., Sun, X., Song, X., et al. (2021). Traditional Chinese Medicine Combined with Pulmonary drug delivery System and Idiopathic Pulmonary Fibrosis: Rationale and Therapeutic Potential. *Biomed. Pharmacother.* 133, 111072. doi:10.1016/j.biopha.2020.111072

Zhao, H., Li, C., Li, L., Liu, J., Gao, Y., Mu, K., et al. (2020). Baicalin Alleviates Bleomycininduced Pulmonary Fibrosis and Fibroblast Proliferation in Rats via the PI3K/AKT Signaling Pathway. *Mol. Med. Rep.* 21, 2321–2334. doi:10.3892/ mmr.2020.11046

Zuo, T., Qian, Y., Zhang, C., Wei, Y., Wang, X., Wang, H., et al. (2019). Data-Dependent Acquisition and Database-Driven Efficient Peak Annotation for the Comprehensive Profiling and Characterization of the Multicomponents from Compound Xueshuantong Capsule by UHPLC/IM-QTOF-MS. *Molecules* 24, 3431. doi:10.3390/molecules24193431

14

Molecular Mechanism of *Gelsemium elegans* (Gardner and Champ.) Benth. Against Neuropathic Pain Based on Network Pharmacology and Experimental Evidence

Wancai Que[1,2†], Zhaoyang Wu[1,2†], Maohua Chen[1†], Binqing Zhang[2], Chuihuai You[3], Hailing Lin[1], Zhichang Zhao[1,2], Maobai Liu[1,2], Hongqiang Qiu[1,2] and Yu Cheng[1,2,4]**

[1]Department of Pharmacy, Fujian Medical University Union Hospital, Fuzhou, China, [2]College of Pharmacy, Fujian Medical University, Fuzhou, China, [3]College of Agriculture, Fujian Agriculture and Forestry University, Fuzhou, China, [4]Department of Pharmacy, Shengjing Hospital of China Medical University, Shenyang, China

***Correspondence:**
Hongqiang Qiu
hongqiangqiu@fjmu.edu.cn
Yu Cheng
chengyu@fjmu.edu.cn

[†]These authors have contributed equally to this work

Gelsemium elegans (Gardner and Champ.) Benth. (Gelsemiaceae) (GEB) is a toxic plant indigenous to Southeast Asia especially China, and has long been used as Chinese folk medicine for the treatment of various types of pain, including neuropathic pain (NPP). Nevertheless, limited data are available on the understanding of the interactions between ingredients-targets-pathways. The present study integrated network pharmacology and experimental evidence to decipher molecular mechanisms of GEB against NPP. The candidate ingredients of GEB were collected from the published literature and online databases. Potentially active targets of GEB were predicted using the SwissTargetPrediction database. NPP-associated targets were retrieved from GeneCards, Therapeutic Target database, and DrugBank. Then the protein-protein interaction network was constructed. The DAVID database was applied to Gene Ontology and Kyoto Encyclopedia of Genes and Genome pathway enrichment analysis. Molecular docking was employed to validate the interaction between ingredients and targets. Subsequently, a 50 ns molecular dynamics simulation was performed to analyze the conformational stability of the protein-ligand complex. Furthermore, the potential anti-NPP mechanisms of GEB were evaluated in the rat chronic constriction injury model. A total of 47 alkaloids and 52 core targets were successfully identified for GEB in the treatment of NPP. Functional enrichment analysis showed that GEB was mainly involved in phosphorylation reactions and nitric oxide synthesis processes. It also participated in 73 pathways in the pathogenesis of NPP, including the neuroactive ligand-receptor interaction signaling pathway, calcium signaling pathway, and MAPK signaling pathway. Interestingly, 11-Hydroxyrankinidin well matched the active pockets of crucial targets, such as EGFR, JAK1, and AKT1. The 11-hydroxyrankinidin-EGFR complex was stable throughout the entire molecular dynamics simulation. Besides, the expression of EGFR and JAK1 could be regulated by koumine to achieve the anti-NPP action. These findings revealed the complex network relationship of GEB in the "multi-ingredient, multi-target, multi-pathway" mode, and explained the synergistic regulatory effect of each complex ingredient of GEB based on the holistic view of traditional Chinese medicine. The present study would provide a scientific approach and strategy for further studies of GEB in the treatment of NPP in the future.

Keywords: ***Gelsemium elegans*** **(Gardner and Champ.) Benth, neuropathic pain, network pharmacology, molecular docking, molecular dynamics simulation**

INTRODUCTION

Chronic pain condition is a major health issue that comprises five of the 11 top-ranking conditions lived with disability and is responsible for economic burden worldwide (Vos et al., 2012; Andrew et al., 2014). The prevalence of neuropathic pain (NPP) as a feature of chronic pain was estimated to range from 1 to 17.9% (van Hecke et al., 2014). NPP is defined as an injury or disease of the somatosensory system involving complex pathogenesis according to the 2011 International Association for the Study of Pain (Jensen et al., 2011). Overall, the current pharmacological interventions in NPP primarily consist of antidepressants or antiepileptics as the first-line treatments (Lunn et al., 2014; Moore and Gaines, 2019), lidocaine plasters, capsaicin high concentration patches, and tramadol as the second-line treatments (van Nooten et al., 2017; Kim et al., 2018), and strong opioids and botulinum toxin A as the third-line treatments (Sommer et al., 2020). Unfortunately, patients with NPP conventional have an inadequate response with only 40–60% of patients achieving partial relief to the current pharmacological therapy and suffering from side effects include sedation, anticholinergic effects, nausea, and orthostatic hypotension (Dworkin et al., 2007; Cavalli et al., 2019). Therefore, there is a necessity to explore more effective analgesics with novel mechanisms and low side effects for the treatment of NPP.

Traditional Chinese medicine (TCM) is an abundant resource for drug development and provides innovative insight into therapeutic approaches. *Gelsemium elegans* (Gardner and Champ.) Benth. (Gelsemiaceae) (GEB) is a toxic plant indigenous to Southeast Asia especially China, which has long been used as Chinese folk medicine for the treatment of various types of pain, such as neuralgia, sciatica, rheumatoid arthritis, and acute pain (Rujjanawate et al., 2003; Lin et al., 2021). Phytochemical studies have revealed that the main active ingredients of GEB are alkaloids, especially the indole alkaloids, such as koumine, gelsemine, gelsenicine, and gelsevirine (Jin et al., 2014). These alkaloids are distributed throughout the whole plant, especially rich in the roots. GEB and its active alkaloids have been studied increasingly and exert promising pharmacological effects in NPP. It was reported that a crude alkaloidal extract solution from GEB could significantly increase the pain thresholds of mice in both hot plate and writhing tests at the dose of 0.5, 1.0, and 2.0 mg/kg (Rujjanawate et al., 2003). As an important active ingredient, previous studies indicated that koumine exhibited a significant analgesic effect *in vitro* and in several animal models of NPP. These studies suggested that koumine alleviated NPP may through a wide variety of mechanisms, including enhancing 3α-hydroxysteroid oxidoreductase mRNA expression and bioactivity (Qiu et al., 2015) in the spinal cord, upregulating allopregnanolone (Xu et al., 2012), and inhibiting astrocyte activation as well as M1 polarization while sparing the anti-inflammatory responses to NPP (Jin et al., 2018a; Jin et al., 2018b). Other active ingredients, gelsemine, gelsenicine, and gelsevirine may produce antinociception by activating the spinal α3 glycine/ allopregnanolone pathway (Zhang and Wang, 2015). However, all the existing studies focused on limited ingredients, targets, and pathways, and lacked the integral thoughts and exploration on TCM with multiple ingredients and targets. Hence, the interactions between ingredients-targets-pathways and other underlying molecular mechanisms of GEB against NPP remain unclear.

Network pharmacology is mostly used to screen the active ingredients, predict the corresponding target, and explore the comprehensive molecular mechanisms of TCM. The key ideas of network pharmacology are based on the theory of system biology and multi-direction pharmacology, which are consistent with the holistic philosophy of TCM (Li and Zhang, 2013). Molecular docking simulation is a computational method for exploring the ligand conformations adopted within the binding sites of receptors in the intermolecular recognition process (Ferreira et al., 2015). Different from traditional pharmacological research methods of TCM, network pharmacology-based analysis combined with molecular docking technology could provide a new perspective for the study of the molecular mechanism of TCM. In the present study, we proposed an "ingredient-target-pathway" network to reveal the potential material basis and compatibility molecular mechanisms of GEB against NPP based on the network pharmacology and experimental evidence. The flowchart of our work is shown in **Figure 1**.

MATERIALS AND METHODS

Identification of Active Ingredients in GEB

The potential active ingredients in GEB were retrieved from the published literature (Jin et al., 2014) and the online public databases, including the Traditional Chinese Medicines Integrated database (TCMID) (http://www.megabionet.org/tcmid/) (Huang et al., 2018), Bioinformatics Analysis Tool for Molecular mechanism of Traditional Chinese Medicine (BATMAN-TCM) (http://bionet.ncpsb.org/batman-tcm/) (Liu et al., 2016), and Traditional Chinese Medicine

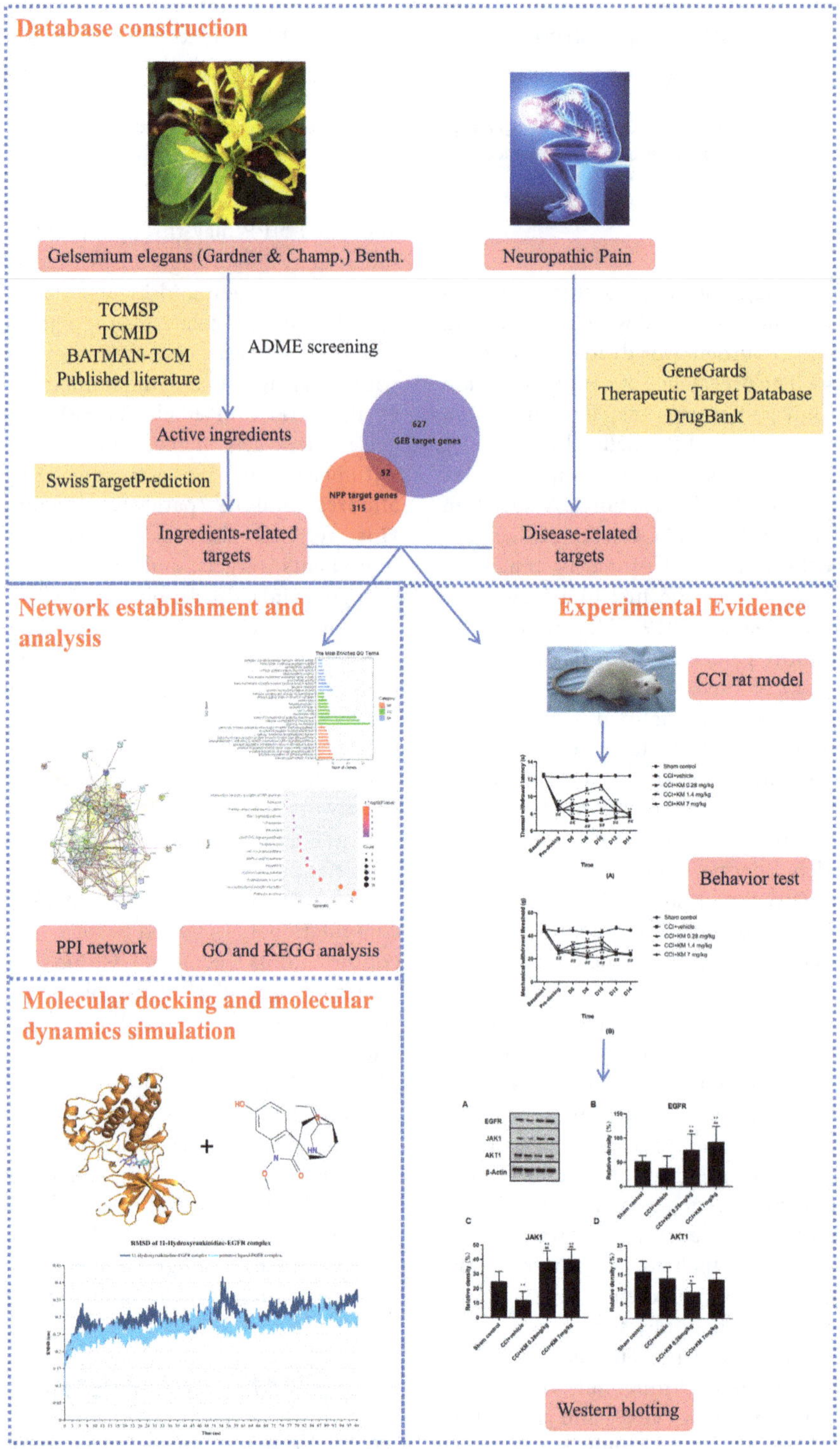

FIGURE 1 | The flowchart of network pharmacology analysis.

database@ Taiwan (http://tcm.cmu.edu.tw/zh-tw/) (Chen, 2011). Active ingredients with oral bioavailability (OB) ≥ 30% and drug-likeness (DL) ≥ two of five features (Lipinski, Ghose, Veber, Egan, and Muegge) were selected, which was recommended by SwissADME (http://www.swissadme.chwebsite) (Daina et al., 2017). The final cluster of chemical ingredients of GEB was determined after removing duplicates.

Identification of Ingredients-Related Targets

Targets of the active ingredients were predicted using SwissTargetPrediction (http://www.swisstargetprediction.ch), a popular online server that could accurately predict the targets of bioactive molecules with known ligands (Gfeller et al., 2014). 3D structural SDF formats (.sdf) of active ingredients of GEB were acquired from the PubChem database (https://pubchem.ncbi.nlm.nih.gov/) and imported into SwissTargetPrediction for identification of potential drug targets in humans. After removing duplicate targets, the targets of ingredients with SwissTargetPrediction probability ≥0.1 were chosen as potential targets, and compounds without target information were excluded.

Identification of Disease-Associated Targets

The disease-associated targets of NPP were collected from GeneCards (https://www.genecards.org/) (Safran et al., 2010), the Therapeutic Target database (https://db.idrblab.org/ttd/) (Wang et al., 2020a), and DrugBank (https://go.drugbank.com) (Wishart et al., 2018). "Neuralgias", "Neuropathic Pain", "Neurodynia", and "Nerve Pain" were used as keywords in the three databases and Homo sapiens targets with a disease relevance score ≥ of three were selected for the study.

Topology Analysis of the Protein-Protein Interaction (PPI) Network

The intersection of ingredients-related targets and disease-associated targets was visualized by overlapping with a Venn diagram. Then, a PPI network was constructed through the String database (https://stringdb.org/) to explore the core regulatory genes (Szklarczyk et al., 2019). PPI information was extracted with an interaction score of 0.4 and the species was only limited to "Homo sapiens". The topology analysis of the PPI was performed with Cytoscape 3.7.2 (http://cytoscape.org/.ver.3.7.2). NetworkAnalyzer analysis was used to screen key targets according to the degree value. The top 15 important proteins with a higher level of degrees in the interaction network were considered as the key targets for GEB in the treatment for NPP. Furthermore, the Molecular Complex Detection (MCODE) plugin was used to detect cluster modules from the complex network with the node score cutoff of 0.2, K-core of 2, and degree cutoff of 2.

Gene Ontology (GO) and Kyoto Encyclopedia Genes Genomes (KEGG) Enrichment Analysis

The GO and KEGG enrichment analysis were performed to explore the signaling pathways and bioprocesses involved in the key targets. The database for Annotation, Visualization, and Integrated Discovery (DAVID, https://david.ncifcrf.gov/.vcr.6.8) was applied to conduct the enrichment analysis (Dennis et al., 2003). The species was limited to "Homo sapiens", and the enrichment of pathway was considered significant when the modified fisher exact false discovery rate (FDR) < 0.01. The results of the KEGG pathway and enriched GO terms of biological processes (BP), cell composition (CC), and molecular function (MF) were visualized by the R software package (3.5.2).

Construction of "Ingredient-Target-Pathway" Network

The "ingredient-target-pathway" networks including the potential ingredients-targets network of GEB against NPP and targets-pathways network of GEB against NPP were constructed by Cytoscape (Shannon et al., 2003). In the network, nodes represent the final active ingredients and targets, while the connections between the nodes represent the interactions between these biological processes and signaling pathways. Three key topological parameters were used to evaluate the topological coefficients between nodes: "degree" (the number of connections between the molecular and target in the core architecture of the network), "betweenness" (the number of shortest paths of a node to the total number of paths through all nodes), and "closeness" (the inverse of the sum of the shortest paths from a node to other nodes in the network).

Ingredients-Targets Molecular Docking

Molecular docking was used to predict the interactions between core active ingredients of GEB and proteins selected from the center targets from a molecular perspective. 3D structures of active ingredients in SDF (.sdf) format were selected from the PubChem database (https://pubchem.ncbi.nlm), and the crystal structures of the target proteins were downloaded from the PDB database (https://www.rcsb.org/) with a crystal resolution of less than 2 Å. Molecular docking was performed by importing the crystal structure into the Pymol 2.4.1 Software (https://pymol.org/2/) for dehydration, hydrogenation, and ligand separation. Thereafter, Autodock Vina 1.1.2 software was used to construct a crystal structure docking grid box for each target. Then the molecules with the lowest binding energy for each active compound in the docking conformation were allowed for semi-flexible docking by comparing with the original ligands and intermolecular interactions (hydrophobicity, cation-π, anion-π, π-π stacking, hydrogen bonding, etc.). Box center coordinates and size of the box were determined for evaluating the interaction. The results were analyzed and visualized using Pymol, and the numbers of grid points in the three dimensions used in this study were 40 40 40 0.375.

Molecular Dynamics Simulation of Ligand Complex

The molecular dynamics simulation study is employed to assess the stability and interaction between the protein and ligands after docking. The simulation run was performed for 100 ns using the NVIDIA RTX 1060 GPU accelerated GROMACS 2020 software molecular dynamics package. In the preliminary stage, the Charmm36 force field was used for the protein parameters.

The CGenFF server was used for the ligand topology, and a TIP3P water model with appropriate Na^+/Cl^- ions was subsequently generated and neutralized the charge of the system. The system converged to a minimum energy level using the steepest descent method of 50,000 steps and <10.0 kJ/mol force. Then, the equilibration process was conducted with 100 ps for constant NVT (number, volume, and temperature) heating to 300 K, followed by 100 ps for constant NPT (number of particles, pressure, and temperature) with a time step of 2 fs. The bonds of atoms were restrained by recruiting the LINCS algorithm. After the processes of energy minimization and equilibration, the molecular dynamics simulation was conducted the leap-frog algorithm for 100 ns with a time step of 2 fs. The geometrical parameters of the systems, such as root mean square deviation (RMSD) and root mean square fluctuation (RMSF), were determined and compared with the primitive ligand complex.

Experimental Verification in Chronic Constriction Injury (CCI) Rat Model

Koumine (99% purity) was isolated from GEB as described by Su et al. (Su et al., 2011), and it was dissolved or diluted in sterile physiological saline (0.9% *w/v* NaCl).

Male Sprague–Dawley rats (180–200 g) were purchased from Shanghai Laboratory Animal Center, Chinese Academy of Sciences. The rats were adapted in the condition of 25 ± 2°C with a 12-h light/dark cycle (lights on at 8:00 am) and free access to standard laboratory food and water. The experiments met the requirements of guidelines for animal care and the use of Fujian Medical University. The experimental protocols were reviewed and approved by the Committee of Ethics of the Fujian Medical University (Fujian, China). Animals were assigned into different groups: the sham control group (rats underwent the surgical procedures without any manipulation related to nerve injury), the CCI model group (rats received the vehicle, 0.28, 1.4, 7.0 mg/kg of koumine). The dose used in the experimental assay was based on the published literature (Jin et al., 2018b), and no adverse effects and sedative effects were observed in the rats. The CCI rat model was performed according to the method described by Bennett et al. (Bennett and Xie, 1988).

Behavior tests consist of thermal hyperalgesia and mechanical allodynia tests. The thermal hyperalgesia test using a commercial thermal paw stimulator (PL-200, Chengdu Technology and Market Co., Ltd., Sichuan, China) was evaluated before operation (baseline), drug administration (pre-dosing), and 6, 8, 10, 12, and 14-days after drug administration (post-dosing), and paw thermal withdrawal latency (TWL) was calculated as described by Hargreaves et al. (Hargreaves et al., 1988). The mechanical allodynia test was measured with a commercially available electronic von Frey apparatus (Model 2390; IITC Life Science Inc., Woodland Hills, CA), and each hind paw and mechanical withdrawal latency (MWL) was calculated 30 min after the TWL measurement according to the published literature (Mitrirattanakul et al., 2006). The observer measuring the behaviors was blind to drug pretreatments in all behavioral tests.

Then, rats were anesthetized by chloral hydrate, and the lumber segments (L5-L6) of the spinal cord were dissected, weighed, and stored at −80°C. Then, the lumber segments were homogenized for 30 min in an ice bath with RIPA lysis buffer (CoWin Biosciences, China) containing phosphatase inhibitor (CoWin Biosciences, China) after ultrasonic crushing. Protein concentrations were determined using an enhanced BCA protein assay kit (Beyotime Biotech Inc., China), and the protein samples were stored at −80°C until use. Total protein samples were separated by sodium dodecyl sulfate polyacrylamide gel electrophoresis and transferred onto the nitrocellulose membrane. The membrane was blocked with 5% non-fat dried milk in tris buffer for 1 h at room temperature and washed with tris-buffered saline and tween 20 every 10 minutes for three times. Then, the membrane was incubated with antibodies (EGFR rabbit pAb: A11577, 1:500, ABclonal; JAK1 rabbit pAb: A5534, 1:500, ABclonal; AKT1 rabbit mAb: A17909, 1:500, ABclonal; β-actin rabbit mAb: AF1186, 1: 1,000, Beyotime) overnight at 4°C. After incubation with the appropriate secondary antibodies (HRP-labeled goat anti-rabbit IgG: A0208, 1:1,000, Beyotime) at room temperature for 1 h, the protein blots were visualized in the ChemiDoc XRS imaging system (Bio-Rad, CA).

RESULTS

Putative Targets of GEB Against NPP

A total of 98 compounds in GEB were retrieved from published literature and online databases, and 57 potentially active ingredients were filtered by OB and DL provided by SwissADME (**Table 1**). 679 potential targets were eventually predicted based on the SwissTargetPrediction after eliminating duplicate targets (**Supplementary Table S1**). 1,047 targets related to NPP were obtained through the Gene Cards database. Out of these targets, 367 potential targets were finally screened out with a disease relevance score ≥3 (**Supplementary Table S2**). Subsequently, as shown in **Figure 2**, 679 GEB ingredients-related targets were intersected with 367 NPP disease-related target genes using Venn diagrams to identify 52 putative targets between GEB and NPP, which were considered candidate targets of GEB against NPP.

PPI Network of Targets for GEB Against NPP

PPI analysis was performed on 52 putative common targets with String database as illustrated in **Figure 3**. The numbers of edges were corresponding to the strength of correlation between two target proteins. The top 15 proteins in the center of the PPI network (**Table 2**), namely AKT1, ENSG00000196689, TNF, CASP3, CXCL8, MAPK8, OPRM1, EGFR, OPRL1, CNR1, PTGS2, CTNNB1, REN, OPRD1, and OPRK1. These proteins were speculated as the core target to play a significant role in the treatment of NPP.

GO Function and KEGG Pathway Enrichment Analysis

The GO and KEGG pathway analysis were performed on the 52 common targets to further explore the possible mechanisms of

TABLE 1 | Information of the active compounds in GEB for network analysis.

NO.	Name	Compound CID	MW	MF	Source
1	N-methoxyanhydrovobasinediol	102004539	338.4	$C_{21}H_{26}N_2O_2$	References
2	Humantenirine	11,132,403	370.4	$C_{21}H_{26}N_2O_4$	TCMID, TCMSP, Reference
3	N-desmethoxyrankinidine	5316594	310.4	$C_{19}H_{22}N_2O_2$	TCMID, TCMSP, References
4	Humantendine	5490912	342.4	$C_{19}H_{22}N_2O_4$	References
5	11-Methoxygelsemamide	5319437	355.4	$C_{21}H_{25}NO_4$	TCM-Taiwan, References
6	Gelsevirine	14217344	352.4	$C_{21}H_{24}N_2O_3$	TCMID, BATMAN-TCM, TCM-Taiwan, References
7	Gelsenicine	21123652	326.4	$C_{19}H_{22}N_2O_3$	References
8	19-Oxogelsenicine	102185549	398.4	$C_{21}H_{22}N_2O_6$	References
9	Gelsedine	21589070	328.4	$C_{19}H_{24}N_2O_3$	TCMID, BATMAN-TCM, TCM-Taiwan, References
10	Gelsemamide	5317542	340.4	$C_{20}H_{24}N_2O_3$	TCMID, TCMSP, References
11	19-Z-akuammidine	44583830	352.4	$C_{21}H_{24}N_2O_3$	References
12	Dihydrokoumine	5316727	308.4	$C_{20}H_{24}N_2O$	BATMAN-TCM, References
13	(19R)-kouminol	NA	324.2	$C_{20}H_{24}N_2O_2$	References
14	(19S)-kouminol	NA	324.2	$C_{20}H_{24}N_2O_2$	References
15	19-(R)-hydroxydihydrokoumine	50278496	324.4	$C_{20}H_{24}N_2O_2$	TCMID, BATMAN-TCM, TCM-Taiwan, References
16	19-(S)-hydroxydihydrokoumine	5318193	324.4	$C_{20}H_{24}N_2O_2$	References
17	20-hydroxydihydrorankinidine	101606432	358.4	$C_{20}H_{26}N_2O_4$	References
18	N-desmethoxyhumantenine	5316593	324.4	$C_{20}H_{24}N_2O_2$	References
19	15-hydroxyhumantenine	101606434	370.4	$C_{21}H_{26}N_2O_4$	TCMID, TCMSP, References
20	Rankinidine	6439112	340.4	$C_{20}H_{24}N_2O_3$	TCMID, TCMSP, References
21	Humantenmine	158212	326.4	$C_{19}H_{22}N_2O_3$	TCMID, BATMAN-TCM, TCM-Taiwan, Reference
22	11-Hydroxyrankinidine	5318332	356.4	$C_{20}H_{24}N_2O_4$	TCMID, References Lin et al. (2021)
23	11-Hydroxyhumantenine	5318224	370.4	$C_{21}H_{26}N_2O_4$	TCMID, References Lin et al. (2021)
24	11-methoxyhumantenine	44583832	384.5	$C_{22}H_{28}N_2O_4$	TCMID, TCMSP, BATMAN-TCM, References Lin et al. (2021)
25	19R-hydroxydihydrogelsevirine	5318192	370.4	$C_{21}H_{26}N_2O_4$	References Lin et al. (2021)
26	19S-hydroxydihydrogelsevirine	5318192	370.4	$C_{21}H_{26}N_2O_4$	References Lin et al. (2021)
27	Gelseoxazolidinine	102297300	428.5	$C_{23}H_{28}N_2O_6$	References Lin et al. (2021)
28	Gelsevanillidine	136811988	460	$C_{27}H_{28}N_2O_5$	References Lin et al. (2021)
29	Gelselegine	10948335	358.4	$C_{20}H_{26}N_2O_4$	TCMID, References Lin et al. (2021)
30	11-Methoxy-19-R-hydroxygelselegine	5319453	404.5	$C_{21}H_{28}N_2O_6$	References Lin et al. (2021)
31	19α-hydroxygelsamydine	102003053	524.6	$C_{29}H_{36}N_2O_7$	References Lin et al. (2021)
32	gelsamydine	5317540	508.6	$C_{29}H_{36}N_2O_6$	TCMID, References Lin et al. (2021)
33	gelegamine E	101467881	370.4	$C_{20}H_{22}N_2O_5$	References Lin et al. (2021)
34	gelegamine C	101467879	514.4	$C_{21}H_{27}IN_2O_5$	References Lin et al. (2021)
35	Gelegamine A	101467877	384.4	$C_{21}H_{24}N_2O_5$	References Lin et al. (2021)
36	Gelegamine B	101467878	384.4	$C_{21}H_{24}N_2O_5$	References Lin et al. (2021)
37	19Z- 16- epi- voacarpine	NA	368.2	$C_{21}H_{24}N_2O_4$	References Lin et al. (2021)
38	11-Methoxyhumantenmine	NA	356.2	$C_{20}H_{24}N_2O_4$	References Lin et al. (2021)
39	GELSENINE	NA	358.19	$C_{20}H_{26}N_2O_4$	References Lin et al. (2021)
40	21 Oxokoumine	NA	320.1	$C_{20}H_{20}N_2O_2$	References Lin et al. (2021)
41	Furanokoumine	NA	322.1	$C_{20}H_{22}N_2O_2$	References (Lin et al., 2021)
42	Koumidine	44584550	294.4	$C_{19}H_{22}N_2O$	TCMID, TCMSP, BATMAN-TCM, References Lin et al. (2021)
43	Gelebolines A	NA	320.15	$C_{20}H_{20}N_2O_2$	References Lin et al. (2021)
44	Gelebolines B	NA	334.2	$C_{21}H_{22}N_2O_2$	References Lin et al. (2021)
45	Gelebolines C	NA	334.1	$C_{20}H_{18}N_2O_3$	References Lin et al. (2021)
46	19E- 16- epi- voacarpine	NA	368.2	$C_{21}H_{24}N_2O_4$	References Lin et al. (2021)
47	19- Z- taberpsychine	5321582	310.4	$C_{20}H_{26}N_2O$	References Lin et al. (2021)
48	Koumicine N- oxide	NA	322.4	$C_{20}H_{22}N_2O_2$	References Lin et al. (2021)
49	Nb-methylgelsedilam	NA	328.14	$C_{18}H_{20}N_2O_4$	References Lin et al. (2021)
50	15-hydroxy-Nb-methylgelsedilam	NA	344.1	$C_{18}H_{20}N_2O_5$	References Lin et al. (2021)
51	Gelsesyringalidine	136704418	490.5	$C_{28}H_{30}N_2O_6$	References Lin et al. (2021)
52	14-Dehydroxygelsefuranidine	1,02417029	404.5	$C_{24}H_{24}N_2O_4$	References Lin et al. (2021)
53	Humantenoxenine	NA	368.17	$C_{21}H_{24}N_2O_4$	References Lin et al. (2021)
54	15-Hydroxyhumantenoxenine	101606434	370.4	$C_{21}H_{26}N_2O_4$	TCMID
55	Kounaminal	102260292	363.5	$C_{22}H_{25}N_3O_2$	References Lin et al. (2021)
56	Dehydrokoumidine	119077162	292.4	$C_{19}H_{20}N_2O$	References Lin et al. (2021)
57	Koumine	91895267	306.4	$C_{20}H_{22}N_2O$	TCMID, TCMSP, BATMAN-TCM, TCM-Taiwan, References Lin et al. (2021)

NA, not applicable.

GEB against NPP. A total of 184 BPs, 34 CCs, and 35 MFs were obtained in GO analysis (**Supplementary Table S3**). The top 10 terms in BPs, MFs, and CCs were shown in **Figure 4A**. It was suggested that GEB attenuated NPP may be through the sensory perception of pain, positive regulation of gene expression/protein phosphorylation/nitric oxide

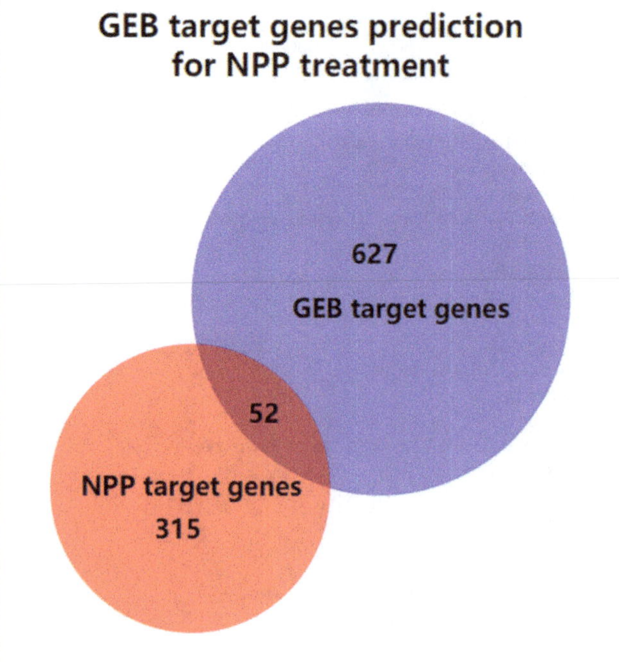

FIGURE 2 | The Venn diagram illustrating the intersection of the GEB target genes and NPP target genes. The blue circle is the GEB target genes, the red circle is the NPP target genes, and the overlap of the two circles indicates GEB target genes prediction for NPP treatment.

biosynthetic/cytosolic calcium ion concentration, and phospholipase C-activating G-protein coupled receptor signaling pathway. Meanwhile, the target protein was mainly distributed in the plasma membrane and involved in protein homodimer activity, enzyme binding, transmembrane receptor protein tyrosine kinase activity, etc.

KEGG pathway analysis identified 73 pathways, including neuroactive ligand-receptor interactions, calcium signaling pathway, MAPK signaling pathway, HIF-1 signaling pathway, cGMP-PKG signaling pathway, Rapl signaling pathway, inflammatory mediators regulating TRP channels, and TNF signaling pathway (**Supplementary Table S4**). The top 15 KEGG pathways based on their *p*-values were selected to generate a bubble chart for visualization (**Figure 4B**).

"Ingredient-Target-Pathway" Network Construction

Based on the active ingredients related to the target genes, the active ingredients–disease targets–pathway network with 114 nodes and 556 edges was constructed (**Figure 5**). Of the 99 nodes, 47 active ingredients nodes, 52 target nodes, and 15 pathways were involved. The top three active ingredient nodes with the most edges were 11-hydroxyrankinidine, 11-hydroxyhumantenine, and gelseoxazolidinine. The average values of the degree values, node betweenness, and closeness of the three topological features of these active ingredients were 13.8, 0.0402, and 0.4424, respectively. The top three target nodes

TABLE 2 | Key targets of the PPI network.

NO.	Common name	Degree
1	AKT1	29
2	ENSG00000196689	27
3	TNF	25
4	CASP3	25
5	CXCL8	24
6	MAPK8	24
7	OPRM1	23
8	EGFR	23
9	OPRL1	20
10	CNR1	20
11	PTGS2	18
12	CTNNB1	18
13	REN	16
14	OPRD1	16
15	OPRK1	16

with the most degrees were EGFR, JAK1, and AKT1. The average values of the degree values, node betweenness, and closeness of the three topological features are 23, 0.0855, and 0.4658, respectively.

Ingredients-Targets Molecular Docking

The molecular docking technology was used to further evaluate the interaction between the ingredients and the targets, and verify the accuracy of the network analysis. The binding strength of the ligand and the receptor depends on the change in the binding energy. The lower the binding energy between the ligand and the receptor, the more stable and greater the possibility of interaction of ligand-receptor binding. The top three core active ingredients and three targets were used as receptors and ligands, respectively. In addition, koumine was also acted as a receptor for target docking simulation since it was one of the most studied ingredients of GEB (**Table 3**). The molecular docking results demonstrated that each ingredient could match well with each target to verify the accuracy of the prediction network construction. 11-Hydroxyrankinidine had the highest affinity for the target of EGFR (PDB: 5HG7), AKT1 (PDB: 3L9M), and JAK1 (PDB: 4E5W), and had the lowest binding energy with EGFR, which indicated that 11-hydroxyrankinidine had a strong affinity with the active pocket of EGFR.

Multi-conformation molecular docking results were visualized using Pymol software in **Figure 5**. The 11-hydroxyrankinidine-EGFR complex was stabilized by three hydrogen bonds with potential residues including MET-793 (2.8 Å) and CYS-797 (3.3 Å) (**Figure 6A**). The 11-hydroxyrankinidine- JAK1 complex was mainly through three hydrogen bonding interactions of ARG-1007 (2.7 Å), LEU-959 (2.8 Å), and LEU-959 (2.5 Å) (**Figure 6B**). The 11-hydroxyrankinidine- AKT1 complex interacted with the residue GLU-170 (2.8 Å) through one hydrogen bond (**Figure 6C**). The results of virtual docking between koumine and the targets EGFR, JAK1, and AKT1 were denoted in **Figure 6D–F** respectively.

Molecular Dynamics Simulation of Ligand Complex

Since 11-Hydroxyrankinidine has the lowest binding energy with EGFR, 11-hydroxyrankinidin-EGFR complex was selected for molecular dynamics simulation to elaborate the dynamic interactions between the protein-ligand complex and confirm the molecular docking results. The system's potential energy converged within 100 ps (**Figure 7A**), which indicated that the simulation system was well prepared. The RMSD graph shown in **Figure 7B** demonstrated that a consistently stable structure of 11-hydroxyrankinidine-EGFR complex throughout the simulation period. The mean (±SD) RMSD of the 11-hydroxyrankinidine-EGFR complex (0.254 ± 0.018 nm) was similar with primitive ligand complex (0.263 ± 0.026 nm), even lower than that of the reference ligand after 26 ns. Meanwhile, the RMSF shows comparatively restricted fluctuation in the protein residues (**Figure 7C**). Mean (±SD) RMSF values of 11-hydroxyrankinidine-EGFR complex and primitive ligand complex were 0.147 ± 0.097 nm and 0.141 ± 0.095 nm, respectively. There were no apparent differences for all complexes in the ligand RMSF. This observation demonstrated that the molecules were capable of forming stable interactions with the protein during simulation.

Anti-NPP Effects of Koumine in CCI Rat Model

In the current study, the TWL to thermal stimulation and the MWL to mechanical stimulation of the CCI rats were significantly decreased compared with the sham group ($p < 0.001$). Koumine attenuated the CCI-induced NPP effect in the dose-dependent and time-dependent manner (**Figure 8**). The results indicated that the maximum anti-NPP effect was reached on day 10 and administration of koumine (7 mg/kg) exhibited the maximum pharmacological effect to reverse NPP.

Validation of Predicted Target Protein With Western Blotting

As shown in **Figure 9**, the relative protein expression of EGFR in koumine treated group was higher than that in sham control and CCI + vehicle groups, which indicated that koumine reversed the CCI-induced downregulation of EGFR in a dose-dependent manner. Similarly, the activation of JAK1 was observed in koumine treated group. In addition, the protein expression of AKT1 in the low-dose group of koumine was lower than that in the sham control group. However, no significance was observed between the sham control group and the low-dose group of koumine. The reason for this may be related to the complex interaction of pathways adjusted by multiple ingredients, which needs to study further.

DISCUSSION

To the best of our knowledge, this is the first systematical study for exploring the potential pharmacological and molecular mechanisms of GEB against NPP from the network pharmacology and experimental perspective. The major findings were as follows: (Vos et al., 2012): a total of 52 proteins were considered as potential targets associated with

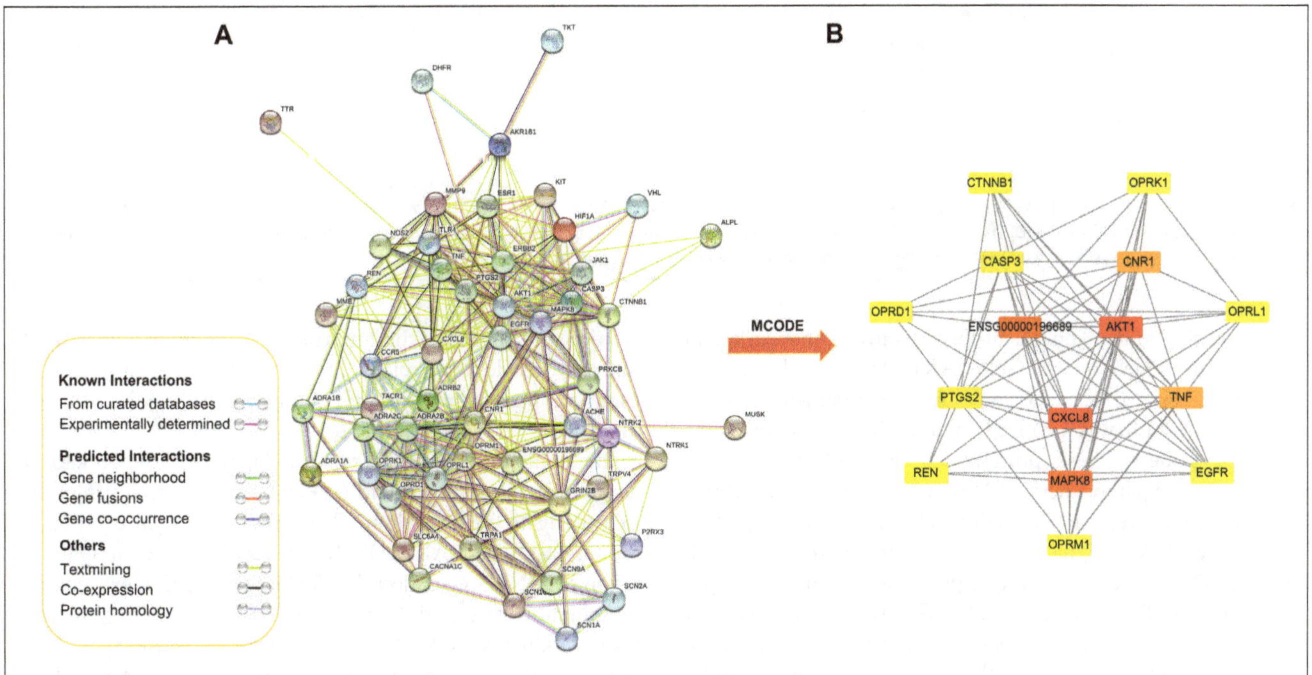

FIGURE 3 | Protein-protein interaction network for GEB in treatment for NPP. **(A)** Protein-protein interactions among the 52 core targets. Network nodes represent proteins, and edges represent protein-protein associations. **(B)** PPI network of the hub genes using MCODE plugin. The color from red/orange/yellow indicated the different importance of the nodes in the whole PPI network. That is, the redder the retangle is, the more important the node is in the PPI network.

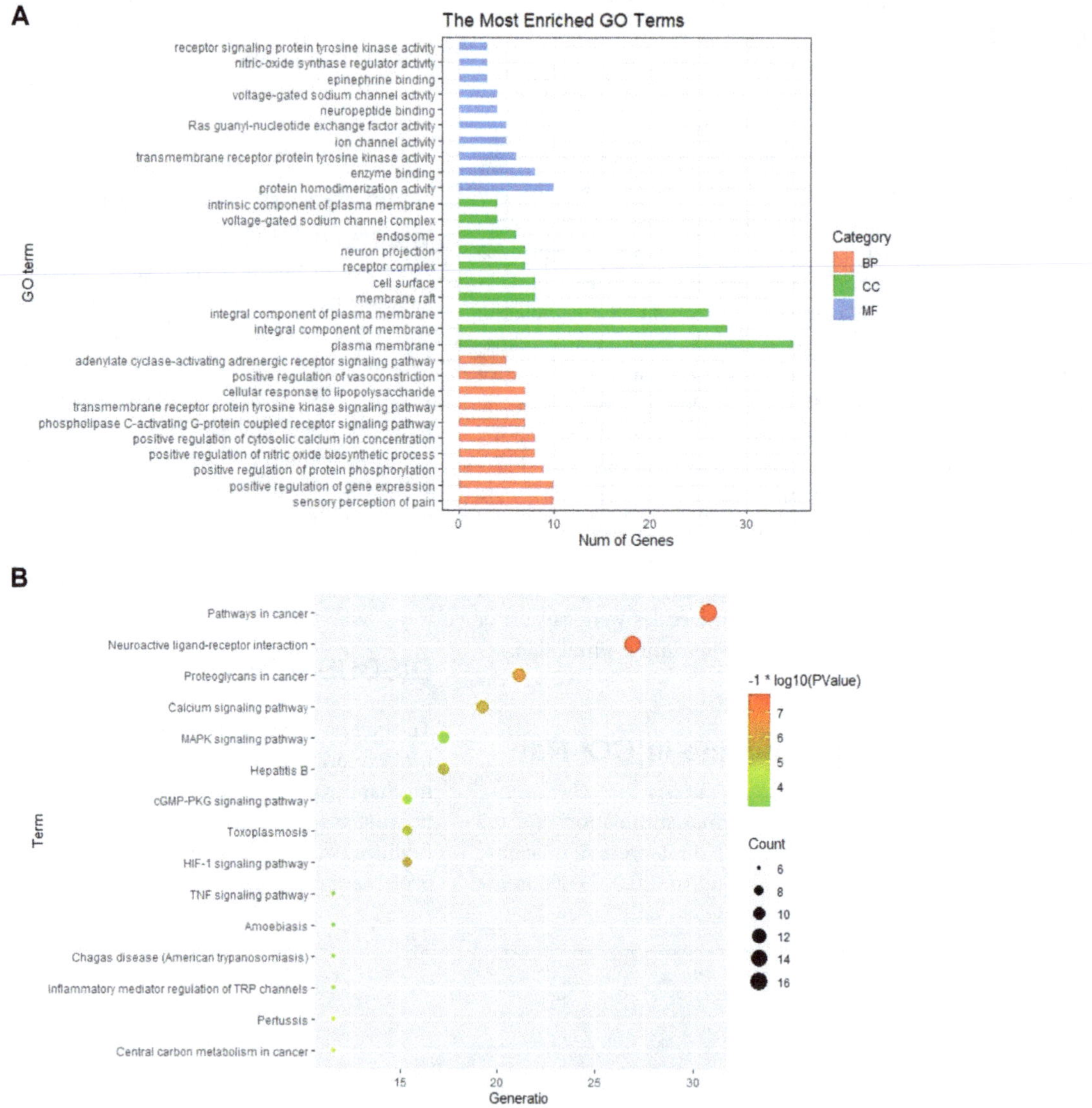

FIGURE 4 | GO and KEGG pathway enrichment analysis of GEB in treatment for NPP. **(A)** GO analysis of significant items of 52 common targets in different functional groups (BPs, CCs, MFs) **(B)** The top 15 KEGG pathways based on their *p*-values. The larger the circle, the greater the number of the target genes in the term. Also, color highlights the size of the FDR: the redder the color, the more significant the value.

NPP according to the "ingredient-target-pathway" network, and the top four targets were EGFR, JAK1, AKT1, and MAPK8; (Andrew et al., 2014); GO and KEGG enrichment analysis revealed that GEB was involved in phosphorylation reactions and nitric oxide synthesis processes. It also participated in 73 pathways in the pathogenesis of NPP, including the neuroactive ligand-receptor interaction signaling pathway, calcium signaling pathway, and MAPK signaling pathway; (van Hecke et al., 2014); a total of 47 active alkaloids might play a synergistic role in the treatment of NPP. Among them, 11-hydroxyrankinidin matched the active pockets of EGFR, JAK1, and AKT1 proteins, with the strongest affinity, suggesting that it may be an essential component of GEB in the treatment of NPP; (Jensen et al., 2011); koumine reversed the CCI-induced downregulation of EGFR and JAK1. These findings revealed the complex network relationship of GEB in the "multi-ingredient, multi-target, multi-pathway" mode, and explained the synergistic regulatory effect of each complex ingredient of GEB based on the holistic view of TCM.

By predicting targets and constructing the PPI network for the common targets of GEB and NPP, 52 targets were distinguished to investigate the possible mechanism of GEB against NPP. The top targets, EGFR, JAK1, AKT1, and MAPK8, were thought to be involved in NPP regulation. The first target, EGFR is expressed on peripheral nerves, and it belongs to the ErbB family of receptor tyrosine kinases (Neto et al., 2017). After nerve injury, EGFR is upregulated in the nervous system and has been proposed as a target for the treatment of NPP (Liu et al., 2006). EGFR also plays a key role in many intracellular signaling pathways, such as phosphatidylinositol 3-kinase, MAPK, and ErbB signaling

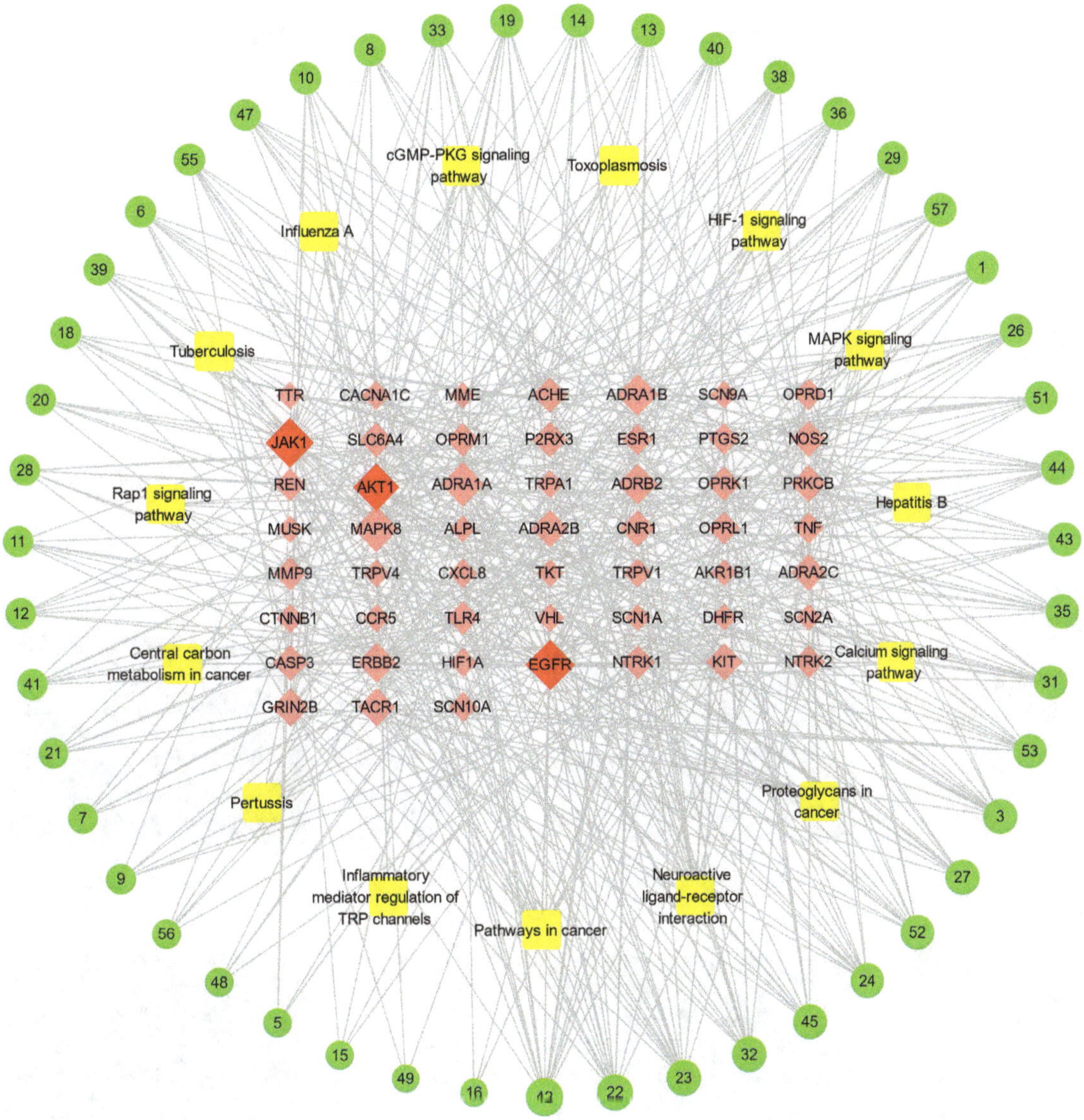

FIGURE 5 | The "ingredient-target-pathway" network for GEB in treatment for NPP. The outer green circle represents active ingredient in GEB, the yellow square indicates the potential pathways, and the red diamond stands for the potential target. For corresponding active ingredient names, refer to Supplementary Table1. the potential target genes shared by GEB and NPP, the orange triangle stands for the active ingredient in GEB, and the green diamond indicates the potential pathways. The size of the node represents the degree values.

pathways (Tao et al., 2013; Borges et al., 2021), which is coherent with the results of KEGG and molecular docking in the present study. Furthermore, treatment of NPP with EGFR-Inhibitors (EGFR-Is) significantly relieved the pain of the majority of patients, which has been reported in clinical and preclinical studies (Kersten et al., 2015; Kersten et al., 2019). The second target, JAK1 is the core member of the JAK family and stimulates the phosphorylation of STAT3 through particular domains (Wang et al., 2020b). The JAK/STAT signaling pathway directly or indirectly affects the action, expression, and regulation of a multitude of cytokines in mediating various mechanisms underlying pain (Simon et al., 2021). JAK1 was increased in spinal nerve ligation triggered NPP rat models (Wang et al., 2020b), which was validated to be a potential therapeutic target of NPP. A previous study revealed that dexmedetomidine had the potential to alleviate NPP by regulating the JAK/STAT pathway in chronic constriction injury rats (Xun and Zheng, 2020). It is suggested that the active ingredients may exert therapeutic effects via regulating JAK1 expression or its function. Another target of AKT, a key downstream substrate in the PI3K pathway, is associated with diverse biological processes (Sun et al., 2006). The phosphorylation of the PI3K/AKT pathway in the spinal cord contributes to the activation of the transcription factor nuclear factor κB and the release of the inflammatory mediators and finally leads to the development of NPP (Chen et al., 2017).

TABLE 3 | Virtual molecular docking of active ingredients of GEB and targets.

Name	The number of hydrogen bond	Amino acid residue	Target	Binding Energy/kcal·mol^{-1}
11-Hydroxyrankinidine	3	MET-793 (2.8) CYS-797 (3.3)	EGFR	−8.7
	3	ARG-1007 (2.7) LEU-959 (2.8) LEU-959 (2.5)	JAK1	−6.5
	1	GLU-170 (2.8)	AKT1	−8
11-Hydroxyhumantenine	1	CYS-797	EGFR	−7.6
	1	GLU-883	JAK1	−5.9
	NA	NA	AKT1	−6.4
Gelseoxazolidinine	1	SER-720	EGFR	−6.4
	NA	NA	JAK1	−5.8
	1	ASN-20	AKT1	−2.5
Koumine	1	CYS-797 (3.2)	EGFR	−7.2
	NA	NA	JAK1	−6.2
	1	ASP-184 (3.1)	AKT1	−7.4

NA, not applicable.

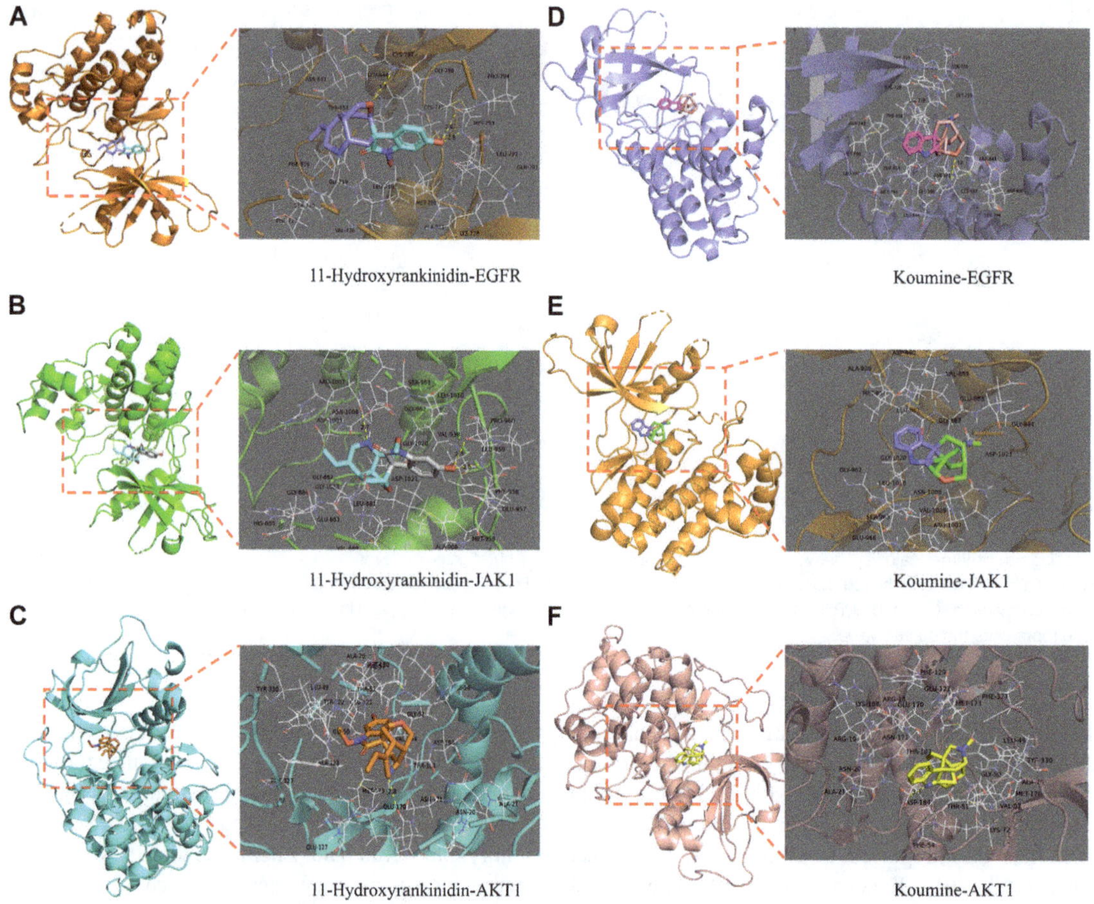

FIGURE 6 | Virtual docking of the binding of EGFR, JAK1, and AKT1 with 11-Hydroxyrankinidine **(A–C)** and koumine **(D–F)** shown as 3D diagrams.

Therefore, the PI3K/AKT pathway is likely a novel target for GEB against NPP. As the potential downstream pathways of the EGFR, accumulating evidence showed that the MAPK family contributes to the regulation of pain hypersensitivity in different injury conditions via phosphorylation activation (Gao et al., 2009; Ji et al., 2009). A slow (>3 days) and persistent (>21 days) activation

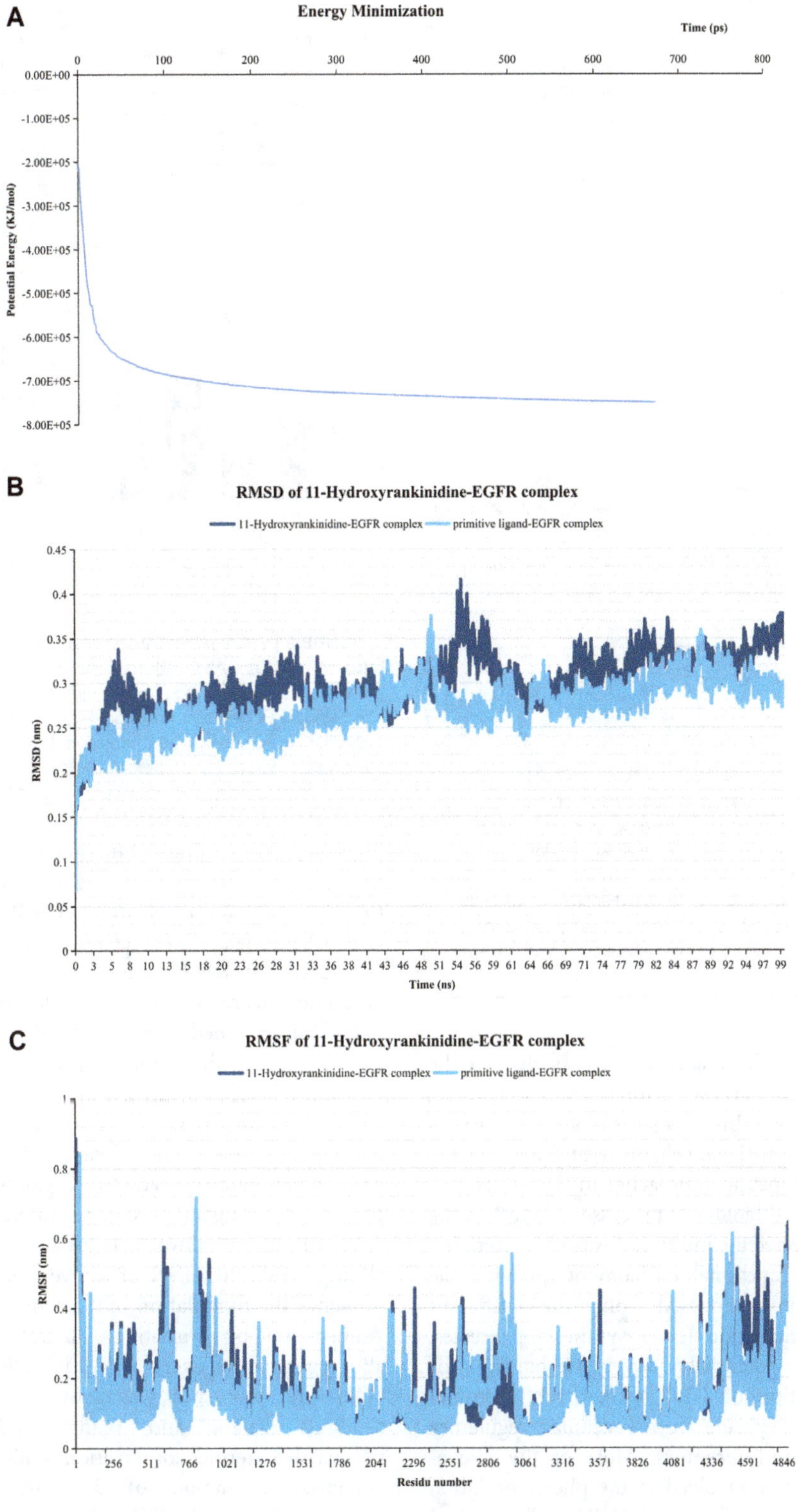

FIGURE 7 | Molecular dynamics simulation of the 11-Hydroxyrankinidine-EGFR complex. **(A)** Energy minimization for molecular dynamics simulation. **(B)** RMSD profiles of complex conducted during 100 ns. **(C)** RMSF profiles of the complex. The primitive ligand of EGFR is ibrutinib.

of MAPK8, known as c-Jun N-terminal kinase 1 (JNK1), could be induced in the spinal nerve ligation model (Zhuang et al., 2006). Although the current evidence was limited, it was reported that the latent mechanism of GEB may be related to the activation of MAPK *in vitro* and *vivo* studies (Yuan et al., 2016; Huang et al., 2021). These pieces of evidence exemplify that the

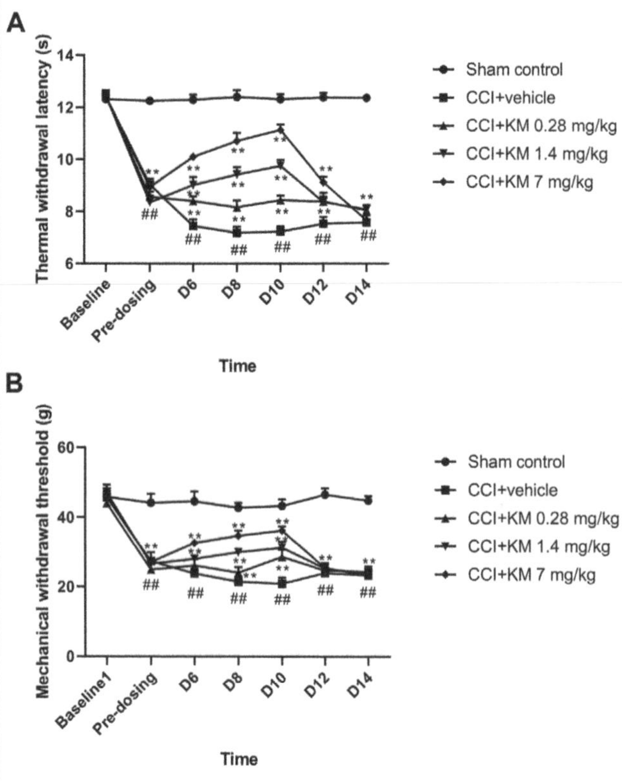

FIGURE 8 | The anti-NPP effect of koumine in sciatic nerve chronic constriction injury rats. **(A)** The time course of the effect of koumine on the thermal withdrawal latency. **(B)** The time course of the effect of koumine on the mechanical withdrawal threshold. The data are presented as the mean ± SD (n = 6) and were analyzed using two-way repeated analysis of variance (ANOVA) followed by Bonferroni's post hoc test, $^{\#\#}p < 0.01$ compared with the sham control group; $^{**}p < 0.01$ compared with the vehicle control group. KM, koumine.

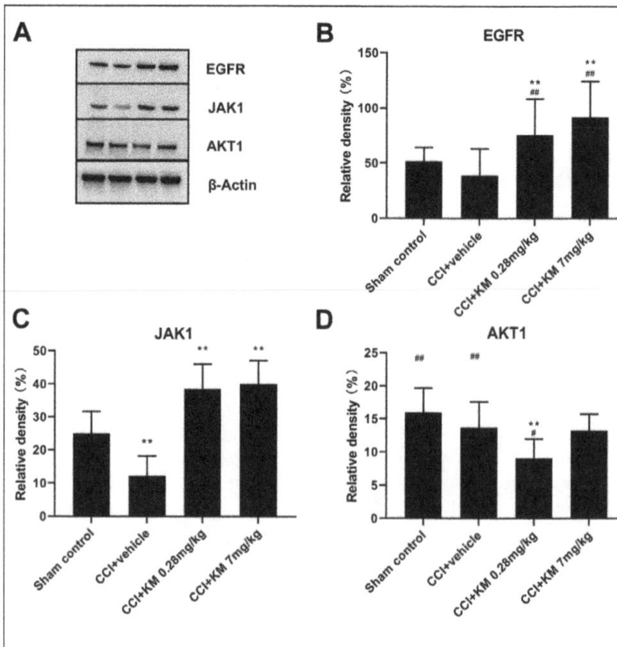

FIGURE 9 | Western blot **(A)** and relative protein expression of EGFR **(B)**, JAK1 **(C)**, and AKT1 **(D)**. The data are presented as the mean ± SD (n = 6) and were analyzed using two-way repeated analysis of variance (ANOVA) followed by Bonferroni's post hoc test, $^{\#\#}p < 0.01$ compared with the sham control group; $^{**}p < 0.01$ compared with the vehicle control group. KM, koumine.

pharmacological activity of GEB against NPP is due to the interaction of these key targets. Moreover, multi-target therapeutics approaches for GEB in control of NPP form a basis for further research on the mechanism of GEB and the development of novel therapeutic approaches in the future.

The related pathways and biological processes of GEB in the treatment of NPP also reflected the multi-pathway characteristics of TCM. Based on GO functional enrichment analysis, the biological process mainly focused on the different phosphorylation and nitric oxide (NO) synthesis processes, which indicated that a potentially novel mechanism for pharmacological intervention of GEB against NPP. Protein phosphorylation plays a key role in the cellular regulatory mechanism of enzymes and receptors. Most of the above-mentioned target activation is involved in the phosphorylation process. For example, phosphorylation of AKT at Thr308 and Ser473 mediate pain behavior through the PI3K/AKT signal pathway (Sun et al., 2006). Notably, GEB reduced the oxidative stress and inflammatory reaction in a phosphorylation state-dependent modulation manner (Yuan et al., 2019; Luo et al., 2020; Wu et al., 2020). In addition, NO is an important neurotransmitter and modulates a wide variety of physiological functions. It has been illustrated that NO mediates the analgesic effect of opioids and other analgesic substances through activation of the cGMP–PKG–ATP-sensitive K^+ channels pathway (Cury et al., 2011), which is consistent with the results of KEGG enrichment. It was also reported that koumine decreases the productions of NO and pro-inflammatory mediators in RAW264.7 cells (Yuan et al., 2016). These findings may partially support our prediction on GO and KEGG pathway enrichment analysis. Furthermore, the KEGG pathway enrichment analysis showed that GEB may participate in neuroactive ligand-receptor interaction, calcium, and inflammatory mediator regulation signaling pathways. Neuroactive ligand-receptor interaction refers to the stereoselectivity between neuroactive steroids and receptors (Wang et al., 2017). Neuroactive steroids act as regulators to influence the modulation of neuronal activity (Smith, 1994). As confirmed by existing literature, the neurosteroid allopregnanolone exert a positive allosteric regulation of the GABA receptor and was activated by GEB and its active alkaloids (Zhang and Wang, 2015). Mirtazapine affects neuroactive steroid composition similarly to koumine with an enhanced formation of 3α-hydroxysteroid dehydrogenase neuroactive steroids (Schüle et al., 2006; Qiu et al., 2015). Based on these, we infer that GEB might serve a crucial role in NPP by influencing the pathway of neuroactive ligand-receptor interaction pathway. In addition, increased expression of voltage-gated calcium channels at dorsal root ganglia and presynaptic terminals increases the excitability of nerve and lead to NPP (Cohen and Mao, 2014).

Inflammatory mediator regulation is another interesting pathway described by KEGG. An increasing number of studies have indicated that inflammatory responses play a key role in the development of NPP (Watkins et al., 2003). Cytokines, which are essential for the induction and maintenance of pain (Zhang and An, 2007), are primarily secreted by immune cells. Pro-inflammatory cytokines (e.g., TNF-α, IL-1β, IL-6, and IL-17) are evoked in inflammatory responses after nerve injury through intracellular mediators, while anti-inflammatory (IL-4, IL-10, TGF-β) signaling molecules show analgesic properties (Hung et al., 2017). The PI3K/AKT signaling pathway is an inflammatory pathway that may be mediated by TNF-α in osteoarthritis, and TNF-α inhibitor treatment significantly reduced the expression of IL-1, IL17a, and IL8 in synovial fibroblasts (Li et al., 2018). In addition, the TNF-induced cutaneous hypersensitivity to mechanical or thermal stimulation is also associated with the cAMP-dependent protein kinase (PKA) pathway and the p38 mitogen-activated protein kinase (MAPK) pathway (Zhang et al., 2002; Schäfers et al., 2003), which are all presented in our network results and provides a systematic and macro perspective to understand their interactions. Another cytokine, IL-17, has shown the potential effect on allodynia. Exogenous IL-17 administration may increase the activity of the transient receptor protein vanilloid 4 (TRPV4) (Hung et al., 2017), which was discovered in network pharmacology. Furthermore, gelsemine and koumine have been shown to inhibit the overexpression of pro-inflammatory cytokines in mice and rats (Jin et al., 2018b; Chen et al., 2020). These above evidenced improve our confidence that GEB can restore the imbalance between pro-inflammatory cytokines and anti-inflammatory cytokines and thus promote its antinociceptive effects.

Based on the "ingredient-target-pathway" network, 47 pivotal active ingredients related to NPP were obtained, such as 11-hydroxyrankinidine, 11-hydroxyhumantenine, gelsamydine, koumidine, and gelebolines C. These ingredients might play a synergistic role in the treatment of NPP. Structurally, the 47 phytochemicals have exhibited diversity. Molecular docking results have disclosed that 11-hydroxyrankinidine, 11-hydroxyhumantenine, gelsamydine, and koumine could bind autonomously with the active pocket of EGFR, JAK1, and AKT1 to form a complex with a relatively stable structure through hydrogen bonds and other interactions. Among them, 11-hydroxyrankinidine has the lowest binding energy and the highest affinity to EGFR. Encouragingly, it was observed that the RSMD and RSMF profiles of the 11-hydroxyrankinidine-EGFR complex were relatively stable, which indicated 11-hydroxyrankinidine showed promising inhibitory activity in NPP. Due to the accessibility, the extracts and monomers derived from GEB have been found to possess anti-NPP biological activity, especially some of the active ingredients, such as koumine (Xu et al., 2012; Qiu et al., 2015; Jin et al., 2018a; Jin et al., 2018b), gelsenicine (Liu et al., 2011), and gelsemine (Zhang et al., 2013; Wu et al., 2015; Chen et al., 2020). To further verify the hypothesis of network pharmacology, that is, the active alkaloids obtained through network pharmacology act on the target to exert an anti-NPP effect, the behavior test and western blotting were applied to evaluate the anti-NPP effects of koumine as well as its molecular mechanism after the analysis of network pharmacology, molecular docking, and molecular dynamics simulation. It was suggested that koumine could upregulate the protein expression of EGFR and JAK1 to achieve the anti-NPP action. Combined with the prediction results, it was reasonable to speculate that koumine or GEB-derived ingredients contributed to the anti-NPP effect through some pain-related targets. Most of the indole alkaloids have a similar skeletal structure. Therefore, it is worthy of further examination for the therapeutic effects of 11-hydroxyrankinidine against NPP both *in vitro* and *in vivo*, though the current data on 11-hydroxyrankinidine is extremely limited. Furthermore, traditional TCM usually is thought to act in synergy to achieve a holistic therapeutic outcome, suggesting the understanding of the synergistic action of these alkaloids with a holistic view.

This present study also has several limitations. Firstly, given the limitations of network pharmacology, the public databases investigated in the study would be constantly updated so some ingredients and targets information has partly lagged. The chemical fingerprint may be a better choice for network construction and mechanism exploration. Secondly, SwissTargetPrediction is a ligand-based tool for predicting the interacting targets of small molecules, which is useful for understanding the molecular mechanisms underlying a specific phenotype or bioactivity, as well as assessing the possibility of repurposing therapeutically-relevant compounds. It is based on the so-called "similarity principle," which states that two similar molecules are likely to have similar properties. However, when there are few (or no) known active ligands for a target of interest, their predictive reliability suffers. Furthermore, when molecules with high structural similarities but different biological activities for the same target coexist, a limitation may also exist. Thirdly, the validation experiment in the current study only provided limited protein, and more targets and pathways may be studied further, especially the possibility of influence and correlations with cytokines. Besides, although 11-hydroxyrankinidine showed promising inhibitory activity in network pharmacology, it is not the most abundant ingredient in GEB. Due its inaccessibility, there has been no report on its pharmacological activities to date. Therefore, koumine was selected in validation in the experiment as a substitute, based on the fact that it is a high-content active alkaloid of GEB that is easily obtained. Furthermore, molecular docking results demonstrated that koumine bonded to the ligand stably. For further study, we can also use pH-zone refining counter-current chromatography to purify the active monomer (Su et al., 2011), for example, 11-hydroxyrankinidine, to determine its analgesic effect in the future.

In the present study, the active ingredient and anti-NPP mechanism of GEB were mapped using network pharmacology, molecular docking, molecular dynamics simulation, and bioinformatics approach. It could promote the understanding of the synergistic action of GEB with a holistic view to explore the key ingredients, targets, and pathways. Different from the current mode of single-target pharmacology in TCM, network pharmacology based on computational prediction could provide broad ideas and be a useful supplement for the mechanism exploration of TCM. In addition, the new potential lead compounds screened in our study, for example, 11-hydroxyrankinidine, may provide a rational direction for future drug discovery and development. With the development of monomer purification technology (Su et al., 2011), it will be hopefully available to identify the anti-NPP effect. What should also be stressed here is that, before experimental validation, network pharmacology prediction could serve as promising, rapid, and cost-effective strategies during the drug discovery and development process in the future.

CONCLUSION

This study revealed the underlying pharmacological mechanisms of GEB on NPP based on network pharmacology and experimental evidence. Forty-seven active alkaloids might play a synergistic role in the treatment of NPP, and 11-hydroxyrankinidin had excellent stability in the active site pocket of EGFR, JAK1, and AKT1, the core targets in network pharmacology. Meanwhile, GEB participates in the regulation of 73 pathways including neuroactive ligand-receptor interaction in the pathogenesis of NPP concentrated mainly on phosphorylation reactions and nitric oxide synthesis processes. Experimental evidence also proved that GEB may regulate the expression of EGFR and JAK1 after the formation of ligand-receptor complexes. In the future, network pharmacology based on computational prediction may provide broad ideas for TCM mechanism exploration as well as cost-effective strategies during the drug discovery and development process.

AUTHOR CONTRIBUTIONS

CY and HQ proposed the project, supervised the study, and reviewed the entire contents of the manuscript. ZW, WQ, and MC performed the study and analyzed the data. ZW drafted the manuscript. WQ, ZW and MC performed animal and western blot experiments. BZ contributed to collecting data from different databases. CY and HL were responsible for the figures and tables. ZZ and ML evaluated the data and amended the manuscript. All authors have read and agree to the published version of the manuscript.

FUNDING

This work was supported by grants from the Natural Science Foundation of Fujian Province (no. 2021J0112), the Youth Project of Health Department of Fujian Province (no. 2020GGB024), the Guiding Project (no. 2021Y0019) and the Innovation Joint Project (no. 2019Y9051, no. 2020Y9066) of Fujian Science and Technology.

ACKNOWLEDGMENTS

We would like to thank Zhang Shuxia for the guidance and help on the experimental part.

REFERENCES

Andrew, R., Derry, S., Taylor, R. S., Straube, S., and Phillips, C. J. (2014). The Costs and Consequences of Adequately Managed Chronic Non-Cancer Pain and Chronic Neuropathic Pain. *Pain Pract.* 14 (1), 79–94. doi:10.1111/papr.12050

Bennett, G. J., and Xie, Y. K. (1988). A Peripheral Mononeuropathy in Rat that Produces Disorders of Pain Sensation like Those Seen in Man. *Pain* 33 (1), 87–107. doi:10.1016/0304-3959(88)90209-6

Borges, J. P., Mekhail, K., Fairn, G. D., Antonescu, C. N., and Steinberg, B. E. (2021). Modulation of Pathological Pain by Epidermal Growth Factor Receptor. *Front. Pharmacol.* 12, 642820. doi:10.3389/fphar.2021.642820

Cavalli, E., Mammana, S., Nicoletti, F., Bramanti, P., and Mazzon, E. (2019). The Neuropathic Pain: an Overview of the Current Treatment and Future Therapeutic Approaches. *Int. J. Immunopathol Pharmacol.* 33, 2058738419838383. doi:10.1177/2058738419838383

Chen, C. Y. (2011). TCM Database@Taiwan: the World's Largest Traditional Chinese Medicine Database for Drug Screening In Silico. *PloS one* 6 (1), e15939. doi:10.1371/journal.pone.0015939

Chen, L., Pan, H., Bai, Y., Li, H., Yang, W., Lin, Z. X., et al. (2020). Gelsemine, a Natural Alkaloid Extracted from Gelsemium Elegans Benth. Alleviates Neuroinflammation and Cognitive Impairments in Aβ Oligomer-Treated Mice. *Psychopharmacology (Berl)* 237 (7), 2111–2124. doi:10.1007/s00213-020-05522-y

Chen, S. P., Zhou, Y. Q., Liu, D. Q., Zhang, W., Manyande, A., Guan, X. H., et al. (2017). PI3K/Akt Pathway: A Potential Therapeutic Target for Chronic Pain. *Curr. Pharm. Des.* 23 (12), 1860–1868. doi:10.2174/1381612823666170210150147

Cohen, S. P., and Mao, J. (2014). Neuropathic Pain: Mechanisms and Their Clinical Implications. *BMJ (Clinical research ed)* 348, f7656. doi:10.1136/bmj.f7656

Cury, Y., Picolo, G., Gutierrez, V. P., and Ferreira, S. H. (2011). Pain and Analgesia: The Dual Effect of Nitric Oxide in the Nociceptive System. *Nitric Oxide* 25 (3), 243–254. doi:10.1016/j.niox.2011.06.004

Daina, A., Michielin, O., and Zoete, V. (2017). SwissADME: A Free Web Tool to Evaluate Pharmacokinetics, Drug-Likeness and Medicinal Chemistry Friendliness of Small Molecules. *Sci. Rep.* 7, 42717. doi:10.1038/srep42717

Dennis, G., Jr., Sherman, B. T., Hosack, D. A., Yang, J., Gao, W., Lane, H. C., et al. (2003). DAVID: Database for Annotation, Visualization, and Integrated Discovery. *Genome Biol.* 4 (5), R60. doi:10.1186/gb-2003-4-5-p3

Dworkin, R. H., O'Connor, A. B., Backonja, M., Farrar, J. T., Finnerup, N. B., Jensen, T. S., et al. (2007). Pharmacologic Management of Neuropathic Pain: Evidence-Based Recommendations. *Pain* 132 (3), 237–251. doi:10.1016/j.pain.2007.08.033

Ferreira, L. G., Dos Santos, R. N., Oliva, G., and Andricopulo, A. D. (2015). Molecular Docking and Structure-Based Drug Design Strategies. *Molecules* 20 (7), 13384–13421. doi:10.3390/molecules200713384

Gao, Y. J., Zhang, L., Samad, O. A., Suter, M. R., Yasuhiko, K., Xu, Z. Z., et al. (2009). JNK-induced MCP-1 Production in Spinal Cord Astrocytes Contributes to central Sensitization and Neuropathic Pain. *J. Neurosci.* 29 (13), 4096–4108. doi:10.1523/jneurosci.3623-08.2009

Gfeller, D., Grosdidier, A., Wirth, M., Daina, A., Michielin, O., and Zoete, V. (2014). SwissTargetPrediction: A Web Server for Target Prediction of Bioactive Small Molecules. *Nucleic Acids Res.* 42, W32–W38. doi:10.1093/nar/gku293

Hargreaves, K., Dubner, R., Brown, F., Flores, C., and Joris, J. (1988). A New and Sensitive Method for Measuring thermal Nociception in Cutaneous Hyperalgesia. *Pain* 32 (1), 77–88. doi:10.1016/0304-3959(88)90026-7

Huang, C.-Y., Yang, K., Cao, J.-J., Wang, Z.-Y., Wu, Y., Sun, Z.-L., et al. (2021). Integration of Metabolomics and Transcriptomicsto Comprehensively Evaluate the Metabolic Effects of Gelsemium Elegans on Pigs. *Animals* 11 (5), 1192. doi:10.3390/ani11051192

Huang, L., Xie, D., Yu, Y., Liu, H., Shi, Y., Shi, T., et al. (2018). TCMID 2.0: A Comprehensive Resource for TCM. *Nucleic Acids Res.* 46 (D1), D1117–d20. doi:10.1093/nar/gkx1028

Hung, A. L., Lim, M., and Doshi, T. L. (2017). Targeting Cytokines for Treatment of Neuropathic Pain. *Scand. J. Pain* 17, 287–293. doi:10.1016/j.sjpain.2017.08.002

Jensen, T. S., Baron, R., Haanpää, M., Kalso, E., Loeser, J. D., Rice, A. S., et al. (2011). A New Definition of Neuropathic Pain. *Pain* 152 (10), 2204–2205. doi:10.1016/j.pain.2011.06.017

Ji, R. R., Gereau, R. W., Malcangio, M., and Strichartz, G. R. (2009). MAP Kinase and Pain. *Brain Res. Rev.* 60 (1), 135–148. doi:10.1016/j.brainresrev.2008.12.011

Jin, G. L., He, S. D., Lin, S. M., Hong, L. M., Chen, W. Q., Xu, Y., et al. (2018). Koumine Attenuates Neuroglia Activation and Inflammatory Response to Neuropathic Pain. *Neural Plast.* 2018, 9347696. doi:10.1155/2018/9347696

Jin, G. L., Su, Y. P., Liu, M., Xu, Y., Yang, J., Liao, K. J., et al. (2014). Medicinal Plants of the Genus Gelsemium (Gelsemiaceae, Gentianales)-Aa Review of Their Phytochemistry, Pharmacology, Toxicology and Traditional Use. *J. Ethnopharmacol* 152 (1), 33–52. doi:10.1016/j.jep.2014.01.003

Jin, G. L., Yue, R. C., He, S. D., Hong, L. M., Xu, Y., and Yu, C. X. (2018). Koumine Decreases Astrocyte-Mediated Neuroinflammation and Enhances Autophagy, Contributing to Neuropathic Pain from Chronic Constriction Injury in Rats. *Front. Pharmacol.* 9, 989. doi:10.3389/fphar.2018.00989

Kersten, C., Cameron, M. G., Bailey, A. G., Fallon, M. T., Laird, B. J., Paterson, V., et al. (2019). Relief of Neuropathic Pain through Epidermal Growth Factor Receptor Inhibition: A Randomized Proof-Of-Concept Trial. *Pain Med.* 20 (12), 2495–2505. doi:10.1093/pm/pnz101

Kersten, C., Cameron, M. G., Laird, B., and Mjåland, S. (2015). Epidermal Growth Factor Receptor-Inhibition (EGFR-I) in the Treatment of Neuropathic Pain. *Br. J. Anaesth.* 115 (5), 761–767. doi:10.1093/bja/aev326

Kim, Y. C., Castañeda, A. M., Lee, C. S., Jin, H. S., Park, K. S., and Moon, J. Y. (2018). Efficacy and Safety of Lidocaine Infusion Treatment for Neuropathic Pain: a Randomized, Double-Blind, and Placebo-Controlled Study. *Reg. Anesth. Pain Med.* 43 (4), 415–424. doi:10.1097/aap.0000000000000741

Li, H., Xie, S., Qi, Y., Li, H., Zhang, R., and Lian, Y. (2018). TNF-α Increases the Expression of Inflammatory Factors in Synovial Fibroblasts by Inhibiting the PI3K/AKT Pathway in a Rat Model of Monosodium Iodoacetate-Induced Osteoarthritis. *Exp. Ther. Med.* 16 (6), 4737–4744. doi:10.3892/etm.2018.6770

Li, S., and Zhang, B. (2013). Traditional Chinese Medicine Network Pharmacology: Theory, Methodology and Application. *Chin. J. Nat. Med.* 11 (2), 110–120. doi:10.1016/s1875-5364(13)60037-0

Lin, H., Qiu, H., Cheng, Y., Liu, M., Chen, M., Que, Y., et al. (2021). *Gelsemium Elegans* Benth: Chemical Components, Pharmacological Effects, and Toxicity Mechanisms. *Molecules* 26 (23), 7145. doi:10.3390/molecules26237145

Liu, B., Chen, H., Johns, T. G., and Neufeld, A. H. (2006). Epidermal Growth Factor Receptor Activation: an Upstream Signal for Transition of Quiescent Astrocytes into Reactive Astrocytes after Neural Injury. *J. Neurosci.* 26 (28), 7532–7540. doi:10.1523/JNEUROSCI.1004-06.2006

Liu, M., Shen, J., Liu, H., Xu, Y., Su, Y. P., Yang, J., et al. (2011). Gelsenicine from *Gelsemium Elegans* Attenuates Neuropathic and Inflammatory Pain in Mice. *Biol. Pharm. Bull.* 34 (12), 1877–1880. doi:10.1248/bpb.34.1877

Liu, Z., Guo, F., Wang, Y., Li, C., Zhang, X., Li, H., et al. (2016). BATMAN-TCM: A Bioinformatics Analysis Tool for Molecular Mechanism of Traditional Chinese Medicine. *Sci. Rep.* 6, 21146. doi:10.1038/srep21146

Lunn, M. P., Hughes, R. A., and Wiffen, P. J. (2014). Duloxetine for Treating Painful Neuropathy, Chronic Pain or Fibromyalgia. *Cochrane Database Syst. Rev.* 1 (1), Cd007115. doi:10.1002/14651858.CD007115.pub3

Luo, Y., Xiong, B., Liu, H., Chen, Z., Huang, H., Yu, C., et al. (2020). Koumine Suppresses IL-1β Secretion and Attenuates Inflammation Associated with Blocking ROS/NF-κB/NLRP3 Axis in Macrophages. *Front. Pharmacol.* 11, 622074. doi:10.3389/fphar.2020.622074

Mitrirattanakul, S., Ramakul, N., Guerrero, A. V., Matsuka, Y., Ono, T., Iwase, H., et al. (2006). Site-Specific Increases in Peripheral Cannabinoid Receptors and Their Endogenous Ligands in a Model of Neuropathic Pain. *Pain* 126 (1-3), 102–114. doi:10.1016/j.pain.2006.06.016

Moore, J., and Gaines, C. (2019). Gabapentin for Chronic Neuropathic Pain in Adults. *Br. J. Community Nurs.* 24 (12), 608–609. doi:10.12968/bjcn.2019.24.12.608

Neto, E., Alves, C. J., Leitão, L., Sousa, D. M., Alencastre, I. S., Conceição, F., et al. (2017). Axonal Outgrowth, Neuropeptides Expression and Receptors Tyrosine Kinase Phosphorylation in 3D Organotypic Cultures of Adult Dorsal Root Ganglia. *PloS one* 12 (7), e0181612. doi:10.1371/journal.pone.0181612

Qiu, H. Q., Xu, Y., Jin, G. L., Yang, J., Liu, M., Li, S. P., et al. (2015). Koumine Enhances Spinal Cord 3α-Hydroxysteroid Oxidoreductase Expression and Activity in a Rat Model of Neuropathic Pain. *Mol. Pain* 11, 46. doi:10.1186/s12990-015-0050-1

Rujjanawate, C., Kanjanapothi, D., and Panthong, A. (2003). Pharmacological Effect and Toxicity of Alkaloids from *Gelsemium Elegans* Benth. *J. Ethnopharmacol* 89 (1), 91–95. doi:10.1016/s0378-8741(03)00267-8

Safran, M., Dalah, I., Alexander, J., Rosen, N., Iny Stein, T., Shmoish, M., et al. (2010). GeneCards Version 3: the Human Gene Integrator. *Database* 2010, baq020. doi:10.1093/database/baq020

Schäfers, M., Svensson, C. I., Sommer, C., and Sorkin, L. S. (2003). Tumor Necrosis Factor-Alpha Induces Mechanical Allodynia after Spinal Nerve Ligation by Activation of P38 MAPK in Primary Sensory Neurons. *J. Neurosci.* 23 (7), 2517–2521. doi:10.1523/jneurosci.23-07-02517.2003

Schüle, C., Romeo, E., Uzunov, D. P., Eser, D., di Michele, F., Baghai, T. C., et al. (2006). Influence of Mirtazapine on Plasma Concentrations of Neuroactive Steroids in Major Depression and on 3alpha-Hydroxysteroid Dehydrogenase Activity. *Mol. Psychiatry* 11 (3), 261–272. doi:10.1038/sj.mp.4001782

Shannon, P., Markiel, A., Ozier, O., Baliga, N. S., Wang, J. T., Ramage, D., et al. (2003). Cytoscape: A Software Environment for Integrated Models of Biomolecular Interaction Networks. *Genome Res.* 13 (11), 2498–2504. doi:10.1101/gr.1239303

Simon, L. S., Taylor, P. C., Choy, E. H., Sebba, A., Quebe, A., Knopp, K. L., et al. (2021). The Jak/STAT Pathway: A Focus on Pain in Rheumatoid Arthritis. *Semin. Arthritis Rheum.* 51 (1), 278–284. doi:10.1016/j.semarthrit.2020.10.008

Smith, S. S. (1994). Female Sex Steroid Hormones: from Receptors to Networks to Performance-Aactions on the Sensorimotor System. *Prog. Neurobiol.* 44 (1), 55–86. doi:10.1016/0301-0082(94)90057-4

Sommer, C., Klose, P., Welsch, P., Petzke, F., and Häuser, W. (2020). Opioids for Chronic Non-Cancer Neuropathic Pain. An Updated Systematic Review and Meta-Analysis of Efficacy, Tolerability and Safety in Randomized Placebo-Controlled Studies of at Least 4 Weeks Duration. *Eur. J. Pain* 24 (1), 3–18. doi:10.1002/ejp.1494

Su, Y. P., Shen, J., Xu, Y., Zheng, M., and Yu, C. X. (2011). Preparative Separation of Alkaloids from *Gelsemium Elegans* Benth. Using pH-Zone-Refining Counter-current Chromatography. *J. Chromatogr. A.* 1218 (23), 3695–3698. doi:10.1016/j.chroma.2011.04.025

Sun, R. Q., Tu, Y. J., Yan, J. Y., and Willis, W. D. (2006). Activation of Protein Kinase B/Akt Signaling Pathway Contributes to Mechanical Hypersensitivity Induced by Capsaicin. *Pain* 120 (1-2), 86–96. doi:10.1016/j.pain.2005.10.017

Szklarczyk, D., Gable, A. L., Lyon, D., Junge, A., Wyder, S., Huerta-Cepas, J., et al. (2019). STRING V11: Protein-Protein Association Networks with Increased Coverage, Supporting Functional Discovery in Genome-Wide Experimental Datasets. *Nucleic Acids Res.* 47 (D1), D607–d13. doi:10.1093/nar/gky1131

Tao, F., Li, Q., Liu, S., Wu, H., Skinner, J., Hurtado, A., et al. (2013). Role of neuregulin-1/ErbB Signaling in Stem Cell Therapy for Spinal Cord Injury-Induced Chronic Neuropathic Pain. *Stem Cells* 31 (1), 83–91. doi:10.1002/stem.1258

van Hecke, O., Austin, S. K., Khan, R. A., Smith, B. H., and Torrance, N. (2014). Neuropathic Pain in the General Population: A Systematic Review of Epidemiological Studies. *Pain* 155 (4), 654–662. doi:10.1016/j.pain.2013.11.013

van Nooten, F., Treur, M., Pantiri, K., Stoker, M., and Charokopou, M. (2017). Capsaicin 8% Patch versus Oral Neuropathic Pain Medications for the Treatment of Painful Diabetic Peripheral Neuropathy: a Systematic Literature Review and Network Meta-Analysis. *Clin. Ther.* 39 (4), 787–e18. doi:10.1016/j.clinthera.2017.02.010

Vos, T., Flaxman, A. D., Naghavi, M., Lozano, R., Michaud, C., Ezzati, M., et al. (2012). Years Lived with Disability (YLDs) for 1160 Sequelae of 289 Diseases and Injuries 1990-2010: a Systematic Analysis for the Global Burden of Disease Study 2010. *Lancet* 380 (9859), 2163–2196. doi:10.1016/s0140-6736(12)61729-2

Wang, J., Cheng, J., Zhang, C., and Li, X. (2017). Cardioprotection Effects of Sevoflurane by Regulating the Pathway of Neuroactive Ligand-Receptor Interaction in Patients Undergoing Coronary Artery Bypass Graft Surgery. *Comput. Math. Methods Med.* 2017, 3618213. doi:10.1155/2017/3618213

Wang, L., Zhu, K., Yang, B., and Cai, Y. (2020). Knockdown of Linc00052 Alleviated Spinal Nerve Ligation-Triggered Neuropathic Pain through Regulating miR-448 and JAK1. *J. Cel Physiol* 235 (10), 6528–6535. doi:10.1002/jcp.29465

Wang, Y., Zhang, S., Li, F., Zhou, Y., Zhang, Y., Wang, Z., et al. (2020). Therapeutic Target Database 2020: Enriched Resource for Facilitating Research and Early Development of Targeted Therapeutics. *Nucleic Acids Res.* 48 (D1), D1031–d41. doi:10.1093/nar/gkz981

Watkins, L. R., Milligan, E. D., and Maier, S. F. (2003). Glial Proinflammatory Cytokines Mediate Exaggerated Pain States: Implications for Clinical Pain. *Adv. Exp. Med. Biol.* 521, 1–21. doi:10.0000/pmid12617561

Wishart, D. S., Feunang, Y. D., Guo, A. C., Lo, E. J., Marcu, A., Grant, J. R., et al. (2018). DrugBank 5.0: A Major Update to the DrugBank Database for 2018. *Nucleic Acids Res.* 46 (D1), D1074–d82. doi:10.1093/nar/gkx1037

Wu, J., Yang, C. L., Sha, Y. K., Wu, Y., Liu, Z. Y., Yuan, Z. H., et al. (2020). Koumine Alleviates Lipopolysaccharide-Induced Intestinal Barrier Dysfunction in IPEC-J2 Cells by Regulating Nrf2/NF-Kb Pathway. *Am. J. Chin. Med.* 48 (1), 127–142. doi:10.1142/s0192415x2050007x

Wu, Y. E., Li, Y. D., Luo, Y. J., Wang, T. X., Wang, H. J., Chen, S. N., et al. (2015). Gelsemine Alleviates Both Neuropathic Pain and Sleep Disturbance in Partial Sciatic Nerve Ligation Mice. *Acta Pharmacol. Sin* 36 (11), 1308–1317. doi:10.1038/aps.2015.86

Xu, Y., Qiu, H. Q., Liu, H., Liu, M., Huang, Z. Y., Yang, J., et al. (2012). Effects of Koumine, an Alkaloid of *Gelsemium Elegans* Benth., on Inflammatory and Neuropathic Pain Models and Possible Mechanism with Allopregnanolone. *Pharmacol. Biochem. Behav.* 101 (3), 504–514. doi:10.1016/j.pbb.2012.02.009

Xun, S., and Zheng, R. (2020). Dexmedetomidine Alleviates Neuropathic Pain by Regulating JAK/STAT Pathway in Rats. *J. Cel Biochem* 121 (3), 2277–2283. doi:10.1002/jcb.29450

Yuan, Z., Liang, Z., Yi, J., Chen, X., Li, R., Wu, J., et al. (2019). Koumine Promotes ROS Production to Suppress Hepatocellular Carcinoma Cell Proliferation via NF-Kb and ERK/p38 MAPK Signaling. *Biomolecules* 9 (10), 559. doi:10.3390/biom9100559

Yuan, Z., Matias, F. B., Wu, J., Liang, Z., and Sun, Z. (2016). Koumine Attenuates Lipopolysaccharide-Stimulated Inflammation in RAW264.7 Macrophages, Coincidentally Associated with Inhibition of NF-Kb, ERK and P38 Pathways. *Int. J. Mol. Sci.* 17 (3), 430. doi:10.3390/ijms17030430

Zhang, J. M., and An, J. (2007). Cytokines, Inflammation, and Pain. *Int. Anesthesiol Clin.* 45 (2), 27–37. doi:10.1097/AIA.0b013e318034194e

Zhang, J. M., Li, H., Liu, B., and Brull, S. J. (2002). Acute Topical Application of Tumor Necrosis Factor Alpha Evokes Protein Kinase A-dependent Responses in Rat Sensory Neurons. *J. Neurophysiol.* 88 (3), 1387–1392. doi:10.1152/jn.2002.88.3.1387

Zhang, J. Y., Gong, N., Huang, J. L., Guo, L. C., and Wang, Y. X. (2013). Gelsemine, a Principal Alkaloid from Gelsemium Sempervirens Ait., Exhibits Potent and Specific Antinociception in Chronic Pain by Acting at Spinal α3 glycine Receptors. *Pain* 154 (11), 2452–2462. doi:10.1016/j.pain.2013.07.027

Zhang, J. Y., and Wang, Y. X. (2015). Gelsemium Analgesia and the Spinal glycine Receptor/allopregnanolone Pathway. *Fitoterapia* 100, 35–43. doi:10.1016/j.fitote.2014.11.002

Zhuang, Z. Y., Wen, Y. R., Zhang, D. R., Borsello, T., Bonny, C., Strichartz, G. R., et al. (2006). A Peptide C-Jun N-Terminal Kinase (JNK) Inhibitor Blocks Mechanical Allodynia after Spinal Nerve Ligation: Respective Roles of JNK Activation in Primary Sensory Neurons and Spinal Astrocytes for Neuropathic Pain Development and Maintenance. *J. Neurosci.* 26 (13), 3551–3560. doi:10.1523/jneurosci.5290-05.2006

15

Transcriptomic Validation of the Protective Effects of Aqueous Bark Extract of *Terminalia arjuna* (Roxb.) on Isoproterenol-Induced Cardiac Hypertrophy in Rats

Gaurav Kumar[1], Nikhat Saleem[1], Santosh Kumar[1†], Subir K. Maulik[2], Sayeed Ahmad[3], Manish Sharma[4] and Shyamal K. Goswami[1]*

[1] School of Life Sciences, Jawaharlal Nehru University, New Delhi, India, [2] Department of Pharmacology, All India Institute of Medical Sciences (A.I.I.M.S.), New Delhi, India, [3] Bioactive Natural Product Laboratory, Department of Pharmacognosy & Phytochemistry, School of Pharmaceutical Education & Research, New Delhi, India, [4] Peptide and Proteomics Division, Defence Institute of Physiology and Allied Sciences (DIPAS), Defence Research and Development Organisation, New Delhi, India

***Correspondence:**
Shyamal K. Goswami
skgoswami@mail.jnu.ac.in

Aqueous extract of the bark of *Terminalia arjuna* (TA) is used by a large population in the Indian subcontinent for treating various cardiovascular conditions. Animal experiments have shown its anti-atherogenic, anti-hypertensive, and anti-inflammatory effects. It has several bioactive ingredients with hemodynamic, ROS scavenging, and anti-inflammatory properties. Earlier we have done limited proteomic and transcriptomic analysis to show its efficacy in ameliorating cardiac hypertrophy induced by isoproterenol (ISO) in rats. In the present study we have used high-throughput sequencing of the mRNA from control and treated rat heart to further establish its efficacy. ISO (5 mg/kg/day s.c.) was administered in male adult rats for 14 days to induce cardiac hypertrophy. Standardized aqueous extract TA bark extract was administered orally. Total RNA were isolated from control, ISO, ISO + TA, and TA treated rat hearts and subjected to high throughput sequence analysis. The modulations of the transcript levels were then subjected to bio-informatics analyses using established software. Treatment with ISO downregulated 1,129 genes and upregulated 204 others. Pre-treatment with the TA bark extracts markedly restored that expression pattern with only 97 genes upregulated and 85 genes downregulated. The TA alone group had only 88 upregulated and 26 downregulated genes. The overall profile of expression in ISO + TA and TA alone groups closely matched with the control group. The genes that were modulated included those involved in metabolism, activation of receptors and cell signaling, and cardiovascular and other diseases. Networks associated with those genes included those involved in angiogenesis, extracellular matrix organization, integrin binding, inflammation, drug metabolism, redox metabolism, oxidative phosphorylation, and organization of myofibril. Overlaying of the networks in ISO and ISO_TA group showed that those activated in ISO group were mostly absent in ISO_TA and TA group, suggesting a global effect of the TA extracts. This study for the first time reveals that TA partially or completely restores the gene regulatory network perturbed by ISO treatment in rat heart; signifying its efficacy in checking ISO-induced cardiac hypertrophy.

Keywords: ***Terminalia arjuna*, cardiac hypertrophy, heart failure, transcriptomics, biological network**

INTRODUCTION

Pathological cardiac hypertrophy (CH) is a major risk factor for heart failure and mortality worldwide. It is characterized by an increase in length and breadth of the cardiac myocytes in association with other physiological/biochemical changes affecting myocardial blood flow, diastolic function, and diminished cardiac output (Shimizu and Minamino, 2016). Being multifactorial in nature, CH is characterized by fibrosis, pro-inflammatory milieu, autophagy, apoptosis, oxidative stress, altered mechanotransduction, and mitochondrial energetics etc. (Marian and Braunwald, 2017; Nakamura and Sadoshima, 2018). At the molecular level, CH is often associated with an extensive re-programing of gene expression in the heart (Raghow, 2016). Such extensive alterations in cardiac functions is presumably not caused due to the perturbation of a single pathway, but rather a cumulative alteration of many signaling modules including cAMP, PKA, PLC, MAPK, PI3K/Akt, m-TOR etc. (Liu and Molkentin, 2016; Wang and Cai, 2017; Gibb and Hill, 2018; Sciarretta et al., 2018). While these signaling networks are highly interactive and complex, the categorical goal of pharmacological science is to target the nodal points and the effectors (Walters et al., 2016; Philipson et al., 2017).

However, the current treatment option available for CH is limited to few drugs like β-blockers, ACE inhibitors, and angiotensin receptor blockers (Talan et al., 2011; Soliman and Prineas, 2017). Although these drugs are being used worldwide for managing CH, they are also associated with various side effects and their efficacy depends upon several variables including pharmacogenomics (Lainscak et al., 2016; Takezako et al., 2017).

In pursuit of finding novel therapy of CH and heart failure, various natural product based preparations are also empirically used due to the evidences of their efficacy, minimal side effects, affordability, and wide acceptability, especially for the people beyond the western hemisphere (Van Galen, 2014; Rastogi et al., 2016). A number of traditional Chinese medicines like QSYQ and Danshensu (*Salvia miltiorrhiza*) have shown cardio-protective effect in many experimental sets up (Zhu et al., 2016; Hao et al., 2017; Layne and Ferro, 2017).

One major impediment of testing the efficacy of phytochemicals in ameliorating diseases is the difficulty in identifying the active ingredient(s) from a complex mixture of bioactive molecules and their targets of actions. While the first can be addressed by standardization of the extracts used in various assays, the latter issue is more complex and ambiguous. It is now acknowledged that the ingredients of many Ayurvedic preparations, traditional Chinese medicines, and even modern pharmacological agents show synergistic as well as antagonistic effects when added together (Zegpi et al., 2009; Parasuraman et al., 2014; Zhang et al., 2014). Therefore, it is more prudent to test the Ayurvedic formulations as the practitioners use it. However, applications of the modern tools of genomics and proteomics that are broad based, quantitative, and largely unbiased, can help us establish the efficacy of phytomedicines in a more unambiguous manner.

In the Indian subcontinent, the stem barks powder of *Terminalia arjuna* (Roxb.) (TA) has been in use as a cardioprotective agent for centuries by Indian system of medicine (Ayurveda) (Mongalo et al., 2016; Amalraj and Gopi, 2017). Studies done in our laboratory have shown that the bark extract of TA has beneficial effects in experimentally induced myocardial ischemia, hypertrophy, fibrosis, and other cardiovascular disorders. It boosts anti-oxidant activities, prevents fibrosis, protects against ischemia reperfusion injury and has anti-hypotensive effects (Kumar et al., 2009; Maulik and Katiyar, 2010; Maulik et al., 2016; Meghwani et al., 2017). In a recent study, arjunolic acid, one of the constituents of the aqueous TA extract, was shown to ameliorate cardiac fibrosis by inhibiting TGF-β signaling (Bansal et al., 2017). Earlier, we had used limited proteomic approach (2D gel based) to establish that TA bark extract substantially modulates the rat cardiac proteome under adrenergic (ISO) stress (Kumar et al., 2017). To further establish the efficacy of TA extract we now have used more robust approach that is global transcriptomic analyses to establish the efficacy of TA extract in modulating various biological pathways and gene networks targeted by ISO. We demonstrate that TA extract reverses ISO induced reprogramming of gene expression in rat heart. Our study for the first time convincingly establishes that the effects of TA are far wider than that is expected for a modern drug usually having a single target.

MATERIALS AND METHODS

Animal Experiments and Ethics Statement

Laboratory bred Wistar male rats (150–200 g, 10–12 weeks) were employed for the study and maintained under standard laboratory conditions (temperature; 25°C ± 2°C, relative humidity; 50% ± 15% and 12-h dark/12-h light period). The study was conducted in accordance with the Institutional Animal Ethics Committee, All India Institute of Medical Sciences, New Delhi, India. All animal care and experimental protocols were performed in compliance with the National Institutes of Health (NIH) Guidelines for the Care and Use of Laboratory Animals (NIH Publication no. 85723, revised 1996).

TA Extract

The material under investigation is a standardized aqueous extract of the bark of TA (made available to us from the Dabur

Research Foundation, Ghaziabad, India). It has been is prepared by extraction as per the literatures of Ayurveda against its traditional claims and as it has been extensively used in the Indian System of Medicine for centuries. For its scientific validation, the extract has been standardized by the fingerprinting using UPLC. All the separated metabolites of the extract have also been characterized by metabolomic profiling using UPLC high resolution mass spectrometry which separated 26 compounds at different Rt with different molecular masses (**Supplemental Figures S1A, B**). The major peaks obtained were at Rt 8.01, 7.80, and at 7.53 with m/z 510.26, 893.46, and 488.25 respectively (**Supplemental Figure S1C**). The major peak at Rt 7.80 was identified as Arjunolic acid with m/z 488.25 (**Supplemental Figure S1D**) which is main marker compound of Arjuna (Kumar et al., 2017).

Administration of TA Extract

The animals were randomly divided into four groups according to drug treatment with5 animals in each group. The groups consisted of control, ISO + saline, ISO_TA, and TA alone. In control group the animals were administered normal saline, 1.0 ml/kg body weight, s.c. once daily for 14 days. In ISO + saline group, rats received both ISO, 5.0 mg/kg body weight s.c. once daily followed by normal saline, 1 ml/kg body weight, orally once daily for 14 days. In the group designated with ISO_TA, rats were administered with ISO, 5.0 mg/kg body weight, s.c. once daily along with the aqueous extract of TA, 125.0 mg/kg body weight, orally once daily for 14 days. In TA group, aqueous extract of TA, 125.0 mg/kg body weight, was administered orally once daily for 14 days. Lyophilized powder of aqueous extract of TA stem bark and ISO was freshly prepared in double distilled water before use.

RNA Isolation

The rats were sacrificed at the end of treatment and the hearts were carefully excised followed by snap freezing at −80°C. The tissues samples from five animals were pooled for each group and total RNA was isolated utilizing TRI Reagent (Sigma Aldrich) as per manufacturer's instructions. The integrity of RNA was checked on 0.8% formaldehyde agarose gel and further purified for gene expression experiments employing RNeasy Mini Kit (Qiagen, Hilden, Germany) with on-column DNAase digestion.

RNA Sequencing

Library Preparation and Sequencing

The respective cDNA libraries were prepared using TruSeq mRNA Sample Prep Kit (Illumina, Inc), as per manufacturer's instructions. Poly-A tail containing mRNA molecules were purified using oligo-dT attached magnetic beads (Illumina, Inc) using two rounds of purification. Purified mRNA were subjected to fragmentation, reverse transcription, end repair, 3′- end adenylation, and adaptor ligation, followed by PCR amplification and bead purification. The unique barcode sequences were incorporated in the adaptors for multiplexed high-throughput sequencing. The final product was assessed for its distribution of size and concentration using 2100 Bioanalyzer (Agilent Technologies), followed by cluster generation and sequencing on HiSeq 2000.

Read Filtering, Processing, and Alignment

The mRNA-Seq reads were aligned to the rat reference genome (downloaded from UCSC) utilizing "Bowtie 2" and "TopHat" as per published method (Langmead and Salzberg, 2012; Ghosh and Chan, 2016). The mapped reads were subsequently fed as input to "Cufflinks" (Langmead and Salzberg, 2012). The assembly files so generated were merged into a unified annotation with the reference transcriptome annotation for further analysis. The merged annotations were quantified using "Cuffdiff" to identify differentially expressed genes (Langmead and Salzberg, 2012). The "FPKM" (fragments per kilobase of transcript per million fragments) parameter was used to quantitate abundance of the transcripts (Li et al., 2017).

Bioinformatics Analysis

Gene Ontology, Pathway Mining, Functional Annotation Clustering was done utilizing various data mining tools. David Bioinformatics resources, which use a previously published gene, list to statistically highlight the most overrepresented (enriched) biological annotation viz., Gene Ontology Terms (Huang et al., 2007; Xing et al., 2016). GeneMANIA, a Cytoscape plug-in were further used for data analysis (Montojo et al., 2010).GeneMANIA, was used to place the data obtained in a functional context and represent it as degree sorted circular view of key networks of statistically significant biological processes. The GeneMANIA integrates association networks from multiple sources into a single composite network using a conjugate gradient optimization algorithm.

RESULTS

Treatment With TA Extracts Blunts the Activated β-Adrenergic Signalling In Heart

In order to understand the molecular mechanisms of cardioprotection by the TA extracts, we analyzed its effects on the overall signatures of β-adrenergic stimulation in rat heart. Rats were injected with ISO (5 mg/kg, once daily, s.c.) and fed with the aqueous TA extract (125 mg/kg, once daily, orally). After 28 days of treatment, the animals were sacrificed and the effects of TA treatment were confirmed at the gross morphological level by weighing the hearts. In reiteration of our previous reports (Kumar et al, 2017), while ISO treatment resulted in an increase in heart to body weight ratio, TA extracts reversed it significantly. As expected, TA alone had no effect on heart to body weight ratio (**Supplemental Figure S2**).

To determine molecular basis of the effects of TA on ISO treatment, we performed RNA sequence based differential gene expression analyses. This is a state of the art technology with tremendous potential for revealing multiple molecular cues associated with diseases and their amelioration by the drugs (Doostparast Torshizi and Wang, 2018). A schematic presentation of the experiment pipeline is shown in **Figure 1A**.

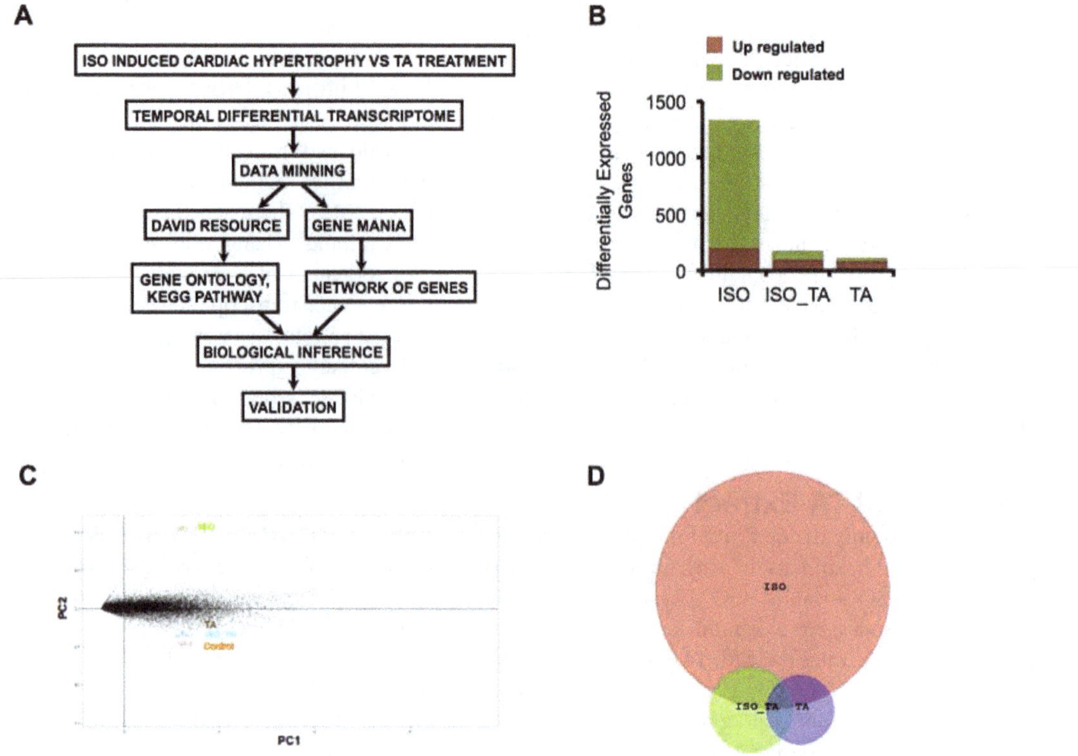

FIGURE 1 | (A) Scheme of data mining workflow for analyzing the transcriptome data. **(B)** The bar graph indicates the number of upregulated and downregulated gene in each condition. **(C)** Principal component analysis (PCA) of gene expression data sets from all three groups represented as two-dimensional plot of PC1 (Component 1) and PC2 (Component 2). **(D)** Venn Diagram representing overlap of differentially expressed Genes in ISO, ISO_TA, and TA groups. (Groups: ISO = ISO treated, ISO_TA = ISO + *T. arjuna* treated, TA, *T. arjuna* treated).

The overall number of differentially expressed genes in all the groups is represented as a bar plot in **Figure 1B** and differentially expressed genes in each group along with log2 fold change are tabulated (**Supplemental Tables S1, S2,** and **S3**). As expected, treatment with ISO generated a wide response with 1,333 genes differentially expressed of which 1,129 were downregulated and 204 were upregulated. In striking contrast, pretreatment of animals with the aqueous TA bark extracts led to a marked reduction of this expression signature, with only 97 genes upregulated and 85 genes downregulated. The TA alone group consisted of 88 upregulated and 26 downregulated genes. Notably, when we subjected the genes modulated by all the groups in principal component analysis, we observed ISO_TA and TA alone groups clustered closely with control group while the ISO group was distinctively separated from this cluster (**Figure 1C**). This analyses showing higher similarity between control, ISO_TA, and TA alone groups thus reiterates our early report that TA suppresses the responses induced by ISO treatment (Kumar et al, 2017). Finally, the intersection of differentially expressed genes between ISO, ISO_TA, and TA group is shown in **Figure 1D**. It is evident from the data that a large number of genes which were induced in ISO group, are missing from the ISO_TA group. Taken together, these results indicate that there are unique gene expression signatures for all groups of animals treated with ISO, TA, or both.

TA Treatment Reverses the Metabolic Reprogramming Induced by ISO Treatment

To elucidate a discernible reversal of ISO-induced differential gene expression pattern by TA, we analyzed the repertoire of regulated genes in different treatment groups using various data mining strategies. We first used "DAVID bioinformatics resources" for systematic and integrative analysis of large data set and extracted key biological pathways (KEGG) that were significantly ($p < 0.1$) regulated. As shown in **Figure 2A** and **Table 1**, the pathways that are downregulated in ISO treated group includes those involved in the metabolism of carbohydrates (71 genes), fatty acids (40 genes), amino acids (34 genes), and nucleic acids (30 genes); receptor activation and cell signaling (105 genes); and cardiovascular and other diseases (160 genes). As shown in **Figure 2A**, among the 71 unique genes involved in carbohydrate metabolism were those associated with glycolysis and gluconeogenesis (Bar A: 15 genes); metabolism of starch and sucrose (Bar B: 10 genes), fructose and mannose (Bar C: six genes), and galactose (Bar D: six genes); TCA cycle (Bar E: 19 genes), pyruvate metabolism (Bar F: 15 genes); pentose phosphate pathway (Bar G: five genes); metabolism of mannose, glyoxylate, and dicarboxylate (Bar H: five genes); and oxidative phosphorylation (Bar I: 28 genes). Similarly, 40 downregulated genes involved in fatty acid metabolism included those associated

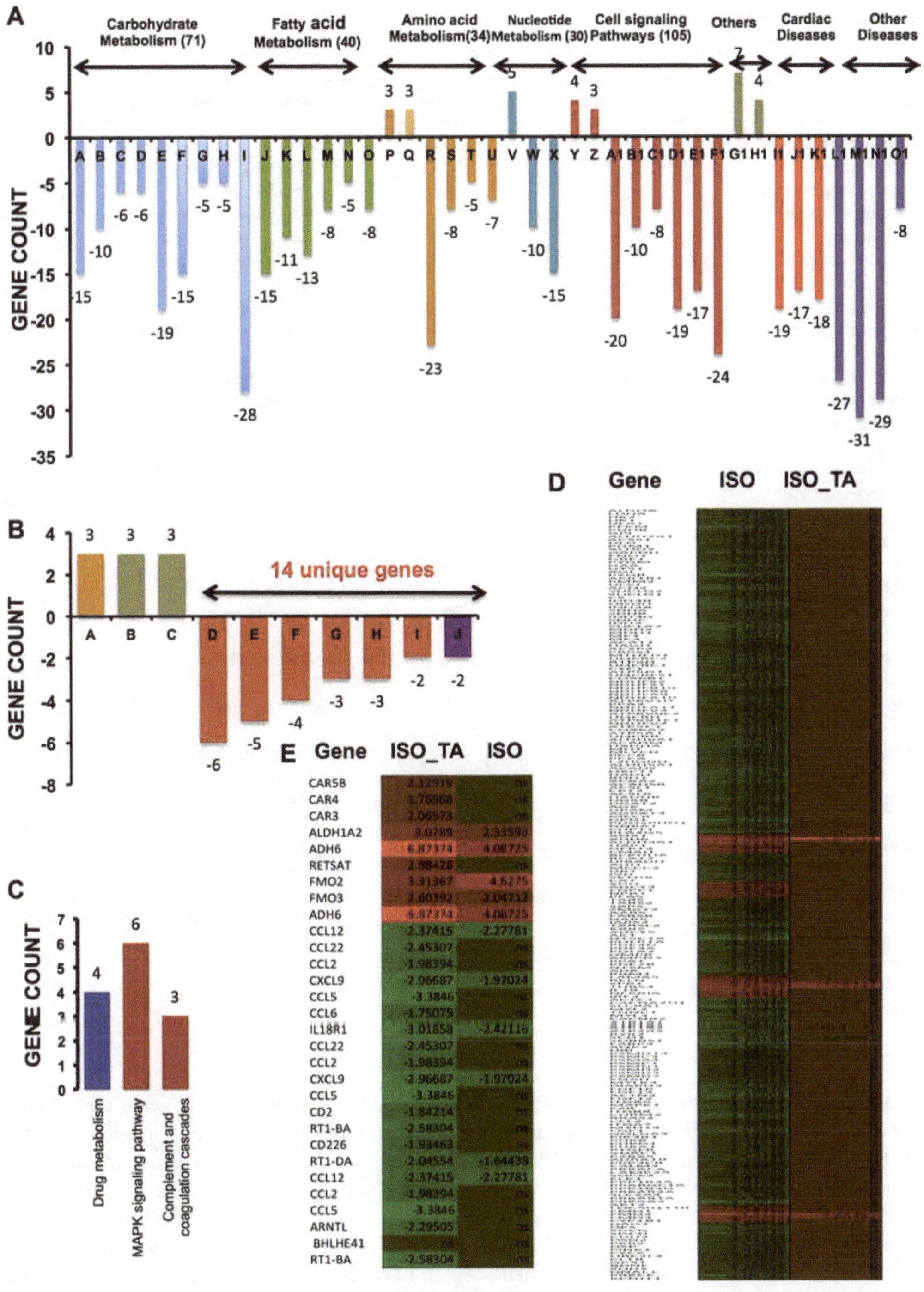

FIGURE 2 | KEGG pathways significantly enriched after multiple testing adjustments ($p < 0.1$) **(A)** Bar graph indicates KEGG pathway upregulated and downregulated after ISO treatment. Pathways under the same group (carbohydrate metabolism, fatty acid metabolism, etc.) are clustered together and marked by the same color. The number of unique genes modulated in each group are shown in parenthesis next to the respective group names. The total number of genes modulated in various pathways under each group is generally larger than the total number of unique genes mentioned in parenthesis. It is due to the occurrence of same genes in multiple pathways and accordingly, those were counted more than once. The individual pathways given in the bar graph (A-O1) is tabulated in **Table 1**. **(B)** Bar graph representing genes upregulated and downregulated by ISO + TA is shown. The total number of unique genes that were downregulated is 14. The total number of genes modulated in various pathways under each group is more than 14 as the same genes might be associated with multiple pathways, hence counted more than once. **(C)** Bar graph representing three different pathways involving 13 unique genes upregulated by TA alone is shown. The individual pathways given in the bar graphs in A and B is tabulated in **Table 1**. **(D)** Heatmap of significantly regulated genes in the ISO group compared to ISO_TA group along with expression value. **(E)** Heatmap of significantly regulated genes in the ISO _TA group compared to ISO group along with expression value. The genes, which are not significantly regulated, are indicated as ns (non-significant). A detail of expression value of heatmap along with p-value is tabulated in **Supplementary Table S5**.

TABLE 1 | List of pathways extracted from "DAVID bioinformatics resources." Codes as indicated in **Figure 2** and respective gene counts are shown. Negative and positive sign indicates downregulation and upregulation respectively.

FIGURE 2A

Code	KEGG Pathways	Gene count	Code	KEGG pathways	Gene count
	Carbohydrate metabolism				
A	Glycolysis/gluconeogenesis	-15	B1	PPAR signaling pathway	-10
B	Starch and sucrose metabolism	-10	C1	Proteasome	-8
C	Fructose and mannose metabolism	-6	D1	Regulation of actin cytoskeleton	-19
D	Galactose metabolism	-6	E1	Calcium signaling pathway	-17
E	Citrate cycle (TCA cycle)	-19	F1	Insulin signaling pathway	-24
F	Pyruvate metabolism	-15		**Others**	
G	Pentose phosphate pathway	-5	G1	Drug metabolism	7
H	Glyoxylate and dicarboxylate metabolism	-5	H1	Metabolism of xenobiotics by cytochrome P450	4
I	Oxidative phosphorylation	-28		**Cardiac disease**	
	Fatty acid metabolism		I1	Dilated cardiomyopathy	-19
J	Propanoate metabolism	-15	J1	Arrhythmogenic right ventricular cardiomyopathy (ARVC)	-17
K	Butanoate metabolism	-11	K1	Hypertrophic cardiomyopathy (HCM)	-18
L	Fatty acid metabolism	-13		**Other disease**	-27
M	Glycerolipid metabolism	-8	L1	Parkinson's disease	
N	Fatty acid elongation in mitochondria	-5	M1	Huntington's disease	-31
O	Glycerophospholipid metabolism	-8	N1	Alzheimer's disease	-29
	Amino acid metabolism		O1	Type II diabetes mellitus 8	-8
P	Tyrosine metabolism	3			
Q	Amino sugar and nucleotide sugar metabolism	3		**FIGURE 2B**	**Gene Count**
R	Valine, leucine and isoleucine degradation	-23	A	Nitrogen metabolism	3
S	Lysine degradation	-8	B	Retinol metabolism	3
T	beta-Alanine metabolism	-5	C	Drug metabolism	3
U	Tryptophan metabolism	-7	D	Chemokine signaling pathway	-6
	Nucleotide metabolism		E	Cytokine-cytokine receptor interaction	-5
V	Purine metabolism	5	F	Cell adhesion molecules (CAMs)	-4
W	Aminoacyl-tRNA biosynthesis	-10	G	NOD-like receptor signalling pathway	-3
X	Purine metabolism	-15	H	Antigen processing and presentation	-3
	Cell signaling pathway		I	Circadian rhythm	-2
Y	ECM-receptor interaction	4	J	Asthma	-2
Z	Cytosolic DNA-sensing pathway	3			
A1	Cardiac muscle contraction	-20			

with the metabolism of propanoate (Bar J: 15 genes) and butanoate (Bar K: 11 genes); fatty acid (Bar L: 13 genes), glycerolipid (Bar M: eight genes); fatty acid elongation in mitochondria (Bar N: five genes); and glycerophospholipid metabolism (Bar O: eight genes). Noticeably, three genes involved in tyrosine metabolism (Bar P) and three genes involved in amino sugar and nucleotide metabolism (Bar Q) were upregulated under ISO treatment. Genes downregulated by ISO were also involved in the anabolism of valine, leucine, isoleucine, and lysine (Bar R: 23 genes); lysine degradation (Bar S: eight genes); and metabolism of beta-alanine (Bar T: five genes) and tryptophan (Bar U: seven genes). Five genes involved in purine metabolism were upregulated under ISO treatment (Bar V). Ten genes involved in aminoacyl-tRNA biosynthesis (Bar W) and seven genes in purine metabolism (Bar X) were also downregulated under ISO treatment. Out of seven genes involved in receptor activation and cell signaling upregulated by ISO, four genes were involved in ECM-receptor interaction (Bar Y) and three in cytosolic DNA-sensing pathway (Bar Z). The largest cluster of genes downregulated by ISO also included those involved in cell signaling and receptor activation. Among the downregulated genes included those involved in cardiac muscle contraction (Bar A1: 20 genes), PPAR signaling (Bar B1: 10 genes), proteostasis (Bar C1: eight genes), regulation of actin cytoskeleton (Bar D1: 19 genes), calcium signaling (Bar E1: 17 genes), and insulin signaling (Bar F1: 24 genes). Out of 160 genes involved in cardiovascular and other diseases modulated by ISO, seven genes involved in drug metabolism (Bar G1) and four genes involved in metabolism of xenobiotics by cytochrome P450 (Bar H1) were upregulated. Among the genes downregulated by ISO, were those associated with hypertrophic, dilated, and arrhythmogenic right ventricular cardiomyopathy (Bar I1: 19 genes, Bar J1: 17 genes, and Bar K1: 24 genes); Huntington's (Bar M1: 31 genes), Parkinson's (Bar N1: 27 genes), and Alzheimer's diseases (Bar O1: 29 genes); type II diabetes (Bar P1: eight genes).

As shown in **Figure 2B**, total of nine genes were upregulated by ISO_TA of which three each were involved in nitrogen, retinol, and drug metabolism respectively (Bar A, B, and C). Total fourteen unique genes were downregulated by the ISO_TA group. Those included genes involved in chemokine and cytokine signaling (Bar D: six genes), cytokine-cytokine receptor interaction (Bar E: five genes), cell adhesion (Bar F: seven genes), NOD-like receptor signaling pathway (Bar G: three genes), antigen processing and presentation (Bar H: three genes), circadian rhythm (Bar I: two genes), and the development of asthma (Bar J: two genes).

Only thirteen genes were upregulated by TA alone as shown in **Figure 2C**. Those were involved in drug metabolism (Bar A: four genes), MAPK signaling (Bar B: six genes), and complement cascade (Bar C: three genes). Taken together, total 316 unique genes were downregulated by ISO, and their levels were restored upon TA treatment (**Figures 2D, E**). This suggests a genome wide effect of TA extract in reversing the pathological effects of ISO.

TA Treatment Ameliorates the Pathological Networks Activated by the Adrenergic Stimulation

We next applied a widely used network extraction tool GeneMANIA to mine various gene networks and associated functions from these data sets (Montojo et al., 2010). Based on the functional similarity or shared topology in the published literature, this tool exhibit networks from the query gene list. The network thus derived were then visualized and analyzed using the visualization software Cytoscape 3.0.2. We derived networks of up- and downregulated genes in all the treatment sets as shown in **Figures 3** and **4** where the extent of modulation are represented by color codes as red: upregulation; green: downregulation; and gray: no significant change. These networks indicate modulation of various key genes, reflecting the diversity of ISO-induced reprogramming of cellular networks and its restoration by TA. In agreement with the data obtained from KEGG pathways, this analysis showed the upregulation of biological networks associated with angiogenesis, extracellular matrix organization, integrin binding, inflammation, drug metabolism, redox metabolism, and corticosteroid response in the ISO-treated group (**Figure 3**). ISO also downregulated the networks like those involved in oxidative phosphorylation, pyrimidine metabolism, myofibril, mitochondrial electron transport chain, and acetyl CoA metabolism (**Figure 4**). The details of the network along with key genes upregulated and downregulated by ISO is given in **Table 2**.

To characterize the impact of pretreatment with TA extracts (ISO_TA) on the metabolic reprogramming elicited by ISO, we overlaid the genes regulated in this groups on the network derived from ISO groups. As shown in **Figures 3** and **4**, nodes in the overlaid network in ISO_TA and TA group showed largely no significantly regulated genes (gray color). Clearly, the metabolic network activated in ISO group was completely absent in ISO_TA (and TA group), suggesting a global effect of the TA extracts. Moreover, TA treatment alone significantly perturbed only a

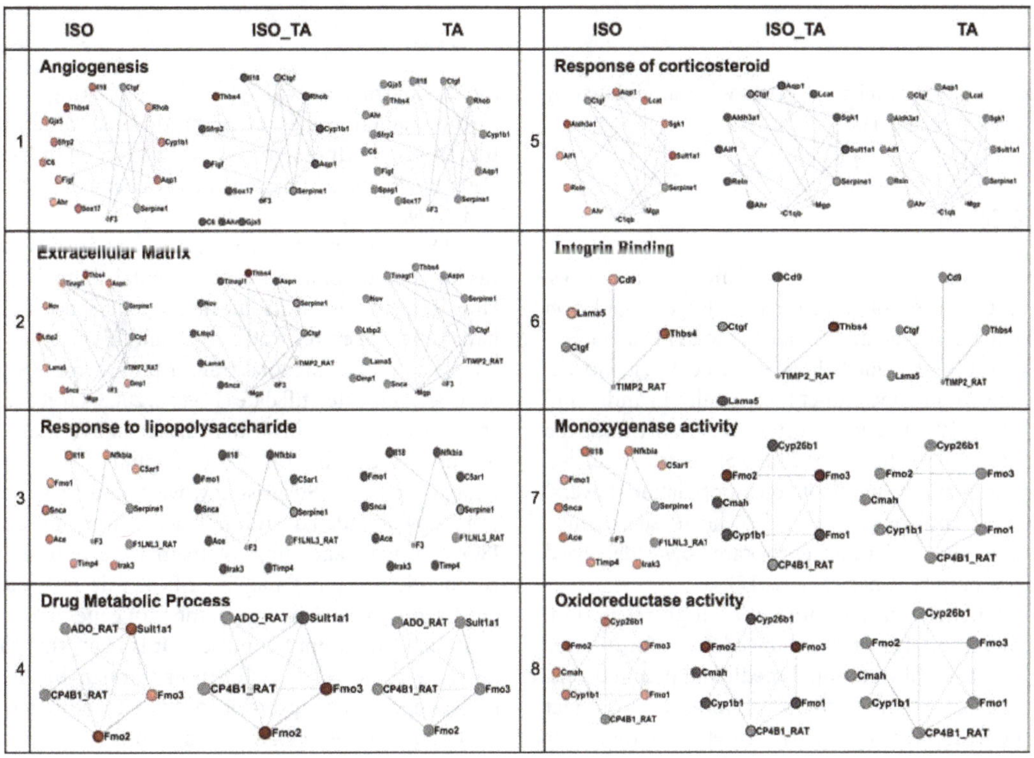

FIGURE 3 | Comparison of enriched non-redundant biological processes represented as "degree sorted circular view" networks of upregulated genes in ISO group extracted from "GeneMANIA" (Cytoscape plugins) along with ISO_TA and TA group overlaid network. Upregulated, downregulated, and undifferentiated gene represented as red node, green node, and gray node respectively.

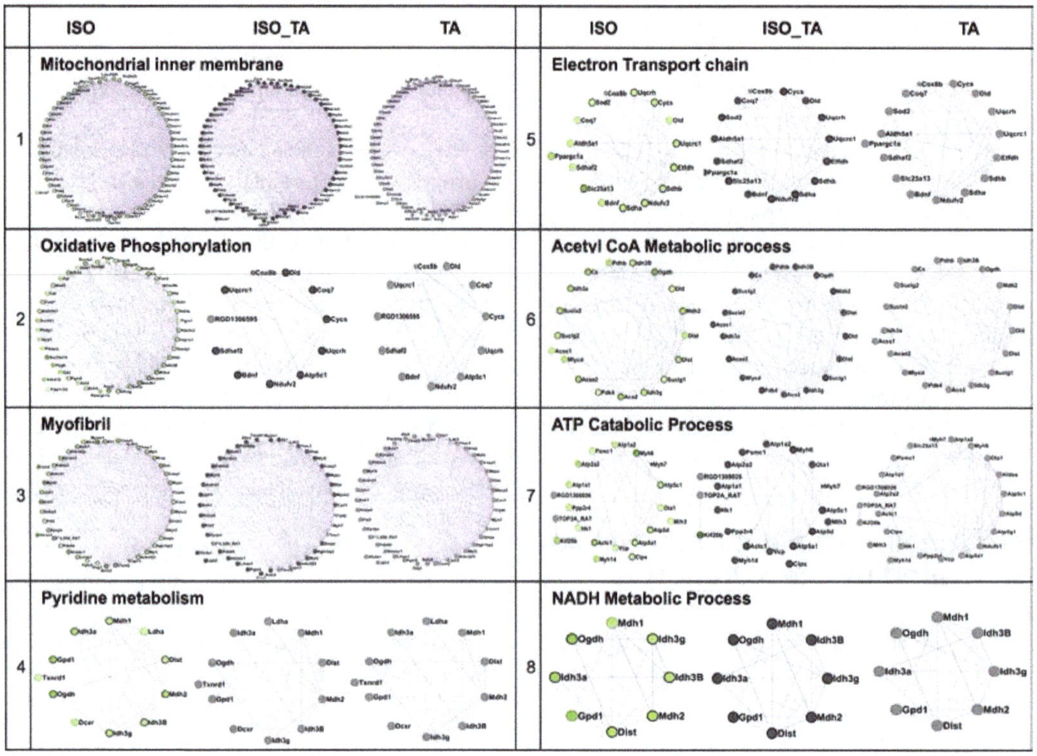

FIGURE 4 | Comparison of enriched non-redundant biological processes represented as "degree sorted circular view" networks of downregulated genes in ISO group extracted from "GeneMANIA" (Cytoscape plugins) along with ISO_TA and TA group overlaid network. Upregulated, downregulated, and undifferentiated gene represented as red node, green node, and gray node respectively.

few networks as a limited number of genes were modulated by TA-treatment (**Figures 3** and **4**).

DISCUSSION

Despite the advancements and availability of modern medicines, especially in past quarter of a century, a large population worldwide still relies upon the traditional medicines (Van Galen, 2014). Although traditional medicines are used worldwide, it is prevalent in the Asian subcontinent, especially in India and China (Jaiswal et al., 2016). Due to sustained support from the government, traditional medicines in China are better regulated and have more acceptability among its own population. Several ancient Chinese formulations have also been successfully exploited for developing modern drugs that are now widely used by the western community (Chao et al., 2017).

Under the ambit of clinical bioinformatics, high-resolution, high-throughput data analyses has enhanced opportunities for examining the efficacies of traditional medicinal preparations. Applications of sophisticated tools of microarray, next generation sequencing, pharmacogenomics etc. enhances our understanding of the mode of actions of various formulations. These advance tools of analytical biology thus provide an opportunity to validate or refute the therapeutic potential of phytomedicines (Beckmann and Lew, 2016). Although the TA extract is widely used for treating various types of cardiovascular ailments by traditional practitioners in the Indian subcontinent, any systematic study of its efficacy using the modern tools of biology has not been done till date (Maulik and Talwar, 2012).

ISO, an adrenergic agonist, is a widely used for studying cardiac pathobiology in experimental animals (Seifert, 2013). However, studies on its effects on gene expression in the heart have largely been restricted to a handful of genes of interest and fewer analyses of the total transcriptome from ISO treated heart have been reported till date (Li et al., 2003; Lu et al., 2012; Talarico et al., 2014). To establish the efficacy of TA in ameliorating CH, we undertook the total transcriptomic analyses of ISO/TA treated rat heart. Surprisingly, we found that total 1129 genes were downregulated and 204 genes were upregulated by the ISO treatment and most of them were restored by TA. Since adrenergic receptors play a critical role in cardiac functions, modulation of such a large number of genes upon sustained ISO treatment might not be unusual. It is likely that the ISO treated heart needs to reset its function through the readjustment of its genome wide expression profile. To be noted that Talarico et al. (2014) have reported change in expression of 493 genes in mouse heart following ISO treatment for an hour. Considering the species difference and experimental parameters like the dose and duration of treatment, our data is largely in tune with theirs (**Supplementary Table S4**).

TABLE 2 | List of networks extracted from GeneMANIA after ISO treatments along with key genes are indicated.

S.no	Network	Key gene
Network upregulated by ISO treatment		
	Angiogenesis	c-fos induced growth factor (Figf)
A		Vascular endothelial growth factor D (Vegf D)
		Connective tissue growth factor (Ctgf)
		Gap junction protein alpha 5 (Gja5)
		Thrombospondin 4 (Thbs4)
B	Extracellular matrix	Laminin subunit alpha 5 (Lma5)
		Latent transforming growth factor beta binding protein 2 (Ltbp2)
	Integrin binding	Metalloproteinase inhibitor 2 (Timp2)
C		Cd9 antigen (Cd9)
	Inflammation	Interleukin-18 (Il18)
D		NFKB inhibitor alpha (Nfkbia)
		Interleukin 1 receptor associated kinase 3 (IRAK3)
	Drug metabolism	Cytochrome P450 (Cyp1b1)
E		Flavin containing monooxygenase 3 (Fmo3)
		TIMP metallopeptidase inhibitor 4 (Timp4)
	Redox metabolism	Sulfotransferase family 1A member 1 (Sulta1)
F		Aminoethanethiol dioxygenase (Ado)
	Corticosteroid response	Serum/glucocorticoid regulated kinase 1 (Sgk1)
G		Aldehyde dehydrogenase 3 family member A1 (Aldh3a1)
Network downregulated by ISO		
H	Oxidative phosphorylation Translocase of inner mitochondrial membrane 44 homolog	ATP synthase (Atp5a1),
		(Timm4)
		Mitochondrial carrier 2 (Mtch2)
		Malate dehydrogenase 2 (Mdh2)
		Ubiquinol-cytochrome c reductase hinge protein (Uqcrh)
		NADH dehydrogenase subunit (NdufV2)
	Pyrimidine metabolism	Oxoglutarate (alpha-ketoglutarate) dehydrogenase (Ogdh)
I		Thioredoxin reductase 1 (Txnrd1)
		Glyceraldehyde-3-phosphate dehydrogenase,(Gpd1)
	Myofibril	Ankyrin repeat domain 23 (Ankrd2)
J		Intracellular hyaluronan binding protein4 (Habp4)
		Junctophilin 1 (Jph1)
	Mitochondrial electron transport	Succinate dehydrogenase flavoprotein subunit (Sdha1)
K	Flavoprotein dehydrogenase (Etfdh)	
	Acetyl CoA metabolism	Acetyl-CoA acyltransferase 1 (Mdh1)
L		NAD-dependent glycerol-3-phosphate dehydrogenase (Gpd1)

In our study, among the 1,333 genes that were modulated by ISO (**Table 2**, **Supplemental Data**) included those involved in metabolism (carbohydrate, fatty acid, and nitrogen; total 105 genes), cell signaling (105 genes), and cardiovascular and other diseases (106 genes). Changes in metabolism such as a shift from oxidative phosphorylation to glycolysis and increased fatty acid oxidation are the hallmarks of heart failure (Fillmore et al., 2014; Fukushima et al., 2015). Since intermediary metabolism involves substantial number of enzymes, modulation of a large number of metabolic genes by ISO is expected, although its significance needs further study. Similarly, adrenergic signaling plays a major role in cardiovascular function and diseases. The mechanisms of adrenoceptor activation, its downstream targets, its signal specificity versus bias and receptor dynamics have been extensively studied for understanding the role of adrenergic system in cardiovascular pathophysiology (Lohse, 2015). Also, the cross talk between adrenergic signaling and that by other receptor viz., insulin, EGF and TGFβ play a critical role in cardiovascular function (Saha et al., 2012; Heger et al., 2016; Fu et al., 2017; Mohan et al., 2017). Signaling by these receptors in heart involve a plethora of kinases, phosphatases, second messengers and gene regulatory proteins. Therefore, changes in expression of more than hundred signaling genes by the sustained adrenergic activation is quite likely.

Although an exhaustive analyses of the role of these diverse group of genes in cardiovascular biology would be desired, it might as well lead to a voluminous but hypothetical compilation of experimental data accumulated over the past several decades. Therefore, we intend to focus onto the relevance of 54 genes that are modulated by ISO treatment and are involved in cardiac diseases. It was quite convincing to find that number of genes downregulated by ISO are involved in Redox-homeostasis/ oxidative stress and noted among them is glutathione-S-transferase (GST, **Table 3**). Glutathione-S-transferase family are Phase II detoxification enzymes that catalyze the covalent conjugation of glutathione (GSH) to electrophilic compounds such as peroxidized lipids, enabling their breakdown. Under oxidative stress, various enzymatic and other proteins susceptible to oxidative damage also undergo S-glutathionylation, a process of covalent conjugation of glutathione to cysteine sulfhydryl or sulfenic acid groups. In a recent study, a member of the GST family, i.e. GSTπ has been shown to catalyze protein S-glutathionylation *in vivo* (Townsend et al., 2009).Downregulation of a number of redox enzymes including GST thus suggest a reduced capacity of the heart to cope up with increased oxidative stress under ISO treatment (Saleem et al., 2018).

Another noticeable observation was the downregulation of expression of a number of contractile proteins viz., Troponin C1, β-Myosin heavy chain, Myosin light chain 2 etc. (**Table 3**). Modulation of expression of contractile proteins have been demonstrated in *ex vivo* cultured myocytes and in experimental rats treated with adrenergic agonists. While in *ex vivo* rat cardiac myocytes, the level of myosin light chain 2 mRNA increases upon treatment with phenylephrine; the mRNA for α-myosin heavy chain decreases in aged spontaneously hypertensive rats with heart failure (Shubeita et al., 1992; Boluyt et al., 1994). In male Sprague-Dawley rats, infusion of NEfor seven days reduce the expression of myosin heavy chain 11, myosin light chain 3 and troponin I. In patients with heart failure, the expression of a number of sarcomeric genes decreases, while their expression is restored in those having left ventricular assisted device (Rodrigue-Way et al., 2005). Taken together, our observation that ISO treatment reduces the mRNA levels of certain sarcomeric

TABLE 3 | Functional class of cardiac disease related genes modulated after ISO treatment.

S.no	Functional class	Gene name
1	Redox homeostasis	1. Glutathione S-transferase A6 (LOC501110) 2. Dimethylaniline monooxygenase (Fmo1, Fmo2, Fmo3) 3. Aldehyde oxidase 1 (Aox1) 4. Alcohol dehydrogenase 6 (Adh6) 5. Aldehyde dehydrogenase (Aldh3a1),
2	Sarcomere function	1. Myosin light chain, phosphorylatable (Mylpf) 2. Myosin regulatory light chain 2 (Mlc2) 3. Myosin light chain kinase 3 (Mylk3) 4. Myosin light chain 3 (Myl3) 5. Troponin C1 (Tnnc1) 6. Myosin-6; Muscle contraction (Myh6) 7. Actinin alpha 2 (Actn2) 8. Actin, alpha cardiac muscle 1 (Acta2) 9. Myosin light chain kinase 3 (Mylk3)
3	Cell/Ca^{++} signaling	1. 5′-AMP-activated protein kinase catalytic subunit alpha-2 (Prkaa2) 2. Protein phosphatase 1E (Ppm1e) 3. Protein phosphatase 1B (Ppm1b) 4. Serine/threonine-protein kinase (STK11) 5. Sarcoplasmic/endoplasmic reticulum calcium ATPase 2 (Atp2a2) 6. Matrix metalloproteinase-24 (Mmp24) 7. Cadherin-2 (Cdh2) 8. 3-phosphoinositide-dependent protein kinase 1 (Pdpk1) 9. Calsequestrin-2 (Casq2) 10. Ryanodine receptor 2 (Ryr2)

genes are in general agreement with studies done by others and the restoration of their levels by TA treatment is significant.

Another set of genes whose expression were downregulated by ISO are involved in cell signaling in general and Ca^{++} signaling in particular. As summarized in **Table 3**, ISO treatment reduced the expression of Ryanodine receptor, Calsequestrin-2, Sarcoplasmic/endoplasmic reticulum calcium ATPase 2 and cardiac phospholamban. Except that of calsequestrin-2, the expression of others decrease in various experimental models of CH and heart failure and in human patients (Nagai et al., 1989; Takahashi et al., 1992; Arai et al., 1996; Kawase and Hajjar, 2008). The mRNA levels of three other genes encoding signaling kinases viz., adenylate cyclase, PKA, and SSTK11 were also downregulated by ISO and restored by TA. The role of adenylate cyclase-PKA in CH has been extensively studied, especially in the context of adrenergic signaling. Available literature suggests that the compartmentalization of cAMP/protein kinase A (PKA) in different subcellular organelles is involved in pathophysiological outcomes under different stimuli (Fields et al., 2016). However, upon extensive literature search, we could not find any report on modulation of expression of these two key enzymes under any pathological context, hence we are unable to correlate our data with that of others. The downregulation of the third kinase, i.e. SSTK11 (Liver Kinase B1/LKB1) in ISO treated heart and its restoration by TA is notable as it prevents CH and dysfunction (Ikeda et al., 2009).

Taken together, above mentioned alteration in the profile of expression of genes involved in metabolism, signaling, and pathology of heart failure are well in conformity of available literature. Further, although substantial literature has shown the beneficial effects of TA in ameliorating various cardiovascular dysfunction, to date no information is available on the modulation of gene expression by TA. Therefore our observation that TA restores a vast majority of genes upregulated and downregulated by ISO in heart is of immense importance. However, TA extract is a mixture of about 26 constituents of which several have been shown to be bioactive (Saha et al, 2012; Kumar et al., 2017). Also, the effects of TA is pleiotropic, as it has anti-atherogenic, hypotensive, inotropic, anti-inflammatory, anti-thrombotic, and antioxidant actions (Maulik and Talwar, 2012). Till date, very little is known about the mechanism of actions of TA at the cellular and molecular levels. Thus, at this point we are unable to offer the mechanistic insight into the global reversal of the effect of ISO by TA. Nevertheless, our present study thus opens up a new window of understanding the beneficial role of TA extract in treating cardiovascular ailments.

ETHICS STATEMENT

The study was conducted in accordance with the Institutional Animal Ethics Committee, All India Institute of Medical Sciences (AIIMS), New Delhi, India. All animal care and experimental protocols were performed in compliance with the National Institutes of Health (NIH) guidelines for the care and use of the Laboratory Animals (NIH Publication no. 85723, revised 1996).

AUTHOR CONTRIBUTIONS

GK has done the data analyses and MS has supervised him. NS has done the animal experiments while SK had done the experimental work at the very early phase. SKM had conceived the entire project. SA had helped in analyzing the TA extract. MS and SKG wrote the manuscript.

FUNDING

The authors thankfully acknowledge funding support from the DST-PURSE awarded by the Department of Science and Technology, Government of India to the Jawaharlal Nehru University. Also, the initial work was done with the support from the Department of Science and Technology under the grant SR/SO/HS-0085/2012 awarded to SKG. GK is a recipient of a NPDF from SERB-DST, Government of India.

REFERENCES

Amalraj, A., and Gopi, S. (2017). Medicinal properties of Terminalia arjuna (Roxb.) Wight & Arn.: a review. *J. Tradit. Complement Med.* 7, 65–78. doi: 10.1016/j.jtcme.2016.02.003

Arai, M., Suzuki, T., and Nagai, R. (1996). Sarcoplasmic reticulum genes are upregulated in mild cardiac hypertrophy but downregulated in severe cardiac hypertrophy induced by pressure overload. *J. Mol. Cell Cardiol.* 28, 1583–1590. doi: 10.1006/jmcc.1996.0149

Bansal, T., Chatterjee, E., Singh, J., Ray, A., Kundu, B., Thankamani, V., et al. (2017). Arjunolic acid, a peroxisome proliferator-activated receptor alpha agonist, regresses cardiac fibrosis by inhibiting non-canonical TGF-beta signaling. *J. Biol. Chem.* 292, 16440–16462. doi: 10.1074/jbc.M117.788299

Beckmann, J. S., and Lew, D. (2016). Reconciling evidence-based medicine and precision medicine in the era of big data: challenges and opportunities. *Genome Med.* 8, 134. doi: 10.1186/s13073-016-0388-7

Boluyt, M. O., O'neill, L., Meredith, A. L., Bing, O. H., Brooks, W. W., Conrad, C. H., et al. (1994). Alterations in cardiac gene expression during the transition from stable hypertrophy to heart failure. Marked upregulation of genes encoding extracellular matrix components. *Circ. Res.* 75, 23–32. doi: 10.1161/01.RES.75.1.23

Chao, J., Dai, Y., Verpoorte, R., Lam, W., Cheng, Y. C., Pao, L. H., et al. (2017). Major achievements of evidence-based traditional Chinese medicine in treating major diseases. *Biochem. Pharmacol.* 139, 94–104. doi: 10.1016/j.bcp.2017.06.123

Doostparast Torshizi, A., and Wang, K. (2018). Next-generation sequencing in drug development: target identification and genetically stratified clinical trials. *Drug Discovery Today* 23, 1776–1783. doi: 10.1016/j.drudis.2018.05.015

Fields, L. A., Koschinski, A., and Zaccolo, M. (2016). Sustained exposure to catecholamines affects cAMP/PKA compartmentalised signalling in adult rat ventricular myocytes. *Cell Signal* 28, 725–732. doi: 10.1016/j.cellsig.2015.10.003

Fillmore, N., Mori, J., and Lopaschuk, G. D. (2014). Mitochondrial fatty acid oxidation alterations in heart failure, ischaemic heart disease and diabetic cardiomyopathy. *Br. J. Pharmacol.* 171, 2080–2090. doi: 10.1111/bph.12475

Fu, Q., Wang, Q., and Xiang, Y. K. (2017). Insulin and beta adrenergic receptor signaling: crosstalk in heart. *Trends Endocrinol. Metab.* 28, 416–427. doi: 10.1016/j.tem.2017.02.002

Fukushima, A., Milner, K., Gupta, A., and Lopaschuk, G. D. (2015). Myocardial energy substrate metabolism in heart failure: from pathways to therapeutic targets. *Curr. Pharm. Des.* 21, 3654–3664. doi: 10.2174/1381612821666150710150445

Ghosh, S., and Chan, C. K. (2016). Analysis of RNA-Seq data using tophat and cufflinks. *Methods Mol. Biol.* 1374, 339–361. doi: 10.1007/978-1-4939-3167-5_18

Gibb, A. A., and Hill, B. G. (2018). Metabolic coordination of physiological and pathological cardiac remodeling. *Circ. Res.* 123, 107–128. doi: 10.1161/CIRCRESAHA.118.312017

Hao, P., Jiang, F., Cheng, J., Ma, L., Zhang, Y., and Zhao, Y. (2017). Traditional chinese medicine for cardiovascular disease: evidence and potential mechanisms. *J. Am. Coll. Cardiol.* 69, 2952–2966. doi: 10.1016/j.jacc.2017.04.041

Heger, J., Schulz, R., and Euler, G. (2016). Molecular switches under TGFbeta signalling during progression from cardiac hypertrophy to heart failure. *Br. J. Pharmacol.* 173, 3–14. doi: 10.1111/bph.13344

Huang, D. W., Sherman, B. T., Tan, Q., Kir, J., Liu, D., Bryant, D., et al. (2007). DAVID bioinformatics resources: expanded annotation database and novel algorithms to better extract biology from large gene lists. *Nucleic Acids Res.* 35, W169–W175. doi: 10.1093/nar/gkm415

Ikeda, Y., Sato, K., Pimentel, D. R., Sam, F., Shaw, R. J., Dyck, J. R., et al. (2009). Cardiac-specific deletion of LKB1 leads to hypertrophy and dysfunction. *J. Biol. Chem.* 284, 35839–35849. doi: 10.1074/jbc.M109.057273

Jaiswal, Y., Liang, Z., and Zhao, Z. (2016). Botanical drugs in Ayurveda and traditional chinese medicine. *J. Ethnopharmacol.* 194, 245–259. doi: 10.1016/j.jep.2016.06.052

Kawase, Y., and Hajjar, R. J. (2008). The cardiac sarcoplasmic/endoplasmic reticulum calcium ATPase: a potent target for cardiovascular diseases. *Nat. Clin. Pract. Cardiovasc. Med.* 5, 554–565. doi: 10.1038/ncpcardio1301

Kumar, S., Enjamoori, R., Jaiswal, A., Ray, R., Seth, S., and Maulik, S. K. (2009). Catecholamine-induced myocardial fibrosis and oxidative stress is attenuated by Terminalia arjuna (Roxb.). *J. Pharm. Pharmacol.* 61, 1529–1536. doi: 10.1211/jpp.61.11.0013

Kumar, S., Jahangir Alam, M., Prabhakar, P., Ahmad, S., Maulik, S. K., Sharma, M., et al. (2017). Proteomic analysis of the protective effects of aqueous bark extract of Terminalia arjuna (Roxb.) on isoproterenol-induced cardiac hypertrophy in rats. *J. Ethnopharmacol.* 198, 98–108. doi: 10.1016/j.jep.2016.12.050

Lainscak, M., Vitale, C., Seferovic, P., Spoletini, I., Cvan Trobec, K., and Rosano, G. M. (2016). Pharmacokinetics and pharmacodynamics of cardiovascular drugs in chronic heart failure. *Int. J. Cardiol.* 224, 191–198. doi: 10.1016/j.ijcard.2016.09.015

Langmead, B., and Salzberg, S. L. (2012). Fast gapped-read alignment with Bowtie 2. *Nat. Methods* 9, 357–359. doi: 10.1038/nmeth.1923

Layne, K., and Ferro, A. (2017). Traditional Chinese medicines in the management of cardiovascular diseases: a comprehensive systematic review. *Br. J. Clin. Pharmacol.* 83, 20–32. doi: 10.1111/bcp.13013

Li, P., Li, J., Feng, X., Li, Z., Hou, R., Han, C., et al. (2003). Gene expression profile of cardiomyocytes in hypertrophic heart induced by continuous norepinephrine infusion in the rats. *Cell Mol. Life Sci.* 60, 2200–2209. doi: 10.1007/s00018-003-3178-5

Li, X., Brock, G. N., Rouchka, E. C., Cooper, N. G. F., Wu, D., O'toole, T. E., et al. (2017). A comparison of per sample global scaling and per gene normalization methods for differential expression analysis of RNA-seq data. *PloS One* 12, e0176185. doi: 10.1371/journal.pone.0176185

Liu, R., and Molkentin, J. D. (2016). Regulation of cardiac hypertrophy and remodeling through the dual-specificity MAPK phosphatases (DUSPs). *J. Mol. Cell Cardiol.* 101, 44–49. doi: 10.1016/j.yjmcc.2016.08.018

Lohse, M. J. (2015). The ins and outs of adrenergic signaling. *J. Mol. Med. (Berl)* 93, 955–962. doi: 10.1007/s00109-015-1323-x

Lu, B., Yu, H., Zwartbol, M., Ruifrok, W. P., Van Gilst, W. H., De Boer, R. A., et al. (2012). Identification of hypertrophy- and heart failure-associated genes by combining in vitro and in vivo models. *Physiol. Genomics* 44, 443–454. doi: 10.1152/physiolgenomics.00148.2011

Marian, A. J., and Braunwald, E. (2017). Hypertrophic cardiomyopathy: genetics, pathogenesis, clinical manifestations, diagnosis, and therapy. *Circ. Res.* 121, 749–770. doi: 10.1161/CIRCRESAHA.117.311059

Maulik, S. K., and Katiyar, C. K. (2010). Terminalia arjuna in cardiovascular diseases: making the transition from traditional to modern medicine in India. *Curr. Pharm. Biotechnol.* 11, 855–860. doi: 10.2174/138920110793262051

Maulik, S. K., and Talwar, K. K. (2012). Therapeutic potential of Terminalia arjuna in cardiovascular disorders. *Am. J. Cardiovasc. Drugs* 12, 157–163. doi: 10.2165/11598990-000000000-00000

Maulik, S. K., Wilson, V., Seth, S., Bhargava, B., Dua, P., Ramakrishnan, S., et al. (2016). Clinical efficacy of water extract of stem bark of Terminalia arjuna (Roxb. ex DC.) Wight & Arn. in patients of chronic heart failure: a double-blind, randomized controlled trial. *Phytomedicine* 23, 1211–1219. doi: 10.1016/j.phymed.2016.02.007

Meghwani, H., Prabhakar, P., Mohammed, S. A., Seth, S., Hote, M. P., Banerjee, S. K., et al. (2017). Beneficial effects of aqueous extract of stem bark of Terminalia arjuna (Roxb.), an ayurvedic drug in experimental pulmonary hypertension. *J. Ethnopharmacol.* 197, 184–194. doi: 10.1016/j.jep.2016.07.029

Mohan, M. L., Vasudevan, N. T., and Naga Prasad, S. V. (2017). Proinflammatory Cytokines Mediate GPCR Dysfunction. *J. Cardiovasc. Pharmacol.* 70, 61–73. doi: 10.1097/FJC.0000000000000456

Mongalo, N. I., Mcgaw, L. J., Segapelo, T. V., Finnie, J. F., and Van Staden, J. (2016). Ethnobotany, phytochemistry, toxicology and pharmacological properties of Terminalia sericea Burch. ex DC. (Combretaceae) - a review. *J. Ethnopharmacol.* 194, 789–802. doi: 10.1016/j.jep.2016.10.072

Montojo, J., Zuberi, K., Rodriguez, H., Kazi, F., Wright, G., Donaldson, S. L., et al. (2010). GeneMANIA Cytoscape plugin: fast gene function predictions on the desktop. *Bioinformatics* 26, 2927–2928. doi: 10.1093/bioinformatics/btq562

Nagai, R., Zarain-Herzberg, A., Brandl, C. J., Fujii, J., Tada, M., Maclennan, D. H., et al. (1989). Regulation of myocardial Ca2+-ATPase and phospholamban mRNA expression in response to pressure overload and thyroid hormone. *Proc. Natl. Acad. Sci. U.S.A.* 86, 2966–2970. doi: 10.1073/pnas.86.8.2966

Nakamura, M., and Sadoshima, J. (2018). Mechanisms of physiological and pathological cardiac hypertrophy. *Nat. Rev. Cardiol.* 15, 387–407. doi: 10.1038/s41569-018-0007-y

Parasuraman, S., Thing, G. S., and Dhanaraj, S. A. (2014). Polyherbal formulation: Concept of ayurveda. *Pharmacognosy Rev.* 8, 73–80. doi: 10.4103/0973-7847.134229

Philipson, D. J., Depasquale, E. C., Yang, E. H., and Baas, A. S. (2017). Emerging pharmacologic and structural therapies for hypertrophic cardiomyopathy. *Heart Fail Rev.* 22, 879–888. doi: 10.1007/s10741-017-9648-x

Raghow, R. (2016). An 'Omics' Perspective on Cardiomyopathies and Heart Failure. *Trends Mol. Med.* 22, 813–827. doi: 10.1016/j.molmed.2016.07.007

Rastogi, S., Pandey, M. M., and Rawat, A. K. (2016). Traditional herbs: a remedy for cardiovascular disorders. *Phytomedicine* 23, 1082–1089. doi: 10.1016/j.phymed.2015.10.012

Rodrigue-Way, A., Burkhoff, D., Geesaman, B. J., Golden, S., Xu, J., Pollman, M. J., et al. (2005). Sarcomeric genes involved in reverse remodeling of the heart during left ventricular assist device support. *J. Heart Lung Transplant.* 24, 73–80. doi: 10.1016/j.healun.2003.10.016

Saha, A., Pawar, V. M., and Jayaraman, S. (2012). Characterisation of Polyphenols in Terminalia arjuna bark extract. *Indian J. Pharm. Sci.* 74, 339–347. doi: 10.4103/0250-474X.107067

Saleem, N., Prasad, A., and Goswami, S. K. (2018). Apocynin prevents isoproterenol-induced cardiac hypertrophy in rat. *Mol. Cell Biochem.* 445, 79–88. doi: 10.1007/s11010-017-3253-0

Sciarretta, S., Forte, M., Frati, G., and Sadoshima, J. (2018). New Insights Into the Role of mTOR signaling in the cardiovascular system. *Circ. Res.* 122, 489–505. doi: 10.1161/CIRCRESAHA.117.311147

Seifert, R. (2013). Functional selectivity of G-protein-coupled receptors: from recombinant systems to native human cells. *Biochem. Pharmacol.* 86, 853–861. doi: 10.1016/j.bcp.2013.07.029

Shimizu, I., and Minamino, T. (2016). Physiological and pathological cardiac hypertrophy. *J. Mol. Cell Cardiol.* 97, 245–262. doi: 10.1016/j.yjmcc.2016.06.001

Shubeita, H. E., Martinson, E. A., Van Bilsen, M., Chien, K. R., and Brown, J. H. (1992). Transcriptional activation of the cardiac myosin light chain 2 and atrial natriuretic factor genes by protein kinase C in neonatal rat ventricular myocytes. *Proc. Natl. Acad. Sci. U.S.A.* 89, 1305–1309. doi: 10.1073/pnas.89.4.1305

Soliman, E. Z., and Prineas, R. J. (2017). Antihypertensive therapies and left ventricular hypertrophy. *Curr. Hypertens. Rep.* 19, 79. doi: 10.1007/s11906-017-0777-3

Takahashi, T., Allen, P. D., Lacro, R. V., Marks, A. R., Dennis, A. R., Schoen, F. J., et al. (1992). Expression of dihydropyridine receptor (Ca2+ channel) and calsequestrin genes in the myocardium of patients with end-stage heart failure. *J. Clin. Invest.* 90, 927–935. doi: 10.1172/JCI115969

Takezako, T., Unal, H., Karnik, S. S., and Node, K. (2017). Current topics in angiotensin II type 1 receptor research: focus on inverse agonism, receptor dimerization and biased agonism. *Pharmacol. Res.* 123, 40–50. doi: 10.1016/j.phrs.2017.06.013

Talan, M. I., Ahmet, I., Xiao, R. P., and Lakatta, E. G. (2011). beta(2) AR agonists in treatment of chronic heart failure: long path to translation. *J. Mol. Cell Cardiol.* 51, 529–533. doi: 10.1016/j.yjmcc.2010.09.019

Talarico, J. A., Carter, R. L., Grisanti, L. A., Yu, J. E., Repas, A. A., and Tilley, D. G. (2014). beta-adrenergic receptor-dependent alterations in murine cardiac transcript expression are differentially regulated by gefitinib in vivo. *PloS One* 9, e99195. doi: 10.1371/journal.pone.0099195

Townsend, D. M., Manevich, Y., He, L., Hutchens, S., Pazoles, C. J., and Tew, K. D. (2009). Novel role for glutathione S-transferase pi. Regulator of protein S-Glutathionylation following oxidative and nitrosative stress. *J. Biol. Chem.* 284, 436–445. doi: 10.1074/jbc.M805586200

Van Galen, E. (2014). Traditional herbal medicines worldwide, from reappraisal to assessment in Europe. *J. Ethnopharmacol.* 158, 498–502. doi: 10.1016/j.jep.2014.07.013

Walters, J. W., Amos, D., Ray, K., and Santanam, N. (2016). Mitochondrial redox status as a target for cardiovascular disease. *Curr. Opin. Pharmacol.* 27, 50–55. doi: 10.1016/j.coph.2016.01.006

Wang, H., and Cai, J. (2017). The role of microRNAs in heart failure. *Biochim. Biophys. Acta Mol. Basis Dis.* 1863, 2019–2030. doi: 10.1016/j.bbadis.2016.11.034

Xing, Z., Chu, C., Chen, L., and Kong, X. (2016). The use of Gene Ontology terms and KEGG pathways for analysis and prediction of oncogenes. *Biochim. Biophys. Acta* 1860, 2725–2734. doi: 10.1016/j.bbagen.2016.01.012

Zegpi, C., Gonzalez, C., Pinardi, G., and Miranda, H. F. (2009). The effect of opioid antagonists on synergism between dexketoprofen and tramadol. *Pharmacol. Res.* 60, 291–295. doi: 10.1016/j.phrs.2009.04.005

Zhang, A., Sun, H., and Wang, X. (2014). Potentiating therapeutic effects by enhancing synergism based on active constituents from traditional medicine. *Phytother. Res.* 28, 526–533. doi: 10.1002/ptr.5032

Zhu, Y. S., Li, Y. L., Ju, J. Q., Du, F., Zang, Y. P., Wang, X. B., et al. (2016). Oral Chinese herbal medicine for treatment of dilated cardiomyopathy: a systematic review and meta-analysis. *Evid. Based Complement Alternat. Med.* 2016, 1819794. doi: 10.1155/2016/1819794

Permissions

All chapters in this book were first published by Frontiers; hereby published with permission under the Creative Commons Attribution License or equivalent. Every chapter published in this book has been scrutinized by our experts. Their significance has been extensively debated. The topics covered herein carry significant findings which will fuel the growth of the discipline. They may even be implemented as practical applications or may be referred to as a beginning point for another development.

The contributors of this book come from diverse backgrounds, making this book a truly international effort. This book will bring forth new frontiers with its revolutionizing research information and detailed analysis of the nascent developments around the world.

We would like to thank all the contributing authors for lending their expertise to make the book truly unique. They have played a crucial role in the development of this book. Without their invaluable contributions this book wouldn't have been possible. They have made vital efforts to compile up to date information on the varied aspects of this subject to make this book a valuable addition to the collection of many professionals and students.

This book was conceptualized with the vision of imparting up-to-date information and advanced data in this field. To ensure the same, a matchless editorial board was set up. Every individual on the board went through rigorous rounds of assessment to prove their worth. After which they invested a large part of their time researching and compiling the most relevant data for our readers.

The editorial board has been involved in producing this book since its inception. They have spent rigorous hours researching and exploring the diverse topics which have resulted in the successful publishing of this book. They have passed on their knowledge of decades through this book. To expedite this challenging task, the publisher supported the team at every step. A small team of assistant editors was also appointed to further simplify the editing procedure and attain best results for the readers.

Apart from the editorial board, the designing team has also invested a significant amount of their time in understanding the subject and creating the most relevant covers. They scrutinized every image to scout for the most suitable representation of the subject and create an appropriate cover for the book.

The publishing team has been an ardent support to the editorial, designing and production team. Their endless efforts to recruit the best for this project, has resulted in the accomplishment of this book. They are a veteran in the field of academics and their pool of knowledge is as vast as their experience in printing. Their expertise and guidance has proved useful at every step. Their uncompromising quality standards have made this book an exceptional effort. Their encouragement from time to time has been an inspiration for everyone.

The publisher and the editorial board hope that this book will prove to be a valuable piece of knowledge for researchers, students, practitioners and scholars across the globe.

List of Contributors

Huanling Lai, Yuwei Wang, Fugang Duan, Ying Li, Zebo Jiang, Lianxiang Luo, Liang Liu, Elaine L. H. Leung and Xiaojun Yao
State Key Laboratory of Quality Research in Chinese Medicines, Macau University of Science and Technology, Taipa, Macau
Macau Institute for Applied Research in Medicine and Health, Macau University of Science and Technology, Taipa, Macau

Ziqing Gao, Gaosong Wu and Jing Zhao
Institute of Interdisciplinary Integrative Medicine Research, Shanghai University of Traditional Chinese Medicine, Shanghai, China

Rui Mi, Zhaoxi Cheng, Huawu Zeng and Ji Ye
School of Pharmacy, Second Military Medical University, Shanghai, China

Xiaofeng Li
School of Pharmacy, Fudan University, Shanghai, China
Institute of Interdisciplinary Integrative Medicine Research, Shanghai University of Traditional Chinese Medicine, Shanghai, China
School of Pharmacy, Second Military Medical University, Shanghai, China

Jiansheng Li
Henan Key Laboratory of Chinese Medicine for Respiratory Disease, Henan University of Chinese Medicine, Zhengzhou, China
Collaborative Innovation Center for Chinese Medicine and Respiratory Diseases Co-constructed by Henan Province and Education Ministry of P.R. China, Zhengzhou, China
Department of Respiratory Diseases, The First Affiliated Hospital of Henan University of Chinese Medicine, Zhengzhou, China

Peng Zhao, Yange Tian, Qingzhou Guan and Yanqin Qin
Henan Key Laboratory of Chinese Medicine for Respiratory Disease, Henan University of Chinese Medicine, Zhengzhou, China
Collaborative Innovation Center for Chinese Medicine and Respiratory Diseases Co-constructed by Henan Province and Education Ministry of P.R. China, Zhengzhou, China
Academy of Chinese Medical Sciences, Henan University of Chinese Medicine, Zhengzhou, China

Kangchen Li, Lanxi Zhang and Xiaofeng Mei
Henan Key Laboratory of Chinese Medicine for Respiratory Disease, Henan University of Chinese Medicine, Zhengzhou, China
Collaborative Innovation Center for Chinese Medicine and Respiratory Diseases Co-constructed by Henan Province and Education Ministry of P.R. China, Zhengzhou, China

Jingxin Xin and Yongbing Yu
Department of Endocrinology, Shandong Provincial Hospital Affiliated to Shandong First Medical University, Jinan, China
Department of Endocrinology, The Second Affiliated Hospital of Shandong First Medical University, Taian, China
Shandong Clinical Research Center of Diabetes and Metabolic Diseases, Jinan, China
Shandong Key Laboratory of Endocrinology and Lipid Metabolism, Jinan, China

Wencong Cheng, Juan Chen and Shanshan Shao
Department of Endocrinology, Shandong Provincial Hospital Affiliated to Shandong First Medical University, Jinan, China
Shandong Clinical Research Center of Diabetes and Metabolic Diseases, Jinan, China
Shandong Key Laboratory of Endocrinology and Lipid Metabolism, Jinan, China

Xinhuan Zhang
Department of Endocrinology, The Second Affiliated Hospital of Shandong First Medical University, Taian, China

Yu Dong
Department of Medicine, Zhejiang Academy of Traditional Chinese Medicine, Hangzhou, China
College of Pharmaceutical Sciences, Zhejiang Chinese Medical University, Hangzhou, China

Ping Qiu, Rui Zhu, Yiqi Wang, Changyu Li and Huajun Zhao
College of Pharmaceutical Sciences, Zhejiang Chinese Medical University, Hangzhou, China

Pinghu Zhang
Institute of Translational Medicine and Jiangsu Key Laboratory of Integrated Traditional Chinese and Western Medicine for Prevention and Treatment of Senile Diseases, Medical College, Yangzhou University, Yangzhou, China

Lisha Zhao and Dan Shou
Department of Medicine, Zhejiang Academy of Traditional Chinese Medicine, Hangzhou, China

Kequn Chai
Department of Medicine, Zhejiang Academy of Traditional Chinese Medicine, Hangzhou, China
College of Pharmaceutical Sciences, Zhejiang Chinese Medical University, Hangzhou, China
Zhejiang Key Laboratory of Tumor Diagnosis and Treatment with Integrated TCM and Western Medicine, Hangzhou, China

Naijun Yuan, Lian Gong, Kairui Tang, Wenzhi Hao, Xiaojuan Li, Qingyu Ma and Jiaxu Chen
Formula-Pattern Research Center, School of Traditional Chinese Medicine, Jinan University, Guangzhou, China

Liangliang He
Formula-Pattern Research Center, School of Traditional Chinese Medicine, Jinan University, Guangzhou, China
College of Pharmacy, Jinan University, Guangzhou, China

Siyuan Zhang, Hua Luo, Zhangfeng Zhong, Yitao Wang, Lin Yang and Dechao Tan
Macau Centre for Research and Development in Chinese Medicine, Institute of Chinese Medical Sciences, University of Macau, Taipa, Macao, China

Shiyi Sun, Yating Zhang, Jiaqi Ma, Yuting Lin and Chaomei Fu
School of Pharmacy, Chengdu University of Traditional Chinese Medicine, Chengdu, China

Leiming Zhang, Yanan Huang, Meiling Wang, Xinlin Wang, Yanfang Wang, Yanfei Hao, Tian Wang, Yuan Du and Fenghua Fu
Key Laboratory of Molecular Pharmacology and Drug Evaluation, Ministry of Education, School of Pharmacy, Yantai University, Yantai, China

Chuanhong Wu
The Biomedical Sciences Institute of Qingdao University (Qingdao Branch of SJTU Bio-X Institutes), Qingdao University, Qingdao, China

Peng Li
College of Arts and Sciences, Shanxi Agricultural University, Taigu, China

Baofeng Fan
Air Force General Hospital, PLA, Beijing, China

Zhuye Gao
Xiyuan Hospital, China Academy of Chinese Medical Sciences, Beijing, China

Siliang Wang, Yun Zhu and Dan Han
Department of Pharmacy, Nanjing Drum Tower Hospital, The Affiliated Hospital of Nanjing University Medical School, Nanjing, China

Cheng Tang
Department of Respiratory Medicine, Affiliated Hospital of Integrated Traditional Chinese and Western Medicine, Nanjing University of Chinese Medicine, Nanjing, China

Heng Zhao
Department of Endocrinology, Jinling Hospital, Medical School of Nanjing University, Nanjing, China

Peiliang Shen
School of Pharmacy, School of Medicine and Holistic Integrative Medicine, Nanjing University of Chinese Medicine, Nanjing, China

Chao Lin
School of Medicine and Holistic Integrative Medicine, Nanjing University of Chinese Medicine, Nanjing, China

Jianling Liu, Meng Jiang, Zhihua Li, Xia Zhang, XiaoGang Li, Yuanyuan Hao, Jinglin Zhu, Chunli Zheng and Yonghua Wang
Key Laboratory of Resource Biology and Biotechnology in Western China, Ministry of Education, School of Life Sciences, Northwest University, Xi'an, China

Xing Su
Pharmacology Department, School of Pharmacy, Shihezi University, Shihezi, China

Wei Xiao
State Key Laboratory of New-tech for Chinese Medicine Pharmaceutical Process, Jiangsu Kanion Parmaceutical, Co., Ltd., Lianyungang, China

Ting Shang, Xin-Tong Wang, Hongyan Zhu, Jia-Ming Gao, Guixiang Pan, Xiumei Gao, Yan Zhu and Yuxin Feng
Tianjin State Key Laboratory of Modern Chinese Medicine, Tianjin University of Traditional Chinese Medicine, Tianjin, China
Research and Development Center of TCM, Tianjin International Joint Academy of Biomedicine, TEDA, Tianjin, China

Neng Wang, Xiaotong Zhang, Shan Liu, Hao Pan, Zhujuan Huang and Fengxue Zhang
The Research Center of Basic Integrative Medicine, Guangdong Provincial Academy of Chinese Medical Sciences, Guangzhou University of Chinese Medicine, Guangzhou, China

Bowen Yang, Shengqi Wang, Yifeng Zheng, Xiong Li and Zhiyu Wang
The Research Center of Basic Integrative Medicine, Guangdong Provincial Academy of Chinese Medical Sciences, Guangzhou University of Chinese Medicine, Guangzhou, China
Integrative Research Laboratory of Breast Cancer, Discipline of Integrated Chinese and Western Medicine, The Second Affiliated Hospital of Guangzhou University of Chinese Medicine, Guangzhou, China

Yingwei Li
The Research Center of Basic Integrative Medicine, Guangdong Provincial Academy of Chinese Medical Sciences, Guangzhou University of Chinese Medicine, Guangzhou, China
Tropical Medicine Institute, Guangzhou University of Chinese Medicine, Guangzhou, China

Lu Ding, Hongyu Qi, Daqing Zhao and Xiangyan Li
Jilin Ginseng Academy, Key Laboratory of Active Substances and Biological Mechanisms of Ginseng Efficacy, Ministry of Education, Jilin Provincial Key Laboratory of Bio-Macromolecules of Chinese Medicine, Changchun University of Chinese Medicine, Changchun, China

Yaxin Li, Siyu Song and Jiachao Zhao
College of Integrated Traditional Chinese and Western Medicine, Changchun University of Chinese Medicine, Changchun, China

Yingying Yang
Graduate College, Beijing University of Chinese Medicine, Beijing, China

Jing Wang
Department of Respiratory, Affiliated Hospital of Changchun University of Chinese Medicine, Changchun, China

Ziyuan Wang
College of Traditional Chinese Medicine, Changchun University of Chinese Medicine, Changchun, China

Wei Zhang and Zeyu Wang
Department of Scientific Research, Changchun University of Chinese Medicine, Changchun, China

Linhua Zhao
Molecular Biology Laboratory, Guang'anmen Hospital, China Academy of Chinese Medical Sciences, Beijing, China

Wancai Que, Zhaoyang Wu, Zhichang Zhao, Maobai Liu and Hongqiang Qiu
Department of Pharmacy, Fujian Medical University Union Hospital, Fuzhou, China
College of Pharmacy, Fujian Medical University, Fuzhou, China

Maohua Chen and Hailing Lin
Department of Pharmacy, Fujian Medical University Union Hospital, Fuzhou, China

Binqing Zhang
College of Pharmacy, Fujian Medical University, Fuzhou, China

Chuihuai You
College of Agriculture, Fujian Agriculture and Forestry University, Fuzhou, China

Yu Cheng
Department of Pharmacy, Fujian Medical University Union Hospital, Fuzhou, China
College of Pharmacy, Fujian Medical University, Fuzhou, China
Department of Pharmacy, Shengjing Hospital of China Medical University, Shenyang, China

Gaurav Kumar, Nikhat Saleem, Santosh Kumar and Shyamal K. Goswami
School of Life Sciences, Jawaharlal Nehru University, New Delhi, India

Subir K. Maulik
Department of Pharmacology, All India Institute of Medical Sciences (A.I.I.M.S.), New Delhi, India

Sayeed Ahmad
Bioactive Natural Product Laboratory, Department of Pharmacognosy & Phytochemistry, School of Pharmaceutical Education & Research, New Delhi, India

Manish Sharma
Peptide and Proteomics Division, Defence Institute of Physiology and Allied Sciences (DIPAS), Defence Research and Development Organisation, New Delhi, India

Index

www.ingramcontent.com/pod-product-compliance
Lightning Source LLC
LaVergne TN
LVHW082138200926
848484LV00008B/2072